To accompany this bestselling textbook
Fundamentals of Anatomy and Physiology Workbook:

A Study Guide for Nurses and Healthcare Students

9781119130093 • 408 pages • March 2017

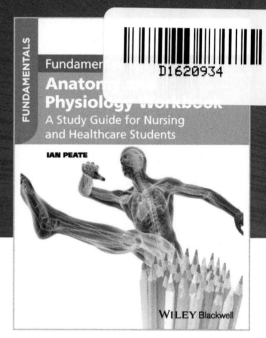

This study guide is a companion to the bestselling textbook *Fundamentals of Anatomy and Physiology for Nursing and Healthcare Students,* and is designed to help and support you with this subject area by testing and consolidating your knowledge of anatomy and physiology. Jam-packed with tips, hints, activities and exercises, this workbook will guide you through the core areas of anatomy and physiology, and provide you with loads of help with your studies.

Designed to support all styles of learning, *Fundamentals of Anatomy and Physiology Workbook* provides you with a wide range of activities including:

- Clear illustrations for tracing, copying, shading and colouring in
- Blank diagrams for labelling
- Multiple choice questions
- Fill in the gap exercises
- Learning tips and hints
- Crosswords
- Word searches

Fundamentals of Anatomy and Physiology

Fundamentals of Anatomy and Physiology

For Nursing and Healthcare Students

Third Edition

Edited By
Ian Peate OBE FRCN

**Gibraltar Health Authority,
St Bernard's Hospital,
Gibraltar**

Suzanne Evans PhD

**University of Newcastle,
New South Wales,
Australia**

WILEY Blackwell

Registered Office(s)
John Wiley & Sons, Inc., 111 River Street, Hoboken, NJ 07030, USA
John Wiley & Sons Ltd, The Atrium, Southern Gate, Chichester, West Sussex, PO19 8SQ, UK

Editorial Office
9600 Garsington Road, Oxford, OX4 2DQ, UK

For details of our global editorial offices, customer services, and more information about Wiley products visit us at www.wiley.com.

Wiley also publishes its books in a variety of electronic formats and by print-on-demand. Some content that appears in standard print versions of this book may not be available in other formats.

Library of Congress Cataloging-in-Publication Data

Title: Fundamentals of anatomy and physiology for nursing and healthcare students / edited by Ian Peate, Suzanne Evans.
Description: Third edition. | Hoboken, NJ : Wiley-Blackwell, 2020. | Includes bibliographical references and index. | Summary: "The third edition of Fundamentals of Anatomy and Physiology is a concise yet comprehensive introduction to the structure and function of the human body. Written with the needs of nursing and healthcare students in mind, this bestselling textbook incorporates clinical examples and scenarios throughout to illustrate how the topics covered are applied in daily practice. Hundreds of full-colour illustrations complement numerous case studies encompassing all fields of nursing practice, alongside learning outcomes, self-assessment tests, chapter summaries, and other effective learning tools"– Provided by publisher.
Identifiers: LCCN 2020017960 (print) | LCCN 2020017961 (ebook) | ISBN 9781119576488 (paperback) | ISBN 9781119576495 (adobe pdf) | ISBN 9781119576518 (epub)
Subjects: MESH: Anatomy | Physiological Phenomena
Classification: LCC QP34.5 (print) | LCC QP34.5 (ebook) | NLM QS 4 | DDC 612–dc23
LC record available at https://lccn.loc.gov/2020017960
LC ebook record available at https://lccn.loc.gov/2020017961

Cover Design: Wiley
Cover Image: © SCIEPRO/Getty Images

Set in 9.5/11pt Minion by SPi Global, Pondicherry, India
Printed and bound by CPI Group (UK) Ltd, Croydon, CR0 4YY

C9781119576488_130223

To all of those nurses and other health and social care staff who have lost their lives as a result of COVID-19.

Contents

Contributors   xvii
Preface   xxi
Acknowledgements   xxv
About the Editors   xxvii
Prefixes, Suffixes   xxix
How to Use Your Textbook   xxxix
About the Companion Website   xli

1   Basic Scientific Principles of Physiology   1

Introduction   2
Levels of Organisation   2
Characteristics of Life   2
Bodily Requirements   3
Life at the Chemical Level   4
Chemical Reactions and Chemical Bonds   6
Acids and Bases   10
Representing Chemical Reactions in Written Form: Chemical Equations   11
Organic Molecules   12
Homeostasis   15
Units of Measurement   16
Conclusion   18
Glossary   18
References   19
Activities   19
Test Your Learning   21
Find Out More   21

2   Cells, Cellular Compartments, Transport Systems, Fluid Movement Between Compartments   23

Introduction   24
Inside the Cell   24
Structure of the Cell Membrane   25
Transport of Substances Across the Cell Membrane   26
How Do Cells Communicate?   30
Fluid Compartments in the Body   31
The Composition of Body Fluids   31
Electrolyte and Water Balance   32
Fluid Movement Between Compartments   34

Bulk Transport Across the Cell Membrane   37
Conclusion   39
Glossary   39
References   40
Further Reading   40
Activities   40
Find Out More   42
Chemical Symbols   42
Conditions   43

3   Genetics   45

Anatomical Map   46
Introduction   46
Deoxyribonucleic Acid (DNA) and Ribonucleic Acid (RNA)   47
The DNA Double Helix   48
Chromosomes   49
From DNA to Proteins   52
Summary of Relationship Between DNA, RNA and Protein   55
The Transference of Genes   56
Inheritance   60
Spontaneous Mutation   70
Disorders of Chromosomes   70
Conclusion   72
Glossary   72
References   73
Further Reading   74
Activities   74
Conditions   76

4   Tissue   77

Introduction   78
Epithelial Tissue   78
Connective Tissue   83
Membranes   89
Muscle Tissue   90
Nervous Tissue   91
Tissue Repair   92
Conclusion   93
Glossary   93
References   94
Activities   94

5   Embryology   97

Introduction   98
Final Maturation of the Oocyte and Sperm   98
Day One: Fertilisation   100
Days 2–5: Pre-Implantation Development   100
Day 6: Implantation   102
Week 2: Early Placental Formation   102

Week 3–8: Post-Implantation Embryonic Development   104
Late Gestation and Birth: Gestational Weeks 13–40 (Embryonic Weeks 11–38)   108
Complications of Pregnancy   111
Conclusion   115
Glossary   115
References   116
Further Reading   116
Activities   117

6   The Muscular System   119

Body Map   120
Introduction   120
Types of Muscle Tissue   120
Functions of the Muscular System   121
Composition of Skeletal Muscle Tissue   122
Gross Anatomy of Skeletal Muscles   122
Microanatomy of Skeletal Muscle Fibre   123
Skeletal Muscle Contraction and Relaxation   127
Energy Sources for Muscle Contraction   130
Aerobic Respiration   130
Organisation of the Skeletal Muscular System   133
The Effects of Ageing   146
Conclusion   146
Glossary   146
References   147
Further Reading   147
Activities   147
Find Out More   149
Conditions   149

7   The Skeletal System   151

Body Map   152
Introduction   152
Bone as a Tissue   154
Other Connective Tissues Closely Associated with the Skeletal System   156
Bone Formation   158
Bone Growth   159
Bone Remodelling   161
Bone Fractures   164
The Axial and Appendicular Skeleton   165
Bone Shapes   166
Joints   170
Conclusion   174
Glossary   175
References   176
Further Reading   176
Activities   177
Match Each Bone to its Correct Shape   178
Find Out More   179
Conditions   179

8   The Circulatory System   181

Body Map   182
Introduction   182
Components of Blood   182
Properties of Blood   184
Plasma   184
Functions of Blood   184
Formation of Blood Cells   186
Red Blood Cells   187
White Blood Cells   191
Platelets   194
Haemostasis   194
Coagulation   194
Blood Groups   197
Blood Vessels   198
Blood Pressure   202
Lymphatic System   203
Lymphatic Organs   207
Conclusion   209
Glossary   209
References   210
Further Reading   210
Activities   211
Find Out More   212
Conditions   212

9   The Cardiac System   215

Body Map   216
Introduction   216
Size and Location of the Heart   216
The Structures of the Heart   217
The Blood Supply to the Heart   223
Blood Flow Through the Heart   228
The Electrical Pathways of the Heart   229
The Cardiac Cycle   233
Factors Affecting Cardiac Output   236
Regulation of Stroke Volume   236
Regulation of Heart Rate   237
Conclusion   239
Glossary   239
References   241
Further Reading   242
Activities   242
Conditions   243

10   The Digestive System   245

Body Map   246
Introduction   246
The Activity of the Digestive System   246
The Organisation of the Digestive System   246

The Digestive System Organs   247
The Structure of the Digestive System   254
The Liver and Production of Bile   264
The Gallbladder   266
The Large Intestine   266
Digestive Tract Hormones   268
Nutrition, Chemical Digestion and Metabolism   268
Conclusion   272
Glossary   273
References   275
Further Reading   276
Activities   276
Find Out More   278
Test Your Learning   278
Conditions   278

11   The Renal System   281

Body Map   282
Introduction   282
Renal System   282
Functions of the Kidney   290
Blood Supply of the Kidney   292
Urine Formation   292
Selective Reabsorption   293
Hormonal Control of Tubular Reabsorption and Secretion   295
Composition of Urine   296
Ureters   298
Urinary Bladder   299
Urethra   300
Micturition   301
Conclusion   302
Glossary   302
References   303
Further Reading   303
Activities   304
Conditions   305

12   The Respiratory System   307

Body Map   308
Introduction   308
Organisation of the Respiratory System   308
The Upper Respiratory Tract   308
The Lower Respiratory Tract   310
Blood Supply   316
Respiration   316
Pulmonary Ventilation   316
Work of Breathing   319
Volumes and Capacities   321
Control of Breathing   323
External Respiration   324
Ventilation and Perfusion   327

Transport of Gases   327
Acid–Base Balance   330
Internal Respiration   330
Conclusion   332
Glossary   332
References   334
Further Reading   335
Activities   335
Conditions   337

13   The Reproductive Systems   339

Body Map   340
Introduction   340
The Male Reproductive System   340
The Female Reproductive System   348
Conclusion   361
Glossary   361
References   363
Further Reading   363
Activities   364
Find Out More   365
Conditions   366

14   The Nervous System   367

Body Map   368
Introduction   368
Organisation of the Nervous System   368
Sensory Division of the Peripheral Nervous System   368
Central Nervous System   369
Motor Division of the Peripheral Nervous System   369
Neurotransmitters   374
Neuroglia   376
The Meninges   376
Cerebrospinal Fluid   377
The Brain   379
The Peripheral Nervous System   383
The Autonomic Nervous System   389
Conclusion   392
Glossary   393
References   394
Further Reading   394
Activities   395
Find Out More   396
Conditions   396

15   The Senses   399

Introduction   400
The Chemical Senses   400
The Senses of Equilibrium and Hearing   408
The Sense of Sight   419

Conclusion   428
Glossary   428
References   430
Further Reading   430
Activities   430
Conditions   432

16   The Endocrine System   433

Body Map   434
Introduction   434
The Endocrine Organs   435
Hormones   437
The Physiology of the Endocrine Organs   439
The Thyroid Gland   443
Glossary   456
References   457
Further Reading   458
Activities   458
Conditions   460

17   The Immune System   461

Body Map   462
Introduction   462
Blood Cell Development   462
Organs of the Immune System   463
The Lymphatic System   464
Lymphoid Tissue   469
Types of Immunity   469
The Innate Immune System   469
Blood Cells   470
The Acquired Immune System   477
Immunoglobulins (Antibodies)   480
Natural Killer Cells   484
Primary and Secondary Response to Infection   485
Hypersensitivity   487
Anaphylaxis   488
Immunisations   488
Conclusion   488
Glossary   489
References   490
Further Reading   491
Activities   491
Find Out More   493
Conditions   493

18   The Skin   495

Body Map   496
Introduction   496
The Structure of Skin   497
The Epidermis   498

Layers of the Epidermis   499
The Dermis   503
The Papillary and Reticular Aspects   503
The Accessory Skin Structures   504
The Functions of the Skin   508
Synthesis of Vitamin D   511
Conclusion   511
Glossary   511
References   512
Further Reading   513
Activities   513
Find Out More   515
Conditions   515

Normal Values   517
Answers   521
Index   529

Contributors

Carl Clare
RN, DipN, BSc (Hons), MSc (Lond), PGDE (Lond)
Carl began his nursing a career in 1990 as a Nursing Auxiliary. He later undertook three years student nurse training at Selly Oak Hospital (Birmingham), moving to The Royal Devon and Exeter Hospitals, then Northwick Park Hospital, and finally The Royal Brompton and Harefield NHS Trust as a Resuscitation Officer and Honorary Teaching Fellow of Imperial College (London). Since 2006 he has worked at the University of Hertfordshire as a Senior Lecturer in Adult Nursing. His key areas of interest are long term illness, physiology, sociology, and cardiac care. Carl has previously published work in cardiac care, resuscitation and pathophysiology.

Suzanne Evans
PhD
Suzanne gained her PhD in neuroscience at the University of Wales in 1989 and has been researching and teaching in universities in the UK, USA, the Caribbean, New Zealand and Australia ever since, receiving numerous teaching awards along the way. She has taught human physiology, pathophysiology and pharmacology at undergraduate and postgraduate level for many years and her special interest is teaching and assessing these subjects in health professional degrees.

Noleen Jones
RN, RNT, Adv. Dip Leadership and Management, BSc (Nursing), FHEA
Noleen's background in nursing is mainly in critical care, where she worked first as a staff nurse, and then as ward manager for a total of 26 years. A subsequent move into practice development identified an interest and aptitude for nursing, health and social care education. Noleen is currently teaching on the Gibraltar BSc (Hons) Adult, BSc (Hons) Mental Health and DipHE nursing programmes.

Jacinta Hope Martin
PhD B. Biotechnology (Honours Class I)
Jacinta's research career began in 2015 following her completion of a Bachelor of Biotechnology Honours program which she followed up with a Doctor of Philosophy (completed in 2019) at the University of Newcastle Australia. She later undertook a role as a research associate at the Hunter Medical Research Institute (also in Newcastle) and has since to McGill University as a Post-Doctoral Research scholar in Montreal, Canada. Jacinta's research interests surround oocyte and embryo development, fertilization, pathophysiological pregnancies and DNA quality.

Karen Mate
BSc (Hons), PhD

Karen started her professional career as a researcher in the area of reproductive physiology; focused on gamete formation, fertilisation, development of assisted reproductive technologies and contraceptive tools for Australian marsupials. After taking a break to spend time with her young family, Karen returned to work as a teaching-focused academic with a research interest in primary care of older adults, dementia and quality use of medicines. Over the past 10 years she has taught human physiology, genetics and biochemistry to a wide range of students in the health professions, including nursing, medicine, pharmacy, physiotherapy, nutrition and dietetics, speech pathology and podiatry.

Louise Mcerlean
RGN, BSc (Hons), MA (Herts)

Louise commenced her nursing career in Glasgow in 1986 and specialised in intensive care nursing. She worked as a Staff Nurse in intensive care and then as a Sister in London. A move to nurse education followed in 2005. Louise has focused on adult nursing and the nursing associate programme and her interests include physiology, clinical skills, simulation and nurse education.

Janet G. Migliozzi
RGN, BSc (Hons), MSc (London), PGDEd., PGCMed.Sim, FHEA, OMS

Janet completed her initial training in London and commenced her career in 1988. She has worked at a variety of hospitals across London, predominately in vascular, orthopaedic and high dependency surgery before specialising in infection prevention and control and communicable disease. Janet has worked in higher education since 1999 and is involved in teaching across a range of healthcare professions programmes both at an undergraduate and post graduate level. She is also involved in the research supervision of students undertaking advanced clinical practice pathways. Her key interests include clinical microbiology, particularly in relation to healthcare associated infections, global communicable disease and public health. Patient safety at a local and global level are also an area of interest. Janet has published in journals and books in areas including immunology, minimising risk in relation to healthcare associated infection and pathophysiology.

Karen Nagalingam
Senior Nurse Lecturer, RN, MSc (Ed), BA (Hons), Pg cert.

Karen qualified as a nurse in 2000 from Sheffield Hallam University. She went on to specialise in renal nursing with experience in inpatients, outpatients, dialysis, transplantation and acute kidney injury. In 2007 she became an Acute Dialysis Nurse Practitioner which involved implementing new innovations, developing the acute kidney injury service as well as managing acutely ill adults.

Karen currently works at the University of Hertfordshire as a Senior Lecturer where she leads modules at undergraduate and post graduate levels relating to the acutely ill adult. Her interests are acute kidney injury, sepsis and simulation. She also has works clinically as an Acute Kidney Injury Nurse Specialist and undertakes acute dialysis. She has published work in various journals and has presented at several conferences.

Jessie Maree Sutherland
PhD (Biological Science), B. Science (Biology Major) Hons Class I

The Sutherland lab research programme incorporates the dissection of the molecular pathways responsible for egg and ovary development in the context of improving the diagnosis of female infertility. Jessie has a strong background in reproduction and fertility, with expertise spanning across the areas of ovarian and testis biology, reproductive toxicology, sexual health, and developmental biology. Jessie's impact in her field has been recognised with the award of a prestigious NHMRC Peter Doherty Biomedical Research Fellowship and the David Healey Award by the Australasian Society of Reproductive Biology. Jessie has an exceptional record in obtaining competitive funding, with more than $1m awarded as a principal investigator since the award of her PhD in 2015. The influence of her research is further recognised through an impressive 30 peer-reviewed publications in esteemed multidisciplinary journals.

Jude Weidenhofer
PhD
Jude begun her career as a laboratory-based medical researcher focusing on understanding the biology of cancer following the completion of her PhD investigating the cellular biology of schizophrenia in 2006. Jude's enthusiasm for education lead her to include the teaching of genetics, biochemistry and cellular biology for undergraduate and post-graduate students alongside her research activities. Since 2014, Jude has focused on the education of nursing and other health professional students in fundamental physiology and biology. Jude has published research findings in both scholarly and laboratory research and is dedicated to improving university education.

Anthony Wheeldon
MSc (Lond), PGDE, BSc(Hons), DipHE, RN
Anthony began his nursing career at Barnet College of Nursing and Midwifery. After qualification in 1995, he worked as a staff nurse and senior staff nurse in the Respiratory Directorate at the Royal Brompton and Harefield NHS Trust in London. In 2000, he started teaching on post-registration cardio-respiratory courses before moving into full-time nurse education at Thames Valley University in 2002. Anthony has a wide range of nursing interests including cardio-respiratory nursing, anatomy and physiology, respiratory assessment, nurse education and the application of bioscience in nursing practice. In 2006, Anthony joined the University of Hertfordshire where he has taught on both pre and post registration nursing courses. He is currently an Associate Subject Group Lead for Adult Nursing.

Preface

Being asked to write a third edition of the well-received *Fundamentals of Anatomy and Physiology for Nursing and Healthcare Students* is an honour. The second edition of the text has received approval by the student community and academics preparing students from the fields of nursing and other healthcare arenas for their careers as healthcare providers.

The third edition of *Fundamentals of Anatomy and Physiology for Nursing and Healthcare Students* has retained many of the attributes in the popular second edition as well as a whole range of new features in this book and also through the companion websites.

For this third edition, those contributing to the text have come from the UK and Australia and are all committed to the provision of high-quality, safe and effective care to a range of communities. The authors are all experienced academics working in higher education, with many years of clinical and educational experience, knowledge and skills, teaching a variety of multidisciplinary student groups at various academic levels. After you have gained a sound understanding of anatomy and physiology we are positive that you will be able to understand better the needs of those people who you have the privilege to offer care to. The provision of high-quality, safe and effective care for all is what each one of us should be striving to provide; however, this will be challenging if we do not fully understand and acknowledge the person in a holistic manner. Those who offer people care and support have to take into consideration the anatomical and physiological elements; they must also, however, take into consideration the psychosocial aspects of the person and their family, addressing the needs of the whole being, the whole person and where appropriate the whole community. We have devised this text in such a way as to encourage learning, understanding and integration. As with previous editions of the text, we hope that you enjoy reading it, and importantly that you are keen to learn more, that you will be interested in delving deeper as you grow and develop into becoming a provider of healthcare that is world class, safe and effective.

We have learnt much from our readers as we have adapted this new edition. We have listened to their comments and responded by making changes and retained those features that are most popular.

The companion to this book, *Fundamentals of Applied Pathophysiology: An Essential Guide for Nursing and Healthcare Students* (Peate, 2017a), also in its third edition, along with the *Fundamentals of Anatomy and Physiology Workbook: A Study Guide for Nursing and Healthcare Students* (Peate 2017b) will help in your development and understanding. Within any programme of study that is related to the provision of care, it is important that you are confident and competent with regards to pathophysiology and anatomy and physiology. It is not enough that you remember all of the facts (of which there are many) that are related to anatomy and physiology; you must also relate these to the people you offer care and support to. Some of those people may be vulnerable and they may be at risk of harm, and it is your responsibility to ensure that you are well informed and that you appreciate the complexities of care provision. This new edition of *Fundamentals of Anatomy and Physiology for Nursing and Healthcare Students* can help you.

It is a requirement of several programmes of study that lead to registration with a professional body that you demonstrate competence and proficiency in a number of areas, and this includes anatomy and physiology.

The human body is as beautiful on the inside as it is on the outside; when synchronised, the mind and body is an astonishing mechanism that has the amazing ability to perform a multitude of astonishingly complex things. Healthcare students practise and study in a variety of healthcare settings, in the hospital and the primary-care setting/pre-hospital care setting and in a person's own home where they are certain to meet and care for people who will have a variety of anatomical and physiological problems. By using a fundamental approach with a sound anatomical and physiological understanding, this has the potential to help the health-care student grow in confidence and competence.

Anatomy and Physiology

In its simplest form, anatomy can be defined as the science related to the study of the structure of biological organisms; there are dictionaries that use such a definition. *Fundamentals of Anatomy and Physiology for Nursing and Healthcare Students* focuses on human anatomy, and the definition of anatomy for the purposes of this text is that it is a study of the structure of the human body. This acknowledges function and also structure; in all biological organisms, structure and function are closely interrelated. The human body will only perform effectively through interrelated systems.

The term anatomy is Greek in origin, meaning 'to cut up' or 'to dissect'. The first scientifically based anatomical studies (attributed to Vesalius, the sixteenth-century Flemish anatomist, doctor and artist) were based on observations of cadavers (dead bodies). More up to date approaches to human anatomy differ, however, as they include other ways of observation; such as the use of a microscope and other complex and technologically advanced imaging tools. Subdivisions are now associated within the broader field of anatomy, with the word anatomy often preceded with an adjective identifying the method of observation; for example, gross anatomy (the study of body parts that are visible to the naked eye, such as the heart or the bones) or microanatomy (where body parts such as cells or tissues are only visible with the use of a microscope).

Living systems can be defined from a number of perspectives:
- At the smallest of levels, the chemical level, atoms, molecules and the chemical bonds connecting atoms provide the structure on which living activity is grounded.
- The cell is the smallest unit of life. Specialised bodies – organelles – within the cell undertake specific cellular functions. Cells can be specialised, such as bone cells and muscle cells. Tissue is a group of cells that are alike, performing a common function. Muscle tissue, for example, is made up of muscle cells.
- Organs are groups of different types of tissues that work together to perform a specific activity. The stomach, is an organ that is made up of muscle, nerve and tissues.
- A system is two or more organs working in unison to carry out a particular activity. The digestive system is an example, it comprises the coordinated activities of a number of organs, these include the stomach, intestines, pancreas and liver.
- Another system having the characteristics of living things is an organism; this has the capacity to obtain and process energy, the ability to react to changes in the environment and the ability to reproduce.

Anatomy is associated with the function of a living organism and because of this it is almost always inseparable from physiology. Physiology can be described as the science that deals with the study of the function of cells, tissues, organs and organisms. Physiology is involved with how an organism carries out its various activities, considering how it moves, how it is nourished, how it adapts to environments that change – human and animal, hostile and friendly. It is in principle the study of life.

Physiology is the foundation upon which we build our knowledge of what life is; it can assist us in deciding how to treat disease as well as helping us to adapt and manage changes that are imposed on our bodies by new and changing surroundings – internal and external. Studying physiology can help in understanding disease (pathophysiology) arising from this; physiologists working with others are able to develop new ways to treat diseases.

There are a number of branches of anatomical study and so too are there a number of physiological branches that can be studied, such as endocrinology, neurology and cardiology.

There are now 18 chapters in this new edition, we have included a new chapter that focuses on embryology. It is not proposed that the text is to be read from cover to cover; however, you may find reading Chapters 1 to 5 first will help you get to grips with some of the more complex concepts; we would encourage you to dip in and out of the book. The chapters use simple and generously sized full-colour artwork to assist you in your understanding and comprehension of the complexities that are associated with the human body from an anatomical and physiological perspective. There are several features contained within each chapter that will assist you to build upon and develop your knowledge base.

The text takes the reader from the microscopic to macroscopic level in the study of anatomy and physiology. The contents demonstrate the movement from cells and tissues through to systems. This approach to learning and teaching is a tried-and-tested approach, especially when helping a learner understand a topic area that may sometimes be seen as complex.

This book has been written with these key principles in mind, to help inform your practice and also to help with your academic work. This third edition retains the features that have helped students bring to life the fascinating subject of human anatomy and physiology; there is also a range of new features provided to further enhance the student experience.

The chapters begin with a number of questions that are offered to test your current knowledge; this permits you to pre-test your knowledge base. Learning outcomes are also provided, covering the content within the chapter; these outcomes are what are expected of you after reading and absorbing the information. This is a minimum of what you can learn; do not be constrained by the learning outcomes, they are only offered so as to guide you.

Another feature in most of the chapters provided to help you consider those people you care for, to help you make clinical links, is the 'Clinical considerations' box. These boxes demonstrate the application to your learning, citing specific care issues that you could come across when working with people in care settings.

The popular feature 'Medicines management', has been retained. In this feature, contributors discuss the administration of medicines, medicine management issues. This can help you appreciate the importance of understanding anatomy and physiology with the intention of administering medicines safely and effectively.

In most chapters, there are Episodes of care boxes. This new addition relates the theory to practice, introducing you to the issues being discussed in a practical way.

At the end of the chapter you are provided with a bank of multiple choice questions. Some of the answers to the questions are not found in the text; in this case, you are encouraged to seek out the answers and in so doing develop your learning further.

The 'Conditions' feature located at the end of the most chapters provides you with a list of conditions associated with the topics that have been discussed. You are encouraged to take some time to write notes about each of the conditions listed; this can help you relate theory to practice. You can make your notes from textbooks or other resources – such as the people you work with – or you could make the notes as a consequence of the people you have cared for. If you are making notes about people you have cared for, it is important that you ensure that you adhere to the rules of confidentiality.

At the end of the chapters is a glossary of terms, presented to enable the learning of difficult words or phrases; understanding these words and phrases is important to your success as a healthcare student. When you have mastered the words your medical vocabulary will have grown and you will be in a better position to develop it further.

There is a list of prefixes and suffixes as well a table of normal values. Normal values (reference values) vary based on a number of factors, including the specific laboratory that supplies them. A patient's blood test values should be interpreted based on the reference value of the laboratory in which the test was done.

A number of features have been assembled to help your learning with two companion websites. The features include an interactive glossary and a series of case studies with the intention of bringing alive the subject matter. The electronic resources associated with this book have been designed to help improve your learning; they are varied and informative and are visually stimulating.

The advantages of these resources are that they can be used in your own place at your own pace, with the aim of encouraging further learning and to build on what it is that you know already. There are also links to other resources via the further reading section at the end of each of the chapters.

Making use of the electronic resources together with the book, as well as the human resources you will encounter in practice, can help to improve the quality of your learning. The electronic resources that are available will not be able to replace the more established face-to-face learning with other students, lecturers, registered practitioners and patients; they do, however, complement it.

Writing this third edition has given us much pleasure and we really hope that you will enjoy reading it. Wishing you much success with your studies: be this in the classroom or in the various care areas that you will find yourself working.

References

Peate, I. (2017a) *Fundamentals of Applied Pathophysiology: An Essential Guide for Nursing and Healthcare Students*, 3rd edn. Oxford: John Wiley & Sons, Ltd.

Peate I. (2017b) *Fundamentals of Anatomy and Physiology Workbook: A Study Guide for Nursing and Healthcare Students*. Oxford: John Wiley & Sons, Ltd.

Acknowledgements

Ian would like to thank his partner Jussi Lahtinen for his encouragement and Mrs Frances Cohen for her unending assistance. I am grateful to the contributors for their ongoing support, the library staff at the Gibraltar Health Authority and the Royal College of Nursing Library London.

Suzanne would like to thank her Australian colleagues Karen Mate, Jude Wiedenhofer, Jessie Sutherland and Jacinta Martin for their enthusiastic support for this edition.

We would like to thank Muralitharan Nair the co-editor for the first and second editions of the book who has decided to take well-earned retirement. Magenta Styles at Wiley has been central in encouraging us to develop this 3rd edition.

About the Editors

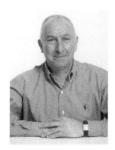

Ian Peate OBE FRCN

Visiting Professor of Nursing St George's University of London and Kingston University, London and Visiting Professor Northumbria University. Visiting Senior Clinical Fellow University of Hertfordshire, Head of School, School of Health Studies, Gibraltar. Editor in Chief British Journal of Nursing.

Ian began his nursing a career at Central Middlesex Hospital, becoming an Enrolled Nurse practising in an intensive care unit. He later undertook three years student nurse training at Central Middlesex and Northwick Park Hospitals, becoming a Staff Nurse then a Charge Nurse. He has worked in nurse education since 1989. His key areas of interest are nursing practice and theory. Ian has published widely. He was awarded an OBE in the Queen's 90th Birthday Honours List for his services to Nursing and Nurse Education and was bestowed a Fellowship from the Royal College of Nursing in 2017.

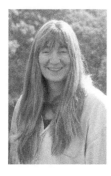

Suzanne Evans PhD

Director of Teaching & Learning and Deputy Head, School of Biomedical Sciences & Pharmacy, Faculty of Health and Medicine, University of Newcastle, New South Wales, Australia.

Suzanne gained her PhD in neuroscience at the University of Wales in 1989 and has been researching and teaching in universities in the UK, USA, the Caribbean, New Zealand and Australia ever since, receiving numerous teaching awards along the way. She has taught human physiology, pathophysiology and pharmacology at undergraduate and postgraduate level for many years and her special interest is teaching and assessing these subjects in health professional degrees.

Prefixes, Suffixes

Prefix: A prefix is positioned at the beginning of a word to modify or change its meaning. Pre means 'before'. Prefixes may also indicate a location, number, or time.

Suffix: The ending part of a word that changes the meaning of the word.

PREFIX OR SUFFIX	MEANING	EXAMPLE(S)
a-, an-	not, without	analgesic, apathy
ab-	from; away from	abduction
abdomin(o)-	of or relating to the abdomen	abdomen
acous(io)-	of or relating to hearing	acoumeter, acoustician
acr(o)-	extremity, topmost	acrocrany, acromegaly, acroosteolysis, acroposthia
ad-	at, increase, on, toward	adduction
aden(o)-, aden(i)-	of or relating to a gland	adenocarcinoma, adenology, adenotome, adenotyphus
adip(o)-	of or relating to fat or fatty tissue	adipocyte
adren(o)-	of or relating to adrenal glands	adrenal artery
-aemia	blood condition	anaemia
aer(o)-	air, gas	aerosinusitis
-aesthesi(o)-	sensation	anaesthesia
alb-	denoting a white or pale colour	albino
-alge(si)-	pain	analgesic
-algia, -alg(i)o-	pain	myalgia
all(o-)	denoting something as different, or as an addition	alloantigen, allopathy
ambi-	denoting something as positioned on both sides	ambidextrous
amni-	pertaining to the membranous foetal sac (amnion)	amniocentesis
ana-	back, again, up	anaplasia
andr(o)-	pertaining to a man	android, andrology
angi(o)-	blood vessel	angiogram
ankyl(o)-, ancyl(o)-	denoting something as crooked or bent	ankylosis
ante-	describing something as positioned in front of another thing	antepartum
anti-	describing something as 'against' or 'opposed to' another	antibody, antipsychotic
arteri(o)-	of or pertaining to an artery	arteriole, arterial

PREFIX OR SUFFIX	MEANING	EXAMPLE(S)
arthr(o)-	of or pertaining to the joints, limbs	arthritis
articul(o)-	joint	articulation
-ase	enzyme	lactase
-asthenia	weakness	myasthenia gravis
ather(o)-	fatty deposit, soft gruel-like deposit	atherosclerosis
atri(o)-	an atrium (especially heart atrium)	atrioventricular
aur(i)-	of or pertaining to the ear	aural
aut(o)-	self	autoimmune
axill-	of or pertaining to the armpit (uncommon as a prefix)	axilla
bi-	twice, double	binary
bio-	life	biology
blephar(o)-	of or pertaining to the eyelid	blepharoplast
brachi(o)-	of or relating to the arm	brachium of inferior colliculus
brady-	'slow'	bradycardia
bronch(i)-	bronchus	bronchiolitis obliterans
bucc(o)-	of or pertaining to the cheek	buccolabial
burs(o)-	bursa (fluid sac between the bones)	bursitis
carcin(o)-	cancer	carcinoma
cardi(o)-	of or pertaining to the heart	cardiology
carp(o)-	of or pertaining to the wrist	carpal tunnel
-cele	pouching, hernia	hydrocele, varicocele
-centesis	surgical puncture for aspiration	amniocentesis
cephal(o)-	of or pertaining to the head (as a whole)	cephalalgy
cerebell(o)-	of or pertaining to the cerebellum	cerebellum
cerebr(o)-	of or pertaining to the brain	cerebrology
chem(o)-	chemistry, drug	chemotherapy
chol(e)-	of or pertaining to bile	cholecystitis
cholecyst(o)-	of or pertaining to the gallbladder	cholecystectomy
chondr(i)o-	cartilage, gristle, granule, granular	chondrocalcinosis
chrom(ato)-	colour	haemochromatosis
-cidal, -cide	killing, destroying	bacteriocidal
cili-	of or pertaining to the cilia, the eyelashes	ciliary
circum-	denoting something as 'around' another	circumcision
col(o)-, colono-	colon	colonoscopy
colp(o)-	of or pertaining to the vagina	colposcopy
contra-	against	contraindicate
coron(o)-	crown	coronary
cost(o)-	of or pertaining to the ribs	costochondral
crani(o)-	belonging or relating to the cranium	craniology
-crine, -crin(o)-	to secrete	endocrine
cry(o)-	cold	cryoablation
cutane-	skin	subcutaneous
cyan(o)-	denotes a blue colour	cyanosis

PREFIX OR SUFFIX	MEANING	EXAMPLE(S)
cyst(o)-, cyst(i)-	of or pertaining to the urinary bladder	cystotomy
cyt(o)-	cell	cytokine
-cyte	cell	leukocyte
-dactyl(o)-	of or pertaining to a finger, toe	dactylology, polydactyly
dent-	of or pertaining to teeth	dentist
dermat(o)-, derm(o)-	of or pertaining to the skin	dermatology
-desis	binding	arthrodesis
dextr(o)-	right, on the right side	dextrocardia
di-	two	diplopia
dia-	through, during, across	dialysis
dif-	apart, separation	different
digit-	of or pertaining to the finger (rare as a root)	digit
-dipsia	suffix meaning '(condition of) thirst'	polydipsia, hydroadipsia, oligodipsia
dors(o)-, dors(i)-	of or pertaining to the back	dorsal, dorsocephalad
duodeno-	duodenum	duodenal atresia
dynam(o)-	force, energy, power	hand strength dynamometer
-dynia	pain	vulvodynia
dys-	bad, difficult, defective, abnormal	dysphagia, dysphasia
ec-	out, away	ectopia, ectopic pregnancy
-ectasia, -ectasis	expansion, dilation	bronchiectasis, telangiectasia
ect(o)-	outer, outside	ectoblast, ectoderm
-ectomy	denotes a surgical operation or removal of a body part; resection, excision	mastectomy
-emesis	vomiting condition	haematemesis
encephal(o)-	of or pertaining to the brain; also see cerebr(o)-	encephalogram
endo-	denotes something as 'inside' or 'within'	endocrinology, endospore
enter(o)-	of or pertaining to the intestine	gastroenterology
eosin(o)-	red	eosinophil granulocyte
epi-	on, upon	epicardium, epidermis, epidural, episclera, epistaxis
erythr(o)-	denotes a red colour	erythrocyte
ex-	out of, away from	excision, exophthalmos
exo-	denotes something as 'outside' another	exoskeleton
extra-	outside	extradural haematoma
faci(o)-	of or pertaining to the face	facioplegic
fibr(o)	fibre	fibroblast
fore-	before or ahead	forehead
fossa	a hollow or depressed area; trench or channel	fossa ovalis
front-	of or pertaining to the forehead	frontonasal
galact(o)-	milk	galactorrhoea
gastr(o)-	of or pertaining to the stomach	gastric bypass
-genic	formative, pertaining to producing	cardiogenic shock
gingiv-	of or pertaining to the gums	gingivitis

PREFIX OR SUFFIX	MEANING	EXAMPLE(S)
glauc(o)-	denoting a grey or bluish-grey colour	glaucoma
gloss(o)-, glott(o)-	of or pertaining to the tongue	glossology
gluco-	sweet	glucocorticoid
glyc(o)-	sugar	glycolysis
-gnosis	knowledge	diagnosis, prognosis
gon(o)-	seed, semen; also, reproductive	gonorrhoea
-gram, -gramme	record or picture	angiogram
-graph	instrument used to record data or picture	electrocardiograph
-graphy	process of recording	angiography
gyn(aec)o-	woman	gynaecomastia
haemangi(o)-	blood vessels	haemangioma
haemat(o)-, haem-	of or pertaining to blood	haematology
halluc-	to wander in mind	hallucinosis
hemi-	one-half	cerebral hemisphere
hepat- (hepatic-)	of or pertaining to the liver	hepatology
heter(o)-	denotes something as 'the other' (of two), as an addition, or different	heterogeneous
hist(o)-, histio-	tissue	histology
home(o)-	similar	homeopathy
hom(o)-	denotes something as 'the same' as another or common	homosexuality
hydr(o)-	water	hydrophobe
hyper-	denotes something as 'extreme' or 'beyond normal'	hypertension
hyp(o)-	denotes something as 'below normal'	hypovolaemia
hyster(o)-	of or pertaining to the womb, the uterus	hysterectomy
iatr(o)-	of or pertaining to medicine, or a physician	iatrogenic
-iatry	denotes a field in medicine of a certain body component	podiatry, psychiatry
-ics	organised knowledge, treatment	obstetrics
ileo-	ileum	ileocaecal valve
infra-	below	infrahyoid muscles
inter-	between, among	interarticular ligament
intra-	within	intramural
ipsi-	same	ipsilateral hemiparesis
ischio-	of or pertaining to the ischium, the hip joint	ischioanal fossa
-ismus	spasm, contraction	hemiballismus
iso-	denoting something as being 'equal'	isotonic
-ist	one who specialises in	pathologist
-itis	inflammation	tonsillitis
-ium	structure, tissue	pericardium
juxta- (iuxta-)	near to, alongside or next to	juxtaglomerular apparatus
karyo-	nucleus	eukaryote
kerat(o)-	cornea (eye or skin)	keratoscope

PREFIX OR SUFFIX	MEANING	EXAMPLE(S)
kin(e)-, kin(o)-, kinesi(o)-	movement	kinaesthesia
kyph(o)-	humped	kyphoscoliosis
labi(o)-	of or pertaining to the lip	labiodental
lacrim(o)-	tear	lacrimal canaliculi
lact(i)-, lact(o)	milk	lactation
lapar(o)-	of or pertaining to the abdomen wall, flank	laparotomy
laryng(o)-	of or pertaining to the larynx, the lower throat cavity where the voice box is	larynx
latero-	lateral	lateral pectoral nerve
-lepsis, -lepsy	attack, seizure	epilepsy, narcolepsy
lept(o)-	light, slender	leptomeningeal
leuc(o)-, leuk(o)-	denoting a white colour	leukocyte
lingu(a)-, lingu(o)-	of or pertaining to the tongue	linguistics
lip(o)-	fat	liposuction
lith(o)-	stone, calculus	lithotripsy
-logist	denotes someone who studies a certain field	oncologist, pathologist
log(o)-	speech	logopaedics
-logy	denotes the academic study or practice of a certain field	haematology, urology
lymph(o)-	lymph	lymphoedema
lys(o)-, -lytic	dissolution	lysosome
-lysis	destruction, separation	paralysis
macr(o)-	large, long	macrophage
-malacia	softening	osteomalacia
mammill(o)-	of or pertaining to the nipple	mammillitis
mamm(o)-	of or pertaining to the breast	mammogram
manu-	of or pertaining to the hand	manufacture
mast(o)-	of or pertaining to the breast	mastectomy
meg(a)-, megal(o)-, -megaly	enlargement, million	splenomegaly, megameter
melan(o)-	black colour	melanin
mening(o)-	membrane	meningitis
meta-	after, behind	metacarpus
-meter	instrument used to measure or count	sphygmomanometer
metr(o)-	pertaining to conditions of the uterus	metrorrhagia
-metry	process of measuring	optometry
micro-	denoting something as small, or relating to smallness	microscope
milli-	thousandth	millilitre
mon(o)-	single	infectious mononucleosis
morph(o)-	form, shape	morphology
muscul(o)-	muscle	musculoskeletal system
my(o)-	of or relating to muscle	myoblast

PREFIX OR SUFFIX	MEANING	EXAMPLE(S)
myc(o)-	fungus	onychomycosis
myel(o)-	of or relating to bone marrow or spinal cord	myeloblast
myri-	ten thousand	myriad
myring(o)-	eardrum	myringotomy
narc(o)-	numb, sleep	narcolepsy
nas(o)-	of or pertaining to the nose	nasal
necr(o)-	death	necrosis, necrotising fasciitis
neo-	new	neoplasm
nephr(o)-	of or pertaining to the kidney	nephrology
neur(i)-, neur(o)-	of or pertaining to nerves and the nervous system	neurofibromatosis
normo-	normal	normocapnia
ocul(o)-	of or pertaining to the eye	oculist
odont(o)-	of or pertaining to teeth	orthodontist
odyn(o)-	pain	stomatodynia
-oesophageal, oesophag(o)-	gullet	gastro-oesophageal reflux
-oid	resemblance to	sarcoidosis
-ole	small or little	arteriole
olig(o)-	denoting something as 'having little, having few'	oliguria
-oma (*sing.*), -omata (*pl.*)	tumour, mass, collection	sarcoma, teratoma
onco-	tumour, bulk, volume	oncology
onych(o)-	of or pertaining to the nail (of a finger or toe)	onychophagy
oo-	of or pertaining to an egg, a woman's egg, the ovum	oogenesis
oophor(o)-	of or pertaining to the woman's ovary	oophorectomy
ophthalm(o)-	of or pertaining to the eye	ophthalmology
optic(o)-	of or relating to chemical properties of the eye	opticochemical
orchi(o)-, orchid(o)-, orch(o)-	testis	orchiectomy, orchidectomy
-osis	a condition, disease or increase	ichthyosis, psychosis, osteoporosis
osseo-	bony	osseous
ossi-	bone	peripheral ossifying fibroma
ost(e)-, oste(o)-	bone	osteoporosis
ot(o)-	of or pertaining to the ear	otology
ovo-, ovi-, ov-	of or pertaining to the eggs, the ovum	ovogenesis
pachy-	thick	pachyderma
paed-, paedo-	of or pertaining to the child	paediatrics
palpebr-	of or pertaining to the eyelid (uncommon as a root)	palpebra
pan-, pant(o)-	denoting something as 'complete' or containing 'everything'	panophobia, panopticon

PREFIX OR SUFFIX	MEANING	EXAMPLE(S)
papill-	of or pertaining to the nipple (of the chest/breast)	papillitis
papul(o)-	indicates papulosity, a small elevation or swelling in the skin, a pimple, swelling	papulation
para-	alongside of, abnormal	paracyesis
-paresis	slight paralysis	hemiparesis
parvo-	small	parvovirus
path(o)-	disease	pathology
-pathy	denotes (with a negative sense) a disease, or disorder	sociopathy, neuropathy
pector-	breast	pectoralgia, pectoriloquy, pectorophony
ped-, -ped-, -pes	of or pertaining to the foot; -footed	pedoscope
pelv(i)-, pelv(o)-	hip bone	pelvis
-penia	deficiency	osteopenia
-pepsia	denotes something relating to digestion, or the digestive tract	dyspepsia
peri-	denoting something with a position 'surrounding' or 'around' another	periodontal
-pexy	fixation	nephropexy
phaco-	lens-shaped	phacolysis, phacometer, phacoscotoma
-phage, -phagia	forms terms denoting conditions relating to eating or ingestion	sarcophagia
-phago-	eating, devouring	phagocyte
-phagy	forms nouns that denotes 'feeding on' the first element or part of the word	haematophagy
pharmaco-	drug, medication	pharmacology
pharyng(o)-	of or pertaining to the pharynx, the upper throat cavity	pharyngitis, pharyngoscopy
phleb(o)-	of or pertaining to the (blood) veins, a vein	phlebography, phlebotomy
-phobia	exaggerated fear, sensitivity	arachnophobia
phon(o)-	sound	phonograph, symphony
phot(o)-	of or pertaining to light	photopathy
phren(i)-, phren(o)-, phrenico	the mind	phrenic nerve, schizophrenia
-plasia	formation, development	achondroplasia
-plasty	surgical repair, reconstruction	rhinoplasty
-plegia	paralysis	paraplegia
pleio-	more, excessive, multiple	pleiomorphism
pleur(o)-, pleur(a)	of or pertaining to the ribs	pleurogenous
-plexy	stroke or seizure	cataplexy
pneumat(o)-	air, lung	pneumatocele
pneum(o)-	of or pertaining to the lungs	pneumonocyte, pneumonia
-poiesis	production	haematopoiesis
poly-	denotes a 'plurality' of something	polymyositis

PREFIX OR SUFFIX	MEANING	EXAMPLE(S)
post-	denotes something as 'after' or 'behind' another	post-operation, post-mortem
pre-	denotes something as 'before' another (in [physical] position or time)	premature birth
presby(o)-	old age	presbyopia
prim-	denotes something as 'first' or 'most important'	primary
proct(o)-	anus, rectum	proctology
prot(o)-	denotes something as 'first' or 'most important'	protoneuron
pseud(o)-	denotes something false or fake	pseudoephedrine
psor-	itching	psoriasis
psych(e)-, psych(o)	of or pertaining to the mind	psychology, psychiatry
-ptosis	falling, drooping, downward placement, prolapse	apoptosis, nephroptosis
-ptysis	(a spitting), spitting, haemoptysis, the spitting of blood derived from the lungs or bronchial tubes	haemoptysis
pulmon-, pulmo-	of or relating to the lungs	pulmonary
pyel(o)-	pelvis	pyelonephritis
py(o)-	pus	pyometra
pyr(o)-	fever	antipyretic
quadr(i)-	four	quadriceps
radio-	radiation	radiowave
ren(o)-	of or pertaining to the kidney	renal
retro-	backward, behind	retroversion, retroverted
rhin(o)-	of or pertaining to the nose	rhinoplasty
rhod(o)-	denoting a rose-red colour	rhodophyte
-rrhage	burst forth	haemorrhage
-rrhagia	rapid flow of blood	menorrhagia
-rrhaphy	surgical suturing	nephrorrhaphy
-rrhexis	rupture	karyorrhexis
-rrhoea	flowing, discharge	diarrhoea
-rupt	break or burst	erupt, interrupt
salping(o)-	of or pertaining to tubes, e.g. Fallopian tubes	salpingectomy, salpingopharyngeus muscle
sangui-, sanguine-	of or pertaining to blood	exsanguination
sarco-	muscular, flesh-like	sarcoma
scler(o)-	hard	scleroderma
-sclerosis	hardening	atherosclerosis, multiple sclerosis
scoli(o)-	twisted	scoliosis
-scope	instrument for viewing	otoscope
-scopy	use of instrument for viewing	endoscopy
semi-	one-half, partly	semiconscious

PREFIX OR SUFFIX	MEANING	EXAMPLE(S)
sial(o)-	saliva, salivary gland	sialagogue
sigmoid(o)-	sigmoid, S-shaped curvature	sigmoid colon
sinistr(o)-	left, left side	sinistrocardia
sinus-	of or pertaining to the sinus	sinusitis
somat(o)-, somatico-	body, bodily	somatic
-spadias	slit, fissure	hypospadias, epispadias
spasmo-	spasm	spasmodic dysphonia
sperma(to)-, spermo-	semen, spermatozoa	spermatogenesis
splen(o)-	spleen	splenectomy
spondyl(o)-	of or pertaining to the spine, the vertebra	spondylitis
squamos(o)-	denoting something as 'full of scales' or 'scaly'	squamous cell
-stalsis	contraction	peristalsis
-stasis	stopping, standing	cytostasis, homeostasis
-staxis	dripping, trickling	epistaxis
sten(o)-	denoting something as 'narrow in shape'	stenography
-stenosis	abnormal narrowing in a blood vessel or other tubular organ or structure	restenosis, stenosis
stomat(o)-	of or pertaining to the mouth	stomatogastric, stomatognathic system
-stomy	creation of an opening	colostomy
sub-	beneath	subcutaneous tissue
super-	in excess, above, superior	superior vena cava
supra-	above, excessive	supraorbital vein
tachy-	denoting something as fast, irregularly fast	tachycardia
-tension, -tensive	pressure	hypertension
tetan-	rigid, tense	tetanus
thec-	case, sheath	intrathecal
therap-	treatment	hydrotherapy, therapeutic
therm(o)-	heat	thermometer
thorac(i)-, thorac(o)-,thoracico-	of or pertaining to the upper chest, chest; the area above the breast and under the neck	thorax
thromb(o)-	of or relating to a blood clot, clotting of blood	thrombus, thrombocytopenia
thyr(o)-	thyroid	thyrocele
thym-	emotions	dysthymia
-tome	cutting instrument	osteotome
-tomy	act of cutting; incising, incision	gastrotomy
tono-	tone, tension, pressure	tonometer
-tony	tension	
top(o)-	place, topical	topical anaesthetic
tort(i)-	twisted	torticollis

PREFIX OR SUFFIX	MEANING	EXAMPLE(S)
tox(i)-, tox(o)-, toxic(o)-	toxin, poison	toxoplasmosis
trache(a)-	trachea	tracheotomy
trachel(o)-	of or pertaining to the neck	tracheloplasty
trans-	denoting something as moving or situated 'across' or 'through'	transfusion
tri-	three	triangle
trich(i)-, trichia, trich(o)-	of or pertaining to hair, hair-like structure	trichocyst
-tripsy	crushing	lithotripsy
-trophy	nourishment, development	pseudohypertrophy
tympan(o)-	eardrum	tympanocentesis
-ula, -ule	small	nodule
ultra-	beyond, excessive	ultrasound
un(i)-	one	unilateral hearing loss
ur(o)-	of or pertaining to urine, the urinary system; (specifically) pertaining to the physiological chemistry of urine	urology
uter(o)-	of or pertaining to the uterus or womb	uterus
vagin-	of or pertaining to the vagina	vagina
varic(o)-	swollen or twisted vein	varicose
vasculo-	blood vessel	vasculotoxicity
vas(o)-	duct, blood vessel	vasoconstriction
ven-	of or pertaining to the (blood) veins, a vein (used in terms pertaining to the vascular system)	vein, venospasm
ventricul(o)-	of or pertaining to the ventricles; any hollow region inside an organ	cardiac ventriculography
ventr(o)-	of or pertaining to the belly; the stomach cavities	ventrodorsal
-version	turning	anteversion, retroversion
vesic(o)-	of or pertaining to the bladder	vesical arteries
viscer(o)-	of or pertaining to the internal organs, the viscera	viscera
xanth(o)-	denoting a yellow colour, an abnormally yellow colour	xanthopathy
xen(o)-	foreign, different	xenograft
xer(o)-	dry, desert-like	xerostomia
zo(o)-	animal, animal life	zoology
zym(o)-	fermentation	enzyme, lysozyme

How to Use Your Textbook

Features Contained within Your Textbook

Learning outcome boxes give a summary of the topics covered in a chapter.

Learning Outcomes

After reading this chapter you will be able to:

- Describe the structure of the heart
- List the arteries that supply blood to the heart muscle
- Describe the electrical excitation of the heart
- Describe the cardiac action potential
- Discuss the cardiac cycle

Your textbook is full of **illustrations and tables.**

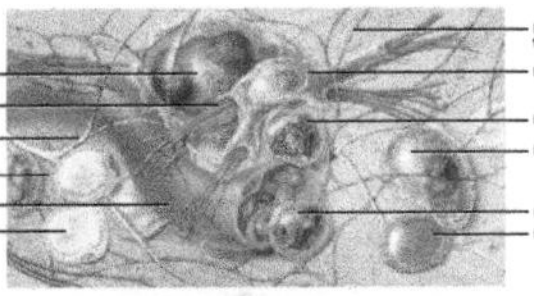

Figure 4.12 **Constituents of connective tissue.** Source Tortora and Derrickson (2017). Reproduced with permission of John Wiley & Sons.

Table 4.2 **Types of connective tissue proper, their main constituents, functions and locations.**

CONNECTIVE TISSUE	MAIN CONSTITUENT	FUNCTIONS	MAIN LOCATIONS
Loose areolar	Collagen, elastic, reticular fibres	Strength Elasticity Support	Subcutaneous layer beneath skin
Loose adipose	Adipocytes	Insulation	Subcutaneous layer beneath skin
		Protection	Tissue surrounding heart and kidneys
		Energy store	Padding around joints
Loose reticular	Reticular fibres	Support	Liver
	Reticular cells	Filtration	Spleen Lymph nodes
Dense regular	Collagen fibres in parallel	Strength Support	Tendons Ligaments
Dense irregular	Collagen fibres arranged randomly	Strength	Skin Heart Tissue surrounding bone Tissue surrounding cartilage
Dense elastic	Elastic fibres	Stretch	Lung tissue Arteries

Loose Connective Tissue

There are three types of loose connective tissue:

- areolar
- adipose
- reticular.

Areolar is the most abundant loose connective tissue. It contains all three fibres (collagen, elastic and reticular) and its primary functions are support, elasticity and strength. Areolar tissue is combined with adipose tissue to form the subcutaneous layer, which connects skin with other tissues and organs.

Clinical considerations demonstrate the practical application to your learning.

Clinical Considerations Magnetic Resonance Imaging (MRI)

Health professional students often question what relevance subatomic particles have to the practice of health care. Magnetic resonance imaging, a widely used diagnostic imaging technique, is one example of how the behaviour of subatomic particles is harnessed for medical purposes. MRI, unlike CT or PET scans, does not involve exposing a patient to ionising radiation, and it is able to produce 3-dimensional images of all body structures, including soft tissue. It is an extremely versatile diagnostic imaging system, and it works by detecting the spin of protons in water molecules. Patients are placed into a powerful magnetic field, which forces the protons contained in the molecules of body water to align with the field (protons have a positive charge, so they will spin round and align when they find themselves in a charge field). When the magnetic field is turned off, those protons all return to their original alignment, but at different speeds, depending on what environment they are in. Capturing these signals released from protons as they realign in various different tissues allows the different tissues to be detected and visualised. Because of the very strong magnetic field, however, metal cannot be placed inside the MRI scanner, so patients with any implants that contain metal cannot be scanned.

Medicines management boxes explore the administration of medicines, allowing you to administer safely and effectively.

> **Medicines Management** Tiny Pumps, Big Consequences ...
>
> Digoxin or a similar drug has been used to manage heart failure for centuries, and is still an important part of the management of congestive heart failure and some cardiac arrhythmias today. The drug makes the heart beat more strongly, by increasing the strength of contraction of the heart muscle – a very beneficial effect for a patient with a failing heart. The drug must be used carefully though, as it has the potential to cause cardiac arrhythmia. Digoxin has its action by inhibiting the sodium/potassium active transporter (sodium-potassium pump) on the cell membranes of heart muscle cells. This transporter pumps sodium ions out of the cell in exchange for potassium ions, thus maintaining the sodium ion concentration gradient across the membrane. This gradient in turn drives an exchange transporter which removes calcium ions from the cell in exchange for sodium ions. When digoxin is used, the inhibition of the sodium-potassium pump reduces the concentration gradient for sodium across the cell membrane, which reduces the transport of calcium out of the cells, resulting in an increased intracellular concentration of calcium in the heart muscle cells. The central role of calcium in muscle contraction means that more calcium equals stronger contraction, so the heart beats harder.

Glossary explaining key terms.

Glossary

Aneuploidy: The presence of an abnormal number of chromosomes in a cell.
Atresia: Degeneration process of the ovarian follicles that do not ovulate.
Colostrum: First secretion from the mammary glands after birth.
Conceptus: Denotes the embryo and its associated extraembryonic structures (i.e. placenta).
Corpus luteum (CL): A hormone-secreting structure that develops in an ovary at the sight of ovulation.
Ectoderm: The outermost of the three primary germ layers of an embryo.
Effacement: Process by which the cervix prepares for delivery (soften, shorten and become thinner) after the baby has repositioned itself in the lower in the abdomen/pelvis region.
Embryogenesis: The formation and development of an embryo.
Endoderm: The innermost of the three primary germ layers of an embryo.
Endometrium: The inner epithelial layer and mucous membrane of the mammalian uterus.
Epididymis: Highly convoluted which connects the testis to the vas deferens.
Fallopian tube (also known as an oviduct or uterine tube): Uterine appendages leading from the ovaries into the uterus.
Fertilisation: The union of the male and female gamete (sperm and oocyte).
Follicle stimulating hormone (FSH): Sex hormone produced by the pituitary gland.
Gametes: Haploid sex cells (eggs and called sperm).
Gastrulation: Phase of early embryonic development during which the single-layered blastula is reorganised into a multilayered structure known as the gastrula.
Gestation: The period of development between conception and birth.
Human chorionic gonadotropin (hCG): Hormone secreted by the placenta which forms the basis of pregnancy tests.
Implantation: The process of attachment and invasion of the uterus endometrium by the blastocyst.
Luteinising hormone (LH): Hormone produced in the anterior pituitary gland which triggers ovulation and corpus luteum development.
Mesoderm: The innermost layer of the three primary germ layers of an embryo.
Miscarriage: Pregnancy loss before 20 weeks of pregnancy.
Oestrogen: Steroid hormones which promote the development and maintenance of female characteristics of the body.
Ovulation: A phase of the female menstrual cycle that involves the release of an egg (ovum) from one of the ovaries.
Preeclampsia: A serious condition of pregnancy, usually characterised by high blood pressure, protein in the urine and severe swelling.
Pre-term: Labour delivery before 37 completed weeks of pregnancy.
Progesterone: Hormone released by the corpus luteum in the ovary.
Stillbirth: Loss of a foetus or baby after 20 weeks' gestation or during birth.
Zygote: Fertilised egg.

Self-assessment review questions help you test yourself before and after each chapter.

Activities

Multiple Choice Questions

1. Which part of the brain is responsible for thinking, reasoning and intelligence?
   (a) cerebellum
   (b) hypothalamus
   (c) cerebrum
   (d) epithalamus
2. Which structures are involved in the control of respiration?
   (a) pons and medulla
   (b) thalamus and epithalamus
   (c) somatic and sensory nervous system
   (d) cerebellum and cerebrum
3. Which neuroglial cell acts as a macrophage?
   (a) oligodendrocyte
   (b) astrocyte
   (c) microglia
   (d) Schwann cell

The website icon indicates that you can find accompanying resources on the book's companion websites.

About the Companion Website

Don't forget to visit the student and instructor companion websites for this book:

www.wileyfundamentalseries.com/anatomy

On this companion website, students will find valuable material designed to enhance their learning, including:
- Case studies
- Glossary terms
- Interactive multiple choice questions
- Interactive true/false questions
- Flashcards
- Links to further reading
- Matching items questions

Scan this QR code to visit the student companion website:

www.wiley.com/go/instructor/anatomy

On this companion website, instructors will find valuable material designed to enhance their teaching, including:
- PowerPoint slides to be used as a complete slide set: including slides with explanatory text combined with figures from the book to cover the main topics for each chapter
- An image bank of all the figures and tables from the book, to download as PowerPoint slides

Scan this QR code to visit the instructor companion website:

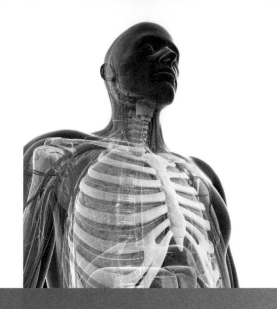

Basic Scientific Principles of Physiology

Suzanne Evans

Test Your Prior Knowledge

- What is the difference between anatomy and physiology?
- What are atoms, ions and electrolytes?
- What is an element?
- How do we distinguish living things from non-living things?
- What is homeostasis?

Learning Outcomes

After reading this chapter you will be able to:

- Outline the levels of organisation of the body.
- Describe the characteristics and the requirements of all living things.
- Interpret chemical symbols and equations and understand the ways in which atoms can bind together.
- Describe the pH scale and its importance to life.
- List the differences between organic and inorganic substances.

Visit the student companion website at www.wileyfundamentalseries.com/anatomy where you can test yourself using flashcards, multiple-choice questions and more. Instructor companion site at www.wiley.com/go/instructor/anatomy where instructors will find valuable materials such as PowerPoint slides and image bank designed to enhance your teaching.

Fundamentals of Anatomy and Physiology: For Nursing and Healthcare Students, Third Edition. Edited by Ian Peate and Suzanne Evans.
© 2020 John Wiley & Sons Ltd. Published 2020 by John Wiley & Sons Ltd.
Student companion website: www.wileyfundamentalseries.com/anatomy
Instructor companion website: www.wiley.com/go/instructor/anatomy

Introduction

Learning about the physiology of the body is very much like learning a foreign language – there are new vocabulary, grammar and concepts to learn and understand. This first chapter introduces you to this new language so that you can then use your knowledge to understand the physiology of the different parts of the body that are discussed in all the other chapters of this book.

First of all there are two terms to learn and understand:

- anatomy, the study of structure;
- physiology, the study of function.

However, structure is always related to function because the structure determines the function, which in turn determines how the body/organ, and so on, is structured – the two are interdependent.

Levels of Organisation

The body is a very complex organism that consists of many components, starting with the smallest of them – the atom – and concluding with the organism itself (Figure 1.1). Starting from the smallest component and working towards the largest, the body operates, and can be studied, on the following levels:

- The chemical level – the atoms, molecules and macromolecules that we are made of.
- The cellular level – the smallest living units in our bodies.
- The tissue level – the groups of cells specialised to perform specific functions, e.g. nerve or muscle tissue.
- The organ level – a structure, consisting of many tissues, specialised to perform a specific function, e.g. the heart.
- The organ system level – a system, consisting of more than one organ, specialised to perform a range of functions, e.g. the cardiovascular system.
- The organism level – the whole individual.

Characteristics of Life

All living organisms have certain characteristics in common, which are considered essential for the maintenance of life. These characteristics are:

- **Sensitivity** – organisms need to be able to sense and respond to changes in their environment such as changes in light levels, temperature, chemical composition, presence of threats, etc.
- **Nutrition** – Seeking out, ingesting and using food to supply energy and the raw materials for growth and development is a very basic requirement.
- **Respiration** – This is the means by which an organism obtains and uses oxygen to release energy from food to power the other activities listed here.
- **Movement** – The ability to change position is essential if an organism is to be able to escape threats, find food, other members of the species, etc.
- **Growth** – This is essential for the development of an organism from birth to adulthood, but also for the renewal and repair of body parts during the life of an organism.
- **Reproduction** – This is an essential process, not for the survival of the individual, but for the survival of the species. Sexual reproduction has the added bonus of continually mixing and re-mixing genetic material to produce genetically unique individuals each time, which increases the ability of a species to adapt and survive over the very long term.
- **Excretion** – the removal of waste substances produced by metabolic processes from the body, to prevent them building up to harmful levels.

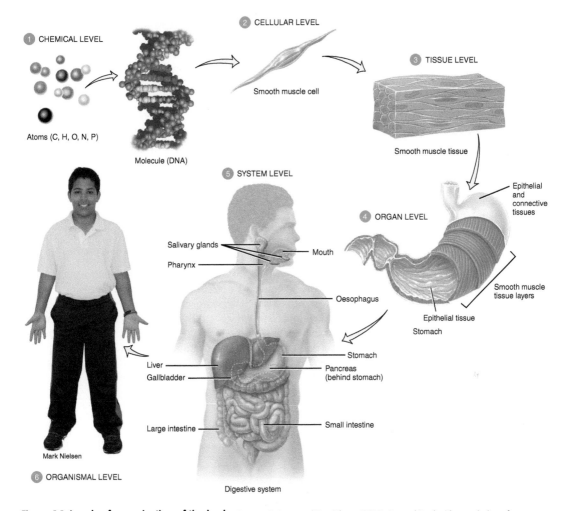

Figure 1.1 **Levels of organisation of the body.** *Source:* Tortora and Derrickson (2014). Reproduced with permission of John Wiley & Sons.

Bodily Requirements

There are five essential requirements that all organisms, including humans, require:

1. **Water:** Water is the most abundant substance found in the body. At birth, our bodies are approximately 78% water. This reduces to 65% at 1 year of age, and to 55–60% in adulthood. Our biochemistry evolved to operate in a watery (aqueous) environment; our cells are filled with a watery, salty solution, in which our cellular processes are carried out, and those cells are also bathed in a watery, salty solution. While it may not look like it, blood is also mainly water, making water important for the transport of substances around our large and complex bodies.

   Body water also helps regulate body temperature, since sweating is an important mechanism for evaporative cooling.

2. **Food:** Food supplies the energy and raw materials for the organism to fulfil all the essential activities of life.

3. **Oxygen:** Oxygen is required for the release of energy from food, by the oxidation of high energy food substances. Oxygen is one of the gases that exists naturally in the air (oxygen makes up approximately 20% of the air).
4. **Sunlight:** All life on earth depends ultimately on sunlight, since plants need this to grow, and other organisms depend directly or indirectly on plants for food.

Life at the Chemical Level

Studying living things at a chemical level reveals a world of 'chemical machinery', carrying out millions of chemical reactions within our cells every minute, which keep us alive, functioning and growing. A living body depends for its continued survival on simple atoms and molecules and also some large and very complex molecules (macromolecules) to carry on the business of living, growing and reproducing. We will cover some of the most biologically important chemicals here.

The Elements

All matter on earth is made up of a range of approximately 100 chemical elements. A chemical element is a pure chemical substance that cannot be broken down into anything simpler by chemical means.

More than 100 elements are thought to exist, but only 98 are known to occur naturally on earth. All the elements are shown in the periodic table of the elements, which sets out the elements in terms of their unique atomic structures and their physical (colour, hardness, density, melting and boiling points) and chemical (the ways in which the element reacts chemically) properties. Based on physical and chemical properties, elements are classified as either metals, metalloids or non-metals. Those classed as metals share the following properties:

- They are solids at room temperature (apart from Mercury, which is liquid!).
- They conduct heat and electricity.
- They donate electrons when forming bonds (see chemical bonding).

Metalloids have some of the properties of metals and some of non-metals. Non-metals share the following properties:

- They may exist as a solid, a liquid or a gas.
- They are poor conductors of heat and electricity.
- They accept electrons from other atoms when forming bonds (see chemical bonding).

Below are some examples of metals and non-metals that are very important in biology:

METALS	NON-METALS
Calcium (Ca)	Chlorine (Cl)
Potassium (K)	Nitrogen (N)
Sodium (Na)	Oxygen (O)
Iron (Fe)	Carbon (C)
	Sulphur (S)
	Phosphorus (P)

The Smallest Unit of Matter: The Atom

Atoms are the building blocks of all matter. Each element in the periodic table consists of its own, unique atoms. The word 'atom' comes from a Greek word meaning 'incapable of being divided'. However, we now know that an atom consists of subatomic particles: electrons, neutrons and protons.

Protons carry a positive electrical charge and electrons carry a negative electrical charge, while the neutron, as its name implies, carries no electrical charge (it is neutral).

As can be seen from Figure 1.2, the protons and neutrons cluster together at the centre of the atom (forming the nucleus), while the electrons orbit constantly around the nucleus, and are kept in orbit by the electromagnetic force exerted by the nucleus.

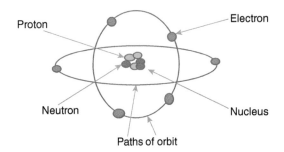

Figure 1.2 **Schematic diagram of an atom.** *Source:* Tortora and Derrickson (2014). Reproduced with permission of John Wiley & Sons.

There are many different types of atoms, differing in the numbers of protons, neutrons and electrons they possess. It is these differences between the various types of atoms that give us the array of chemical elements you will see on the periodic table of the elements.

Regardless of the type of atom, the atomic structures all obey the following rules:

- The nucleus is always central.
- The number of protons an atom possesses in its nucleus is known as the atomic number of that atom.
- The total number of particles in the nucleus of an atom (i.e. the number of protons and neutrons added together) is the atomic mass number. The mass of an atom is almost all in its nucleus – the electrons orbiting around the nucleus have virtually no weight – they are really just electrical charges in motion, but they are extremely important to the behaviour of the atom, as you will see.
- As the number of electrons an atom possesses increases, the electrons form layers of orbits, or shells, which get larger and further from the nucleus. The inner shell can contain a maximum of two electrons and the second and third shells shell can contain a maximum of eight electrons. The electrons in the outermost shell of an atom determine whether and how the atom forms bonds with other atoms to make new chemicals. The electrons in the outermost shell are known as the valence electrons, as they are able to take part in bonding reactions with other atoms (see chemical bonds section).

Figure 1.3 shows the atomic structure of some of the most biologically important substances, or elements, with their atomic numbers and mass numbers.

If you look closely at the number of electrons in the various atoms shown in Figure 1.3, you will see that in each atom, the number of electrons is equal to the number of protons. Since each proton carries a positive charge and each electron carries a negative charge, having an equal number of each will mean that the atom has an overall neutral charge. For example, the carbon atom has six electrons, six protons and six neutrons. The equal and opposite electrical charges of the electrons and protons cancel each other out, so that the atom is electrically neutral and it is said to be in a state of equilibrium.

When referring to these different elements, we use symbols to represent each one, rather than writing out their names each time. For example, the symbol for sodium is Na (after its Latin name natrium), the symbol for potassium is K (after its Latin name kalium), Chlorine is Cl, and the symbol of Carbon is C.

Clinical Considerations Magnetic Resonance Imaging (MRI)

Health professional students often question what relevance subatomic particles have to the practice of health care. Magnetic resonance imaging, a widely used diagnostic imaging technique, is one example of how the behaviour of subatomic particles is harnessed for medical purposes. MRI, unlike CT or PET scans, does not involve exposing a patient to ionising radiation, and it is able to produce 3-dimensional images of all body structures, including soft tissue. It is an extremely versatile diagnostic imaging system, and it works by detecting the spin of protons in water molecules. Patients are placed into a powerful magnetic field, which forces the protons contained in the molecules of body water to align with the field (protons have a positive charge, so they will spin round and align when they find themselves in a charge field). When the magnetic field is turned off, those protons all return to their original alignment, but at different speeds, depending on what environment they are in. Capturing these signals released from protons as they realign in various different tissues allows the different tissues to be detected and visualised. Because of the very strong magnetic field, however, metal cannot be placed inside the MRI scanner, so patients with any implants that contain metal cannot be scanned.

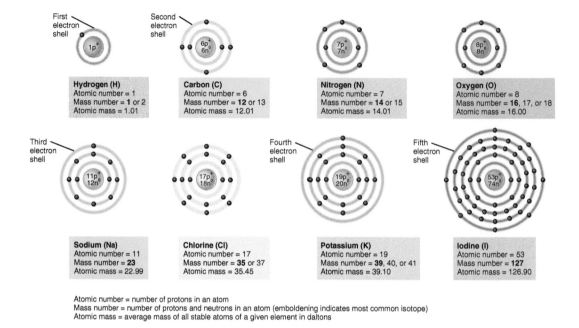

Atomic number = number of protons in an atom
Mass number = number of protons and neutrons in an atom (emboldening indicates most common isotope)
Atomic mass = average mass of all stable atoms of a given element in daltons

Figure 1.3 The structure of some biologically important atoms. *Source:* Tortora and Derrickson (2014). Reproduced with permission of John Wiley & Sons.

Chemical Reactions and Chemical Bonds

If atoms remained in their neutral state of equilibrium, then the world might be very different – it might contain only the 100 or so species of atom that are known to exist on earth. However, when the conditions are right, atoms react with other atoms to form molecules and compounds. A molecule, therefore, is formed when two or more of the same atoms bond chemically to each other, and a compound is formed when two or more different types of atoms bond chemically. This ability of different atoms to combine creates a huge variety of possible molecules and compounds, each of which possess their own physical and chemical properties. Why do these reactions occur? Remember that atoms achieve a lower energy, more stable state when they have a full outer shell of electrons. Accordingly, a joining together of two or more atoms that results in a more stable, lower energy state for all of them will be a reaction that will readily occur.

There are a couple of different types of chemical bonds:

Ionic Bonds

Ionic bonding involves the exchange of electrons from one atom to another. Because this exchange will alter the charge on any atom giving or receiving an electron (remember that the electron has a negative charge), it will create charged substances. Look for example, at the sodium atom depicted in Figure 1.4a. The sodium atom has a single electron in its outer shell. Since that shell needs 8 electrons to be full, then it must pick up another 7 electrons to achieve a lower energy state – a tall order! It could, however, lose that one electron, leaving the full second shell as the outer shell, thus achieving a full outer shell by 'donating' an electron to any atom that might be in need of an extra one. Of course, having donated its one electron, the number of protons in the sodium atom will exceed the number of electrons by one, giving the atom a net positive charge. At that point, it becomes known as a sodium ion (Na+), and since it has a net positive charge, it is a positive ion, also known as a cation.

You don't have to look far to find a suitable electron acceptor; chlorine has an outer shell containing 7 electrons, so accepting an extra electron would allow it to achieve a lower energy state:

By the same token, though, the chlorine atom now has one more electron than it has protons, and so gains a net negative charge, and is now known as a chloride ion (Cl−), and is a negative ion, also known as an anion (Figure 1.4b).

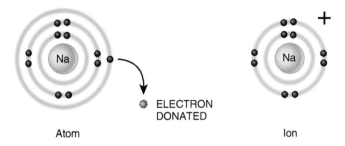

Figure 1.4a **The single electron in the outer shell of the sodium atom can be donated during a chemical reaction, leaving a positively charged, sodium ion.** *Source:* Tortora and Derrickson (2014). Reproduced with permission of John Wiley & Sons.

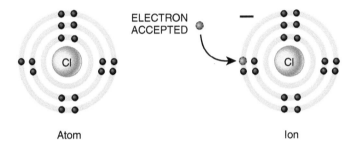

Figure 1.4b **A chlorine atom needs only one electron to complete its outer shell, so will readily react with electron donors like sodium, and accept the donated electron. This creates a negatively charged, chloride ion.** *Source:* Tortora and Derrickson (2014). Reproduced with permission of John Wiley & Sons.

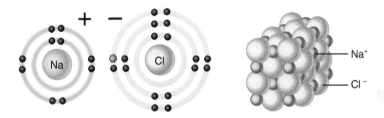

Figure 1.4c **The ionic bonding between a sodium and a chloride ion results in a neutral molecule, sodium chloride. Sodium chloride molecules pack together to form a regular, lattice, crystalline structure.** *Source:* Tortora and Derrickson (2014). Reproduced with permission of John Wiley & Sons.

Having exchanged electrons, the newly formed sodium and chloride ions are now oppositely charged. Opposite charges attract one another, while similar charges repel. The attractive forces between the two ions therefore 'bond' them together, since together, they form a neutral molecule, sodium chloride (NaCl) (Figure 1.4c).

Since the chemical bond is the result of the attractive force between the two ions, this bond is known as an ionic bond. Ionic bonds, therefore, are those that form between ions because of the attraction between opposite charges. These are not the strongest of chemical bonds because, in the presence of other ions, the individual components of an ionically bonded molecule may be more strongly attracted to other charged substances around them, thus breaking the ionic bond and freeing the two ions from each other. This often happens when ionically bonded substances are placed in water, since the water molecule, while not an ion, is a polar molecule, which can set up weak ionic bonds between itself and ions (see polar molecules section).

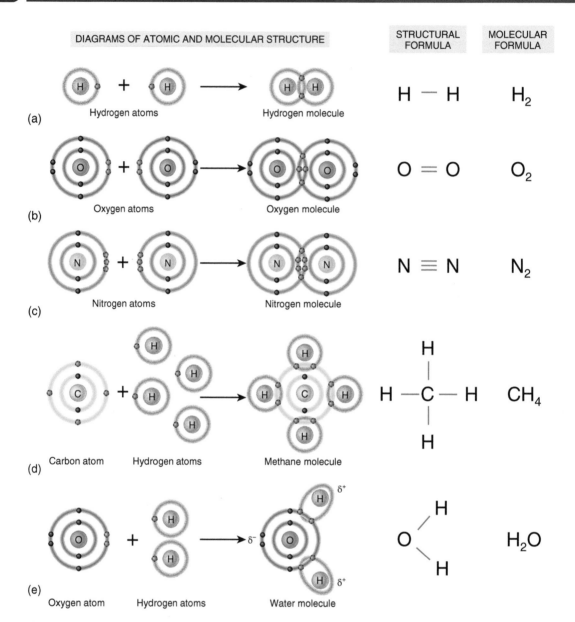

Figure 1.5 (a–e) Some covalently bonded substances, showing the sharing of electrons between the atoms.
Source: Tortora and Derrickson (2014). Reproduced with permission of John Wiley & Sons.

There is a second way in which atoms can bond, and this is known as covalent bonding. This form of bonding involves the sharing of valence electrons rather than the complete donation and accepting of electrons.

Electrons rapidly orbit the nucleus of an atom, and if two atoms are so close together that their electron outer shells overlap at the closest point, one electron can orbit both atomic nuclei (Figure 1.5).

Notice that some of the common covalent compounds shown in Figure 1.5 contain double and triple covalent bonds, in which four or six electrons are shared to create the bonds.

Polar Molecules

Sometimes, covalently bonded molecules do not share their electrons equally and the shared electron may spend more time orbiting one end of the covalent bond than the other, giving a more negative charge to that part of the molecule. This difference in charge between one end of a molecule and the other is called polarity, and a molecule that has a charge disparity between its two ends is known as a polar molecule. Water is a polar molecule because the two shared electrons that form each of the bonds between the oxygen atom and the hydrogen atoms spend more time orbiting the oxygen nucleus, thereby making the oxygen end of the molecule more negative than the hydrogen end. When we illustrate the molecule (Figure 1.6), the polarity is indicated by the Greek letter delta (δ) followed by a plus or minus sign to indicate the relative charge at each end of the molecule.

Because of this charge difference within the molecule, polar molecules can attract ions or other polar molecules of the opposite charge, just like ions, and this attraction forms weak bonds. Polar molecules will often swing round and line up with their more negative ends towards a positive charge, or away from a negative charge. The most important weak bond of this type occurs between water and other polar molecules or ions. Because the weak attraction is between the more positive hydrogen end of one water molecule and the more negative end of another water molecule, this type of bond is known as a hydrogen bond (Figure 1.7).

Electrolytes

When ionically bonded substances are placed in water, the ionic bonds break, and the ionically bonded substances 'dissociate' or fall apart, and the ions are released into the water as separate entities, no longer bound to each other. If you were to apply an electrical potential to a solution like this, by placing electrodes attached to a battery into the water, the ions in solution would respond by moving through the solution – the positively charged ions would move in one direction (towards the negatively battery pole) and the negatively charged

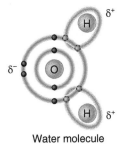

Water molecule

Figure 1.6 **Water, a polar molecule, with its positive and negative poles shown.** *Source:* Tortora and Derrickson (2014). Reproduced with permission of John Wiley & Sons.

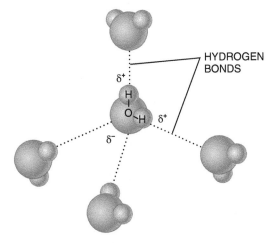

Figure 1.7 **Hydrogen bonds and water. The weak bonds between the hydrogen of one water molecule and the oxygen of a neighbouring water molecule are known as hydrogen bonds, and account for the cohesion, or 'stickiness' of water, for surface tension effects and for its tendency to mix well with other polar molecules and ions.** *Source:* Tortora and Derrickson (2014). Reproduced with permission of John Wiley & Sons.

ions in the other (towards the positively charged battery pole). By this movement, the ions would effectively carry their charge through the solution, thereby allowing electrical current to pass through the solution. Because of this, ions in solution are known as electrolytes, and an electrolyte solution will allow current to pass through it.

Acids and Bases

The concept of acidity is an extremely important one to understand, as maintaining acid-base balance in the body is essential for life. The acidity of a solution is a measure of the number of hydrogen ions in that solution; the more hydrogen ions in a solution, the more acidic it is. Acids are compounds, which when placed in water, dissociate into hydrogen ions and a second ion (which will vary depending on the acid). Any substance, therefore, which releases free hydrogen ions when it is put into a solution, is an acid. The more hydrogen ions it releases, the stronger the acid it is. Conversely, an alkali (or base), is a substance which removes hydrogen ions from solution, usually by releasing hydroxyl ions (OH^-), into a solution. Hydroxyl ions are attracted to and readily bind with H^+ ions, resulting in water.

A substance, therefore, which removes free hydrogen ions from a solution by providing another ion to bind them up, is an alkaline substance.

Acidity and alkalinity are measured on the pH scale, which extends between 0 and 14, the most acidic being 0 (many more hydrogen ions than hydroxyl ions in solution) and the most alkaline being 14 (many more hydroxyl ions than hydrogen ions in solution). Halfway between these two extremes, 7 on the pH scale, is the neutral point (an equal number of hydrogen ions and hydroxyl ions), as indicated on the pH scale accompanied by hydrogen and hydroxyl ion concentrations in Figure 1.8.

The pH scale is a logarithmic scale, which means that each unit on the scale corresponds to a 10-fold change in the concentration of hydrogen ions. For example, a solution with a pH 3 is 10 times more acidic than a solution of pH 4, 100 times (10×10) more acidic than solution of pH 5, and 1000 times ($10 \times 10 \times 10$) more acidic than a solution of pH 7. The same applies to pH values that are above 7 (i.e. alkaline solutions).

Blood and pH Values

The normal pH range in blood is slightly above 7 on the pH scale, it is therefore slightly alkaline. However, for the purposes of physiology, a blood pH lower (more acidic) than 7.35 is considered to be too acidic, and one greater than 7.45 is too alkaline, and when either of these events occurs it can have a serious effect on physiological function – as is discussed in other chapters within this book. The pH range for blood may seem very narrow, but because the scale is a logarithmic one, just a small change in pH indicates a very significant

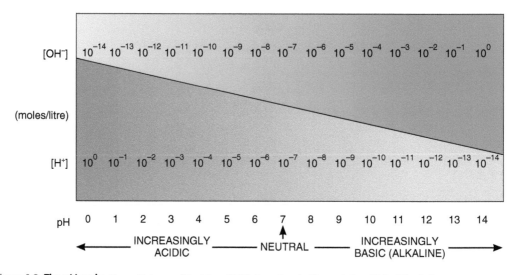

Figure 1.8 **The pH scale.** *Source:* Tortora and Derrickson (2014). Reproduced with permission of John Wiley & Sons.

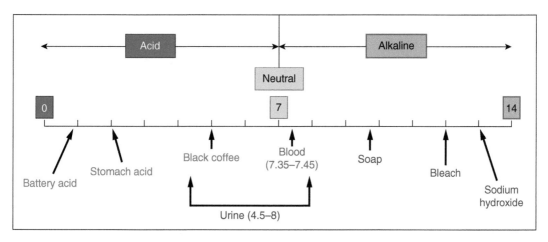

Figure 1.9 **The pH of some common household substances and some body fluids.**

alteration in H^+ concentration. An alteration of pH from pH 7.4 to pH 7.3 actually represents a doubling of the H^+ ion concentration (Figure 1.9).

Representing Chemical Reactions in Written Form: Chemical Equations

As already mentioned, to make writing chemistry quicker and easier, we use symbols to represent each element in the periodic table. When one element reacts with another to form a new compound, we can represent that reaction using the same symbols, showing the compounds reacting (the reactants) and the new compounds resulting from the reaction (the products).

As an example, let us look at a reaction which produces water, one of the most important and ubiquitous compounds on earth. We all know water as a liquid at room temperature, yet it is formed by the reaction between the gases hydrogen and oxygen. Two atoms of hydrogen bond with one atom of oxygen to create the new molecule we know as water. However, because in nature hydrogen gas exists as a hydrogen molecule (two hydrogen atoms bound together) as does oxygen gas (two oxygen atoms bound together), this means that two hydrogen molecules will actually react with one oxygen molecule, producing two water molecules. That equation is represented as:

$$2H_2 + O_2 \rightarrow H_2O$$

Since each water molecule contains two hydrogen atoms and only one oxygen atom, the chemical formula indicates this by placing a subscript 2 after the symbol for hydrogen, and since two hydrogen molecules are required for the reaction, a large 2 before hydrogen indicates this.

Chemical reactions can also be shown in a more graphical way, using not only the chemical symbols, but also diagrams of the atoms and molecules themselves, to give a better idea of their structure, as shown in Figure 1.10.

So, a chemical equation is just a shorthand way of showing a chemical reaction.

It is important to understand that chemical reactions involve a rearrangement of atoms and molecules to form different molecules and compounds – nothing can be created and nothing destroyed in these reactions, so the total number of atoms and molecules must be the same on each side of a chemical equation. Remember that chemical bonds form in the first place to allow atoms and molecules to achieve a lower energy, more stable, state, so it follows that if a chemical rearrangement is to take place, then the rearranged form of the chemicals must be a still lower energy state. When these reactions occur, therefore, energy is released as heat when chemical bonds are broken and different ones formed. This means that heat is one of the products of the reaction, along with the chemical products. Chemical reactions which

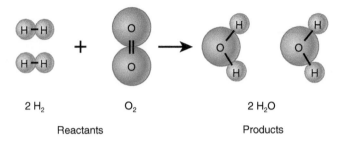

2 H$_2$ O$_2$ 2 H$_2$O

Reactants   Products

Figure 1.10 Pictorial depiction of the reaction between two hydrogen molecules and one oxygen molecule to produce two water molecules. *Source:* Tortora and Derrickson (2014). Reproduced with permission of John Wiley & Sons.

produce heat as a by-product of the reaction are known as exothermic reactions. Humans often put exothermic reactions to good use – the best example being the crackling fire that keeps us warm in winter – the heat from the fire is in fact the heat produced by the exothermic chemical reaction between the cellulose (in the fire wood) and oxygen (in the air). The arrow in the middle of the chemical equation indicates the direction of the reaction; in other words, it points towards the products of the reaction. This is not to say that the reaction cannot also reverse and proceed from right to left as written, but it does mean that if the reaction from left to right is exothermic, then energy will need to be supplied in order to get it to go back the other way. Take the example shown earlier, of the gases hydrogen and oxygen combining to form water; that reaction is exothermic. It is also possible for the reaction to proceed in the opposite direction, and water to break apart to yield hydrogen and oxygen, but energy would have to be supplied to drive this reaction, so it would not happen spontaneously.

In a chemical equation, the reactants and the product may be separated by a single arrow ($\rightarrow$) as in the earlier example of H$_2$O. This indicates that the reaction occurs only in the direction that the arrow is pointing. If a reaction can proceed in either direction, it is known as a reversible reaction, and is written with arrows pointing in both directions.

An example of a reversible reaction, and one which is a very important reaction in the control of acid-base balance in the body, is the reaction between carbon dioxide and water to form carbonic acid.

$$CO_2 + H_2O \rightleftharpoons H_2CO_3 \rightleftharpoons HCO_3^- + H^+$$

Carbonic   Bicarbonate   Hydrogen
acid   ion   ion

Not only does the reaction take place in two stages, but, as the arrows indicate, the reactions can also proceed in both directions, with bicarbonate and hydrogen ions combining to form carbonic acid, which then rearranges to produce carbon dioxide and water. Reactions like this, which can proceed in either direction, will create an equilibrium, a point at which there is a mix of products and reactants. This means that changes in the balance between the reactants and the products would therefore be expected to 'tip' the reaction in one direction or the other. This behaviour is very important in the rapid buffering of acids and alkalis in the blood, to help maintain normal blood pH.

Organic Molecules

Chemicals can be classified as being either organic or inorganic. These terms derive from the observation that the molecules that make up living things are large, carbon-containing compounds, and these became known as organic compounds, because they formed living (organic) material. Organic molecules contain carbon, often in long chains, with hydrogen, and are usually very large molecules. Inorganic molecules, on the other hand, do not contain carbon and hydrogen atoms arranged in long chains, although some do contain carbon (carbon dioxide, for example, is an inorganic compound) and some contain hydrogen (water, for example). Inorganic molecules tend to be much smaller.

There are other characteristics which set organic and inorganic compounds apart:

- **Organic** molecules:
  - contain carbon (C) and hydrogen (H);
  - are usually larger than inorganic molecules;
  - dissolve in water and organic liquids;
  - include carbohydrates (sugars), proteins, lipids (fats) and nucleic acids (part of DNA) – see Chapter 3, Genetics. Organic molecules are sometimes known as the 'molecules of life' for this reason.
- **Inorganic** molecules:
  - include water (H_2O), carbon dioxide (CO_2) and inorganic salts.
  - are usually smaller than organic molecules;
  - usually dissolve in water or react with water to produce ions;

Examples of Organic Substances

Carbohydrates

This group of organic molecules, also known as saccharides, makes up one of our major food groups, and includes sugars, starch and cellulose. The smallest and simplest members of the group, the monosaccharides, provide energy to cells as well as forming part of some of the structures in cells (see Chapter 2). They contain carbon (C), hydrogen (H) and oxygen (O), usually in the proportion CH_2O; that is, with two hydrogen atoms to every one oxygen and carbon atom.

Carbohydrates are classified into three groups based on their molecular size:

Monosaccharides $\begin{cases} \text{Glucose (dextrose), formula } C_6H_{12}O_6 \\ \text{Fructose (fruit sugar), formula also } C_6H_{12}O_6 \end{cases}$

Disaccharides $\begin{cases} \text{Sucrose (table sugar), formula } C_{12}H_{22}O_6 \\ \text{Lactose (milk sugar), formula } C_{12}H_{22}O_{11} \end{cases}$

Polysaccharides $\begin{cases} \text{Starch (amylose), formula } (C_6H_{10}O_5)n \\ \text{Glycogen, formula } (C_6H_{10}O_5)n \\ \text{Cellulose, formula } (C_6H_{10}O_5)n \end{cases}$

Monosaccharides and disaccharides can be referred to collectively as simple sugars or simple carbohydrates. Disaccharides, as the name suggests, consist of two monosaccharides bonded together – a sucrose molecule is one molecule of glucose bound to one molecule of fructose. The much larger polysaccharides are referred to as complex sugars or complex carbohydrates. It is the foods containing complex carbohydrates that are often listed as having a low glycaemic index, since, as larger sugars that require digestion before they can be absorbed, they arrive in the bloodstream more gradually.

Fats

Fats are one part of a larger group of chemicals known as lipids. They form another major food group, and are used in the diet to provide energy, but cell membranes are made of lipids and the group of hormones known as the steroids are also lipids, so this group plays a range of important roles in human function. Like carbohydrates, they consist of carbon (C), hydrogen (H) and oxygen (O), but because the relative proportions of these atoms are different from the carbohydrates, the lipids have different properties. They are only soluble in non-polar solvents like alcohol, for example, and not in water.

There are several types of lipids, but some of the most common are the following:

Fatty acids. These molecules are the 'building blocks' of larger, more complex lipids, and do not often exist on their own. They consist of long chains of carbon and hydrogen, with an organic acid group at the end (Figure 1.11). There are many different types of fatty acid, three common examples being oleic acid – found in olive, sunflower, peanut and palm oil, palmitic acid – found in palm oil, meat and dairy and stearic acid – found most commonly in animal fats.

Triglycerides (triacylglycerols). These molecules consist of three fatty acid molecules attached to a glycerol molecule (Figure 1.12). The long chains of the fatty acid molecules anchored to the glycerol molecule make the triglycerides look a little like three ties on a hanger.

These are the lipids that our cells can use for energy, and we often measure triglycerides circulating in the blood when checking a person's blood lipid profile.

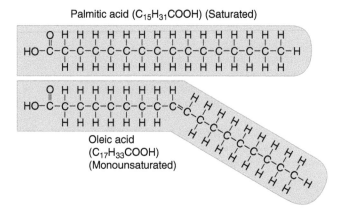

Figure 1.11 **The fatty acids palmitic acid and oleic acid, indicating the general structure of fatty acids.** *Source:* Tortora and Derrickson (2014). Reproduced with permission of John Wiley & Sons.

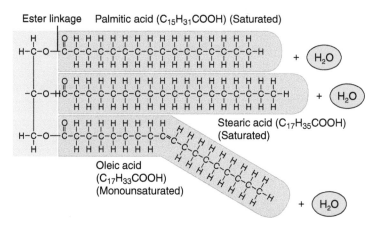

Figure 1.12 **Triglyceride molecule.** *Source:* Tortora and Derrickson (2014). Reproduced with permission of John Wiley & Sons.

Clinical Considerations Cholesterol, Blood Lipids and Health

Routine measurement of blood lipids includes measurement of a number of lipids carried in the blood stream, and usually includes triglycerides, low density lipoprotein (LDL), high density lipoprotein (HDL) and total cholesterol. While fats are an excellent source of energy, excessively high levels of triglycerides, LDL and total cholesterol are linked with an increased risk of cardiovascular disease. High levels of HDL, on the other hand, are associated with reduced risk of cardiovascular disease. Improving blood lipid profiles to improve health can be achieved by dietary changes and increasing physical activity, but the use of drugs known as statins has a more powerful effect on cholesterol levels, and these drugs have been widely prescribed for this purpose. As with any drug, the benefits of taking it have to be carefully weighed against the risks. The data seem to suggest that raising HDL to provide a protective effect is just as, or perhaps more, important than reducing LDL, so refinements to the way the problem of high blood lipids are managed are on the way.

Phospholipids. As the name suggests, these lipids have a phosphate group as a component of their molecules. A double layer of these molecules makes up the basis of our cell membranes, as will be discussed in Chapter 2 (Figure 1.13).

Steroids. Steroids are substances that are quite different chemically from lipids, but are considered lipids because they are insoluble in water. A number of very important hormones are steroids, as is cholesterol, which is a vital component of cell membranes. The names of these substances usually indicate the chemical group they belong to, by including -sterol or -sterone in the name, e.g. cholesterol, corticosterone, aldosterone, progesterone, testosterone.

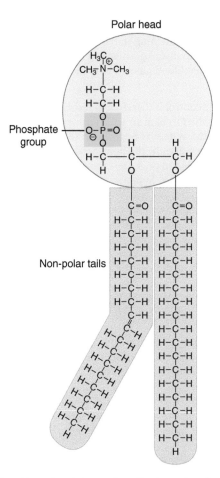

Figure 1.13 **Phospholipid molecule. This molecule has a 'head', where the phosphate group is located, and two 'tails', consisting of two fatty acid molecules.** *Source: Tortora and Derrickson (2014). Reproduced with permission of John Wiley & Sons.*

Proteins

Proteins are large molecules built from amino acids strung together to form long chains. The body makes many different proteins, each one with a different sequence and number of amino acids strung together. The structural material that makes up the body is protein, and many vital molecules such as hormones receptors, enzymes and antibodies are proteins. It is useful to think of protein function in two major categories: structural proteins (make up our structures) and functional proteins (part of our biochemical machinery, including receptors, enzymes and antibodies). Proteins will be discussed in much greater depth in Chapter 3.

Homeostasis

Homeostasis is the maintenance of a relatively stable internal environment in the face of a constantly changing external environment – from cold to hot, from dry to wet, from acid to alkaline and so on. Homeostatic mechanisms are continuously monitoring and controlling variables in the body such as blood pH, core temperature, blood pressure, blood glucose levels and many others. Regardless of the variable being controlled, homeostatic systems all follow a general scheme:

1. A detector system to monitor changes in the variable. These detectors are collectively known as receptors, and we have many types – each one specialised to detect a particular variable, e.g. baroreceptors detect pressure changes in blood vessels, chemoreceptors detect changes in the concentration of some chemicals and thermoreceptors detect temperature changes.

2. A control centre to receive the messages from the detectors about changes, and to organise a response to counteract the change, thereby maintaining stability.
3. Effectors, to bring about the response, e.g. shivering and 'goosebumps' when a drop in temperature is detected, increased insulin when blood glucose level increases or an increase in heart rate when a drop in blood pressure is detected.

Since the tendency of homeostatic control is therefore to resist, or at least limit, the size of changes occurring within the internal environment, the mechanism which achieves this is often referred to as a negative feedback loop, since the response of the system is opposite to (a negative of) the change that triggered it. For example, if the blood pressure drops slightly, the homeostatic mechanism that controls blood pressure will respond by producing an increase in blood pressure – the response is therefore opposite to the change, hence the feedback to the change is negative to it. Systems that work like this are inherently stable, as they tend to resist change within the system.

Much of the study of human function is the study of these complex homeostatic control mechanisms, and the maintenance of good health depends on their effectiveness. It is important to remember that homeostasis does not 'lock' a variable at one setting, but limits the degree to which a variable can change, so that our systems are flexible enough to adapt to changing demands and conditions, but stable enough to maintain an internal environment that is consistent with healthy function of our body systems.

Units of Measurement

To conclude this chapter, which introduces certain scientific concepts and prepares the reader for the remaining chapters, just some brief notes about units of measurement. This is an important section because the ability to identify and understand units of measurement will enhance the understanding of the complex human organism.

A unit is a standardised, descriptive word that specifies the dimension of a measured property. Traditionally there have been seven properties of matter that have been measured independently of each other, namely:

- **time** – measures the duration that something occurs;
- **length** – measures the length of an object;
- **mass** – measures the mass (commonly taken to be the weight) of an object;
- **current** – measures the amount of electric current that passes through an object;
- **temperature** – measures how hot or cold an object is;
- **amount** – measures the amount of a substance that is present;
- **luminous intensity** – measures the brightness of an object.

Originally, each country had its own units of measurement. In the UK, for example, there were such units as furlongs, miles, poles, gallons, quarts, bushels, pecks and so on. This made it difficult for people, particularly scientists, from other countries to work with each other, so several years ago an international system of units was agreed upon by most major countries (however, a notable exception to this agreement is the USA). This new agreed system became known as the Système International d'Unités (or SI units for short). It is a system of units that relates present scientific knowledge to a unified system of units. Tables 1.1, 1.2, 1.3, 1.4, 1.5, 1.6 and 1.7 give the SI units, unit prefixes and some Imperial unit equivalents that will be useful as reference while working through this book.

Table 1.1 **The fundamental SI units.**

QUANTITY	NAME	SYMBOL
Length	metre	m
Mass	kilogram	kg
Time	second	s
Current	ampere	A
Temperature	Kelvin	K
Amount of substance	mole	mol
Luminous intensity	candela	cd

Table 1.2 **Other common SI units.**

PHYSICAL QUANTITY	NAME	SYMBOL
Force	Newton	N
Energy	Joule	J
Pressure	Pascal	Pa
Potential difference	Volt	V
Frequency	Hertz	Hz
Volume	litre	L

Table 1.3 **Multiples of SI units.**

PREFIX	SYMBOL	MEANING	SCIENTIFIC NOTATION
tera	T	one million million	10^{12}
giga	G	one thousand million	10^{9}
mega	M	one million	10^{6}
kilo	k	one thousand	10^{3}
hecto	h	one hundred	10^{2}
deca	da	ten	10^{1}
deci	d	one tenth	10^{-1}
centi	c	one hundredth	10^{-2}
milli	m	one thousandth	10^{-3}
micro	μ	one millionth	10^{-6}
nano	n	one thousandth of a millionth	10^{-9}
pico	p	one millionth of a millionth	10^{-12}
femto	f	one thousandth of a pico	10^{-15}
atto	a	one millionth of a pico	10^{-18}

Table 1.4 **Measures of weight.**

1 kg = 1000 g

1 g = 1000 mg

1 mg = 10^{-3} g

1 μg = 10^{-6} g

1 pound = 0.454 kg/454 g

1 ounce = 28.35 g

25 g = 0.9 ounce

1 ounce = 8 dram

Table 1.5 **Measures of volume.**

1 L = 1000 mL

100 mL = 1 dL

1 mL = 1000 μL

1 UK gallon = 4.5 L

1 pint = 568 mL

1 fluid ounce = 28.42 mL

1 teaspoon = 5 mL

1 tablespoon = 15 mL

Table 1.6 **Measures of length.**

1 m = 10^{-3} km

1 cm = 10^{-2} m

1 mm = 10^{-3} m

1 m = 39.37 inches

1 mile = 1.6 km

1 yard = 0.9 m

1 foot = 0.3 m

1 inch = 25.4 mm

Table 1.7 **Measures of energy.**

1 calorie = 4.184 J

100 calories = 1 dietary Calorie or kilocalorie

1 dietary Calorie = 4184 J or 4.184 kJ

1000 Calorie = 4184 kJ

1 kJ = 0.238 Calories

Conclusion

This concludes this brief introduction to some of the basics of chemistry and biology. As you will appreciate, the study of body function at any level, whether it be at the level of molecules reacting or at the level of the whole person, is extremely complicated, but also fascinating.

Learning something about how bodies function and how they respond to the challenges placed upon them in both health and disease can equip you with power to save lives in your future practice. It is only through gaining an understanding of the wonderful machines we inhabit that we can learn how to best care for them. Enjoy the discoveries that await you.

Glossary

Acid: A chemical substance with a pH below 7.

Acid-base balance: The maintenance of pH within controlled limits. This is essential for good health. See pH.

Alkali: A chemical substance with a pH above 7.

Anatomy: The study of the structures of the body.

Anion: An ion with a negative charge.

Antibody: Proteins that recognise and attach to specific infectious agents in the body.

Atomic number: The number of protons in the nucleus of an atom.

Atoms: The smallest unit of matter.

Base: An alkaline substance.

Bonds: The joining together of various substances, particularly atoms and molecules. See chemical bond, covalent bonds, ionic bonds, and polar bonds.

Cation: An ion with a positive charge.

Chemical bond: The 'attractive' force that holds atoms together.

Chemical reaction: A process in which chemical substances react together to produce a different chemical form. This is usually expressed by a chemical equation.

Compound: A substance that is made up of two or more elements chemically bonded together.

Covalent bonds: Bonds between atoms formed by the sharing of electrons between the atoms.

Electrolyte: Substance that produces a solution that conducts electricity when placed in water. Physiologically important electrolytes include sodium and potassium ions.

Electrons: The parts of an atom that orbit the atomic nucleus and carry a negative electrical charge. See also neutrons and protons.

Elements: A chemical substance that cannot be broken down into anything simpler by chemical means.

Enzymes: Proteins produced by cells that increase the rate of biochemical reactions in the body.

Homeostasis: The maintenance of a stable internal environment by the use of systems of detectors, control centres and effectors.

Inorganic substances: Substances that do not contain long chains of carbon and hydrogen molecules (although they may contain carbon and hydrogen).

Ionic bonds: Bonds that form between ions with opposite charges.

Ions: The entities formed when atoms lose or gain electrons, thereby becoming positively or negatively charged.

Mole: The unit of measurement of the amount of a substance.

Molecules: Electrically neutral group of two or more atoms bonded together.

Neutral substance: A chemical substance that is neither acidic nor alkaline.

Neutron: The parts of an atom that carry a neutral electrical charge (i.e. they have no electrical charge). See also electrons and protons.

Organelles: Structural and functional parts of a cell.

Organic substances: Substances that contain carbon molecules (e.g. carbohydrates, lipids, proteins).

pH: A measure of the acidity or alkalinity of a solution. See acid–base balance.

Physiology: The study of the way in which the body structures function.

Polar bonds: Bonds that form between polar molecules, in which the increased negativity of one pole of a polar molecule is attracted to the increased positivity of the opposite pole of another molecule. Hydrogen bonds are polar bonds.

Product (chemical reactions): The new substance/s formed following a chemical reaction.

Protons: Subatomic particles found in the atomic nucleus which carry a positive electrical charge. See also electrons and neutrons.

Reactant (chemical reactions): The individual substances involved in a chemical reaction.

Shell (of an atom): The name given to the orbits of electrons moving around the nucleus of an atom.

Valency: The number of hydrogen atoms an element is able to combine with. This is the bond-forming power of an element, and depends on the number of electrons in its outermost shell.

References

Tortora, G.J. and Derrickson, B.H. (2014) *Principles of Anatomy and Physiology*, 14th edn. Hoboken, NJ: John Wiley & Sons.

Activities

Multiple Choice Questions

1. The characteristics of life include:
   (a) digestion, excretion, irritation
   (b) absorption, bleeding, circulation
   (c) excretion, perspiration, reproduction
   (d) respiration, growth, responsiveness

2. The four essential requirements for all organisms are:
   (a) respiration, digestion, excretion and circulation
   (b) oxygen, water, sunlight, food
   (c) food, low temperatures, carbon dioxide, oxygen.
   (d) pressure, sight, water, food

3. Protons possess:
   (a) a stable electrical charge
   (b) no electrical charge
   (c) a negative electrical charge
   (d) a positive electrical charge

4. An atom contains five electrons in its outermost shell. Which of the following is it most likely to do when it reacts?
   (a) donate 5 electrons to another atom, becoming a more stable, neutral atom
   (b) donate three electrons to another atom, becoming a negatively charged ion
   (c) accept three electrons from another atom, becoming a negatively charged ion
   (d) accept one electron from another atom, becoming a neutral, more stable atom
5. Which of the following is not a type of chemical bond?
   (a) polar
   (b) equatorial
   (c) ionic
   (d) covalent
6. There are three classes of elements, namely:
   (a) metals, non-metals, metalloids
   (b) metals, oxidants, electrons
   (c) carbons, non-metals, metalloids
   (d) metalloids, non-metals, atomic
7. Which of the following is both an anion and a compound?
   (a) NaCl
   (b) Cl⁻
   (c) Na⁺
   (d) HCO_3^-
8. Which of the following are organic substances?
   (a) carbohydrates, proteins, lipids
   (b) carbohydrates, water, oxygen
   (c) water, proteins, lipids
   (d) lipids, oxygen, proteins
9. Which of these pH values is the least acidic?
   (a) 1.0
   (b) 0.8
   (c) 11
   (d) 6.5
10. Homeostasis is:
    (a) the effective use of receptors
    (b) a measurement of acidity in the body
    (c) maintenance of a stable internal environment
    (d) a combination of physical properties
11. A molecule of water is a combination of these atoms:
    (a) 1 × hydrogen, 1 × oxygen, 1 × carbon
    (b) 2 × oxygen, 1 × carbon
    (c) 2 × oxygen, 1 × hydrogen
    (d) 1 × oxygen, 2 × hydrogen
12. In biochemistry, a 'mole' is a unit of:
    (a) intensity of radiation
    (b) luminosity of light
    (c) pH of a solution
    (d) amount of a substance
13. The pH of a solution depends on:
    (a) the number of ions in the solution
    (b) the number of electrolytes in the solution
    (c) the number of hydrogen ions in the solution
    (d) the number of organic ions in the solution
14. Which of the following is a complex carbohydrate?
    (a) a polysaccharide
    (b) a protein
    (c) a monosaccharide
    (d) a triglyceride

15. An atom has an atomic number of 20. That means it has:
    (a) 10 electrons
    (b) 10 protons and 10 neutrons
    (c) 20 protons
    (d) 10 protons and 10 electrons

True or False
1. An ion is an atom that is in an electrically neutral state.
2. Molecules are combinations of atoms.
3. Many electrolytes are essential minerals.
4. Organic substances contain carbon and hydrogen.
5. Lipids are examples of inorganic substances.
6. Proteins are built up from amino acids and provide the structural material for the body.

Test Your Learning

1. What is the importance of respiration for the body?
2. Why is water essential for all organisms, including humans?
3. How is the atomic number of an atom calculated?
4. What is an ion, and what is its importance for us?
5. Make a list of some of the common elements found in the body.
6. Explain what is happening in the chemical reaction as depicted by this chemical equation:

$$C_6H_{12}O_6 + 6O_2 + 6H_2O + ATP\,(\text{cellular energy})$$

7. Discuss the importance of the pH of blood.
8. Discuss the importance of carbohydrates to the body.

Find Out More

1. Look at a copy of the periodic table of elements and mark off the ones you have come across in this chapter and that are important for humans.
2. Many electrolytes are essential minerals for the body. Find out which these are.
3. Find out about, and make notes on, the process of osmosis and its importance for human functioning and health.
4. Discuss the acid-base balance and its importance for maintaining good health – and, indeed, for life itself.
5. Discuss what is happening in these two equations – you will need to have access to chemical abbreviations to help you understand the symbols:

$$N_2 + 3H_2 \rightarrow 2NH_3$$
$$H_2CO_3 \rightarrow H^+ + HCO_3^-$$

6. Find out the normal range of human pH and then discuss why it is important for the nurse to alert medical staff if a patient's pH is found to be outside the normal range.
7. Find out more about the importance of homeostasis to health.
8. Lipids/fats can be either saturated on unsaturated – find out from the foodstuffs that you normally eat which of them contain either or both of these types of lipids and their role(s) in healthy nutrition.
9. Take one day, and on that day look at your breakfast, lunch and tea/dinner (as well as snacks, etc.) and try to find out the contents of them all in terms of carbohydrates, lipids and proteins.
10. How can a nurse help to provide a healthy diet for their patients while they are in hospital and/or the community?

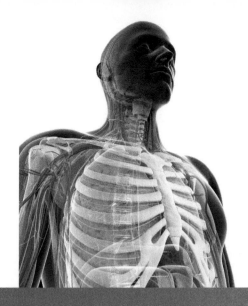

2

Cells, Cellular Compartments, Transport Systems, Fluid Movement Between Compartments

Suzanne Evans

Test Your Prior Knowledge

- **Where do cells come from?**
- **What, approximately, is the average size of a human cell?**
- **What are the various forms human cells can take?**
- **How are human cells taken and examined for diagnostic purposes?**
- **An understanding of cell biology is particularly vital for finding a cure for which group of diseases?**

Learning Outcomes

After reading this chapter you will be able to:

- **Describe the functions of the major cell organelles.**
- **Describe how the structure of the plasma membrane determines its permeability.**
- **List the various ways in which substances move into and out of cells.**
- **Based on the circumstances, predict the movements of water by osmosis and explain the reason for its importance to living organisms.**
- **List the major differences in ionic composition between intracellular and extracellular compartments.**

Visit the student companion website at www.wileyfundamentalseries.com/anatomy where you can test yourself using flashcards, multiple-choice questions and more. Instructor companion site at www.wiley.com/go/instructor/anatomy where instructors will find valuable materials such as PowerPoint slides and image bank designed to enhance your teaching.

Fundamentals of Anatomy and Physiology: For Nursing and Healthcare Students, Third Edition. Edited by Ian Peate and Suzanne Evans.
© 2020 John Wiley & Sons Ltd. Published 2020 by John Wiley & Sons Ltd.
Student companion website: www.wileyfundamentalseries.com/anatomy
Instructor companion website: www.wiley.com/go/instructor/anatomy

Introduction

Cells are the basic structural and functional units that make up all living organisms. Some organisms, such as bacteria and protozoans, are unicellular, consisting of a single cell, but many are multicellular, made up of billions of cells sometimes, as in the case of humans. Multicellular animals possess a range of cells that are specialised to perform various special functions (Figure 2.1).

Regardless of the specialisation though, all cells contain the same structures and organelles that perform the basic functions of the cell, such as growth, metabolism and reproduction. Each cell (with the exception of mature red blood cells) also contains its own complete set of instructions for carrying out these activities in the form of genetic material or DNA (Figure 2.2).

Inside the Cell

Cells are filled with a jelly-like fluid known as cytosol, in which the cell's organelles are suspended. The cytosol is 90% water, with various dissolved ions, amino acids, sugars and lipids. The entire cell is bounded by a protective cell membrane, which maintains the integrity of the cell. In order to carry out their activities, however, cells need to obtain a supply of nutrients and water from their surroundings, and they need to be able to expel waste products from the cell into their surroundings, so there is a requirement for transport of selected substances across the membrane.

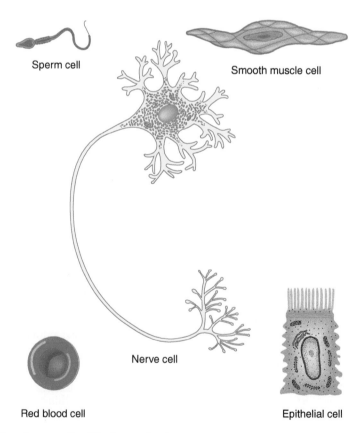

Sperm cell

Smooth muscle cell

Nerve cell

Red blood cell

Epithelial cell

Figure 2.1 **Examples of some cells of the human body.** *Source:* Tortora and Derrickson (2009). Reproduced with permission of John Wiley & Sons.

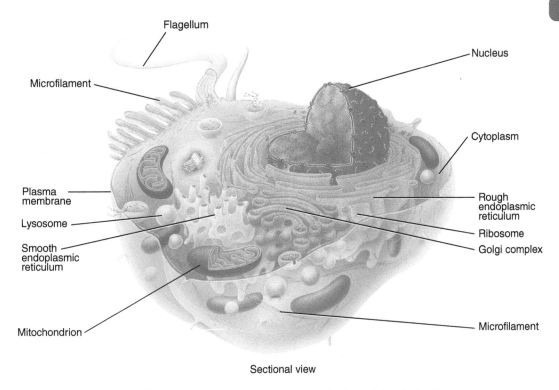

Figure 2.2 **Structure of a cell.** *Source:* Nair and Peate (2009). Reproduced with permission of John Wiley & Sons.

Structure of the Cell Membrane

The cell membrane consists of a double layer (bilayer) of phospholipid molecules, which forms a stable barrier between the two aqueous compartments, i.e. the inside and the outside of the cell. The phospholipid molecule, as discussed in Chapter 1, has a globular head and two thin tails, which are the fatty acids (see also O'Connor and Adams, 2010). While the charge on the fatty acid tails is evenly distributed, the charge on the head of the molecule is unevenly distributed, making just the head of this molecule polar. As was also described in Chapter 1, polar molecules tend to mix with other polar molecules and ions, whereas non-polar molecules do not. The polar heads of the phospholipid molecules therefore mix with water, in other words they are hydrophilic (water-loving). The fatty acid 'tails' of the molecules, on the other hand, do not mix with water, so they are hydrophobic (water-hating). When placed in water, therefore, phospholipid molecules line up so that their heads are in contact with the water, and their tails are not. The only way this can be achieved, of course, is for the molecules to form a double layer, with the molecules effectively 'back to back', with their heads orientated outwards, in contact with the water, and the tails orientated inwards, away from the water (see Figure 2.3). This means that the bilayer is self-sealing. This also means that water and water-soluble substances cannot pass through the cell membrane, because they would be repelled by the water-hating tails in the middle of the bilayer. However, since the cell needs to receive nutrients and other vital substances from its surroundings, there must be ways to transport certain substances across the membrane. This special transport is carried out by protein molecules embedded in the membrane (Figure 2.3). These proteins form channels through which water and selected ions can cross the lipid bilayer, they form transporters that carry certain substances across the membrane, and they form receptors, responsible for cell–cell recognition and cell–cell signalling.

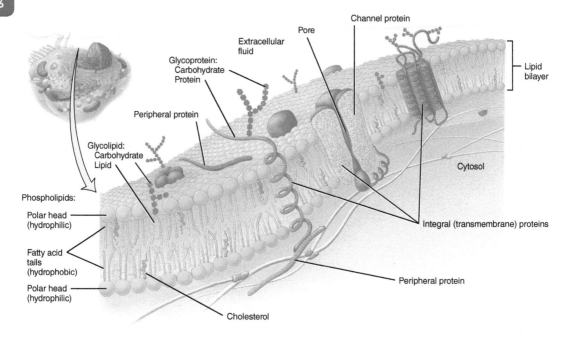

Figure 2.3 **Cell membrane.** *Source:* Tortora and Derrickson (2009). Reproduced with permission of John Wiley & Sons.

Transport of Substances Across the Cell Membrane

All organisms, whether single-celled or multicellular, need to be able to obtain essential nutrients and oxygen from their surroundings, and the bigger and more complex the organism, the greater the need for transport mechanisms to quickly and efficiently get substances to where they are needed in the body. Because all cells are surrounded by the cell membrane, transport into a cell requires that substances can get across the cell membrane somehow.

Transport can occur via passive or active mechanisms. Passive transport does not require the input of energy in order to drive the process (equivalent to rolling a car down a hill), but active transport does (equivalent to driving a car up a hill).

Passive Transport

The simplest form of passive transport is a process known as diffusion. Diffusion comes about because all atoms and molecules are in constant motion – the molecules in a gas can move more freely than those of a liquid, which in turn move more freely than molecules in a solid, but all are constantly vibrating. The speed of this movement is related to the temperature; as the temperature of a substance increases, the molecules will vibrate more rapidly, and as temperature drops, the molecular movement slows down. Because of this constant motion, molecules do not stay exactly where they have been placed and will move and spread out by the process of diffusion. For example, if you carefully place some crystals of solid dye at the bottom of a flask of water and do not stir it, you will find that over time the dye will gradually spread throughout the water in the flask, until the water is evenly coloured (Figure 2.4).

Diffusion therefore results in the distribution of a substance being 'evened out'. Another way of expressing this would be to say that diffusion is the passive movement of a substance from where it is in high concentration to where it is in lower concentration, or the passive movement of a substance down its concentration gradient. The rate at which diffusion occurs depends on a number of factors:

i. Whether the substance is a gas, a liquid or a solid. Because the random movement of the molecules is much greater in a gas then a liquid or a solid, diffusion will occur more rapidly in gases, than in liquids, and diffusion in liquids will be much faster than in solids.

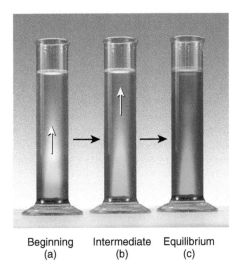

Beginning   Intermediate   Equilibrium
(a)   (b)   (c)

Figure 2.4 **Diffusion in a fluid. At the beginning of our experiment, a crystal of dye placed in a cylinder of water dissolves (a) and then diffuses from the region of higher dye concentration to regions of lower dye concentration (b). At equilibrium (c), the dye concentration is uniform throughout, although random movement continues.** *Source:* Tortora and Derrikson (2009). Reproduced with permission of John Wiley & Sons.

ii. The temperature – diffusion becomes more rapid as temperature increases.
iii. Molecular size – small molecules will move faster than large ones.
iv. Steepness of the concentration gradient – the bigger the difference in concentration, the faster the diffusion will occur to even out that difference.
v. Distance over which diffusion is occurring – molecules will even out their concentration over a small area more rapidly than over a large area.

Diffusion does not only occur in a single compartment though; molecules will also diffuse across a cell membrane if their concentration on the other side of the membrane is different (and provided, of course, that the molecule can get through the membrane). Small, hydrophobic molecules and gases such as oxygen and carbon dioxide readily cross cell membranes by diffusion (Figure 2.5). The exchange of respiratory gases in the lungs occurs by simple diffusion and occurs rapidly enough to provide enough oxygen for our needs and remove the carbon dioxide we produce, even when we are working hard.

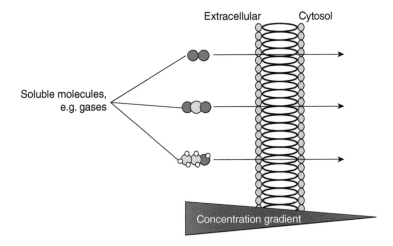

Figure 2.5 **Simple diffusion.** *Source:* Nair and Peate (2009). Reproduced with permission of John Wiley & Sons.

Osmosis – A Special Case of Simple Diffusion

Imagine a container that is divided in the middle by a structure that is similar to a cell membrane. A weak salt solution is placed on one side of this membrane, and a strong salt solution is placed on the other. According to the principle of diffusion, therefore, we would expect the salt molecules to diffuse down their concentration gradient in order to even out their concentration. However, water will be present at a greater concentration in the weaker salt solution than the stronger solution, so we should also expect that water will diffuse down its own concentration gradient just like any other molecule. In this scenario, therefore, salt should be moving from the more concentrated salt solution to the weaker solution, and water should be moving from the less concentrated salt solution into the more concentrated one. This is indeed what would happen if the membrane dividing the two halves of the container were permeable to both salt and water, but in fact, it is not. Cell membranes, as already mentioned, are semi-permeable, that is, they only allow certain substances to cross them. Water is able to cross the membrane relatively freely by means of pores or water channels created by proteins in the membrane, but ions and larger molecules cannot cross freely.

Going back to our imaginary scenario therefore, since the salt would not be able to cross the membrane, then only water would be moving, and it would be moving from the weaker to the more concentrated solution. Over time, we would see water accumulating on the side of the container that had the stronger salt solution in it. The water level on this side would increase above the water level on the other side, and of course, the solution would be diluted so that its concentration was closer to that of the weaker solution on the other side. Whether the two solutions could ever reach a situation where their concentrations were exactly the same would depend on a number of things: how different the concentrations were to start with, how much room there was for water to accumulate on the side with the stronger solution, and whether the movement of water was being opposed by any other force (e.g. an increasing pressure due to more and more water arriving on one side of the membrane).

The presence of a semi-permeable membrane, such as a cell membrane, therefore prevents the simple diffusion of many substances down their concentration gradients, by virtue of the simple fact that they cannot get across, but it does not prevent water from diffusing. This means that where cell membranes are involved, it is the diffusion of water across these membranes that will dominate above all else. It is this movement of water down its concentration gradient across a semi-permeable membrane that is termed osmosis.

Osmosis is an incredibly important process for living things, since the inside and outside of their cells, and their various body compartments, are separated by semi-permeable membranes. This means that whenever there is a difference in the concentration of solutions between the inside and the outside of cells, or between one body compartment and another, the movement of water by osmosis will inevitably occur.

Understanding and being able to predict the process of osmosis is a vital skill for nurses, and yet it is one that students of nursing often struggle to grasp. Remember that osmosis is quite simply the diffusion of water across a membrane from where it is present in higher concentration to where it is present at a lower concentration. Because water is one of the few molecules that is able to cross the membrane freely, and because our body fluids are watery, osmosis plays a central role in our normal function. Osmosis dictates that any change in total solute concentration in any of our fluid compartments will trigger a flow of water between compartments to even out this change.

An often-used example of the importance of osmosis that is highly relevant for nursing is what happens when the concentration of the solution outside red blood cells does not match the concentration inside the cells. Red blood cells spend their lives circulating in the blood, suspended in plasma. The plasma is, like all body fluids, a watery solution. The composition of the blood plasma may be very different to the composition of the intracellular fluid of the red blood cell in terms of the actual solutes, but because most solutes cannot freely cross the membrane, they will not be able to diffuse down their concentration gradients, and so those differences in composition will be maintained. However, if the concentration of water in the plasma is different from that inside the red blood cell, then water will move to even the concentration out. The experiment illustrated in Figure 2.6 shows us how an imbalance in the water concentration between the intracellular and extracellular compartments can result in damage to, or destruction of, cells. If this were allowed to happen in a person's bloodstream to any great extent, the person could die as a result.

Facilitated Diffusion

Highly charged molecules, such as ions, and large molecules, such as sugars and amino acids, cannot cross the membrane by simple diffusion, so special transport arrangements are needed for these substances if they

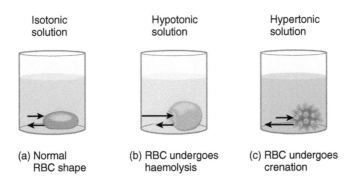

Figure 2.6 **(a–c) Osmotic effects of the concentration of a solution on a red blood cell. In (a) a cell is placed in a solution that has the same total solute and therefore water concentration as the intracellular fluid (an isotonic solution), in (b) a cell is placed in a solution that has a lower total solute and therefore higher water concentration than the inside of the cell (a hypotonic solution), and in (c) a cell is placed in a solution that has a higher total solute concentration and therefore lower water concentration than the inside of the cell (a hypertonic solution).** *Source:* Tortora and Derrikson (2009). Reproduced with permission of John Wiley & Sons.

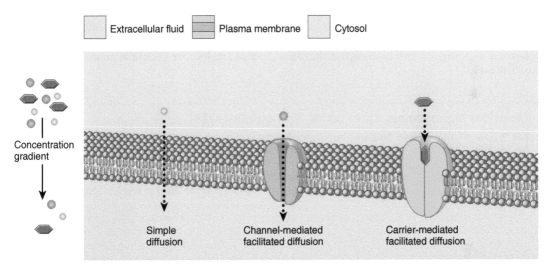

Figure 2.7 **Passive transport mechanisms.** *Source:* Nair and Peate (2009). Reproduced with permission of John Wiley & Sons.

are to gain access to cells down their concentration gradient. In these cases, transport is 'facilitated' by proteins that span the cell membrane and provide a passageway for these substances.

Ions pass through specific proteins that create channels for them to pass through (known as ion channels). The ions still diffuse passively, but they do so through the channel rather than through the lipid bilayer directly. These channels are usually specific to one ion, and they are usually gated, so that ions can only pass through the channels under conditions which cause the channels to open. Larger molecules, including organic molecules such as glucose, bind to specific protein 'carrier' molecules, located in the membrane. These more complex passive processes are known as facilitated diffusion (Figure 2.7). Note, though, that these are still passive transport processes, because the substances are moving down their concentration gradients, i.e. from an area of where they are at higher concentration to one where they are at a lower concentration.

Active Transport

In some situations, for example when taking up glucose or other nutrients, cells need to concentrate substances, which will mean those substances will need to be moved from an area of lower concentration to an area

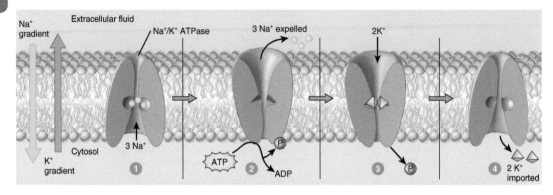

Figure 2.8 **The Na⁺/K⁺ pump.** *Source:* Tortora and Derrikson (2009). Reproduced with permission of John Wiley & Sons.

of higher concentration, or up their concentration gradient. In these situations, active transport is required, and this transport requires energy to drive it. Examples of active transport include the glucose transporter which moves glucose into cells for use or storage, and the sodium-potassium (Na+/K+) pump – a transport system present in all cell membranes, which actively transports sodium ions out of the cell and potassium ions into the cell (Figure 2.8). These ions are both being moved up their concentration gradients, as sodium ions are at a greater concentration outside the cell and potassium ions are present at greater concentration inside the cell.

Medicines Management Tiny Pumps, Big Consequences …

Digoxin or a similar drug has been used to manage heart failure for centuries, and is still an important part of the management of congestive heart failure and some cardiac arrhythmias today. The drug makes the heart beat more strongly, by increasing the strength of contraction of the heart muscle – a very beneficial effect for a patient with a failing heart. The drug must be used carefully though, as it has the potential to cause cardiac arrhythmia. Digoxin has its action by inhibiting the sodium/potassium active transporter (sodium-potassium pump) on the cell membranes of heart muscle cells. This transporter pumps sodium ions out of the cell in exchange for potassium ions, thus maintaining the sodium ion concentration gradient across the membrane. This gradient in turn drives an exchange transporter which removes calcium ions from the cell in exchange for sodium ions. When digoxin is used, the inhibition of the sodium-potassium pump reduces the concentration gradient for sodium across the cell membrane, which reduces the transport of calcium out of the cells, resulting in an increased intracellular concentration of calcium in the heart muscle cells. The central role of calcium in muscle contraction means that more calcium equals stronger contraction, so the heart beats harder.

The Energy to Power Active Transport Comes from the Cell's Mitochondria

The mitochondria take in oxygen and nutrients such as glucose and fatty acids, and from these raw materials produce a supply of a high energy molecule, adenosine triphosphate (ATP). This molecule contains high-energy bonds with the phosphate groups which, when broken, release energy that can power cellular functions. Once the ATP has been split and the resulting energy released for use, adenosine diphosphate (ADP) and phosphate remain, and the ATP molecule can be regenerated by the mitochondria to supply more energy.

How Do Cells Communicate?

Large multicellular organisms require a lot of organisation and coordination between cells in order for the organism to be able to function as a whole, which means that cells must be able to send and receive chemical messages. Incoming messages are received and converted into action in the cell by proteins in the membrane that recognise specific signalling molecules. The 'docking' of the molecule with its protein receptor in the membrane triggers a cellular response, which may be the synthesis and release of a specific protein or lipid, the opening or closing of certain ion channels, or the activation of an enzyme, for example.

Fluid Compartments in the Body

Humans are filled with water, and in fact, 50–60% of our body weight is water. The water is not, of course, pure – it contains many dissolved substances (solutes) and larger suspended particles. In addition, the watery solutions in our bodies are separated into a number of compartments, and the composition of the solutions in each compartment can differ significantly. We can divide these body compartments firstly into the intracellular compartment (the fluid contained inside cells) and the extracellular compartment (the fluid outside cells). The extracellular compartment is then further divided into the interstitial (between the cells) and the intravascular (blood and lymph) compartments.

The intracellular compartment is the largest of the body's fluid compartments, containing around 67% of the total body water, distributed in millions of tiny volumes in the cells. The next largest is the extracellular interstitial fluid containing about 25% of total body water, and the smallest, at around 7%, is the blood plasma and lymph in the intravascular compartment (Figure 2.9).

The major fluid compartments in the body have been discussed but it should also be noted that a very small portion of extracellular fluid is represented by body fluids such as cerebrospinal fluid, gastrointestinal tract fluids, aqueous humour in the eye and joint fluid. These fluids, which are produced by epithelial tissue lining the spaces in which they are found, are collectively known as transcellular fluid. While small in volume, these fluids are vitally important to the normal function of the tissues and organs in which they are found, as you will discover.

The Composition of Body Fluids

The composition of the intracellular fluid differs from that of extracellular fluid in a number of ways, but the most important differences are in the ions. Extracellular fluid contains a high concentration of sodium and chloride ions, and a relatively low concentration of potassium and organic ions, and the reverse is true for intracellular fluid (Table 2.1).

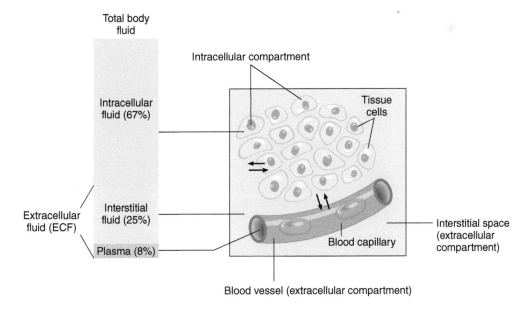

Figure 2.9 **Body fluid compartments.** *Source: Nair and Peate (2009). Reproduced with permission of John Wiley & Sons.*

Table 2.1 Important points of comparison between the ionic composition of intracellular vs extracellular fluids.

	ICF	ECF
Most abundant cation	Potassium (K⁺)	Sodium (Na⁺)
Most abundant anion	Organic phosphate (HPO_4^{3-}) Proteins	Chloride (Cl⁻) Bicarbonate (HCO_3^-)
Total solute concentration	280–300 mmoL L⁻¹	280–300 mmoL L⁻¹
Cations vs anions	Equal numbers	Equal numbers

The differences between intracellular and extracellular fluid composition will mean that for the various solutes, concentration gradients exist between the intracellular and extracellular compartments. However, as already mentioned, ions and large molecules such as proteins do not have free passage across cell membranes, so they are not free to diffuse down their concentration gradients and equalise the fluid compositions. In order to ensure that there is no net movement of water between these compartments, though, the intracellular and extracellular compartments must contain the same concentration of water, or put another way, they must have the same total concentration of solutes. It does not matter that the solutes are not of the same type – it just matters that they are present in the same total concentration in both compartments. Notice also that both extracellular and intracellular compartments contain an equal number of positive and negative ions, making each compartment electrically neutral.

Electrolyte and Water Balance

Both intracellular and extracellular fluids contain several electrolytes, such as sodium chloride and sodium bicarbonate, which dissociate to yield ions in solution, shown in Table 2.1. These ions, since they carry charge and can move through the solution, carry current when they move (this is where the term electrolyte originated). In fact, they perform this function in our nerve and muscle cells, which are electrically powered, as you will see in Chapters 7 and 14.

Table 2.2 provides a summary of the most important electrolytes and their main functions.

Table 2.2 Principal electrolytes and their functions.

ELECTROLYTES	FUNCTION	DISTRIBUTION
Sodium (Na⁺)	Important extracellular cation, which is key to the generation of action potentials in nerve cells. As the most abundant extracellular cation, it plays an important role in maintaining extracellular fluid volume.	Mainly in ECF
Potassium (K⁺)	Important intracellular cation, which is key to establishing the resting membrane potential of a cell, and in the activity of nerve and muscle cells.	Mainly in ICF
Calcium (Ca^{2+})	Physiologically, a very important ion. It is a vital factor for coupling stimulus to response in many functions, e.g. release of neurotransmitter from activated nerve cells, activation of clotting factors, muscle contraction after activation of muscle cells and many more.	Mainly in ECF
Magnesium (Mg^{2+})	Helps to maintain normal nerve and muscle function.	Mainly in ICF
Chloride (Cl⁻)	Abundant anion in ECF, therefore important for fluid balance. Used to produce hydrochloric acid in the stomach.	Mainly in ECF
Bicarbonate (HCO_3^-)	Important in acid-base balance, as buffer of hydrogen ions in plasma.	Mainly in ECF
Phosphate (HPO_4^-)	Essential for bone formation and maintenance.	Mainly in ICF

Table 2.3 Homeostatic control mechanisms for the major body fluid ions and water.

	MONITORED BY	CONTROLLED BY	ACTION OF HORMONE
Plasma Na^+	Specialised cells in the kidney detect Na^+ concentration and blood volume	Aldosterone	Works at the kidneys to increase the retention of Na^+ and the excretion of K^+. Therefore increases Na^+ and decreases K^+ in body fluids
Plasma K^+	No specialised cells known	Aldosterone	
Plasma Ca^{2+}	Specialised cells in the parathyroid gland detect plasma Ca^{2+}, concentration	Parathyroid hormone	Works at the gut to increase the absorption of Ca^{2+}, the kidneys to reduce the excretion of Ca^{2+}, and the bones to release calcium to replace deficits in the plasma
Water	Specialised cells in the brain (osmoreceptors) detect shrinkage due to dehydration and kidney cells detect blood volume changes	Antidiuretic hormone (ADH)	Works at the kidneys to increase the retention of water. Increases water in body fluids, thereby also increasing volume of body fluids

Because of the central roles of many of these ions in physiological functions, it is important that their levels are maintained within narrow limits, as too much or too little of any of them could cause a number of failures, in nerve and muscle function, body fluid maintenance, blood clotting, bone health and so forth. In addition, water in the body is inextricably linked to electrolyte balance, thanks to osmosis: if the concentration of electrolytes in any fluid compartment increases, then by definition the concentration of water in that same fluid compartment will be decreased, and water will move by osmosis from another fluid compartment. In this way, water can be said to 'follow' electrolytes in the body. This means that electrolyte and fluid levels are locked together by osmosis. The levels of the most important electrolytes and water are separately controlled to keep them all within physiological limits. The major hormones involved in their homeostatic control are shown in Table 2.3.

Episode of Care Adult

Meria, aged 65, presented to the emergency department with severe hyponatraemia. According to her daughter, the patient was falling frequently and unable to walk and her speech was difficult to understand. Despite these symptoms, she was also observed to be conversing with her daughter in the room.

The patient had been suffering flu-like symptoms for about 2 weeks and had been vomiting for the previous 4 days. She complained of abdominal pain on one occasion during the emergency doctor's assessment. The doctor carried out a blood test for electrolytes, which showed Meria's plasma sodium level was 100 mmol L^{-1}. During the assessment, Meria revealed that she had been drinking large amounts of water to flush toxins from her system.

She was given an intravenous bolus of 100 mL 3% saline solution and fluid intake was restricted. A series of blood tests was carried out at intervals to check her electrolytes. Three hours after admission, the patient's serum sodium had risen to 107 mmol L^{-1}, and two hours after this, serum sodium had risen to 114 mmol L^{-1}. Meria's serum sodium level continued to return to normal over the next 12 hours

Over the course of her stay in the hospital, Meria continued to make a steady recovery and was discharged following dietary assessment and advice from the dietician.

Hyponatraemia is the most commonly seen type of electrolyte imbalance. It is defined as a serum sodium level of below 135 mmol L^{-1}. It can result from the effects of drugs, excessive secretion of antidiuretic hormone, heart failure, renal failure or excessive diarrhoea, vomiting or sweating accompanied by drinking water. Severe hyponatraemia is defined as serum sodium below 125 mMol L^{-1}, so Meria had a very severe imbalance, which required urgent correction. The presence of symptoms confirms the severity, as milder forms of hyponatraemia do not often produce significant symptoms. Dilutional hyponatraemia is a relatively common form of this imbalance, and can result from consistent excessive intake of water, which, when added to the fluid compartments of the body, dilutes the sodium concentration in the extracellular fluid to below normal levels. Meria will also have been losing sodium (and fluids) through vomiting. The obvious answer to the problem is to administer sodium in a solution, but, if Meria has been drinking a lot of water, she may already have a high fluid volume due to excessive drinking, so adding more fluids may not be the best move. On the other hand, restricting fluid intake and waiting for the water and sodium balance to normalise might take a long time, and Meria would be at risk during this time. A bolus of hypertonic saline can be given to correct this severe deficit more quickly. This will provide additional sodium but not too much additional water. The aim would be to increase the serum sodium level by about 0.5 mM L^{-1} every hour, as raising the level too rapidly can cause damage to the central nervous system.

See American College of Emergency Physicians (n.d.).

Multiple Choice Questions

1. Which of the following is not an electrolyte?
   (a) albumin
   (b) sodium
   (c) magnesium
   (d) calcium
2. Consistent excessive intake of water can lead to:
   (a) renal cysts
   (b) dilutional hyponatraemia
   (c) renal colic
   (d) dilutional hypernatraemia
3. The ability of an extracellular solution to make water move into or out of a cell by osmosis is known as:
   (a) tonicity
   (b) energy potential
   (c) clonicity
   (d) membrane potential
4. With regards to Meria, the following factors may increase the risk of hyponatraemia:
   (a) young age, hypertension, presence of renal disease, increase in physical activity and fluid intake
   (b) older age, some drugs, presence of renal disease, decrease in physical activity and dehydration
   (c) older age, some drugs, presence of renal disease, increase in activity and fluid intake
   (d) older age, some drugs, presence of renal disease, increase in physical activity and dehydration
5. In acute hyponatraemia, sodium levels drop rapidly. This can result in:
   (a) starvation and hyperpyrexia
   (b) rapid cerebral oedema
   (c) slow onset brain swelling
   (d) over-excitability

Fluid Movement Between Compartments

Movement of fluid between the intracellular and the extracellular compartments will be by osmosis and will therefore occur if there is a concentration gradient for water (a solute concentration difference) across the cell membrane. Normally this gradient does not exist, as there is an equal total solute concentration between inside the outside the cell, as shown in Table 2.1, but if such a gradient were introduced by changes in the water or solute concentration in one of the compartments, then osmotic movement of water would occur. How much water would move would depend on the size of the gradient. We use the term osmotic pressure to give us an idea of the size of any concentration gradient for water across a cell membrane, since this gives us a sense of how much water would move. The osmotic pressure is in fact the pressure that would have to be exerted on a solution to resist the movement of water due to osmosis. This is useful because it allows us to measure and therefore put a number to the water-driving power of osmosis.

The movement of extracellular fluid between the intravascular and the interstitial compartments is determined by two forces: the osmotic pressure and the hydrostatic pressure that the blood exerts against the walls of the vessel (we usually just call this blood pressure). The hydrostatic pressure in blood vessels is at its highest in the arteries, and gradually decreases as the blood travels through the network of blood vessels; from arteries to arterioles to capillaries, then to venules and finally to veins. As blood enters a

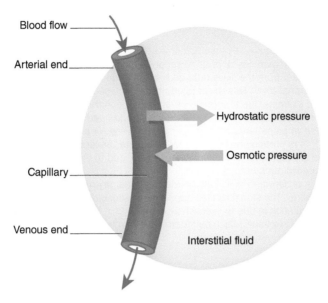

Figure 2.10 **Capillary hydrostatic and osmotic pressures.** *Source:* Peate and Nair (2011). Reproduced with permission of John Wiley & Sons.

capillary from an arteriole, it is therefore at a higher pressure at that point than when it reaches the end of the capillary just before it enters a venule. Capillaries, of all the blood vessels in the circulatory system, are the ones that are adapted to allow exchange of substances between the blood and the interstitial fluid, and their walls are perforated to allow this to happen. Changes in pressure inside and outside the capillary will therefore determine whether substances will move out of or into the capillary. There is a greater tendency for fluid to move out of the blood vessel and into the interstitial fluid at the start of the capillary (the arterial end), because the hydrostatic pressure is greater there, and a tendency for fluid to move into the capillary at the venous end of the capillary where the hydrostatic pressure is lower. Fluid and solutes therefore leave the arterial end of the capillaries and move into the interstitial fluid, whereas they return to the capillaries at the venous end. It is important to note that although a bulk flow of fluid and its solutes occurs at the capillary level, the process of diffusion is also continuing, so that as oxygen-rich blood flows into the capillary at the arterial end, the oxygen in the plasma will diffuse rapidly down its concentration gradient out of the capillary and into the surrounding interstitial fluid, and from there into the cells in the area, and carbon dioxide will move into the blood in the same way. Glucose will also be able to diffuse from the capillaries into interstitial fluid because, unlike the cell membrane, the capillary wall is readily permeable to solutes, which means that the osmotic pressure within the capillary is principally determined by only the largest molecules, the plasma proteins, that cannot leave the capillaries. The osmotic pressure exerted by the proteins in capillaries is referred to as 'oncotic' or 'colloid osmotic' pressure and is typically 25–30 mmHg. It increases as the blood flows along the capillary from the arterial to the venous end, because the fluid and smaller solutes leaving the capillary as a result of the hydrostatic pressure leave behind proteins in the blood and less water, which results in an increased protein concentration (and therefore a lower water concentration). Water will therefore move into the capillary at the venous end as a result of osmosis (Figure 2.10).

In normal conditions, therefore, the flow of fluid out of the capillary at the arterial end would be balanced by the subsequent flow back into the capillary at the venous end, and there would be no net gain or loss of fluid by the intravascular or interstitial compartments. However, if anything occurs to alter the hydrostatic or osmotic pressures in either compartment, the situation may rapidly change. For example, higher than normal hydrostatic pressure in the blood vessels can increase the tendency of fluid to move out of the capillaries into the interstitial fluid and remain there, leading to oedema (excess fluid in tissues).

Clinical Considerations Dehydration

Dehydration may be caused by insufficient water intake, excessive water loss or a combination of both. The most common cause of dehydration is failure to drink enough liquid. The average person loses water from the body on a daily basis in urine, in expired air, through perspiration and from the gastrointestinal tract. This water needs to be replaced to prevent dehydration. If water loss is greatly increased, for example due to intense perspiration, and the water lost is not replaced by drinking, dehydration will occur, which could result in shock and death within only a few hours. The risk of this is greatly increased when patients have difficulty swallowing, or a reduced sense of thirst or capacity to respond to thirst. This is particularly true in elderly patients. Severe vomiting or diarrhoea can result in loss of a large volume of body water and electrolytes which need to be consistently replaced as long as the illness persists if dehydration is to be avoided.

Signs and symptoms of dehydration include headache, thirst, dry mouth, low volume of very concentrated urine, dizziness and lethargy. The skin may also appear shrunken, blood pressure may drop and the heart rate increase. If the dehydration is due to excessive perspiration in high temperatures, the loss of fluid can result in a shutting down of sweating, which can then allow core temperature to rise dangerously.

Episodes of Care Adult

Boon Sew, a 48-year-old male, was rushed to the emergency department after being rescued from his burning house. He was asleep when a spark from the fireplace started a fire, leaving him trapped in his bedroom. By the time the fire rescue team arrived, he had suffered severe burns and smoke inhalation.

On arrival at the emergency department, he was unconscious. He had second-degree burns over 5% of his body and third-degree burns over 20% of his body – both covering his thoracic and abdominal regions and his right elbow. His vital signs were quite unstable: blood pressure was 53/35 mmHg; heart rate was 200 beats per minute; and respiratory rate was 38 breaths per minute. He was deteriorating from circulatory failure. Two intravenous lines were inserted and fluids and electrolytes were administered. His vital signs stabilised and he was admitted to the intensive care unit.

Burnt skin no longer functions as an adequate body covering, and fluid and solutes escape at a rapid rate from the extracellular fluid compartment through the burnt areas (heat also escapes from the blood at the burn site and the person with burns can get very cold very quickly as a result). The loss of fluid from the burns would result in a large drop in blood volume and therefore blood pressure, which would explain Boon's low arterial pressure, despite the heart beating rapidly in an attempt to maintain it. The resulting poor circulation would mean that the supply of oxygen and nutrients to the cells and the removal of waste products would be compromised at the same time that the airways themselves were damaged by heat and smoke. This would explain the elevated respiratory rate. The administration of intravenous fluids would help to restore the lost volume in the blood, thereby improving blood pressure and circulation, but intravenous fluids with electrolytes would need to be maintained for some time, as extracellular fluid will continue to seep from the burns. While fluids will help to stabilise vital signs, consideration will need to be given to how much damage the blood tissue has sustained – burns over a large area can result in the destruction of large numbers of blood cells as they are carried to the burnt area and destroyed by heat or lost from the body through the open burn. Boon will probably need red blood cells or whole blood before long, to ensure his blood is able to transport enough oxygen. Boon will also need pain medication, as burns can be extremely painful. Another consideration for Boon's care will be in the prevention of infection, since third degree burns will readily allow the entry of bacteria and other disease-causing organisms, so care will need to be taken to ensure that his burns are clean and sterile.

Boon Sew regained consciousness the following day and was able to respond verbally. Once his condition was stable and he was able to respond to treatment, he was transferred to the ward where he continued to make a good recovery. He was then discharged after making a full recovery, due in no small part to the skillful care he received.

Multiple Choice Questions

1. Boon has experienced a third-degree burn, which is characterised by:
   (a) destruction of epidermis only
   (b) destruction of epidermis, dermis and underlying subcutaneous tissue
   (c) destruction of epidermis and dermis, leaving only skin and appendages
   (d) destruction of epidermis and some dermis

2. Initial response to severe burn injury or early shock state is characterised by:
   (a) an increase in cardiac output and metabolic rate
   (b) a decrease in cardiac output and hyperthermia
   (c) a decrease in cardiac output and metabolic rate
   (d) an increase in cardiac output and decrease in metabolic rate
3. At what point post-burn may Boon experience hypokalaemia?
   (a) as soon as the injury has occurred
   (b) during the late recovery phase
   (c) during fluid remobilisation
   (d) during the fluid shift
4. Boon's blood pressure was 53/35 mmHg and his heart rate was 200 beats per minute. Why might this be?
   (a) as a result of severe pain
   (b) because of an overwhelming infection
   (c) due to fluid shift
   (d) as a result of haemorrhage
5. Which clinical manifestations might indicate that Boon is moving into the fluid remobilisation phase of recovery?
   (a) an increase in peripheral oedema and a decreased blood pressure
   (b) decreased sodium and increased haematocrit
   (c) increased urine output, decreased urine specific gravity
   (d) none of the above

Bulk Transport Across the Cell Membrane

So far, this chapter has covered the ways in which individual molecules of a substance can cross cell membranes, either by active or passive processes. However, there are many situations in which larger amounts of a substance need to be moved into or out of a cell quickly. For this to occur, the items to be transported are bundled up in a membrane of their own, forming a small, membrane-bound package called a vesicle. On contact with the cell membrane, the membrane of the vesicle melts into (fuses with) the cell membrane, and the contents are released into or outside the cell, depending on the direction of transport. This kind of bulk transport is used to remove unwanted substances from cells and to secrete substances such as hormones, enzymes or neurotransmitters from cells, and to bring large items into cells.

Endocytosis: Bulk Transport into Cells

Endocytosis is the process by which cells take in molecules such as proteins from outside the cell by engulfing them with their cell membranes (Figure 2.11). It is used by all cells of the body to bring polar and large molecules into the cell in bulk. The cell membrane folds around the substances to be transported and a vesicle is formed, containing the substance. Endocytosis may involve small droplets of a substance, in which case it is known as pinocytosis (from the Greek meaning 'cell drinking'). All cells use pinocytosis to supply their needs. Certain cells of the immune system are also able to carry out another form of endocytosis, phagocytosis (from the Greek meaning 'cell eating'). In phagocytosis, whole cells, such as bacteria, or large pieces of cells can be ingested by a cell. The object in this case though, is to engulf and destroy something harmful as a protective measure, rather than to obtain nutrients or useful substances. Our immune systems are equipped with a number of phagocytic cells which perform a vital role in defending us against bacteria and other disease-causing organisms by engulfing and destroying those organisms.

Exocytosis: Bulk Transport Out of Cells

Exocytosis is the process by which the cell moves packages of substances from the inside of the cell to the outside. Newly synthesised products, such as hormones or enzymes to be secreted, are packaged into vesicles by the Golgi apparatus, and transported to the cell membrane. At the cell membrane, the vesicle membrane fuses with the cell membrane and the contents of the vesicle are deposited outside the cell (Figure 2.12).

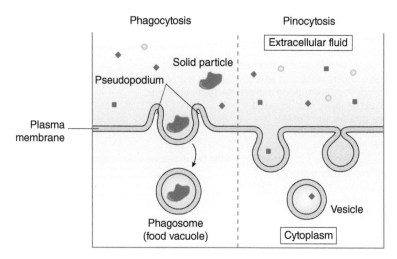

Figure 2.11 **Phagocytosis and pinocytosis.** *Source:* Peate and Nair (2011). Reproduced with permission of John Wiley & Sons.

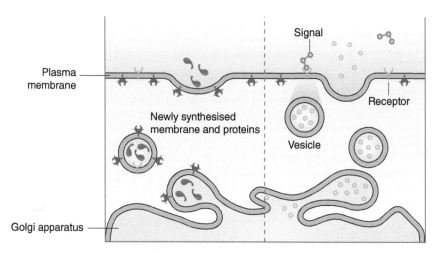

Figure 2.12 **Exocytosis. Proteins, lipids and other products produced in the cell are packaged into vesicles by the Golgi apparatus to be moved out of the cell. Exocytosis can be stimulated by an incoming signal.** *Source:* Nair and Peate (2009). Reproduced with permission of John Wiley & Sons.

Clinical Considerations Administration of Intravenous Fluids

Administration of fluids and electrolytes in situations where body fluids have been lost and blood volume is low can save lives. The aim is to expand the circulating plasma volume, thereby increasing blood pressure. The fluid solution used must be isotonic and non-toxic. A crystalline solution such as sodium chloride is often used at a concentration of 0.9% (this is known as normal saline), but other solutes such as sodium lactate (Ringer's lactate and Hartmann's solutions) can also be used. Crystalline fluids given intravenously will not remain in the bloodstream, however, since the solutes will leave the capillaries and move into the interstitial space along with water. This will mean that a much greater volume of fluids will need to be given, to compensate for the volume of fluid that moves out of the intravascular compartment (third spacing). Colloid solutions provide an alternative, as they contain large molecules such as the protein albumin (5% solution), or the polysaccharide dextran that cannot escape from the capillaries. Since the molecules cannot leave the blood, the water will not either, as a result of the osmotic pull of the colloids trapped in the blood vessel. This means that less fluid is needed to expand the plasma volume. Colloidal solutions are much more expensive, however, and can produce an allergic response in some patients.

Although fluid replacement is necessary for a patient who has low blood volume (hypovolaemia), over-zealous administration of fluids, or administration when fluids are not needed can be detrimental to a patient's health. If fluids are administered to a patient with normal blood volume, fluid overload may occur, causing fluid to enter lung spaces, increased excretory demands to be placed on the kidneys, and increased workload on the heart. Nurses need to be aware of this and monitor patients carefully for signs of fluid overload, such as respiratory difficulty, abnormal lung sounds, high blood pressure and oedema (see Hilton *et al.*, 2008).

Conclusion

The cell, as the smallest living unit in the body, represents the smallest scale on which we are able to study physiological function; at higher levels – tissue, organ, organ system and organism levels – we are observing the concerted and coordinated functions of cells working together. Everything the organism is able to do is due to the correct functioning of billions of cells. How the cell does what it does is therefore a fundamental part of the study of physiology. The health and life cycle of individual cells also comes to the fore in cancer research, as the search for ways to cure cancer focuses around the study of the mysteries of individual cells, and what makes them start to divide in an uncontrolled manner. The fluids which our cells are filled with and bathed in are also vital to normal function. Our bodies are filled with salty solutions, and the semi-permeable nature of our plasma cell membranes ensures that those salty solutions cannot mix freely. This control of what can and cannot cross cell membranes explains the various specific transport mechanisms that cells have developed in order to be able to supply their needs, and it explains the electrical potentials that are created between one side of the membrane and the other, due to the distribution of electrolytes between the intracellular and extracellular fluids. This electrical potential can be converted to electrical current by the membrane opening ion channels and allowing ions to flow, carrying their charge, and this is the basis of our electrically operated nerve and muscle cells.

For the nurse, a sound understanding of osmosis and electrolyte and fluid balance is absolutely essential. All patients, regardless of their age or health status, can become vulnerable to dehydration, overhydration or electrolyte imbalance as a result of drugs, stress, infection, renal problems or inappropriate fluid intake. Being aware of what water and electrolytes do and where they go in the body is the first step to understanding how watery creatures like humans function, and to ensuring that they are safe when in your care.

Glossary

Active transport: The energy-requiring process by which substances are moved up their concentration gradient (i.e. from an area with lower concentration to one with a higher concentration).

Adenosine diphosphate (ADP): The product produced when Adenosine triphosphate (ATP) is metabolised with the breaking of its high energy phosphate bond to release energy.

Adenosine triphosphate (ATP): High-energy compound which provides energy for the cell when its high energy bonds with phosphate groups are broken.

Compartments: Spaces within the body that are separated by living membranes.

Cytoplasm: The fluid and contents of a cell.

Diffusion: The movement of substances down their concentration gradients from a higher to a lower concentration.

Electrolytes: Substances that dissociate in water to form ions.

Endocytosis: Bulk movement into a cell.

Extracellular: Outside cells.

Exocytosis: Bulk movement out of a cell.

Facilitated diffusion: Diffusion with the aid of a transport protein.

Hydrophilic: Water-loving, soluble in water.

Hydrophobic: Water-hating, insoluble in water and soluble in lipids

Hypertonic: A solute concentration higher than that of intracellular fluid. Cells placed in a hypertonic solution would shrink, as water would flow out into the hypertonic solution by osmosis.

Hypotonic: Solute concentration lower than that of intracellular fluid. Cells placed in a hypotonic solution would swell, as water would flow from the hypotonic solution into the cells by osmosis.

Interstitial: Between cells.

Intracellular: Inside the cell.

Organelles: 'Mini organs' that perform the vital functions of the cell.

Osmosis: Movement of water through a selectively permeable membrane to even out the solute concentration on either side of the membrane.

Osmotic pressure: The pressure that must be exerted on a solution into which water is flowing by osmosis in order to completely oppose that osmotic movement.

Passive transport: The process by which substances move down a concentration gradient without requiring energy.

Plasma membrane: Outer layer of the cell.

Transport protein: Large protein molecules that move specific substances across a cell membrane.

References

American College of Emergency Physicians (n.d.) Hyponatremia case review. https://www.acep.org/life-as-a-physician/ethics--legal/standard-of-care-review/hyponatremia-case-review/ (accessed 20 June 2019).

Hilton, A.K, Pellegrino, V.A. and Scheinkestel, C.D. (2008) Avoiding common problems associated with intravenous fluid therapy. *Medical Journal of Australia* **189**(9): 509–513.

Nair, M. and Peate, I. (2009) *Fundamentals of Applied Pathophysiology: An Essential Guide for Nursing Students*. Oxford: John Wiley & Sons, Ltd.

O'Connor, C.M. and Adams, J.U. *(2010) Essentials of Cell Biology*. Cambridge, MA: NPG Education, 2010. https://www.nature.com/scitable/ebooks/essentials-of-cell-biology-14749010/122997196 (accessed June 2019).

Peate, I. and Nair, M. (2011) *Fundamentals of Anatomy and Physiology for Student Nurses*. Chichester: John Wiley & Sons, Ltd.

Tortora, G.J. and Derrickson, B.H. (2009) *Principles of Anatomy and Physiology*, 12th edn. Hoboken, NJ: John Wiley & Sons, Inc.

Further Reading

Diabetes Insipidus

NHS Choices (2019) *Introduction*. http://www.nhs.uk/conditions/diabetes-insipidus/Pages/Introduction.aspx (accessed 19 June 2019).
Useful NHS website for up-to-date information on diseases you may come across in practice.

Electrolytes and Electrolyte Balance

Best Practice Advocacy Centre New Zealand (2011) *A primary care approach to sodium and potassium imbalance*. https://bpac.org.nz/BT/2011/September/docs/best_tests_sep2011_imbalance_pages_2-14.pdf. (accessed 20 June 2019).

Felman, A. (2017) *Medical News Today, Everything you need to know about electrolytes*. https://www.medicalnewstoday.com/articles/153188.php (accessed 25 February 2020).

Lederer, E., Nayak, V., Alsauskas, Z.C. and Mackelaite, L. (2018) *Hyperkalemia Treatment and Management*. http://emedicine.medscape.com/article/240903-treatment (accessed 20 June 2019).

Activities

Multiple Choice Questions

1. A solution containing a higher concentration of solutes than the cytosol of a cell is:
   (a) hypotonic
   (b) isotonic
   (c) hypertonic
   (d) osmotonic

2. Which structure controls the movement of materials into and out of cells?
   (a) the nucleus
   (b) the cytoplasm
   (c) the plasma membrane
   (d) the endoplasmic reticulum

3. Which of the following is true of diffusion?
   (a) diffusion is faster at lower temperature
   (b) diffusion is faster when the concentration gradient is greater
   (c) the molecular weight of the molecule will not affect the diffusion rate
   (d) the more ATP in the cell, the faster the diffusion

4. Which organelles act as the cell's 'post office' by sorting, processing and packaging materials to be transported within the cell or sent outside the cell?
   (a) Golgi complex
   (b) mitochondria
   (c) rough endoplasmic reticulum
   (d) smooth endoplasmic reticulum

5. Cells from a gland were examined under a microscope and found to contain a lot of smooth endoplasmic reticulum. What are these cells most likely to be making?
   (a) protein hormones
   (b) transport proteins
   (c) digestive enzymes
   (d) steroid hormones

6. Which of the following transport systems requires energy?
   (a) simple diffusion
   (b) osmosis
   (c) sodium / potassium pump
   (d) facilitated diffusion

7. The main structural component of a cell membrane is:
   (a) phospholipids
   (b) cholesterol
   (c) proteins
   (d) complex carbohydrates

8. Which organelles are sometimes referred to as the powerhouse of the cell due to the fact that they produce ATP for the cell?
   (a) Golgi complex
   (b) mitochondria
   (c) rough endoplasmic reticulum
   (d) smooth endoplasmic reticulum

9. A drop of food colouring that spreads out after being placed in a jar of water is an example of:
   (a) osmosis
   (b) mixing
   (c) diffusion
   (d) bulk flow

10. If a molecule is hydrophobic, it means that:
    (a) it will break water molecules into H+ and OH- ions.
    (b) it will repel hydrogen
    (c) it will not mix with water
    (d) it will dry out readily

11. How do cells get glucose from the extracellular fluid?
    (a) by diffusion
    (b) by osmosis
    (c) via an active transporter
    (d) via facilitated diffusion

12. Which of the following electrolytes is the most abundant extracellular cation?
    (a) calcium
    (b) potassium
    (c) chloride
    (d) sodium

13. Which of the following is the most abundant intracellular anion?
    (a) chloride
    (b) organic phosphate

(c) potassium
(d) bicarbonate

14. A patient is suffering from a condition that results in blockage of small veins, resulting in oedema. The oedema would be due to:
    (a) reduced flow of fluid out of capillaries at the arterial end of the capillary
    (b) reduced blood pressure in the arteries
    (c) reduced flow of fluid back into capillaries at the venous end
    (d) increased flow of fluid into capillaries at both ends

15. What effect would giving a patient with normal fluid and electrolyte balance an intravenous infusion of very hypotonic saline have?
    (a) the blood cells would become crenated
    (b) the blood volume would increase and remain elevated for several days
    (c) the blood cells would swell and burst
    (d) the blood volume would decrease due to water loss to the interstitial compartment

True or False

1. A molecule will move from where it is at a lower concentration to where it is at greater concentration, i.e. down its concentration gradient.
2. Facilitated diffusion does not require energy.
3. The interstitial compartment is part of the extracellular compartment.
4. The cell membrane contains cholesterol.
5. Potassium is the principal extracellular ion.
6. Chloride ions are negatively charged.
7. Hyponatraemia means high sodium levels.
8. 0.9% normal saline is a hypertonic solution.
9. ADH reduces the loss of water in the urine.

Find Out More

1. What are organelles and their functions?
2. What are the factors affecting diffusion?
3. Discuss the effects of low potassium level on the cardiovascular system.
4. What do you understand by the term 'third fluid space'? What role does it play in fluid balance?
5. Explain what happens to fluid in the fluid compartments when a person is
   a. dehydrated
   b. overhydrated.
6. What do you understand by the term secondary active transport?
7. Do mitochondria contain DNA?
8. In an active transport system, from where do the cells get their energy?

Chemical Symbols

Write the correct chemical symbols for the following electrolytes:

Potassium _____
Sodium _____
Bicarbonate _____
Chloride _____
Organic phosphate _____
Sulphate _____
Calcium _____

Conditions

The following is a list of conditions that are associated with the subjects discussed in this chapter. Take some time and write notes about each of the conditions. You may make the notes taken from textbooks or other resources (e.g. people you work with in a clinical area) or you may make the notes about people you have cared for. If you are doing this, you must ensure that you adhere to the rules of confidentiality.

Water intoxication

Pulmonary oedema

Nausea and vomiting

Acidosis

Alkalosis

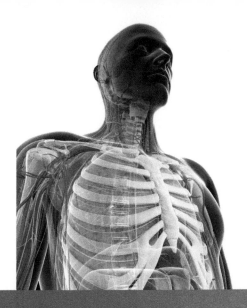

3

Genetics

Jude Weidenhofer

Test Your Prior Knowledge

- What are the four bases that are found in DNA and what is their role in the double helix?
- If we have a DNA base sequence of ACATGGCTA, what would the corresponding RNA bases be?
- What is happening during the interphase stage of the cell cycle?
- What do we mean by Mendelian inheritance?
- What is the difference between autosomal recessive inheritance and autosomal dominant inheritance?

Learning Outcomes

After reading this chapter you will be able to:

- Explain what genes and alleles are and their importance to our health.
- Describe the basics of the DNA double helix and chromosomes.
- Understand and describe protein synthesis, including transcription and translation.
- Explain the cell cycle and cell division.
- Understand Mendelian inheritance patterns: autosomal dominant, recessive and X-linked.
- Describe the basics of non-Mendelian inheritance patterns.

Visit the student companion website at www.wileyfundamentalseries.com/anatomy where you can test yourself using flashcards, multiple-choice questions and more. Instructor companion site at www.wiley.com/go/instructor/anatomy where instructors will find valuable materials such as PowerPoint slides and image bank designed to enhance your teaching.

Fundamentals of Anatomy and Physiology: For Nursing and Healthcare Students, Third Edition. Edited by Ian Peate and Suzanne Evans.
© 2020 John Wiley & Sons Ltd. Published 2020 by John Wiley & Sons Ltd.
Student companion website: www.wileyfundamentalseries.com/anatomy
Instructor companion website: www.wiley.com/go/instructor/anatomy

Anatomical Map

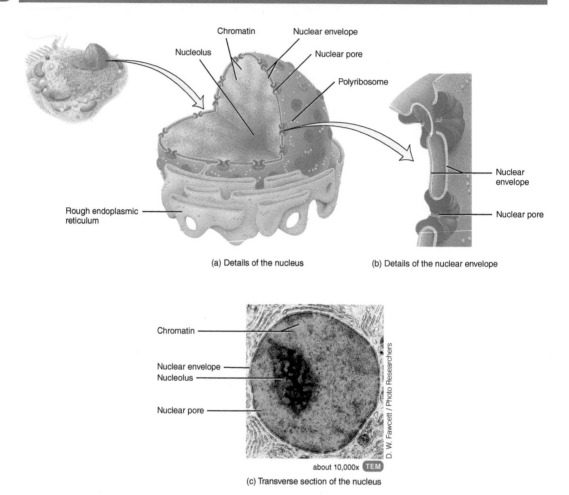

(a) Details of the nucleus

(b) Details of the nuclear envelope

(c) Transverse section of the nucleus

Figure 3.1 **(a–c) The cell nucleus.** *Source:* Tortora and Derrickson (2014). Reproduced with permission of John Wiley & Sons.

Introduction

Genetics is an area of rapid knowledge expansion, which makes it fascinating and increasingly complex. Genetics is also incredibly important as it includes the understanding of what makes us human; our DNA and the genes it carries. In addition, many health problems are directly caused by errors to genes and other health problems are influenced by our genetics.

So, what are genes? Genes are sections of deoxyribonucleic acid (DNA) that are carried within our chromosomes. Genes contain sets of instructions to make particular proteins, which allow us to function. Your genes direct all your activities including growth, development and ageing, reproduction, general health and functioning, in conjunction with the environmental influences you experience. Our genetic material is inherited from our parents, who in turn inherited theirs from their parents. So, although we share many similar features with our biological relations, each of us is genetically unique. In this chapter we will understand the role our genes play in these similarities and differences and how this is important to health and disease.

Deoxyribonucleic Acid (DNA) and Ribonucleic Acid (RNA)

Genes are sections of DNA that contain the information for making the proteins that are vital to normal function. To assist in understanding how DNA determines our individuality and function, let's start by defining a few terms:

DNA	Deoxyribonucleic acid – part of the double helix/chromosome
RNA	Ribonucleic acid, transcribed from DNA
mRNA/tRNA	Messenger RNA/transfer RNA – these work along with ribosomes to assemble proteins from amino acids that have been coded for by the DNA/gene

The capacity of our cells to replicate their own DNA constitutes the basis of all hereditary transmission. This is because it allows us to produce new cells that have the identical information to existing cells, and to make the reproductive cells, the gametes (eggs and sperm), that create new life. We will examine these processes in more detail later. The other major function of DNA is as a template for the synthesis of RNA. There are many types of RNA, with mRNA holding the message from DNA that provides the instructions to synthesise proteins with the assistance of tRNA, rRNA and some enzymes. Proteins perform many of the functions of cells and hence are important in determining our own unique features.

DNA is contained within the nucleus of our cells as a molecular structure known as chromatin – a complex of DNA wound around a particular type of protein (histone protein). Each length of chromatin, known as a chromosome, houses a proportion of the roughly 30,000 genes that are needed to make a human. Each nucleated cell has 23 pairs of chromosomes within its nucleus. Chromosomes are considered a pair if they have the same genes on them. As each pair has a different number and set of genes, each pair is unique and so we can identify each of the 23 pairs of human chromosomes by their nucleic acid structure. The human chromosomes are designated as chromosomes 1 through 22, known as autosomal chromosomes, and the 23rd pair are the sex chromosomes, X and Y: either two X chromosomes in females or one X chromosome and one Y chromosome in males. The only exception to this is the cells involved in reproduction. These cells, called gametes – ova (eggs) from the mother and spermatozoa (sperm) from the father, have just one copy of each chromosome (i.e. 23 chromosomes in total).

Some people do not have 46 chromosomes. These individuals have an aneuploidy, which is an abnormal number of chromosomes in cells. People with Down syndrome, for example, have 47 chromosomes, with three copies of chromosome 21 (a condition known as trisomy 21), while people with Turner syndrome (also known as 45, X), have only 45 chromosomes, as they have only one sex chromosome, an X chromosome (Crespi, 2008). There are also instances where people have extra or missing parts of chromosomes. We will consider this and other gross chromosomal abnormalities later in this chapter.

Episodes of Care Learning Disability

Turner Syndrome is a genetic condition that affects 1 in 2500 girls. Females with this condition experience a variety of symptoms that vary in severity with the degree of chromosomal abnormality. Girls with Turner syndrome may be missing a complete X chromosome, or just part of one, and it may be missing from all their cells, or only some cells (a phenomenon known as mosaicism). A diagnosis of Turner syndrome is made by counting the chromosomes in the nuclei of white blood cells from a sample of the child's blood; a procedure known as a karyotype analysis.

Girls with this syndrome display a number of characteristics including short stature, a neck that is thickened towards the base, swollen hands and feet, an inability to straighten their elbows completely, congenital heart defects, infertility and delayed or absent puberty. Some children also experience difficulty with maths and map reading due to poor spatial awareness. Some of these issues can be resolved with medical interventions such as providing growth hormone to increase stature, assisted reproductive techniques and taking oestrogen to assist puberty.

Carly is a regular visitor to the school nurse, as she has frequent ear infections. On her most recent visit the nurse made a comment about this and Carly responded that it was a feature of Turner syndrome (small ear canals lead to repeat infections). This was the first the nurse had heard about Carly having

Turner syndrome and she was a little surprised as Carly did not show many of the other common signs. Carly told her she had been taking growth hormone to help her grow taller. The nurse asked her if she had told any of her teachers that she had this condition. Carly replied that she wanted to be as normal as possible and that her parents felt she had the best chance of this if few people knew about her condition. The nurse, knowing that about 80% of girls with Turner syndrome have a learning disability in maths, suggested she at least speak with her maths teacher. As a result of the discussion, Carly was offered assistance with learning in situations where her spatial deficit was an issue. Carly also had her hearing tested and found that her frequent infections were beginning to affect her hearing, which was further contributing to her learning issues. These simple changes made as a result of awareness of this genetic condition may also assist Carly with her self-esteem and motivate her to persevere with her learning.

Multiple Choice Questions

1. Turner syndrome is
   (a) a genetic condition where the female only has one X chromosome
   (b) a genetic condition where an individual only has one sex chromosome, either an X or Y
   (c) a genetic condition caused by a mutation in a single gene on the X chromosome
   (d) a genetic condition in which any one of the 46 chromosomes is missing.
2. Which of these would be the best description of a genetic mosaic?
   (a) an individual who is infertile
   (b) an individual who displays a number of common symptoms of a disease but does not have that disease
   (c) someone with the incorrect number of chromosomes
   (d) someone who has variability in the number of chromosomes in their cells: some cells have the correct number whereas others do not.
3. Which of the following is NOT a common symptom of Turner syndrome?
   (a) spatial learning difficulties
   (b) hearing impairment
   (c) hair loss
   (d) short stature and non-straightening elbows
4. Turner syndrome would be diagnosed:
   (a) by a karyotype analysis
   (b) solely off the height of the individual
   (c) through having one of more of the common symptoms
   (d) by ultrasound looking for the common heart defects
5. Turner syndrome is often treated with oestrogen. The oestrogen assists with:
   (a) obtaining a normal height
   (b) improving intellectual performance
   (c) triggering the onset of puberty
   (d) preventing hearing impairment

The DNA Double Helix

The structure of the DNA double helix was determined in the 1950s by James Watson and Francis Crick, following the work of Rosalind Franklin. The structure is vital to our cellular functioning, as it allows cells to make exact copies of their DNA and assists in repairing small errors. The double helix is made up of two strands of DNA, which consists of chemical complexes known as nucleotides strung together. A nucleotide consists of three chemical groups:

- **deoxyribose** – a five-carbon cyclic sugar;
- **phosphate** – an inorganic, negatively charged phosphorous-containing molecule;
- **base** – a nitrogen-carbon ring structure, of which there are 4 types found in DNA:
  adenine (A)
  thymine (T)
  guanine (G)
  cytosine (C).

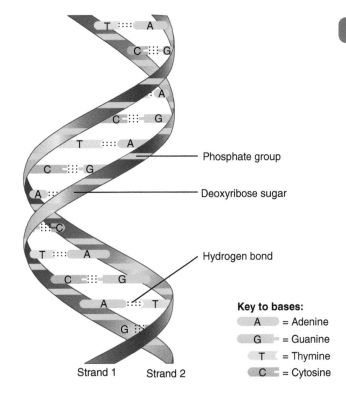

- DNA is made of two strands twisted in a spiral staircase-like structure called a double helix.
- Each strand consists of nucleotides bound together.
- Each nucleotide consists of a deoxyribose sugar bound to a phosphate group and one of 4 nitrogenous bases [adenine (A), thymine (T), guanine (G), cytosine (C)].
- The nitrogenous bases pair together through hydrogen bonding to form the 'steps' of the double helix.
- Adenine pairs with thymine and guanine pairs with cytosine.

Phosphate group

Deoxyribose sugar

Hydrogen bond

Key to bases:
A = Adenine
G = Guanine
T = Thymine
C = Cytosine

Strand 1   Strand 2

Figure 3.2 **A pictorial representation of a portion of the double helix.** *Source.* Tortora and Derrickson (2014). Reproduced with permission of John Wiley & Sons. This spiraling structure would continue so that each piece of DNA contained millions of nucleotides. Note the interaction of the bases is selective, so that A only pairs with T and C only pairs with G. These pairings are held by hydrogen bonds which hold the two strands of DNA together.

These strings of nucleotides twist around forming a spiral molecule resembling a ladder. The sides of the ladder are formed by the deoxyribose-phosphate groups of the nucleotides. The rungs are formed by the bases of one strand interacting with the bases of the other strand and therefore hold the sides of the ladder together. It is the sequence of these nucleotides and their specific bases (the rungs) along the length of the ladder-like DNA molecule that holds the genetic code. There is a strict rule governing which bases will interact with each other to form the rungs of the DNA ladder, and it is that Adenine (A) will only bind to Thymine (T), and Guanine (G) will only bind to Cytosine (C). So, if, for example, one strand of DNA has a base sequence AGGCAGTGC, then the opposite strand will have the complementary base sequence, which will be TCCGTCACG; you can see this in Figure 3.2.

The complementary bases are held together by hydrogen bonds, whereas each nucleotide is held to the next with covalent bonds (these bonds were discussed in Chapter 1). Of the two types of chemical bonds, hydrogen bonds are weaker, which has implications for the processes of DNA replication and transcription, as you will see.

Chromosomes

As stated earlier the DNA of eukaryotes (organisms, including humans, whose cells contain a nucleus and other organelles enclosed within membranes) is contained within the nucleus as lengths of chromatin known as chromosomes. As shown in Figure 3.3, the DNA winds around the histones forming a nucleosome. Many nucleosomes are required to package one strand of DNA. If the DNA inside the nucleus of a human cell were stretched out, it would be approximately 2 meters long, but because it is so tightly coiled it fits into the nucleus, which is about six micrometers in diameter. Chromatin can either be loosely structured to allow the

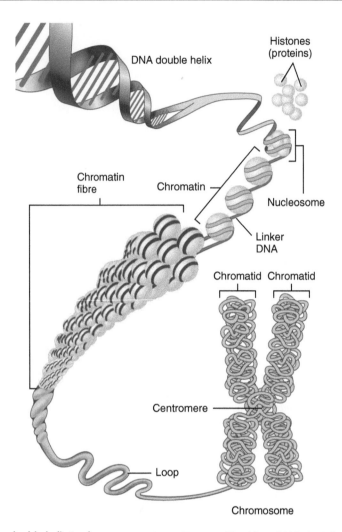

Figure 3.3 **DNA from double helix to chromosome.** *Source:* Tortora and Derrickson (2009). Reproduced with permission of John Wiley & Sons. The combination of DNA and histones is known as chromatin, which is arranged as a series of nucleosomes. Each nucleosome contains a histone protein which the DNA is wound around to keep it neatly organised and allow it to be tightly packaged to fit inside the nucleus. At certain times of the cell cycle the chromatin becomes even more tightly packaged into the typical chromosome shape, with each chromatid in the chromosome containing the exact same sequence of bases.

cell to expose the sequence of bases and use these instructions for making proteins, or at other times, tightly packaged into the 'X' structure, of the chromosome, which is the form it takes during cell division, which will be explained later.

The term chromosome can be confusing because it refers to each length of double stranded DNA found in the nucleus (remember we have 46 in total), and also to a couplet of two strands of DNA, one a copy of the other, after the DNA has been replicated. The chromosome structure shown in Figure 3.3 depicts DNA, that has already been copied, so each chromosome is made up of two chromatids joined together at the centromere. DNA is replicated just before a cell needs to divide itself to make two new cells. This process occurs as part of the cell cycle, which we will look at later in this chapter.

In most humans, each nucleated cell (i.e. each cell with a nucleus) has 46 chromosomes, which occur as 23 pairs (Figure 3.4). Of those 23 pairs, one pair determines the gender of the person.

- Females have a matched homologous (the same) pair of X chromosomes.
- Males have an unmatched heterologous (different) pair – one X and one Y chromosome.

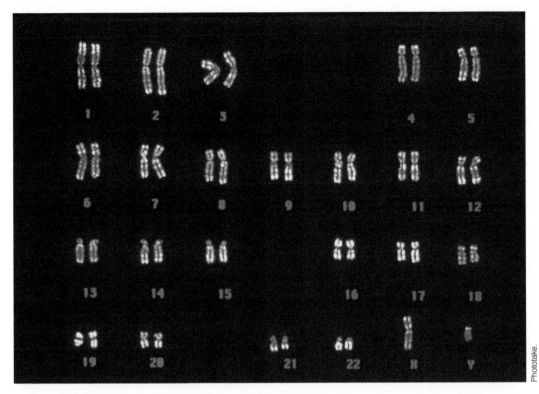

Phototake.

Figure 3.4 **The chromosomes of a human male – a karyotype. Chromosomes only take on this particular shape during cell division. The assessment of karyotype can be performed to identify the presence of some genetic disorders. Each chromosome is identified by its size and 'banding' pattern following staining with particular dyes.** *Source:* Snustad and Simmons (2012). Reproduced with permission of John Wiley & Sons.

- The remaining 22 pairs of chromosomes are known as autosomes (each pair is homologous as they have the same genes on them). In biology, the suffix 'some' means body, so autosome means 'self body'. Thus, 'autosomes' can be defined as the chromosomes that determine physical characteristics – in other words, all the characteristics of a person that are not connected with gender. This is not to say that the X and Y chromosomes only have genes for gender determination. The X chromosome contains hundreds of genes, including those for red/green colour vision, blood clotting and tooth enamel, to name a few. In contrast, the Y chromosome has only 70 genes or so, most of which are involved in determining male gender. So the majority of the genes of the X chromosome are not matched by a corresponding gene on the Y chromosome. This means that although the Y chromosome contains some of the same genes as the X chromosome, such as that for tooth enamel, most do not match the X chromosome genes, which has important implications for the inheritance of some genetic conditions, as discussed later in this chapter.

The position a gene occupies on a chromosome is called a locus, and there are different loci for eye colour, height, hair type, and so on ('loci' is the plural of 'locus'). Think of the locus as the address of that particular gene on Chromosome Street in the same way that a house number signifies where you live on your street.

Our autosomes occur in pairs, which means we have two pieces of DNA for each autosomal gene. Each version of a gene is known as an allele. So, we can say that alleles for each gene occur at the same loci on homologous chromosomes. As you inherited one of the chromosomes in the homologous pair from your mother and the other from your father, you therefore received one allele for each gene from your mother and one from your father. Alleles do not have to have exactly the same sequence of bases, although they will be very similar, but they do provide information for alternative forms of proteins that perform a particular function. Eye colour is a good example – if we consider that eyes are either brown or blue (there are other alternatives but these are governed by more complex factors that we will not consider here), then we know that there is one gene that determines eye colour located at the same place on each of the two chromosomes of a homologous pair. One allele of this gene will come from the father and the other from the mother. If a child's mother has blue eyes and the father brown eyes, the child may have blue or brown eyes, depending upon factors that will be discussed later.

In the human population, a gene may have more than two possible alleles, but each individual person will only have two. A person with a pair of identical alleles for a particular gene locus is said to be homozygous for that gene, whereas someone with two different alleles is heterozygous for that gene. Whether you are homozygous or heterozygous for one gene will not influence whether you are homozygous or heterozygous for another gene. The alleles you have for a gene determines your genotype for that gene, so each individual has thousands of genotypes (one for each gene).

The allele combinations for a particular gene can interact in different ways to produce variations on the characteristic the gene is coding for. This is because some alleles are recessive and some are dominant.

- A dominant allele exerts its effect and is physically manifested (the phenotype) when present on at least one of the chromosomes of the pair (so you could have two dominant alleles (homozygous genotype) or have one dominant and one recessive allele (heterozygous genotype) and still show the same physical characteristic (phenotype).
- A recessive allele has to be present on both chromosomes to manifest itself physically (phenotype). So, to see the effect of a recessive allele, you have to have a homozygous genotype for that gene (or lack the dominant allele).

This will be explained more fully later in this chapter, but it is very important because of the significance that it has in hereditary disorders.

From DNA to Proteins

DNA is a nucleic acid with two major functions; to direct protein synthesis and to faithfully carry genetic information from one generation of cells to the next, and from one generation of individuals to the next.

Protein Synthesis

Synthesis simply means 'production'; hence, the production of protein from raw materials. The instructions for making proteins are found in DNA, so to synthesise proteins the genetic information encoded in the DNA has to be turned into a corresponding sequence of protein building blocks (amino acids).

This occurs in two processes: transcription and translation. The process of transcription creates a messenger RNA (mRNA) copy of the DNA. Transcription of a gene is similar to transcribing information from a textbook onto a piece of paper that we can take with us, leaving the book in the library. During translation, the mRNA code is 'read' and turned into a protein molecule.

Transcription

DNA has to be transcribed into RNA, because DNA is 'stuck' in the nucleus due to its size. Whereas proteins need to be synthesised in the ribosomes, within the cell's cytoplasm (Chapter 2). Using a specific portion of DNA (a gene) as a template, the genetic information stored in the sequence of bases of DNA is rewritten so that the same information appears in the bases of RNA. To do this, the two strands of the DNA have to separate (Figure 3.5). This is achieved by momentarily breaking the hydrogen bonds that pair each of the bases in the double helix strands together. The exposed bases are now available to pair with their complementary bases by hydrogen bonding (remember the base-pairing rule), but this time the bases are on RNA nucleotides, so the new molecule is RNA, specifically messenger RNA (mRNA).

As with DNA, guanine can only pair with cytosine in RNA. But while the thymine in DNA only binds to adenine in the RNA, there is no thymine in RNA, so adenine binds to the RNA base uracil (U), which does not occur in the DNA molecule.

DNA		mRNA
guanine (G)	–	cytosine (C)
cytosine (C)	–	guanine (G)
thymine (T)	–	adenine (A)
adenine (A)	–	uracil (U)

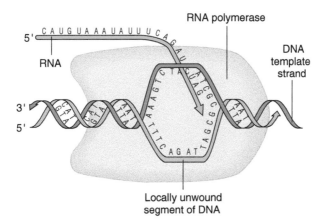

Figure 3.5 The separation of DNA for transcription. A small segment of DNA containing the gene to be transcribed opens up as the hydrogen bonds between complementary bases are temporarily broken. A strand of RNA is then formed and when finished it is released and the DNA bonds reform. *Source:* Snustad and Simmons (2012). Reproduced with permission of John Wiley & Sons.

For example, if DNA has a base sequence AGGCAGTGC, then the complementary base sequence on mRNA will be UCCGUCACG. Figure 3.5 demonstrates the way in which the DNA separates to allow the RNA to be formed with the same information as one of the DNA strands in that region.

In addition to the sequence of bases in DNA that provide the code for the body's proteins, some regions of DNA provide important regulatory information. DNA can therefore be loosely classified as being part of an exon or an intron (also referred to as coding or non-coding regions, respectively). Bases within exons provide the amino acid order for the protein and bases in introns direct regulation of protein synthesis activities, such as when and how much of each protein should be made. Other non-exon parts of DNA determine where each individual gene starts and finishes. The interspersing of introns amongst the exons of a gene also allows alternate forms of mRNA to be generated from the same gene, and this partly explains why we have over 100,000 proteins but only around 30,000 genes.

The removal of introns following transcription is known as splicing and results in the formation of the mature mRNA molecule. The mRNA is therefore a copy of a section of a chromosome small enough to be transported out of the nucleus ready for the next step: translation. However, in addition to serving as the template for the synthesis of mRNA, DNA also provides the information for the synthesis of other kinds of RNA (more research continues to find new types of RNA), two of which, ribosomal RNA (rRNA) and transfer RNA (tRNA) are also essential for the translation step of protein synthesis. rRNA, together with the ribosomal proteins, makes up the ribosomes, and tRNA matches the code on the mRNA with the correct amino acids.

Translation

In genetics, translation is the process by which the specific sequence of bases in mRNA is used to specify the amino acid sequence of a protein. There are 20 different amino acids from which our proteins are assembled.

Translation occurs in the cell's cytoplasm and involves all three types of RNA, as well as ribosomal proteins. The following is the sequence of the major steps of protein synthesis, also shown in Figures 3.6 and 3.7.

- In the cytoplasm, a small and a large ribosomal subunit assemble around the start of the mRNA molecule to provide the platform where the mRNA is decoded into amino acids.
- Each amino acid is attached to a specific tRNA molecule. Each tRNA has a unique sequence of three bases, known as an anti-codon, which determines the particular amino acid it is attached to.
- Each tRNA also matches by complementary base-pairing to a group of three bases (codon) in mRNA. In this way the mRNA is decoded by tRNAs and the correct amino acids added to the growing protein molecule, as determined by the sequence of codons in the mRNA. Sequences of three bases in DNA (known as triplets) therefore relate to the sequence of codons in mRNA.

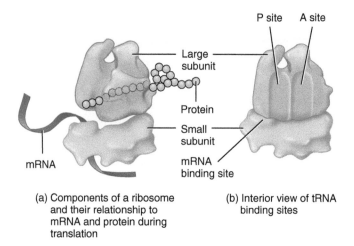

(a) Components of a ribosome and their relationship to mRNA and protein during translation

(b) Interior view of tRNA binding sites

Figure 3.6 (a, b) Translation begins with the mRNA associating with the small and large ribosomal subunits. The ribosome is therefore important in ensuring the mRNA is decoded as the correct groups of three bases (codons). *Source:* Tortora and Derrickson (2009). Reproduced with permission of John Wiley & Sons.

Let's look at this process in a little more detail as shown in Figure 3.7:

- The tRNAs attach to their associated amino acids.
- The ribosome attaches to the mRNA at the site that designates the start of the protein.
- The ribosome has 'sites' within it that line up with the codons of the mRNA.
- The tRNAs attempt to bond their anti-codons with the codon that is lined up with the ribosome. Only the tRNA with the complementary anti-codon to the codon will be able to bind (because of complementary base pairing). For example, only the tRNA with the anticodon UAC can bind if the mRNA codon is AUG. As a result, the 'correct' amino acid is put into the right place in the amino acid chain. Note this base pairing of codon and anticodon only occurs when the mRNA is attached to a ribosome.
- The ribosome now moves along the mRNA strand so the next codon is lined up in the ribosome, now the second tRNA anticodon moves into position.
- The adjacent amino acids on the two tRNAs are joined to each other by a peptide bond (through the action of the ribosome). The first tRNA detaches itself from the mRNA strand and binds a new molecule of its specific amino acid.
- Meanwhile, the ribosome continues moving along the strand of mRNA, and the process repeats, creating a progressively larger protein chain until the protein specified by the mRNA strand (which was initially specified by the genes on the DNA strand) is complete – in other words, the correct number of amino acids have been joined together in the correct order.
- The addition of amino acids is stopped by the termination codon, a combination of three bases that signals the protein is complete. The newly assembled protein and the mRNA are released from the ribosome.

Although understanding the process of protein synthesis may take a while, the process itself is very quick. In fact, protein synthesis progresses at the rate of about 15 amino acids per second. In addition, as the ribosome moves along the mRNA strand it vacates the starting point of the mRNA allowing another ribosome to assemble at that place (Figure 3.7). In this way, many molecules of the same protein are made from a single strand of mRNA at one time. Hence, more protein will be made than the amount of mRNA that was made.

In genetics, the concept of mutation is an important one, with many implications for health. Mutation is a permanent change to the sequence of bases in the DNA double helix. Mutations can be brought about by external agents (like UV radiation from the sun) or internal agents (like highly reactive free radicals) that damage the DNA. They can also result from a copying error when DNA is replicating (making a copy of itself) prior to a cell dividing. Fortunately, cells are equipped to repair much of the damage that occurs, but major errors may be irreparable. A mutation that causes a change to the sequence of DNA bases will flow on and result in an incorrect mRNA and amino acid sequence, resulting in an incorrect protein structure. This can lead to dysfunctional proteins and genetic disease. Further, if a mutation is present in one of our gametes, then it can be passed on to our children.

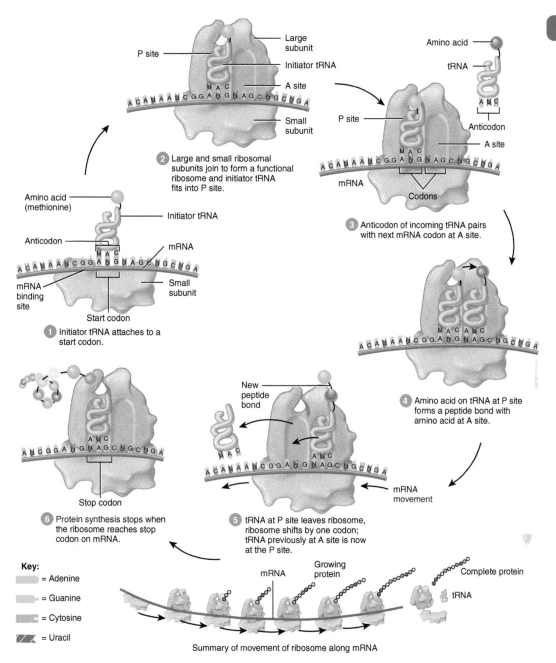

Figure 3.7 **Summary of the movement of the ribosome along mRNA.** *Source:* Tortora and Derrickson (2009). Reproduced with permission of John Wiley & Sons.

Summary of Relationship Between DNA, RNA and Protein

We can now define a gene as a sequence of nucleotides on a DNA molecule that serves as the master recipe for manufacturing a specific protein.

- Genes are on average about 1000 pairs of nucleotides long.
- The base sequence of the gene determines the base sequence of the mRNA.
- The base sequence of the mRNA determines the amino acid sequence of the protein coded by that gene.

- No two genes have exactly the same sequence of nucleotides. Each gene has a number of possible alleles (slight variations in nucleotide sequence) that will produce variation in the mRNA and therefore in the protein sequence and this is the fundamental reason for variation between individuals in our population.

Medicines Management Three-Parent Babies!

This is a very new procedure aimed at preventing mitochondrial disorders being passed on to new generations. Mitochondria, the ATP-producing organelles, also contain their own piece of DNA that houses the genes required for the cell's energy production. Mutations in mitochondrial DNA can result in serious, often fatal, diseases resulting in muscle wastage, nerve damage, loss of sight or heart failure. These diseases are passed on to offspring from the mother, as the mitochondria in the cells of any offspring come from the mother. Approximately 1 in 4000 women are clinically affected or are at risk for developing a mitochondrial mutation in their eggs.

In January 2015, the UK became the first country to allow what have become known as 'three-parent babies'. The DNA from the mother's egg is placed into a donor egg that has had its nuclear DNA removed. This egg is then fertilised *in vitro* by the father's sperm, (so the nuclear DNA is the usual combination of maternal and paternal DNA). The mitochondria of the donor egg remain and will be the source of new mitochondria in the cells of the child. The resulting child will have three biological parents – the mother and father (who supplied the nuclear DNA), and the woman who supplied the mitochondria and other organelles. The child will be the genetic offspring of the mother and father as the nuclear DNA is the major determinant of a person's phenotype. But, as a result of the donor mitochondria, which are free of mutations, the child, and, if a girl, her descendants, will not suffer the effects of mutations carried in the DNA of her mother's mitochondria.

Since this procedure introduces genetic changes that will be passed on from female three-parent babies, there are ethical concerns about the use of this process. There are also health concerns, as this technology is still in its infancy and the long-term effects of manipulating an egg in this way have not yet been established. Therefore, more research and tight regulatory controls around procedures such as these need to be in place, to ensure that the risks of the procedure do not outweigh the benefits.

See The conversation (28 September 2016) 'World's first three-parent baby raises questions about long-term health risks'.

The Transference of Genes

This section explains how genetic information is transferred from existing cells to new cells, and also from parents to children. First, we will look at how cells pass on genetic information to new cells.

Cells must be able to divide and create new cells for growth and to replace dead and damaged cells. The new cells must all contain a complete set of the genetic information (the DNA) that was in the first cell, which means cells must replicate their DNA accurately prior to dividing into two cells. The process by which cells divide their DNA to produce two new cells is known as mitosis. All human cells undergo a cell cycle, during which they are either actively undergoing mitosis, or undertaking their normal functions and preparing for mitosis.

While cells reproduce themselves by simple mitotic division, individuals reproduce by sexual reproduction, a process which involves the joining and mixing of genetic material from two different individuals (the father and the mother). In order to mix the chromosomes from two individuals and not end up with twice the normal amount of chromosomes, gametes (sperm and eggs) which contain only half the normal number of chromosomes are used. The process by which gametes are produced is known as meiosis.

Whether mitosis or meiosis is occurring, an exact copy of the cell's DNA must first be made (replication). During this process the two strands of the DNA separate, exposing the bases, which can now pair with their complementary bases on free nucleotides, and a new copy of each strand of the DNA is made, see Figure 3.8.

At the end of DNA replication, each of the 46 chromosomes will have an exact duplicate of itself. Each chromosome will exist as two identical chromatids joined by a centromere. This process occurs in the stage of the cell cycle known as interphase. Interphase is also the stage during which the cell will undertake its normal everyday functions. At the end of interphase, the cell will commence mitosis if it is one of the bodies somatic cells or meiosis if it is one of the bodies gamete-producing cells. Note that once mitosis/meiosis is

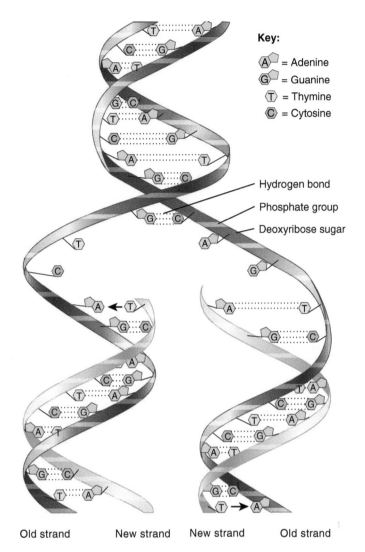

Key:
- Ⓐ = Adenine
- Ⓖ = Guanine
- Ⓣ = Thymine
- Ⓒ = Cytosine

Hydrogen bond
Phosphate group
Deoxyribose sugar

Old strand   New strand   New strand   Old strand

Figure 3.8 **DNA replication. To make additional chromosomes to distribute to new cells, DNA has to be replicated by first separating the two strands, and then creating a new complementary strand for each of the original strands. At the end of this process the cell will have two identical chromatids each consisting of an 'old' and a 'new' strand.** *Source:* Tortora and Derrickson (2009). Reproduced with permission of John Wiley & Sons.

complete, the cell will again be in interphase. Indeed, if we look at the cell cycle (Figure 3.9), we see that the cell spends the majority of time in interphase. During this period, in addition to producing the extra DNA, the cell must also increase the number of organelles such as mitochondria.

Mitosis

The process of mitosis produces two identical cells, each with 46 chromosomes, from one cell. This process occurs in four stages: prophase, metaphase, anaphase and telophase, with specific events occurring in each stage (shown in Figure 3.10). Note that for simplicity, only a few chromosomes are shown.

During interphase, the individual chromosomes in the nucleus are difficult to see because they are in the form of uncoiled threads so that they can be replicated and used for transcription. However, during mitosis the chromosomes are tightly packaged into discrete units (chromosomes, depicted in Figure 3.3) so they can be accurately divided equally amongst the daughter cells and not damaged during the process. During this first step in mitosis the cell also produces spindle fibres, specialised structures that attach to the chromosomes and assist in aligning them along the center of the cell.

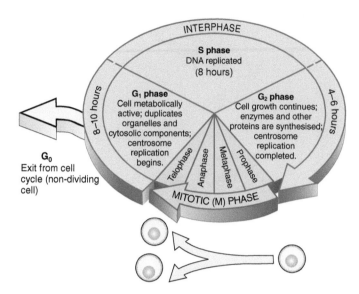

Figure 3.9 **The cell cycle.** *Source:* Tortora and Derrickson (2009). Reproduced with permission of John Wiley & Sons. Note the indicated timing of each stage is a guide and the exact timings depend on the particular cell type involved. In fact, the timing of interphase varies from one day to many months or even years dependent on the cell and the bodies requirements. The mitotic phase, however, is generally quick, taking only a few hours once it begins.

During the early stages of mitosis the nuclear envelope dissolves, leaving the chromosomes temporarily in the cytoplasm. The spindle fibres extend from opposite sides of the cell (poles) and attach to each chromosome, one from each pole. The spindle fibres then contract back towards the poles, pulling the chromatids apart and towards each pole. The spindle fibres disappear, and a nuclear envelope forms around each set of 46 chromosomes. Finally, the cytoplasm is also divided (cytokinesis) to produce two separate, identical cells each containing 46 chromosomes.

Meiosis

Meiosis is the form of cell division used only to produce the gametes, i.e. male sperm and female ova.

The cells of the human body that contain 23 pairs of chromosomes (46 in total) are referred to as diploid cells. Gametes, on the other hand, possess only 23 chromosomes, and are referred to as haploid cells. Therefore, when gametes fuse during reproduction the combined DNA from both gametes equals 46 chromosomes. Gametes develop from cells with 46 chromosomes, and through the process of meiosis end up with 23 chromosomes.

Meiosis is divided into eight stages, in contrast to the four of mitosis, occurring as two meiotic divisions: meiosis I and meiosis II. The stages have the same names as those occurring during mitosis, since they describe similar events. There are, however, some important differences between the two meiotic divisions, so to distinguish these we identify the four stages of meiosis I as prophase I, metaphase I, anaphase I, telophase I, and the four stages of meiosis II as prophase II, metaphase II, anaphase II and telophase II. As with mitosis, these stages occur in a sequential fashion with the progression from one stage to the next tightly controlled.

Meiosis I

Prior to the first meiotic division the cell is in interphase, just as it is prior to mitosis, and would have replicated all its chromosomes. The early events of the first meiotic division are similar to mitosis with the tight coiling of the chromosomes, dissolution of the nuclear envelope and generation of the spindle fibres. However, instead of lining up along the middle of the cell as 46 individual chromosomes (as in mitosis), the chromosomes line up in their pairs so that there are 23 pairs of chromosomes lying side by side across the equator of the cell. While next to each other this way, the paired chromosomes are able to swap some of their DNA. Each chromosome pair includes one maternal and one paternal chromosome, containing the same genes (but not

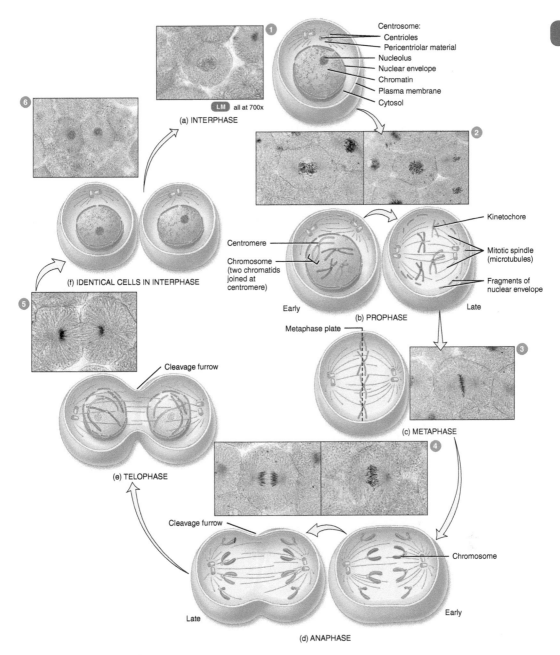

Figure 3.10 **The stages of the somatic cell cycle. Somatic cells are all the cells of the body except the gametes. When we need a new somatic cell, the DNA is replicated during interphase (a), the nucleus is divided by mitosis (b-e) resulting in the formation of two identical daughter cells (f).** *Source:* Tortora and Derrickson (2009). Reproduced with permission of John Wiley & Sons.

necessarily the same alleles). Some of the DNA can be swapped between the maternal and paternal versions of the genes at this point, in a process called 'crossing over' or recombination (see Figure 3.11). The genes still remain in the correct loci, but some alleles that were originally on the paternal chromosome may swap to the maternal one, and vice versa. This creates entirely new versions of the chromosomes with a mix of alleles that did not exist in the parent – a process which adds genetic variation to the offspring.

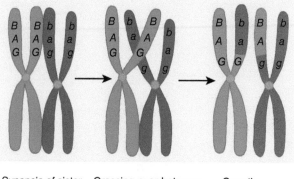

Synapsis of sister chromatids   Crossing-over between non-sister chromatids   Genetic recombination

Details of crossing-over during prophase I

Figure 3.11 **Gene crossover (recombination). During meiosis I homologous chromosomes pair together. The chromatids can then exchange information between non-sister chromatids in the homologous pair (sister chromatids are the exact copies made by DNA replication). This creates chromosomes that have a mix of alleles of the genes of the original chromosomes.** *Source:* Tortora and Derrickson (2009). Reproduced with permission of John Wiley & Sons.

As in mitosis, the spindles extend from the poles of the cell, but instead of connecting and pulling single chromatids (as in mitosis), they connect with and pull whole chromosomes to the poles. Each pole now has 23 chromosomes contained in a new nuclear envelope. The division of the cytoplasm completes meiosis I producing two haploid cells (but still with replicated sister chromatids) from the original diploid cell.

Meiosis II

During the second meiotic division, both of the cells produced by the first meiotic division divide again. However, as there is no interphase between meiosis I and meiosis II, the DNA is not replicated prior to this division. Meiosis II is similar to mitosis, the main difference being that there are only 23 chromosomes to line up at the equator. The individual chromatids of these 23 chromosomes are pulled apart and moved to the poles during this division. The resulting cells each contain 23 single chromatids. Note that at the end of this process there are four haploid cells from one original parent cell. If an egg (ovum) was being produced, then each cell would contain 22 autosomes and one X chromosome. If sperm (spermatozoa) were being produced, then two of the four sperm cells would contain Y chromosomes along with the 22 autosomes, and two would contain an X chromosome along with their 22 autosomes. It is therefore the sperm that determines the gender of the child, since all ova contain an X chromosome, but a sperm cell can contain an X or a Y chromosome.

Inheritance

We are a product of our genes, or perhaps more precisely a product of our genes acted on and influenced by our environment. Our environment in this context includes factors such as time, space, relationships, education, nutrition, physical activity, sun exposure, air quality and so on.

We inherit our genes from our parents through the direct transfer of their chromosomes into the gametes that fused to produce us. But why are we still unique? The answer lies in the behavior of the alleles of each gene. This concept was first investigated in the 1860s by the monk Gregor Mendel. Mendel was assigned to care for the monastery garden. Mendel was very curious and began to wonder why the offspring of plants differed from their parents. He carried out controlled experiments in crossbreeding of plants and used statistics to interpret his results (the use of statistics was not common in biology at that time).

In 1866, Mendel published a paper of his work and the response from the scientific community was a deafening silence – his observations and theories were completely ignored until their 'rediscovery' in the early 1900s. It is this work that forms the basis of the science of inheritance that we now understand. Any human characteristic or genetic disorder that fits with his theories is said to follow a Mendelian (or classical/ simple) inheritance pattern, with characteristics/disorders that fit the more recently identified inheritance patterns referred to as being non-Mendelian (or complex).

Without any knowledge of DNA or genes, Mendel was able to postulate that there were factors that controlled an organism's characteristics. He determined that these occur in pairs and he discovered that within the pair, the information could be identical (what we now call homozygous) or the pieces of information could be slightly different (heterozygous). This allowed him to explain the concepts of dominance and recessivity that was explained earlier in this chapter. Mendel derived two laws of inheritance from his experimental work, the law of independent assortment and the law of segregation.

The law of segregation states that the members of a gene pair separate equally into the gametes. This law means that during meiosis I, when the homologous chromosomes pair up together and separate into the daughter cells, the paired alleles for each gene (i.e. the paternal and maternal chromosomes) will separate into two separate cells – both chromosomes of a pair will not end up in the same cell. Therefore, the offspring will have new 'pairings' created from the single sets of chromosomes contained in the egg and sperm when they fused together.

The law of independent assortment states that the chromosomes contained in each gamete will contain a random mix of maternally and paternally derived chromosomes – the pairs of chromosomes that line up on the cell equator prior to separation do not have paternal chromosomes on one side and maternal on the other – they are randomly assorted, and so each new cell/gamete will receive an unpredictable number of maternal and paternal chromosomes as each chromatid is pulled into its new cell. The diagrams in Figure 3.12 illustrate these concepts with cells that have two pairs of chromosomes instead of 23.

Mendelian Inheritance

We inherit our DNA from our parents, who inherited theirs from their parents. So we share some of our DNA with our grandparents and great grandparents, etc. The phenotypes which result from our inherited DNA will depend on the inheritance patterns of the genes. For characteristics that follow a Mendelian inheritance pattern, genes can be autosomal dominant, autosomal recessive or X-linked recessive.

Remember, that at each locus (gene), the alleles can be either dominant or recessive. If a dominant allele is present, then it will always be reflected in the phenotype, regardless of the other allele, but a recessive allele will only appear in the phenotype if there is no dominant allele. Note that when we represent these alleles in written form, dominant alleles are usually given capital letters, while recessive alleles are usually given lowercase letters.

In genetics we are often interested in calculating the probability of inheriting certain dominant or recessive alleles. We do this by considering the possible alleles that any gamete produced by the parents could have for a particular gene, and then work out the possible combinations that could come together in the offspring. When calculating the probability of inheriting any particular genotype, it is important to remember that the probability applies independently to each child born. For example, if the risk of inheriting a particular pair of alleles of a gene is 25% or 1 in 4, it does not mean that the couple have to have 4 children before they are likely to have a child with those alleles; it means that each child will have a 25% chance of having the alleles in question. So, whilst we report a risk as a percentage, all of the children of a couple may inherit the same pair of alleles for a locus or they may have different combinations.

Using our knowledge of dominant and recessive alleles and probability we can also identify which traits are dominant and which recessive. If a man with red hair and a woman with brown hair have many children, and all of them have brown hair, then this would suggest that the brown allele is dominant and the red allele recessive. If this is true, the father must be homozygous for the red allele in order to have red hair. Therefore, he only has a red allele to pass to his children. So, what can we say about his children's genotype? Since they all have brown hair, they must all have at least one dominant (brown) allele, and we also know they must all have a recessive (red) allele, as they had to get one allele from their father. Therefore, they must be heterozygous for this particular gene.

If one of these children goes on to have a child with red hair, like their grandfather, then we know that the child must have inherited a red allele from their mother to complement the red allele from their brown haired father, since the child would have to possess two red alleles to have red hair. Both parents must therefore have been heterozygous for hair colour. This is often referred to as a trait 'skipping a generation' and is something that we can only see with recessive traits.

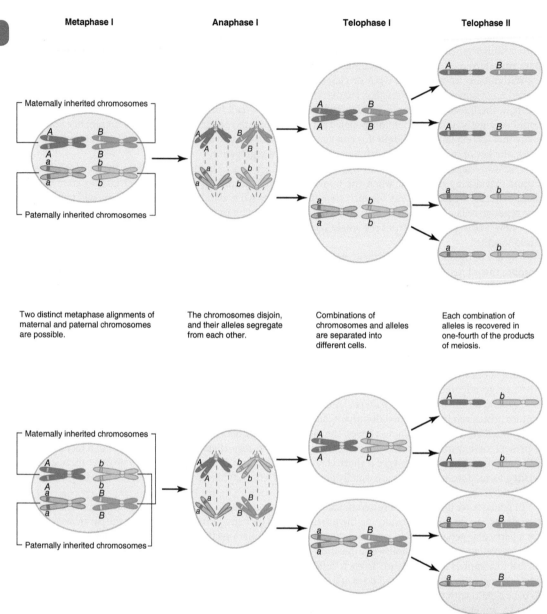

| Metaphase I | Anaphase I | Telophase I | Telophase II |

Two distinct metaphase alignments of maternal and paternal chromosomes are possible.

The chromosomes disjoin, and their alleles segregate from each other.

Combinations of chromosomes and alleles are separated into different cells.

Each combination of alleles is recovered in one-fourth of the products of meiosis.

Figure 3.12 **Mendel's laws of genetic inheritance. The two diagrams show the effects during meiosis of random assorting of chromosomes on the combinations of chromosomes in the gametes. The law of segregation is also shown as for each chromosome pair of the original cell, only one is found in each gamete.** *Source:* Snustad and Simmons (2012). Reproduced with permission of John Wiley & Sons.

Autosomal Dominant Inheritance and Ill Health

If a person has one dominant allele that causes disease, such as Huntington's disease or neurofibromatosis, the person will have the disease, since the allele is dominant and will therefore determine the phenotype, but what is the risk of any of the person's children having the disease?

To determine the probability, we need to know the genotypes of both parents. If we assume the other parent does not have the disease, they are homozygous for the recessive allele, and therefore cannot possess

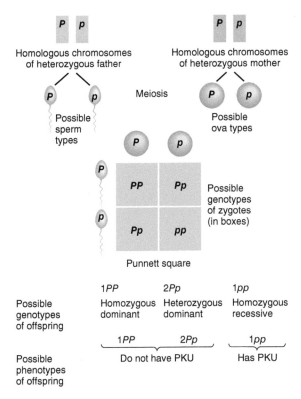

Figure 3.13 Punnet squares are used to assess risk of offspring having a particular condition. The interpretation relies upon knowing whether the condition is dominant or recessive. The punnet square is created by putting together the alleles carried by both parents from the column and row that forms the boxes of the square. This then offers four possible genotype combinations, which, depending on the original parental alleles, may include the same genotype repeated. The number of combinations resulting in disease can then be determined. *Source:* Tortora and Derrickson (2009). Reproduced with permission of John Wiley & Sons.

the dominant disease-causing allele. This parent can therefore only pass on a recessive allele to his or her children. However, the parent with the disease has a 50% chance of passing the dominant allele to their children, as this person has one dominant and one recessive allele. There is therefore a 50% probability that a child will have the autosomal dominant disorder. If the affected parent was homozygous for the dominant allele, the risk of it being passed to any offspring would be 100% (as all offspring would get one of the dominant alleles). Alternatively, if both parents were heterozygous for the dominant condition the risk of a child inheriting the condition would be 75%. We can use a device known as a punnet square to show us why. Figure 3.13 shows an example for parents who are heterozygous for the gene involved in the disorder phenylketonuria (PKU). The dominant allele for this gene is the normal allele that protects the individual from having PKU.

Autosomal Recessive Inheritance and Ill Health

Autosomal recessive diseases occur when a disease-causing allele is recessive, which means an individual must have two of these alleles to have the disease. The parents of that individual must each have passed on one recessive allele to their child, and they would each have been heterozygous (or homozygous) for the condition. When a person is heterozygous for a recessive disease they are said to be a carrier, as the disease allele is present in their genotype (and could possibly be passed to their offspring) but they do not have the disease themselves. A genetic disease can be carried through many generations and not seen until a carrier has children with someone who is also a carrier for the same condition (or suffers from the condition). The approach to calculating the probability of inheriting an autosomal recessive disease is the same as that used for dominant disease-causing traits.

Let's consider an example of a couple who are both carriers of the mutant allele that causes cystic fibrosis. As both parents are carriers then they have the same genotype, Cc (remember upper case is used for dominant alleles), which means that half of each parent's gametes will have the C allele and the other half the c allele. To determine the likelihood that these parents have a child with cystic fibrosis or who is a carrier we can use a punnet square (see Figure 3.13 for how to construct one). From this we see that there is a 25% chance of the child inheriting the C allele from both of their parents. Any child with this genotype (CC) would be phenotypically normal (since the dominant allele in this case is not the disease-causing one) and, in the future, cannot pass on the disease-causing allele to their children, since they do not possess it. There is also a 25% (or 1 in 4) chance that the child would inherit the c allele from both their parents. This child would have cystic fibrosis. The other two possible combinations result in the same Cc genotype (but with the C allele coming from a different parent in each case) therefore there is a 50% (or 1 in 2) chance that they will have a child who is a carrier of the cystic fibrosis allele. Any child with the cc (affected) or Cc (carrier) genotype has a possibility of having affected children in the future, depending on their partner's genotype. It is important to remember that the calculated probabilities apply to each pregnancy separately (LeMone *et al.*, 2015). So, if these parents have four children it does not mean that they will have one child with each of the possible genotypes in the punnet square. Each pregnancy has the same chances of inheriting one of the genotypes as the other pregnancies.

Medicines Management Gene Replacement Therapy

Gene therapy is one way in which genetic disorders can be treated, or at least ameliorated, by:
- replacing the mutated or malfunctioning gene;
- manipulating or turning off the gene that is causing the disease;
- stimulating other bodily functions to fight the disease.

The most common form of gene therapy is replacement of a malfunctioning or missing gene with a healthy one. There have been many attempts to cure diseases using this form of therapy. In the late 1990s, unsuccessful attempts were made to treat cystic fibrosis. Whereas, in the early 2000s, gene replacement therapy for the immune deficiency, adenosine deaminase deficiency severe combined immunodeficiency, was successfully carried out. Despite many refinements, gene therapy still poses a risk of serious complications, partly due to the method of using modified viruses to 'carry' and insert the 'new' corrective genes into the DNA of the body cells. Insertion of a healthy gene, essentially a length of DNA, into an existing genome at exactly the correct point to override the abnormal gene is a difficult and complex maneouvre. In the earliest gene therapy trials, despite the therapy being initially successful, two children went on to develop leukaemia as a result of the 'new' gene inserting into the wrong place in the genome. Fortunately, this problem has now been largely eliminated, and gene replacement for this and other primary immunodeficiencies is regularly carried out in specialist centres.

In addition to the risk of cancer developing, other problems can arise with this therapy. For instance, the inserted virus could be perceived as a foreign invader by the immune system, which could lead to the body attacking the virus and with it its own organs. So far, in the case of children with specific severe primary immunodeficiencies, this has not been a problem, but it is an ever-present risk. These risks must be weighed against the fact that there are no completely effective alternative treatments. Like every advance in medical science, both failures and small successes spurs on researchers and doctors to refine, correct and improve the treatments for these and other genetic conditions.

Clinical Considerations Genetic Counselling

Generally, the clinical application of genetics in health is the responsibility of doctors and scientists. However, genetic counselling is an extremely important aspect of genetics that is within the nurse's scope of practice. While there are professionals who are specially trained in genetics and genetic counselling, on a day-to-day basis the nurse is the health practitioner that spends the greatest time with a patient and builds rapport. The nurse is therefore in an ideal position to offer counselling to individuals and their families regarding risk associated with genetic diseases. This, of course, places a responsibility on the nurse to be well informed about genetic inheritance patterns.

Genetic counselling involves providing information and support to patients and their family and answering their specific questions. The inclusion of the family is very important when dealing with inherited disease, as there are ramifications for the whole family. If requested, counselling may occur privately with individual family members who have questions that are particularly relevant to them.

For a consultation, a genetic counsellor will need:

- knowledge of genetics, genetic diseases and current treatment options;
- respect for the patient and family;
- time, patience and empathy.

During a consultation, the genetics counsellor will:

- begin building rapport and trust;
- provide information in appropriate language so the patient and family can make informed and independent decisions;
- allow the patient/family time to process the information, being patient and innovative in repeat explanations so they can absorb and understand the situation;
- allow the patient and family time to think things over, arrange for them to be seen again in the near future, and be available to answer questions as they arise;
- maintain privacy and confidentiality;
- be truthful about potential consequences, discuss the positives and negatives and clearly explain the risks of passing on a genetic disease;
- respect the patient's/family member's beliefs and feelings rather than imposing their own;
- not make decisions for the individuals involved; for example, do not tell a couple to end a pregnancy, or have a specific treatment.

Whilst most hospitals now have specialist genetics counsellors, they are not always available to patients or their families, which is where the nurse on the ward or in the clinic comes into their own. The nurse will be trusted and available to discuss these matters without the formality of an appointment and official consultation. Consequently, the nurse needs to have knowledge of the conditions and their treatments and outcomes, especially when it comes to genetic inheritance medical problems. The nurse plays a vital role in providing patients with the support and information they require, as they become ready to receive it. Much of what the genetics counsellor has discussed with the patient/family may need to be repeated and reinforced during the patient's stay in hospital.

Skills in Practice Constructing a Family Pedigree to Assess Risk

When guiding a couple on the risk of having a child with a genetic condition present in their family, it can be useful to construct a family pedigree chart. This is a family tree which includes the pertinent genetic information required to study inheritance patterns. It is important to advise the family involved that they need to be as honest as they can with the answers to the questions you will need to ask in order to construct the pedigree.

So that a pedigree can be understood by all health care professionals, conventional symbols are used to indicate biological relationships and the presence of the condition in question. It is very important to display genetic relationships as accurately as possible. For instance, identical (monozygotic) twins share near 100% genetics, whereas non-identical (dizygotic) twins have no more similarity in their genetics than any other siblings from the same parents. However, non-identical twins may share many more common environmental influences than non-twin siblings. These considerations are often important in determining risk.

Many families may not differentiate biological relatives from non-biological relatives, and this may become apparent as the pedigree is constructed, as the biological inheritance lines are shown for their family. An example of a pedigree is shown in Figure 3.14. Men are identified by squares, women by circles, and offspring connected to their parents by lines. The circles or squares of individuals with the condition in question are filled in to allow the inheritance pattern to be seen.

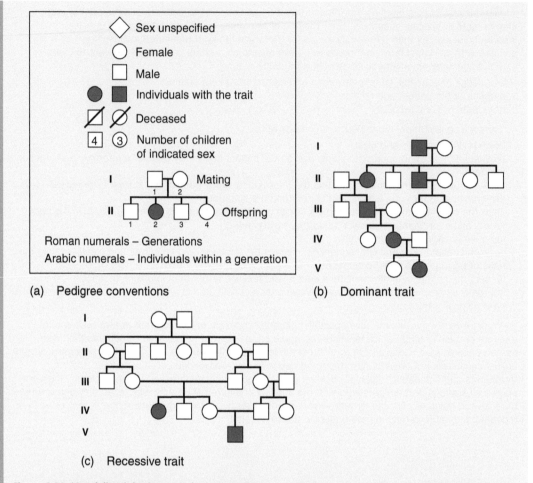

Figure 3.14 **Mendelian inheritance in human pedigrees. (a) Pedigree conventions. (b) Inheritance of a dominant trait. The trait appears in each generation. (c) Inheritance of a recessive trait. In this instance, the two affected individuals are the offspring of relatives, although this is not required to inherit a recessive trait.** *Source*: Snustad and Simmons (2012). Reproduced with permission of John Wiley & Sons.

Morbidity and Mortality of Dominant Versus Recessive Disorders

Autosomal dominant disorders are generally less severe than recessive disorders, because everyone with the disease allele also has the disease. If an autosomal dominant disorder produced severe or fatal effects, then people with the allele would be more likely to die before reaching an age to reproduce. In this way, the alleles for severe autosomal dominant disorders cease to exist in the population. The only ones that remain are those that do not cause the death of the sufferer before they reach sexual maturity. Huntington's disease is a fatal autosomal dominant disorder that survives in the population because the disease does not tend to show itself until adulthood, giving time for the sufferer to have unknowingly passed the affected gene on to the next generation. Autosomal recessive disorders on the other hand, are often severe as a person can be a carrier of the allele and pass it on to their offspring without having any disease at all.

X-linked Recessive Disorders

Disorders can be inherited on the sex chromosomes in addition to the autosomes. The sex chromosomes determine gender, as possession of two X chromosomes results in a female, while one X and one Y results in a male. Since most of the genes on the X chromosome do not have an equivalent on the Y chromosome, and

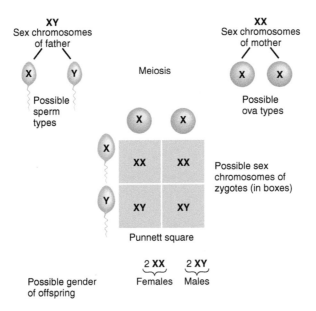

Figure 3.15 **Determination of gender in offspring.** *Source:* Tortora and Derrickson (2009). Reproduced with permission of John Wiley & Sons.

males and females have different X and Y combinations, inheritance patterns of genes located on the sex chromosomes require different interpretation to autosomal gene inheritance.

In order to be male, a person needs just one Y chromosome, so maleness is similar to a dominant trait, since it is not opposed by an alternative allele on the paired chromosome. Using the punnet square approach, we see that the chances of having a boy or a girl are 50% (Figure 3.15).

A male child must of course have received his Y chromosome from his father, since his mother doesn't have one. So, it also follows that a boy must have got his X chromosome from his mother (Figure 3.15).

Some serious genetic disorders are due to mutations in genes located on the X chromosome. Examples are X-linked haemophilia and Duchenne muscular dystrophy. These disorders are recessive, which means that to have the condition there must not be a dominant (normal) allele present. Females have two X chromosomes, so can be heterozygous and therefore only a carrier. Whereas males that have the affected X are always affected as their Y chromosome does not have the same genes, so there is no chance of a dominant allele. Therefore, males are more commonly affected with these diseases than females. For a female to have a disease of this kind, her father would have to be a sufferer, and her mother would have to be (at least) a carrier of the disease. This is much less likely to occur, particularly since the diseases are often fatal before the sufferer reaches reproductive age.

With X-linked recessive conditions, therefore, the risk is completely dependent on gender. To indicate this in pedigrees, X chromosomes bearing mutated (recessive) alleles are marked with a superscript lower case letter (eg X^h, Figure 3.16). Using this example of red green colour blindness, the possible genotypes of offspring from these parents are:

- a girl who does not carry the affected allele, so is neither a carrier nor affected;
- a boy who does not carry the abnormal allele, so has a normal X and a Y and is neither a carrier nor affected;
- a girl who carries the abnormal allele (X^c), but the action of that gene is blocked by her other X allele, so she is not affected, but is a carrier;
- a boy who carries the abnormal X allele (X^c). As the Y chromosome does not have this gene it is unable to block the action of the abnormal gene, so he is affected (and can of course pass the allele on to any female offspring he produces).

Consequently, we can say that:

- 50% (or 1 in 2) female children will be carriers;
- 50% (or 1 in 2) male children will have the disease.

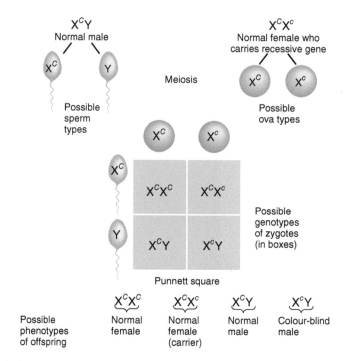

Meiosis

Possible sperm types

Possible ova types

Punnett square

Possible genotypes of zygotes (in boxes)

Possible phenotypes of offspring | Normal female | Normal female (carrier) | Normal male | Colour-blind male

Figure 3.16 **X-linked inheritance.** *Source:* Tortora and Derrickson (2009). Reproduced with permission of John Wiley & Sons.

Non-Mendelian (Complex) Inheritance

This chapter is mainly concerned with understanding Mendelian inheritance patterns. However, there are many human traits and diseases that do not follow these simple inheritance patterns. We will not consider these in great detail but do need to be aware of them. One very well-known example is that of our blood groups. Our red blood cells have proteins on their surface that are antigenic, meaning that they will cause an immune response if introduced into the bloodstream of a person with a different blood group. This will cause the destruction of the red blood cells and severe illness or death. Blood transfusions can therefore only be from donors with compatible blood groups. Humans have one of four 'blood types', named A, B, AB and O. These types result from the different possible alleles of a single gene, so there is an A allele, a B allele and an O allele. Both A and B alleles are dominant over the O allele: so if you inherit an A and an O allele then you will have blood type A, just as if you inherited two A alleles. This is what we have seen previously with Mendelian inheritance. However, some people have blood type AB, having inherited an A and a B allele and because these two alleles are co-dominant with each other both are expressed in the phenotype of a person with this genotype.

Some genes have alleles that show incomplete dominance, in which case the phenotype is a mixture roughly half way between the phenotype of one allele and the other; for example, the gene for flower colour might have a red allele and a white allele, which, if the alleles showed incomplete dominance, might result in a pink flower if they were both present.

Many of our traits are the result of not one but many genes, and are also influenced by our environment. With these complexities of inheritance it is often much harder to determine a causative gene or genes for any disorder, which makes predicting inheritance risk much more difficult.

Xeroderma pigmentosum is an inherited condition that is strongly influenced by the environment. The condition is autosomal recessive and results in skin that is hypersensitive to ultraviolet light and its damaging effects. Sufferers are very prone to skin cancers and skin damage, and the disease shortens life expectancy considerably. If the sufferer can be completely protected from ultraviolet light from the sun, then the effects of the disease can be reduced or eliminated. The inherited disease phenylketonuria (PKU) is also environmentally influenced. In many countries, babies are screened for the mutant allele for this condition at birth, because if they can avoid phenylalanine in the diet from birth, they are spared the neurological degeneration that occurs with this condition (this is also why food and beverages have to clearly state if they contain phenylalanine). These conditions are also said to be 'modifiable' genetic diseases because the disease outcome can be modified by environmental changes.

Episodes of Care Mental Health

Schizophrenia is a mental illness involving disorders of thought and mood, affecting about 1% of the population. Individuals with schizophrenia experience periods of psychosis (delusions and hallucinations) as well as social withdrawal, poor self-care and a range of cognitive impairments. The severity of any of these symptoms varies greatly between individuals. Therefore, not all patients will receive the same treatments, nor will they all respond the same way to these treatments. Unfortunately, many of the current treatments for schizophrenia also have severe side-effects that greatly affect compliance.

Although the exact cause of schizophrenia is still an area of intense research, it is clear that genetics plays a large role in its development. Schizophrenia is therefore considered a complex genetic disorder as it does not follow a simple Mendelian inheritance pattern. The identical twin of a schizophrenia sufferer has a 50–80% chance of developing the condition also, but it is not a certainty, which highlights the complexity of its inheritance pattern. This makes it difficult to counsel individuals and families about their risk of inheriting this disorder as there are so many factors to consider. There is a slightly higher incidence of schizophrenia in males and onset is typically around puberty.

Mark has recently been diagnosed with schizophrenia. He has been struggling to maintain a job for the past year, he was looking more and more dishevelled and becoming withdrawn from society. He was brought into emergency by his friend who found him behaving in a strange manner, mumbling to himself and expressing concerns about the safety of his family, who were not with him. Mark was admitted to the psychiatric care ward where his medication was reviewed, and he received psychiatric care. His family visited him regularly and his wife shared her concerns about whether their children would also develop schizophrenia with the nurse. The nurse explained that the inheritance of schizophrenia was poorly understood so it was hard to determine, but that the family should look out for early signs, as the best outcomes are achieved with early diagnosis and intervention. The nurse also explained some environmental triggers (such as illicit drug use) and suggested they attempt to avoid these, as there is certainly an environmental influence on the development of schizophrenia in individuals whose genetics make them more susceptible to this disorder. Fortunately, Mark received the treatment he needed and was able to go home with a medication plan.

Multiple Choice Questions

1. Schizophrenia is a condition that:
   (a) affects 1% of the population
   (b) affects females more commonly than males
   (c) has a typical age of onset over 50
   (d) all of the above
2. What is the inheritance pattern of schizophrenia?
   (a) autosomal dominant
   (b) autosomal recessive
   (c) complex non-Mendelian
   (d) non-heritable and only influenced by the environment
3. Mark has an identical twin. This means that Mark's twin:
   (a) has the same risk as anyone else in the population of developing schizophrenia
   (b) will definitely develop schizophrenia
   (c) will develop schizophrenia if he uses illicit drugs
   (d) has a high risk of developing schizophrenia
4. Which of these would be considered symptoms of schizophrenia?
   (a) lack of self-care
   (b) clarity of thought
   (c) periods of extreme enthusiasm and impulsive behaviour
   (d) childhood learning difficulties
5. The treatments for schizophrenia:
   (a) are 100% successful with early intervention
   (b) include medications and psychiatric care
   (c) only involve medications which have severe side-effects
   (d) are not usually successful so patients require hospitalisation

70 Spontaneous Mutation

There is another way for an unusual or abnormal gene to occur and cause genetic disorders. This is by spontaneous mutation. Because of the great speed and precision needed for replication of DNA, it is possible for mistakes to occur, and in this way genetic mutations arise. There is no way of predicting or preventing this, as the first sign will be disease manifestation.

Mutations that can cause disease due to their effects on various genes may also be brought about by chemicals or trauma.

Skills in Practice Genetic Screening of Newborns (Heel Prick or Guthrie Test)

 This is a genetic blood test that is performed on newborn babies at 2–5 days of age. Typically, the test is performed before the baby leaves hospital with the results provided on a subsequent visit with either the baby health nurse or the GP.

An explanation of the test procedure and purpose should be provided and consent obtained prior to the test. The procedure itself is quite straightforward, but it is essential that it is done in sterile conditions. The nurse should wear gloves to prevent any transfer of body fluids to the baby or to the test sample. The heel of the baby is cleaned with an appropriate agent and a small sharp needle (similar to those used for sampling blood glucose from a finger) is used to draw a drop of blood from the baby. Two blood drops are then squeezed onto a special piece of filter paper known as a Guthrie card. The blood is allowed to dry on the card and it is then packaged and sent to a pathology lab for testing. The infant may cry during this procedure, so it is important that the parents are on hand ready to cuddle and console the baby.

As consent is needed it is important that the purpose of the test is adequately explained. The blood taken by this test will be extracted from the Guthrie card and the DNA from the white blood cells extracted. An analysis of specific genes within the DNA will be conducted to identify if the baby has any of the alleles for a number of rare but serious genetic and metabolic conditions. The conditions screened for vary between countries, but will typically include cystic fibrosis, phenylketonuria (PKU), congenital hypothyroidism and galactosaemia. The reason these rare conditions are screened in this way is that prompt intervention provides the best outcome for individuals with these conditions. For PKU and galactosaemia, a simple early alteration to diet can prevent the onset of severe illness or fatality. Because they are inherited in a recessive fashion, the parents may not be aware of any family history of these conditions, so it is important to counsel them on the risks that they may be carriers of any of these conditions, based on your understanding of genetics and the incidence of the alleles involved in the population. It is also important to counsel them that this test is only a screening test, not a diagnostic test.

The conditions screened for in this test are continually being expanded. Australia added the genetic condition spinal muscular atrophy (SMA), one of Australia's leading causes of infant death to the screening in 2018.

Disorders of Chromosomes

We have so far focused on mutations to a gene which cause disease. A mutation represents a tiny change to our DNA (as little as one base may be changed), but it is also possible for large sections of a chromosome (and therefore many genes) to be affected through errors in the chromosome structure. These may involve duplication of large portions (so an individual has three alleles for all of the genes involved); deletions of large portions (so an individual only has one allele for many genes); rearrangements in which the order of the genes on the chromosome changes or a gene even moves between chromosomes; and also the addition or loss of an entire chromosome, as mentioned earlier in this chapter.

Rearrangements of chromosomes have varying effects, and typically do not cause serious problems for the individual, as all the genetic information is still present in their cells. However, the offspring of these individuals can be greatly affected, because of the separation of the homologous chromosomes into different gametes, which means that some gametes will not contain a complete set of genetic information or will contain too much. For example, if part of chromosome 21 had broken and attached to chromosome 14, when gametes are produced one of them will have a 'short' chromosome 21 that is missing information. The other gamete will have a chromosome 14 with some chromosome 21 attached plus a normal chromosome 21.

A child produced from this gamete would end up with three alleles for genes on this segment of chromosome 21. This is one way in which a baby can end up with too many alleles for the genes of chromosome 21 resulting in Down syndrome.

Episodes of Care Child

Acute lymphoblastic leukaemia (ALL) is a cancer of white blood cells in which mutations in one type of white blood cell causes them to divide uncontrollably, leading to potentially fatal disturbances in the blood. ALL is one of the most common cancers in children. One rare genetic alteration, occurring in 2–10% of childhood ALL cases (Ph+ALL), is a reciprocal translocation between chromosomes 22 and 9. The swapping of information between these chromosomes effectively creates two different chromosomes, one of which is known as the Philadelphia chromosome. This chromosome contains new genes, created form the fusion of genes from the original chromosomes, which encode for abnormal proteins, produced in an uncontrolled way. This results in cancerous changes to any white blood cell containing this fusion gene.

Casey is an 8-year-old girl recently diagnosed with Ph+ALL. Casey's parents are very concerned about her prognosis as they remember a child they went to school with died from ALL. They are also very concerned that Casey is not being offered the same chemotherapy that they have heard other children with ALL are receiving. They talk with the nurse caring for Casey about their concerns.

The nurse explains about the Philadelphia chromosome, and the production of a protein that is causing Casey's cancer. The nurse also explained that other ALL cases are caused by different genetic effects that respond well to chemotherapy, but that Casey's genetic alteration does not. Fortunately, research had discovered a new drug that specifically 'turns off' the activity of the abnormal protein causing Casey's ALL and that this was therefore able to halt the division of these ALL cells. The nurse also explained that if the treatment stopped working there were other drugs that could be tried.

Casey's ALL was successfully treated with the first drug that targeted the mutation in her white blood cells and she made a full recovery. However, Casey's father is worried that her children will also get Ph+ALL The nurse uses her knowledge of genetics to explain to the family that this change has occurred only in Casey's white blood cells and not in the other cells in her body. The nurse explains that the eggs Casey will make will not come from her blood cells and that there is little chance that this mutation is also in those cells. Therefore, Casey is unlikely to pass this on to her future children.

Multiple Choice Questions

1. ALL:
   (a) is a cancer occurring in all cells within the blood
   (b) is the most common childhood cancer
   (c) has a high mortality rate
   (d) is always caused through the formation of fusion genes
2. Children with Ph+ALL receive a different treatment from children with ALL because:
   (a) they have the best prognosis so can be spared toxic therapies
   (b) they have a high risk of passing it on to their children
   (c) they have a specific gene change that causes an abnormal protein that can be stopped with a particular drug
   (d) the gene fusion in their white blood cells causes them to be able to fight infections better
3. The abnormal fusion gene is formed by:
   (a) a translocation between chromosomes 9 and 22
   (b) the addition of chromosome 21
   (c) the insertion of new genetic information into chromosome 22
   (d) a virus changing the sequence of the gene
4. The chance of Casey having a child in the future with Ph+ALL is:
   (a) 100%, because this mutation will also have occurred in her gametes
   (b) very high, because the treatment she received will cause mutations in her DNA
   (c) 50%, because the fusion gene is dominant
   (d) very low, because the change in her white blood cells will not affect her gametes
5. Ph+ALL can also occur in adults. These adults would:
   (a) have inherited it from their parents
   (b) all be female as the chromosomes involved are sex chromosomes
   (c) receive the same treatment as Casey as the underlying gene defect is the same
   (d) all of the above

72 Conclusion

This completes the chapter on basic genetics. Although genetics may appear complicated, it is a very important subject because our genes not only make us what we are, but also leave us susceptible to certain diseases and have a say in how we respond to treatment for diseases, how we live our lives, work, develop relationships, and indeed survive in the world.

Glossary

Adenine (A): One of the four bases of **DNA and RNA**.

Allele: One of the possible DNA sequences that a particular gene can have.

Amino acid: The building blocks of proteins, there are 20 that are used for the synthesis of proteins as directed by the sequence of nucleotides.

Anticodon: A group of three bases on tRNA. The 20 amino acids have a particular anticodon so that it puts the right amino acid in the protein as identified by the DNA and mRNA sequence.

Autosome: Chromosomes that are not one of the two sex chromosomes. Humans have 22 pairs of autosomes.

Autosomal dominant disorder: A medical disorder caused by a faulty version (allele) of dominant gene that is inherited from one of the parents.

Autosomal recessive disorder: A medical disorder caused when two faulty alleles for a gene are inherited: one from each parent.

Base: Component of nucleotides that form the code that specifies the cell's proteins. There are four bases used in DNA: A, C, T, G; and four in RNA: A, C, U, G.

Cell cycle: The process by which a cell prepares for, and undertakes, cell growth and division.

Chromatid: One of the DNA double helix strands of a replicated **chromosome**.

Centromere: The point at which two **chromatids** are attached in a **chromosome**.

Chromosome: Mixture of **DNA** and protein (chromatin) – contains our genetic make-up.

Codon: A triplet of **bases** on **mRNA** that encodes for a particular **amino acid**.

Cytosine (C): One of the bases of **DNA** or **RNA**.

Deoxyribose: A major part of **DNA**, deoxyribose is derived from a sugar known as ribose but has lost an atom of oxygen.

Diploid cell: Cell that contains two of each **chromosomes**. See **haploid cell**.

DNA: Deoxyribonucleic acid, found in the cell nucleus and is the molecule that houses the information in our genes.

Dominant allele: Allele of a **gene** that can exert its effects on the body on its own. In other words, it dominates a **recessive allele** at the same **locus**.

Double helix: Two strands of **DNA** joined together in a spiral formation.

Equator of the cell: The centre of the cell during cell division.

Gamete: A reproductive cell; spermatozoon **(spermatozoa, sperm)** or ovum **(ova, egg)**.

Gene: A portion of DNA that codes for a protein. A unit of **heredity** in a living organism.

Gene crossover (Recombination): The process at the commencement of **meiosis** whereby genetic material may be transferred between chromatids of homologous **chromosomes**. Contributes to genetic diversity.

Genotype: The two particular alleles that an individual has for a gene. The genotype of a person will determine their **phenotype**.

Guanine (G): One of the four bases of **DNA** or **RNA**.

Haploid cell: A cell that contains just one of each **chromosome**. See **diploid cell**.

Heredity: The passing down of **genes** from generation to generation.

Heterologous: 'Different', see **homologous**.

Heterozygous: A pair of dissimilar **alleles** for a particular **gene locus**. See **homozygous**.

Histone Proteins: Found in cell nuclei, package and order the **DNA** into **nucleosomes** – so making it possible for the **chromosomes** to fit into a cell without becoming tangled.

Homologous: 'Same' – see **heterologous**.

Homozygous: A pair of identical **alleles** for a particular **gene locus**. See **heterozygous**.

Interphase: The longest stage of the **cell cycle**, during which the cell is growing and preparing to divide.

Locus: A **gene's** position on a **chromosome**.

Meiosis: Process of cell division that allows for the production of **haploid gametes** from **diploid cells**, so ensuring the correct number of **chromosomes** are passed to the offspring.

Mendelian genetics: The concepts of inheritance associated with characteristics (phenotypes) that are governed by a single gene (named after Gregor Mendel).

Mendel's law of segregation: Only one **allele** from each parent can be inherited by their child.

Mendel's law of independent assortment: Members of different pairs of **alleles** are randomly sorted into the **gametes**.

Mitosis: The process of cell division undertaken by somatic cells (not gametes) that ensures each cell obtained by this process has an exact copy of the chromosomes of the original cell.

mRNA: **(messenger ribonucleic acid)** provides a means to get the information (genes) held in DNA out of the nucleus into the cytoplasm to provide the information to synthesise proteins.

Nucleic acid: A mixture of phosphoric acid, sugars, and organic **bases**, nucleic acids direct the course of protein synthesis (or production), so regulating all cell activities. **DNA** and **RNA** are nucleic acids.

Nucleosome: A unit of packaged DNA in a cell's nucleus; it consists of a segment of **DNA** wound around a **histone**.

Nucleotide: The building block of **DNA** and **RNA**, consisting of sugar (deoxyribose in DNA, ribose in RNA), phosphate and one of the four **bases**.

Ova (Ovum, eggs): Female reproductive cells, these cells are haploid.

Phenotype: The expressed features of a person, derived from the interaction of the **genotype** of a person with the environment.

Poles: Opposite ends of a cell during some stages of cell division.

Recessive allele: Requires another recessive allele at the same **locus** before it can have an effect on the body. In other words, it is not **dominant** over another allele of that **gene**.

Ribosomes: Small structures made from protein and ribosomal RNA involved in making proteins (see Chapter 2).

RNA: Ribonucleic acid – **transcribed** from DNA (there are several types of RNA with mRNA, tRNA and rRNA essential for protein synthesis).

Spermatozoa (spermatozoon, sperm): Male reproductive cells, these cells are haploid.

Spontaneous mutation disorder: A medical disorder caused by a new fault that has developed on a **gene sequence**; that is, neither of the parents carries the faulty version (allele) of that **gene**.

Strand: The long parts of the **double helix**, consisting of **deoxyribose** and **phosphate**.

Termination codon: A **triplet** of **bases** that stops the joining of **amino acids** once the specified protein of that sequence has been produced.

Thymine (T): One of the bases of **DNA** (not used in RNA).

Transcription: In genetics, the generation of **RNA** from **DNA** such that they hold the same information.

Translation: In genetics, the process by which information in the bases of **mRNA** is used to specify the **amino acid sequence** of a protein.

Triplet: Sequence of three **DNA bases** that code for an amino acid.

tRNA: Transfer ribonucleic acid; important in the production of proteins as it decodes the message found in **mRNA** to provide the correct order of **amino acids** for the protein being produced.

Uracil (U): One of the four bases of RNA (not used in DNA).

X-linked recessive disease: A medical disorder caused by a fault in a gene of the X **chromosome** (one of the sex chromosomes), inherited in a recessive pattern.

References

Crespi, B. (2008) Turner syndrome and the evolution of human sexual dimorphism. *Evolutionary Applications* **1**(3): 449–461.

LeMone, P., Burke, K., Bauldoff, G. and Gubrud, P. (2015) *Medical–Surgical Nursing: Critical Thinking in Client Care*, 6th edn. Upper Saddle River, NJ: Pearson Prentice Hall.

Snustad, D.P. and Simmons, M.J. (2012) *Principles of Genetics*, 6th edn. Hoboken, NJ: John Wiley & Sons, Inc.

Tortora, G.J. and Derrickson, B.H. (2009) *Principles of Anatomy and Physiology*, 12th edn. Hoboken, NJ: John Wiley & Sons, Inc.

Tortora, G.J. and Derrickson, B.H. (2014) *Principles of Anatomy and Physiology*, 14th edn. Hoboken, NJ: John Wiley & Sons.

Further Reading

UK: https://www.nhs.uk/conditions/pregnancy-and-baby/newborn-blood-spot-test/
Australia: https://www.betterhealth.vic.gov.au/health/conditionsandtreatments/newborn-screening
Ph+ALL: https://www.stbaldricks.org/blog/post/what-is-philadelphia-chromosome-positive-all
Bartels, D. (2010) *Genetic Counseling: Ethical Challenges and Consequences*. Piscataway, NJ: Transaction Publishers.
Fletcher, H. and Hickey, I. (2012) *BIOS Instant Notes in Genetics*, 4th edn. Abingdon: Taylor & Francis.
Jones, S. and Van Loon, B. (2014) *Introducing Genetics: A Graphic Guide*. London: Icon Books Ltd.
Jorde, L.B., Carey, J.C., Bamshad, M.J. and White, R.L. (2009) *Medical Genetics*, 4th edn. St Louis, MO: Mosby.
Lister Hill National Center for Biomedical Communications (2010) *Genetics Home Reference: Your Guide to Understanding Genetic Conditions*. Bethesda, MD. http://ghr.nlm.nih.gov.
Robinson, T.R. (2010) *Genetics for Dummies*. Chichester: John Wiley & Sons, Ltd.
Skirton, H. and Patch, C. (2013) *Genetics for Healthcare Professionals*. New York: Garland Science.
Vipond, K. (2013) *Genetics: A Guide for Students and Practitioners of Nursing and Health Care*, revised edn. Banbury: Scion Publishing Ltd.

Activities

Multiple Choice Questions

1. With regard to DNA bases, adenine in DNA pairs with:
   (a) guanine
   (b) uracil
   (c) cytosine
   (d) thymine

2. The two strands of the DNA double helix are held together by:
   (a) hydrogen bonds between deoxyribose and phosphate
   (b) hydrogen bonds between complementary bases
   (c) covalent bonds between deoxyribose sugars in the opposite strands
   (d) covalent bonds between like bases

3. Normally, humans have:
   (a) 44 chromosomes
   (b) 46 chromosomes
   (c) 47 chromosomes
   (d) 45 chromosomes

4. The position that a gene occupies on a chromosome is known as:
   (a) the allele
   (b) the locus
   (c) the autosome
   (d) the histone

5. The reason that changes to the DNA sequence can cause genetic disease is that:
   (a) proteins are translated directly from the DNA
   (b) proteins are translated from the mRNA which was transcribed from the DNA
   (c) proteins are transcribed from the mRNA which was translated from the DNA
   (d) proteins are made of nucleotides like DNA

6. If DNA has a base sequence of ATAGCGAC, then the corresponding sequence of mRNA will be:
   (a) UAUCGCUG
   (b) TATCGCTG
   (c) AUAGCGUG
   (d) ATAGCGAC

7. The difference between meiosis and mitosis is:
   (a) that meiosis produces four diploid cells from one parent whereas mitosis only produces two
   (b) mitosis is used for the production of gametes, whereas meiosis is for the generation of new somatic cells

(c) during meiosis homologous chromosomes are divided into separate daughter cells, whereas in mitosis they stay together

(d) meiosis produces sperm, whereas mitosis produces eggs

8. Which important events happen during interphase of the cell cycle?
   (a) the cell obtains and processes nutrients required for making new organelles
   (b) the cell replicates (duplicates) its chromosomes
   (c) the cell becomes larger
   (d) all of the above

9. Gene crossover (recombination) is a process that:
   (a) is a major cause of genetic disease
   (b) allows for increased variation in the alleles of a couple's children
   (c) causes children of homozygous parents to be heterozygous
   (d) allows recessive alleles to dominate over dominant alleles

10. In Mendelian genetics, Mendel's law of segregation states that:
    (a) alleles are different sequences of genetic material occupying the same locus
    (b) humans have 46 chromosomes
    (c) only one allele from each parent can be inherited by a child
    (d) different pairs of alleles sort independently of each other

11. If both parents are carriers of a faulty allele for cystic fibrosis (an autosomal recessive condition), what is the chance that their child has cystic fibrosis?
    (a) 75%
    (b) 50%
    (c) 25%
    (d) 0%

12. A man has haemophilia (X-linked recessive) and is concerned that his son will have haemophilia as well. His wife is homozygous for the normal allele for this gene. What is the risk of his son having haemophilia?
    (a) 50%
    (b) 25%
    (c) 100%
    (d) 0%

13. Laura has the autosomal dominant genetic disorder Huntington's disease and is concerned that her three girls will also develop this disorder. Which of these options would be the best advice for Laura?
    (a) the condition is related to a gene defect on the X chromosome and therefore it would only affect boys
    (b) each child will need to decide for themselves whether they will be tested to see if they also have the dominant allele and will therefore develop this disorder
    (c) there is a 50% chance of her passing on the disorder and therefore at least one of her children will develop Huntington's disease
    (d) as the disease is dominant all her children will develop the disorder

14. A couple have just received their results for their prenatal screening test for the risk of their baby being born with Down Syndrome. They have high risk and so have been offered further genetic testing. If the baby has Down syndrome the test would show:
    (a) 46 chromosomes with three of them being chromosome 21
    (b) 47 chromosomes with three of them being chromosome 21
    (c) 45 chromosomes with only one chromosome 21
    (d) 45 chromosomes with 22 normal autosome pairs but only one sex chromosome

15. A couple both have brown hair and their baby is born with red hair. The father questions you privately over this as neither of his parents or any of his siblings have red hair. You advise him:
    (a) that it is very common for spontaneous mutations to occur in the locus for hair colour resulting in red hair
    (b) red hair only occurs when an individual has two alleles for red hair and as such it is very common for it to be carried through a family and not seen for many generations
    (c) he should consider a paternity test as having red hair is the result of a dominant allele
    (d) having red hair is the result of environmental insults during pregnancy such as having an infection

True or False

1. Males have 46 chromosomes, 22 pairs of autosomes an X and a Y.
2. A person with a heterozygous genotype would have a phenotype associated with the recessive allele.
3. Homologous chromosomes can exchange information between chromatids during meiosis.
4. The two strands of the double helix are held together by covalent bonds between complementary bases.
5. Having a blood group of AB is an example of non-Mendelian genetics.

Conditions

The following is a list of common genetic conditions. Take some time and write notes about each of the conditions. You may make the notes taken from textbooks or other resources (e.g. people you work with in a clinical area), or you may make the notes as a result of people you have cared for. If you are making notes about people you have cared for, you must ensure that you adhere to the rules of confidentiality.

Motor neurone disease

Prader–Willi syndrome

Alzheimer disease, type 2

Neurofibromatosis

Down syndrome

Turner syndrome

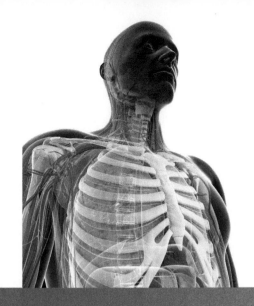

4

Tissue

Anthony Wheeldon

Test Your Prior Knowledge

- List the four main types of body tissue.
- What are the main functions of epithelial tissue?
- Name the four types of connective tissue.
- Which types of muscle are involuntary?
- What are the main steps of tissue repair?

Learning Outcomes

After reading this chapter you will be able to:

- Describe the characteristics of epithelial tissue.
- List the classifications of epithelial tissue.
- Discuss the functions of connective tissue.
- List the classifications of connective tissue.
- Describe the process of tissue repair.

Visit the student companion website at www.wileyfundamentalseries.com/anatomy where you can test yourself using flashcards, multiple-choice questions and more. Instructor companion site at www.wiley.com/go/instructor/anatomy where instructors will find valuable materials such as PowerPoint slides and image bank designed to enhance your teaching.

Fundamentals of Anatomy and Physiology: For Nursing and Healthcare Students, Third Edition. Edited by Ian Peate and Suzanne Evans.
© 2020 John Wiley & Sons Ltd. Published 2020 by John Wiley & Sons Ltd.
Student companion website: www.wileyfundamentalseries.com/anatomy
Instructor companion website: www.wiley.com/go/instructor/anatomy

Introduction

The human body consists of around 50 trillion to 106 trillion individual structural working units called cells (Marieb and Hoehn, 2018). Cells work together to ensure that homeostasis is maintained. Cells come in many different shapes, sizes and life spans; however, they can be categorised depending on their structure and functions. A group of cells that have a similar structure and function are called tissue, and within the human body there are four distinct types of tissue. Cells that provide a covering for organs and structures, for example, are referred to as epithelial tissue, whereas cells that provide support for structures are called connective tissue. Cells that govern body movement are muscle tissue, and cells that help control homeostasis are nervous tissue. Most organs of the body contain a selection of all four tissue types. The heart, for example, contains muscle tissue, is controlled by nervous tissue, lined by epithelial tissue and supported by connective tissue. Tissue also has the capacity to repair itself. This chapter examines all four types of tissue and the process of tissue repair.

Epithelial Tissue

Epithelial tissue is essentially a sheet of cells that covers an area of the body. Epithelial tissue covers or lines body surfaces (i.e. skin), or it lines the walls and the organs within body cavities. The major role of epithelial tissue is as an interface; indeed, nearly all the substances absorbed or secreted by the body must pass through epithelial tissue. Broadly speaking, epithelial tissue has six main functions:

- absorption
- protection
- excretion
- secretion
- filtration
- sensory reception.

Not all epithelial tissue carries out all six functions. In many areas of the body epithelial tissue specialises in just one or two functions. Epithelial tissue in the digestive system, for example, specialises in absorption of nutrients, whereas epithelial tissue within skin provides a protective layer.

Epithelial tissue cells are closely bonded together in continuous sheets, which have an apical and a basal surface. The apical surface faces outwards, towards the exterior of the organ it covers. Apical surfaces can be smooth, but most have hair-like extensions called microvilli. Microvilli dramatically increase the surface area of the epithelial tissue and therefore increase its ability for absorption and secretion. Some areas, within the respiratory tract, for example, possess larger hair-like extensions called cilia, which are also capable of propelling substances. Lying close to the basal surface is a thin sheet of glycoproteins that acts as a selective filter, governing which substances can enter epithelial tissue. Epithelial tissue is innervated by neurons, but it has no blood supply as such. Rather than being served by a network of capillaries, epithelial tissue receives a supply of nutrients from nearby blood vessels. Owing to its protective role, epithelial tissue needs to endure a great deal of abrasion and environmental damage, and epithelial cells need to be very hardy and tough. This hardiness is generated by their ability to divide and regenerate rapidly, resulting in the swift replacement of damaged epithelial cells. However, this regenerative capacity is reliant upon a plentiful supply of nutrients.

Epithelial tissue can be categorised into the following three distinct types:

- simple
- stratified
- glandular.

Simple epithelium consists of a single layer of cells bound into a continuous sheet. Stratified epithelium is also arranged into a continuous sheet but is thicker with numerous layers of cells. Glandular epithelium forms the glands of the body.

All epithelial cells have six sides; indeed, under a microscope a cross-section of epithelial tissue looks like a honeycomb. Epithelial cells can be subdivided further into the following three different six-sided shapes:

- cuboidal
- columnar
- squamous.

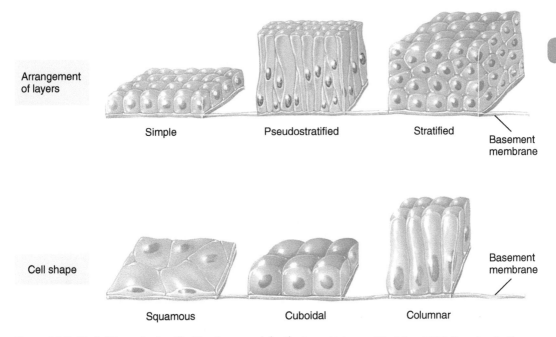

Figure 4.1 **Epithelial tissue is classified by shape and depth.** *Source:* Tortora and Derrickson (2017). Reproduced with permission of John Wiley & Sons.

As their names suggest, cuboidal and columnar epithelial cells are square and tall respectively, whereas squamous epithelial cells are rather flat and scaly (see Figure 4.1). When examining the many different types of epithelial cell, it is easy to work out its size and shape by its name. For instance, simple squamous epithelium is thin, flat and scale-like.

Simple Epithelium

Because simple epithelia consist of a single cellular layer it specialises in absorption, secretion and filtration rather than protection.

Simple squamous epithelium is quite often very permeable and is found where the diffusion of nutrients is essential. Capillary walls, the alveoli of the lungs and the glomeruli in the kidneys are all lined with simple squamous epithelium, which facilitates the rapid diffusion of nutrients. Simple squamous epithelium is also found within the heart and blood and lymph vessels. Simple squamous epithelium found within the heart and blood and lymph vessels is called endothelium (see Figure 4.2).

Simple cuboidal epithelium specialises in secretion as well as absorption. Simple cuboidal epithelium is found in the lining of the ovaries, the kidney tubules and the ducts of smaller glands. It also forms part of the secretory portions of glands such as the thyroid and pancreas (see Figure 4.3).

Simple columnar epithelium can be ciliated or non-ciliated. As its name suggests, ciliated simple columnar epithelium has cilia on its apical surface. It is found in areas of the body where movement of fluids, mucus or other substances is required. Ciliated simple columnar epithelial tissue, for example, lines the passageways of the central nervous system and helps propel cerebrospinal fluid. It also lines the Fallopian tubes and helps move oocytes recently expelled from the ovaries (see Figure 4.4). A common location for non-ciliated simple columnar epithelium is the lining of the digestive tract from the stomach to the rectum (see Figure 4.5). Non-ciliated simple columnar epithelium performs two broad functions. Some possess microvilli, greatly increasing their surface area for absorption; others specialise in the secretion of mucus. Such cells are referred to as goblet cells owing to their cup-like shape. Simple columnar epithelial cells are generally of equal size. However, in some instances simple columnar epithelial cells vary in height, with only the tallest reaching the apical surface. This gives the illusion that the tissue has many layers, like stratified epithelium. Such examples of columnar epithelial tissue are called pseudostratified columnar epithelium. Pseudostratified columnar epithelium is found within the lining of the male reproductive system; however, the most common location is the lining of the respiratory tract (see Figure 4.6).

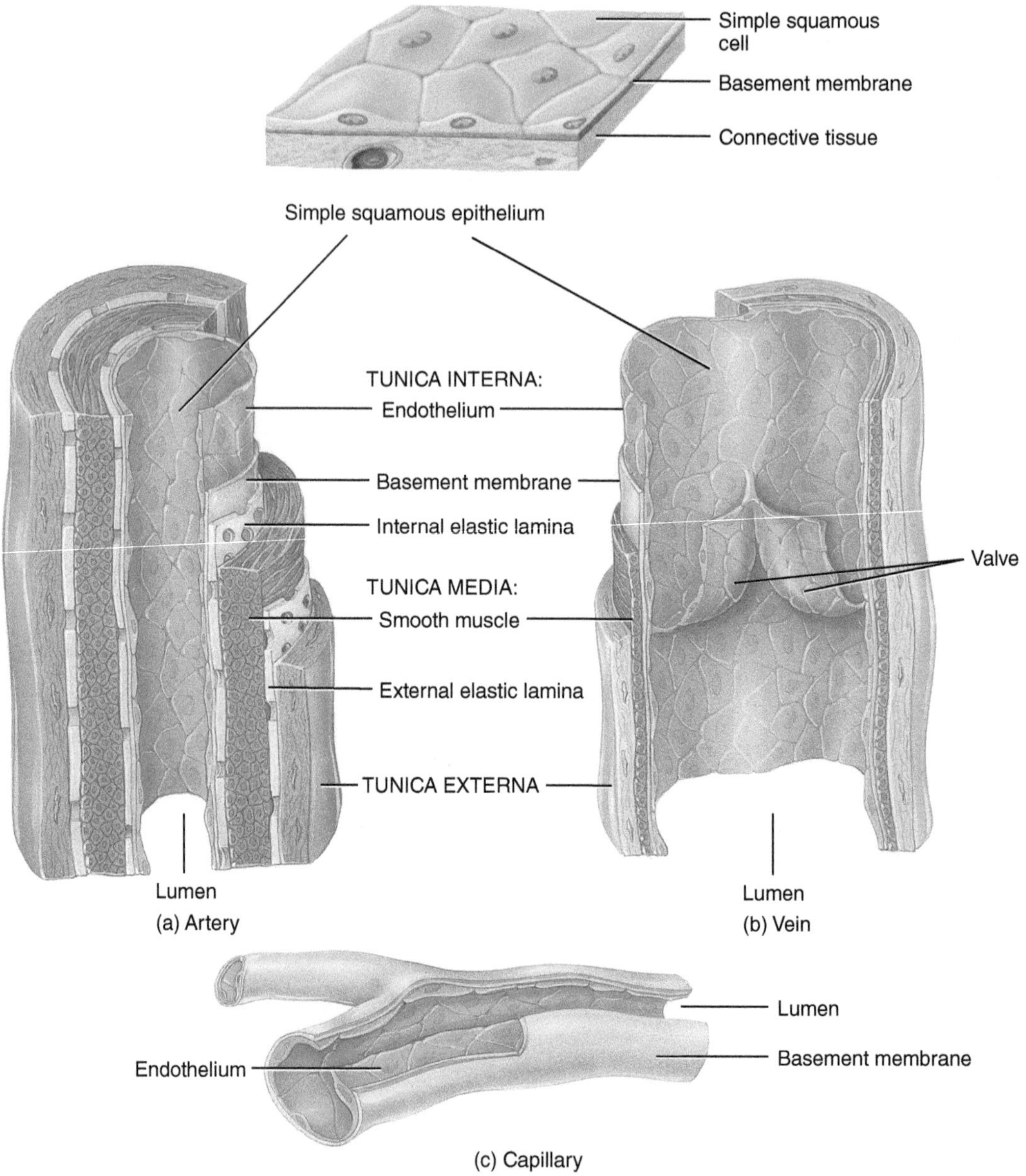

Figure 4.2 (a–c) **Simple squamous epithelium forms the endothelial layer of blood vessels.** *Source:* Tortora and Derrickson (2017). Reproduced with permission of John Wiley & Sons.

Stratified Epithelium

Unlike simple epithelia, stratified epithelia have many layers. The cells regenerate from below, with new cells dividing on the basal layer pushing the older cells towards the surface. As stratified epithelium is thicker, its principal function is protection.

Stratified squamous epithelium is the most common stratified epithelium and forms the external part of skin (see Chapter 18). Stratified squamous epithelial tissue is keratinised, toughened by the presence of keratin, a special tough fibrous protein. Non-keratinised stratified squamous epithelial tissue lines wet areas of the body – the mouth, the tongue and the vagina for example (see Figure 4.7). Only the outer layers of stratified squamous epithelium are squamous in shape; the basal layers may be cuboidal or columnar.

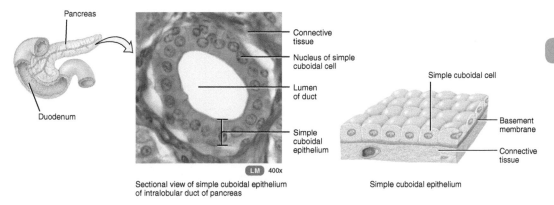

Sectional view of simple cuboidal epithelium
of intralobular duct of pancreas

Simple cuboidal epithelium

Figure 4.3 Simple cuboid epithelium forms part of the secretory portion of the pancreas. *Source:* Tortora and Derrickson (2017). Reproduced with permission of John Wiley & Sons.

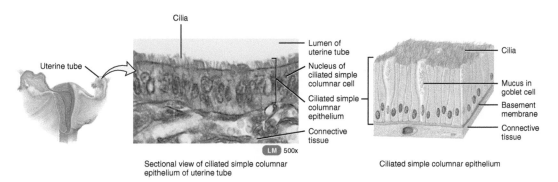

Sectional view of ciliated simple columnar
epithelium of uterine tube

Ciliated simple columnar epithelium

Figure 4.4 Ciliated simple columnar epithelium lines the Fallopian tubes. *Source:* Tortora and Derrickson (2017). Reproduced with permission of John Wiley & Sons.

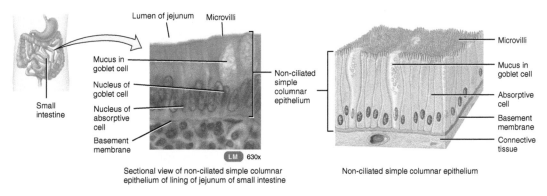

Sectional view of non-ciliated simple columnar
epithelium of lining of jejunum of small intestine

Non-ciliated simple columnar epithelium

Figure 4.5 Non-ciliated columnar epithelium lines the digestive tract. *Source:* Tortora and Derrickson (2017). Reproduced with permission of John Wiley & Sons.

Stratified cuboidal epithelium is found in the oesophagus, sweat glands and in the male urethra (see Figure 4.8). Stratified columnar epithelium, however, is quite rare. Small amounts can be found in the male urethra and in the ducts of some glands. Another common example of stratified epithelium is transitional epithelium, which may have both squamous and cuboidal cells in its apical surface. The basal surface may contain both cuboidal and columnar cells. Transitional epithelium can withstand a great deal of stretch and is found in organs such as the bladder, which is subject to considerable distension (see Figure 4.9).

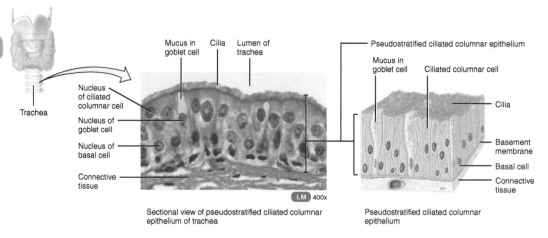

Figure 4.6 Pseudostratified ciliated columnar epithelium lines the trachea. *Source:* Tortora and Derrickson (2017). Reproduced with permission of John Wiley & Sons.

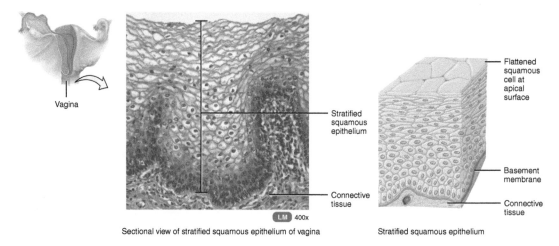

Figure 4.7 Non-keratinised stratified squamous epithelial tissue lines the vagina. *Source:* Tortora and Derrickson (2017). Reproduced with permission of John Wiley & Sons.

Glandular Epithelia

The glands of the body are formed by glandular epithelia. All glands are classified as *endocrine* or *exocrine*. Glands that secrete their products internally are called endocrine glands. Endocrine glands release hormones, regulatory chemicals for use elsewhere in the body (see Chapter 16). Exocrine glands release their products onto the surface of epithelial tissue. Exocrine glands are either *unicellular* or *multicellular*. Unicellular exocrine glands consist of a single cell type and the main example is the goblet cell, which releases a glycoprotein called mucin. Once dissolved in water mucin forms mucus, which lubricates and protects surfaces. Multicellular exocrine glands are far more complex, coming in several shapes and sizes. Some exocrine glands are simple and consist of a single branched duct, whereas others are more complex with multibranched ducts (see Figure 4.10). However, they all contain two distinct areas: an epithelial duct and secretory cells (acinus). Exocrine glands that are tubular in shape can be found within the digestive system and stomach. Other exocrine glands are spherical and referred to as alveolar or acinar. The oil glands within skin and mammary glands are two examples of spherical- or acinar-shaped exocrine glands. Glands that are both tubular and acinar are referred to as tubulacinar. The salivary glands, for example, are tubulacinar.

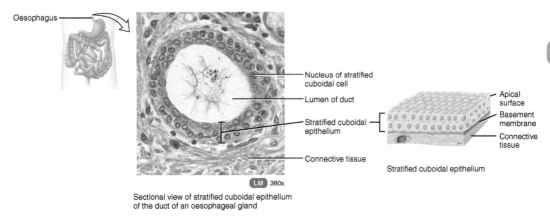

Oesophagus

Nucleus of stratified cuboidal cell

Lumen of duct

Stratified cuboidal epithelium

Connective tissue

Apical surface

Basement membrane

Connective tissue

Stratified cuboidal epithelium

LM 380x

Sectional view of stratified cuboidal epithelium of the duct of an oesophageal gland

Figure 4.8 Cuboidal epithelial tissue is found in the oesophagus. *Source:* Tortora and Derrickson (2017). Reproduced with permission of John Wiley & Sons.

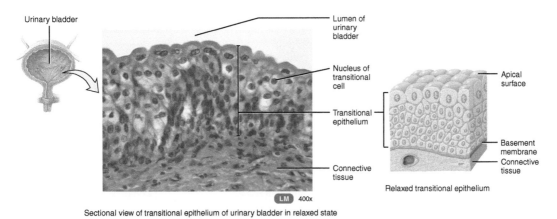

Urinary bladder

Lumen of urinary bladder

Nucleus of transitional cell

Transitional epithelium

Connective tissue

Apical surface

Basement membrane

Connective tissue

Relaxed transitional epithelium

LM 400x

Sectional view of transitional epithelium of urinary bladder in relaxed state

Figure 4.9 Transitional epithelium lines the bladder and allows for distension. *Source:* Tortora and Derrickson (2017). Reproduced with permission of John Wiley & Sons.

Connective Tissue

Connective tissue is the most abundant tissue in the human body. Its main functions are to bind tissues together, reinforcement, insulation, protection and support. All epithelial tissue is reinforced by the connective tissue base it rests upon (see Figure 4.11). There are four types of connective tissue:

- connective tissue proper
- cartilage
- bone
- liquid connective tissue.

Connective tissue is not present on body surfaces and, unlike epithelial tissue, is highly vascular and receives a rich blood supply.

The following types of cell are present in connective tissue:

- adipocytes
- primary blast cells
- macrophages
- plasma cells
- mast cells
- leucocytes (white blood cells).

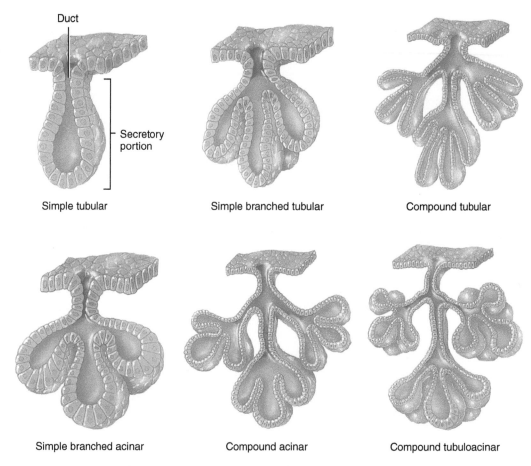

Duct

Secretory
portion

Simple tubular   Simple branched tubular   Compound tubular

Simple branched acinar   Compound acinar   Compound tubuloacinar

Figure 4.10 **Exocrine glands classified by shape, with examples of location.** *Source:* Tortora and Derrickson (2017). Reproduced with permission of John Wiley & Sons.

Adipocytes are fat cells. Within connective tissue adipocytes store triglycerides (fats). Primary blast cells continually secrete ground substance and produce mature connective tissue cells. Each type of connective tissue contains its own unique primary blast cells (see Table 4.1). Macrophages, plasma cells and white blood cells form part of the body's immune system. Their functions are as follows:

- Macrophages engulf invading substances and plasma cells produce antibodies.
- White blood cells are not normally found in significant numbers within connective tissue; however, they do migrate into connective tissue during inflammation.
- Mast cells produce histamine, which promotes vasodilatation during the body's inflammatory response.

Connective tissue cells are surrounded by a collection of substances referred to as the extracellular matrix. The function of the extracellular matrix is to ensure that connective tissue can bear weight and withstand tension, abuse and abrasion. As a result, connective tissue can cope with stresses and strains other tissues would not be able to tolerate. The two main elements of extracellular matrix are:

- ground substance
- fibres.

Ground substance: This consists of interstitial fluid, cell adhesion proteins and glycosaminoglycans. Cell adhesion proteins act as connective glue, keeping the tissue cells together. Glycosaminoglycans trap water and ensure ground substance has a jelly-like constitution. The higher the amount of glycosaminoglycans present the harder the ground substance will be.

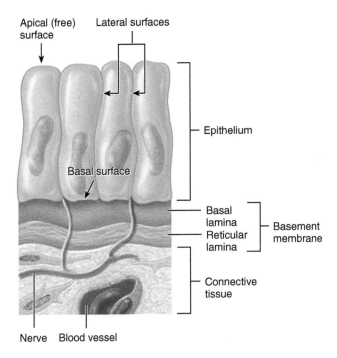

Figure 4.11 Connective tissue reinforces epithelial tissue. *Source:* Tortora and Derrickson (2017). Reproduced with permission of John Wiley & Sons.

Table 4.1 The major primary blast cells and their connective tissue type.

CONNECTIVE TISSUE TYPE	PRIMARY BLAST CELL	CONNECTIVE TISSUE CELL
Connective tissue proper	Fibroblast	Fibrocyte
Cartilage	Chondroblast	Chondrocyte
Bone	Osteoblast	Osteocyte

Fibres: There are three types of fibre found within extracellular matrix:

- collagen
- elastic
- reticular.

Collagen fibres are the most abundant fibre found within the extracellular matrix and are essentially the protein collagen. Collagen is very tough; indeed, collagen fibres are stronger than similar-sized steel fibres (Marieb and Hoehn, 2018). Reticular fibres are much thinner but also contain bundles of collagen. They provide support and strength and are found in greater numbers in soft organs such as the spleen and lymph nodes. Elastic fibres contain the rubberlike protein called elastin, which facilitates stretch and recoil. Elastic fibres are found in greater numbers in tissue that must endure stretch, such as skin and blood vessel walls (see Figure 4.12).

Connective Tissue Proper

Aside from cartilage, bone and blood, all connective tissue belongs to this class. Connective tissue proper is subdivided further into:

- loose connective tissue
- dense connective tissue.

Loose connective tissue contains fewer fibres than dense connective tissue (see Table 4.2).

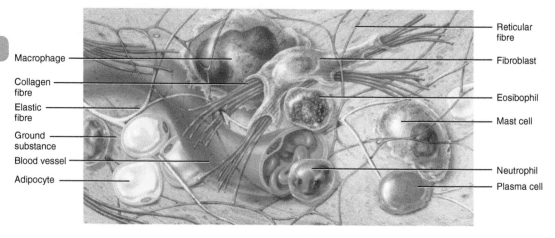

Reticular fibre
Macrophage
Fibroblast
Collagen fibre
Eosibophil
Elastic fibre
Mast cell
Ground substance
Blood vessel
Neutrophil
Adipocyte
Plasma cell

Figure 4.12 **Constituents of connective tissue.** *Source:* Tortora and Derrickson (2017). Reproduced with permission of John Wiley & Sons.

Table 4.2 **Types of connective tissue proper, their main constituents, functions and locations.**

CONNECTIVE TISSUE	MAIN CONSTITUENT	FUNCTIONS	MAIN LOCATIONS
Loose areolar	Collagen, elastic, reticular fibres	Strength Elasticity Support	Subcutaneous layer beneath skin
Loose adipose	Adipocytes	Insulation	Subcutaneous layer beneath skin
		Protection	Tissue surrounding heart and kidneys
		Energy store	Padding around joints
Loose reticular	Reticular fibres	Support	Liver
	Reticular cells	Filtration	Spleen Lymph nodes
Dense regular	Collagen fibres in parallel	Strength Support	Tendons Ligaments
Dense irregular	Collagen fibres arranged randomly	Strength	Skin
			Heart Tissue surrounding bone Tissue surrounding cartilage
Dense elastic	Elastic fibres	Stretch	Lung tissue Arteries

Loose Connective Tissue

There are three types of loose connective tissue:

- areolar
- adipose
- reticular.

Areolar is the most abundant loose connective tissue. It contains all three fibres (collagen, elastic and reticular) and its primary functions are support, elasticity and strength. Areolar tissue is combined with adipose tissue to form the subcutaneous layer, which connects skin with other tissues and organs.

Adipose tissue contains adipocytes, whose primary function is to store triglycerides (fat). The primary functions of adipose tissue are to provide insulation, protection and an energy store.

Reticular tissue only contains reticular fibres. Its main function is to form a protective framework or stroma that surrounds the liver, spleen and lymph nodes. Within the spleen, reticular connective tissue can also filter blood, assisting with the removal of old blood cells.

Dense Connective Tissue

Dense connective tissue contains more collagen or elastic fibres. Dense connective tissue that is made primarily from collagen is said to be either regular or irregular depending on the organisation of the collagen fibres. Dense regular connective tissue contains collagen fibres that are arranged in parallel rows. It has a silvery appearance and is both tough and pliable. Dense, irregular connective tissue is found in ligaments and tendons. Its collagen fibres are randomly arranged but closely knitted together. Dense irregular tissue can withstand pressure and pulling forces and is found in skin and the heart as well as the membranes that surround cartilage and bone. Dense elastic connective tissue consists of elastic fibres. Dense elastic connective tissue is found in areas of the body that must withstand great amounts of stretch, such as arteries and lung tissue.

Cartilage

Cartilage contains a compact network of collagen fibres and is stronger than both loose and dense connective tissue. It has the ability to return to its original shape after stress and movement. Its strength and resilience are provided by a gel-like substance called chondroitin sulphate, which is found in cartilage ground substance. Cartilage is surrounded by a layer of dense irregular tissue called perichondrium. Perichondrium is the only area of cartilage that is served by blood and nervous tissue. There are three types of cartilage:

- hyaline
- fibrocartilage
- elastic.

Hyaline cartilage is the most common cartilage in the human body. It mainly comprises collagen fibres with cartilage cells, with chondrocytes accounting for around 10% of its volume. The collagen fibres are so fine they are almost invisible, giving hyaline cartilage a bluish appearance. Because hyaline cartilage is both strong and flexible it can act as a shock absorber, reducing friction around joints. Hyaline cartilage is also found in the rib cage and airways.

Elastic cartilage is almost identical to hyaline cartilage. The major difference between hyaline and elastic cartilage is the greater presence of elastic fibres. Elastic cartilage can withstand greater movement and bending and is found in areas of the body where stretchability is required, the outer ear for example.

Fibrocartilage is the strongest of the three cartilages. Its strength is provided by rows of chondrocytes and collagen. Because it can withstand great pressure it is found where hyaline cartilage meets tendons or ligaments, between the discs of the vertebrae for example (see Figure 4.13).

Bone

Along with cartilage, bones make up the human skeletal frame. Bone is similar to cartilage but contains even greater amounts of collagen. For this reason, bone is harder and more rigid, facilitating greater protection and support for body structures. However, unlike cartilage, bone receives a rich supply of blood. Bone also stores fat and plays an important role in the production of blood cells. A more detailed examination of bones can be found in Chapter 6.

Liquid Connective Tissue

Connective tissue that has a liquid extracellular matrix includes:

- blood
- lymph.

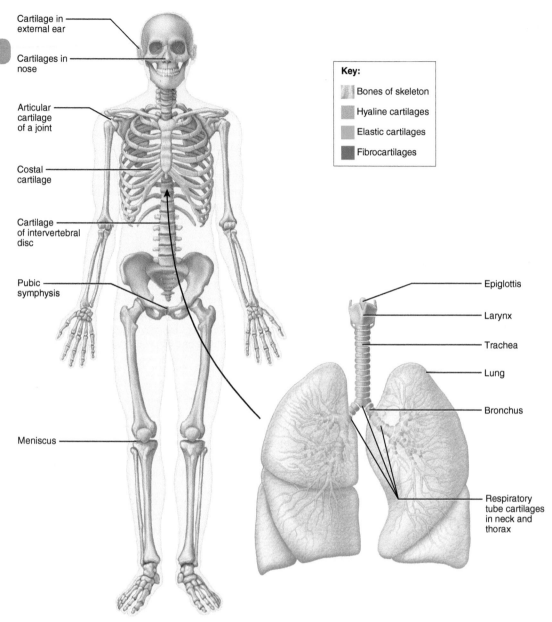

Cartilage in external ear

Cartilages in nose

Articular cartilage of a joint

Costal cartilage

Cartilage of intervertebral disc

Pubic symphysis

Meniscus

Key:

Bones of skeleton

Hyaline cartilages

Elastic cartilages

Fibrocartilages

Epiglottis

Larynx

Trachea

Lung

Bronchus

Respiratory tube cartilages in neck and thorax

Figure 4.13 **Where cartilage is found within the body.** *Source:* Jenkins *et al.* (2009). Reproduced with permission of John Wiley & Sons.

Blood and lymph are said to be atypical connective tissues because, strictly speaking, they do not connect tissues or provide mechanical support. The extracellular matrix of blood is plasma. Blood cells include erythrocytes, leucocytes and platelets. Blood and plasma perform many important functions. For a detailed explanation of blood, see Chapter 8. Lymph has a clear extracellular matrix very similar to plasma. The primary function of lymph is defence against invading pathogens. A more detailed exploration of lymph can be found in Chapter 17.

Membranes

Membranes are sheets of tissue that cover or line areas of the human body. Structurally, membranes consist of an epithelial tissue layer that is bound to a basement layer of connective tissue. There are four major types of membrane:

- cutaneous
- mucous
- serous
- synovial.

Cutaneous Membranes

The principal example of a cutaneous membrane is skin. It consists of an outer stratified squamous epithelial layer, which sits on top of a thick layer of dense irregular connective tissue. Chapter 18 is dedicated to the functions and structure of skin.

Mucous Membranes

Mucous membranes line the external surfaces of body cavities. Examples include hollow organs of the digestive tract, the respiratory system and the renal system. All mucous membranes are wet or moist, but not all secrete lubricating mucus. The mucous membranes of the renal system, for example, are wet due to the presence of urine. Most mucous membranes contain stratified squamous or simple columnar epithelium supported by a layer of connective tissue referred to as lamina propria.

Serous Membranes

Serous membranes or a serosa cover internal body cavities. They consist of areolar connective tissue that is covered by a special kind of simple squamous epithelium called mesothelium. Mesothelium secretes a watery substance referred to as serous fluid, which allows organs to slide against one another with ease. Serous membranes consist of an outer or parietal layer and an inner or visceral layer. The largest example is the peritoneum, which lines the organs of the abdominopelvic cavity. The protective lining of the lungs, the parietal and visceral pleura, provides another example of an important serous membrane. The parietal and visceral pleura glide over one another when the thorax expands on inspiration.

Synovial Membranes

Unlike serous, mucous and cutaneous membranes, synovial membranes do not contain any epithelial tissue. Synovial membranes are mainly found in moving joints and consist of areolar connective tissue, adipocytes, and elastic and collagen fibres. They secrete synovial fluid, which bathes, nourishes and lubricates the joints. Synovial fluid also contains macrophages, which destroy invading microbes and remove debris from the joint cavity. Synovial membranes are also found in cushion-like sacs in the hands and feet that ease the movement of tendons (see Figure 4.14).

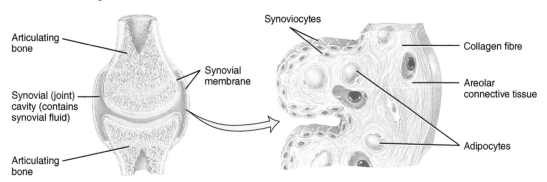

Figure 4.14 **Synovial membranes fill joint cavities.** *Source:* Tortora and Derrickson (2017). Reproduced with permission of John Wiley & Sons.

Clinical Considerations Peritonitis

Peritonitis is the inflammation of the peritoneum, the serous membrane that lines both the digestive organs and the wall of the abdominopelvic cavity. The causes of peritonitis are either chemical or bacterial. Chemical peritonitis results from damage to neighbouring structures; that is, a piercing wound or ulcer that leaks digestive juices into the peritoneum. Bacterial peritonitis results from the direct contamination of the peritoneum; that is, a ruptured appendix or perforated bowel. If left unaddressed, chemical peritonitis will lead to bacterial peritonitis.

Peritonitis is an acute medical emergency and is associated with high mortality. Survival rates have increased since the use of prophylactic antibiotics (Hubert and VanMeter, 2018).

Clinical Considerations Pneumothorax

A pneumothorax or collapsed lung occurs when air accumulates in the pleural cavity, the small space between the visceral and parietal pleura. It most often occurs as the result of trauma but can also occur in chronic lung disease. In a small number of cases the pleura separates spontaneously due to a congenital defect. In small pneumothoraces the lungs will reinflate over time, but large pneumothoraces are potentially life threatening. Chest drains are often inserted to remove the air from the pleura and allow the lungs to re-inflate (Woodrow, 2013).

Muscle Tissue

Muscle tissue contains long muscle fibres whose primary function is to generate force. Muscle tissue is found where there is a need for movement and maintenance of posture. Muscle is classified in three ways:

- skeletal
- smooth
- cardiac.

Skeletal muscle is found adjacent to the skeleton and its function is twofold: the movement of the skeleton and the maintenance of body posture. The structure of the muscle fibres within skeletal muscle gives a striped or striated appearance. Skeletal muscle is also voluntary, meaning its movement can be controlled by conscious control (see Figure 4.15).

(a)

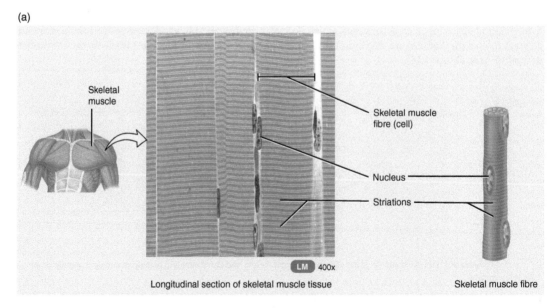

Figure 4.15 **The major muscle types with examples of their location: (a) skeletal muscle; (b) cardiac muscle; (c) smooth muscle.** *Source:* Tortora and Derrickson (2017). Reproduced with permission of John Wiley & Sons.

(b)

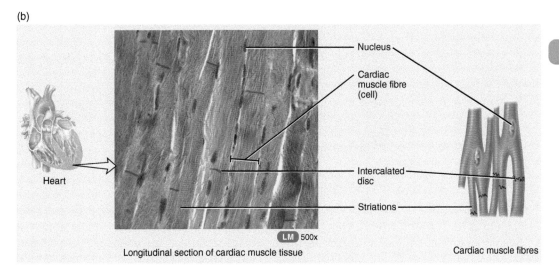

Longitudinal section of cardiac muscle tissue   Cardiac muscle fibres

(c)

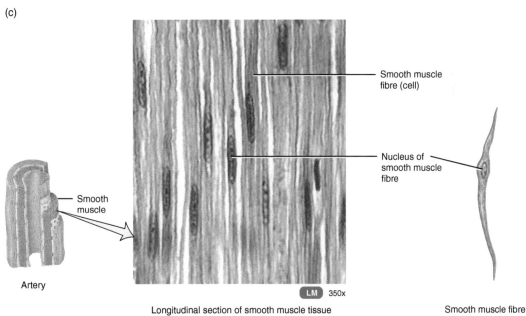

Longitudinal section of smooth muscle tissue   Smooth muscle fibre

Figure 4.15 (Continued)

Smooth muscle, on the other hand, is both involuntary and non-striated. Smooth muscle is found in hollow internal structures where fluid or solid substances need to be propelled from one area to another. Smooth muscle is found in blood vessels, where blood is propelled through the vascular system, and the gastrointestinal tract, where chyme is moved from the stomach through the intestines towards the rectum.

Cardiac muscle muscle is striated, but it is also involuntary. As its name suggests, cardiac muscle is only found in the heart and provides the driving force of contraction. A more detailed examination of muscle can be found in Chapter 7.

Nervous Tissue

Nervous tissue is found within the nervous system (see Chapter 14). There are two types of nervous tissue cells:

- neurones
- neuroglia.

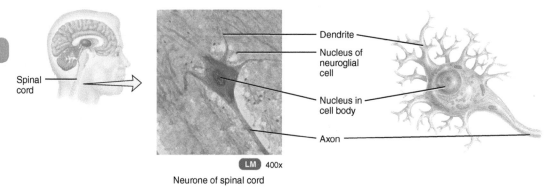

LM 400x

Neurone of spinal cord

Figure 4.16 **An example of nervous tissue.** *Source:* Tortora and Derrickson (2017). Reproduced with permission of John Wiley & Sons.

Neurones are the functioning unit of the nervous system. They consist of three basic parts: the cell body, an axon and dendrites (see Figure 4.16). Their primary function is the propagation of nerve signals within the central and peripheral nervous systems.

Neuroglia do not propagate nerve signals; rather, they nourish, protect and support neurones.

Tissue Repair

Tissue repair occurs in order to replace cells that are damaged, worn out or dead. Each of the four tissue types has the capacity to regenerate and replace cells injured by trauma, disease or other events. However, the tissue types have differing success rates. Because epithelial cells have to withstand large amounts of wear and tear, they have great capacity for renewal. Epithelial tissue often contains immature cells called stem cells, which can divide and replace lost cells easily. Most connective tissue also has great capacity for renewal; however, owing to the lack of blood supply, cartilage can take a long time to heal.

Muscle and nervous tissue by comparison have poor regeneration properties. Skeletal muscle and smooth muscle fibres divide very slowly, and mitosis does not occur in cardiac muscle tissue. Stem cells migrate from blood to the heart where they divide and produce a small number of new cardiac muscle fibres. Nervous tissue does not normally undergo mitosis to replace damaged neurones.

Tissue repair involves the proliferation of new cells, which stem from cell division in the parenchyma (tissue cells/organ cells) or from the stroma (supporting connective tissue). The replenishing of tissue by parenchymal and stroma cells is called regeneration. If parenchymal cells are solely responsible for tissue repair, then a near-perfect regeneration may occur. If fibroblasts from stroma are involved in tissue repair, new connective tissue is generated to replace the damaged tissue. This new connective tissue, primarily consisting of collagen, is referred to as scar tissue. The process of scar tissue generation is called fibrosis. Unlike cells regenerated from parenchymal cells, scar tissue cells are not designed to perform the original functions of the damaged cells. Therefore, any organ or structure with scar tissue will have impaired function.

In open or large wounds granulation occurs. Granulation describes the formation of granulation tissue, which covers the healing tissue and secretes bacterial fluid. During this process both parenchymal and stromal cells are active in the repair. Fibroblasts provide new collagen tissue to strengthen the area, and new blood capillaries sprout new buds and bring the necessary nutrients to the area.

Clinical Considerations Diabetic Foot Ulcers

Between 12 and 25% of patients with diabetes develop leg and foot ulcers. This is because diabetes can cause macroangiopathy, which obstructs blood flow in large arteries. The slower flow of blood through the arteries in the legs results in the development of leg and foot ulcers. Patients with diabetes also experience lengthy recovery times from leg and foot injuries. The lack of blood flow also reduces the tissue's ability to fight off infection. Those patients with diabetes are therefore at increased risk of developing gangrene and amputation (Hubert and VanMeter, 2018).

Conclusion

All human cells can be categorised into four classifications: epithelial tissue, connective tissue, muscle tissue and nervous tissue. Epithelial tissue covers or lines structures and organs. It specialises in absorption, secretion, protection, excretion, filtration and sensory reception. Almost every substance that passes in and out of the body travels through epithelial tissue. Connective tissue not only connects tissues, it also protects, supports and insulates them. Connective tissue is dense and strong; examples include cartilage and bone. Muscle tissue provides movement and posture, whereas nervous tissue forms the major part of the nervous system. Tissue has the ability to regenerate and renew itself; however, epithelial and connective tissues have a greater capacity for repair than other tissues.

Glossary

Abdominopelvic cavity: Body cavity that encompasses the abdominal and pelvic cavities. The abdominal cavity contains the stomach, intestines, spleen, liver and other associated digestive organs. The pelvic cavity contains the bladder and some reproductive organs.

Apical surface: Surface of body organ that faces outwards, towards the surface.

Avascular: Structure that does not contain blood vessels.

Basal surface: Surface that forms the base of a body organ.

Cartilage: Strong form of connective tissue that contains a dense network of collagen and elastic fibres.

Chyme: A fluid substance consisting of partially digested food and digestive enzymes, which is found travelling through the digestive tract.

Connective tissue: Tissue that binds, reinforces, insulates, protects and supports structures.

Diffusion: The movement of particles from areas of high concentration to low concentration.

Endocrine gland: Glands that release hormones.

Epithelial tissue: Tissue that lines or covers body surfaces.

Exocrine glands: Glands that secrete their products externally (i.e. mucus, sweat).

Extracellular matrix: A collection of largely non-living substances that separate the living cells of connective tissue.

Gland: A structure that manufactures a product (e.g. hormones, mucus, sweat).

Glycoproteins: Special proteins that contain simple sugar chains. Glycoproteins play an important role in cell-to-cell communication.

Hormones: Regulatory chemicals released by endocrine glands for use elsewhere in the body (e.g. thyroxine, insulin).

Innervated (innervate): Stimulated by nerve cells.

Interstitial fluid: The fluid that bathes cells.

Keratin: A special tough fibrous protein found in skin.

Lymph nodes: Small lymphatic structures that filter lymphatic fluid.

Macrophages: White blood cells that specialise in the destruction and consumption of invading pathogens.

Membrane: A sheet of tissue that covers or lines an area of the body.

Mitosis: The division and replication of cells.

Neuroglia: Cells of the nervous system that support and nourish neurones.

Neurone: A nerve fibre.

Parenchyma: The cells that constitute the function part of an organ.

Prophylactic antibiotics: Antibiotics prescribed to prevent infection.

Oocytes: Female reproductive cell.

Spleen: Large lymph organ, responsible for production of lymphocytes, immune response and the cleansing of blood.

Stroma: The internal framework of an organ.

Subcutaneous: Underneath the skin.

Vertebrae: The disc-shaped bones that make up the spinal column.

References

Hubert, R.J. and VanMeter K.C. (2018) *Gould's Pathophysiology for the Health Professions*, 6th edn. St Louis: Elsevier.

Jenkins, G.W., Kemnitz, C.P. and Tortora, G.J. (2009) *Anatomy and Physiology from Science to Life*. Hoboken, NJ: John Wiley & Sons, Inc.

Marieb, E. and Hoehn, K. (2018) *Human Anatomy and Physiology – Global Edition*, 11th edn. Harlow: Pearson Education.

Tortora, G.J. and Derrickson, B.H. (2017) *Principles of Anatomy and Physiology*, 15th edn. Hoboken, NJ: John Wiley & Sons, Inc.

Woodrow, P. (2013) Interpleural chest drainage. *Nursing Standard* **27**(40): 49–56.

Activities

Multiple Choice Questions

1. Which of the following epithelial tissues has a single layer of square-shaped cells?
   - (a) pseudostratified columnar epithelium
   - (b) ciliated simple columnar epithelium
   - (c) simple cuboidal epithelium
   - (d) stratified cuboidal epithelium
2. Which of the following epithelial tissue's structure gives the illusion of multiple layers?
   - (a) pseudostratified columnar epithelium
   - (b) ciliated simple columnar epithelium
   - (c) simple cuboidal epithelium
   - (d) stratified cuboidal epithelium
3. Which of the following is not a function of simple epithelium?
   - (a) protection
   - (b) secretion
   - (c) absorption
   - (d) filtration
4. What is the primary function of transitional epithelium?
   - (a) absorption
   - (b) stretch
   - (c) secretion
   - (d) protection
5. Which of the following statements on connective tissue is false?
   - (a) connective tissue is the most abundant in the human body
   - (b) connective tissue is present only on body surfaces
   - (c) all epithelial tissue is supported by connective tissue
   - (d) its main functions are to prevent the binding of tissues, to insulate, protect and support
6. Which fibres ensure that connective tissue is strong and tough?
   - (a) collagen fibres
   - (b) reticular fibres
   - (c) elastic fibres
   - (d) plasma fibres
7. Which of the following connective tissues stores triglycerides?
   - (a) areolar tissue
   - (b) adipose tissue
   - (c) dense regular connective tissue
   - (d) reticular tissue
8. Which of the following statements on cartilage is true?
   - (a) fibrocartilage is found within the ears
   - (b) elastic cartilage is almost identical to fibrocartilage
   - (c) hyaline cartilage is the most abundant in the human body
   - (d) the weakest cartilage tissue is fibrocartilage cartilage

9. Blood is an example of _____ connective tissue.
   (a) liquid
   (b) loose
   (c) avascular
   (d) dense

10. Bone is an example of …
   (a) Connective tissue
   (b) Muscle tissue
   (c) Nervous tissue
   (d) Supportive tissue

11. Which of the following areas does not contain mucous membranes?
   (a) the urinary tract
   (b) the respiratory system
   (c) the pericardium
   (d) the digestive tract

12. Smooth muscle is both
   (a) involuntary and striated
   (b) involuntary and non-striated
   (c) voluntary and striated
   (d) voluntary and non-striated

13. Which of the following statements is true?
   (a) skeletal muscle is involuntary
   (b) cardiac muscle is found in the heart
   (c) smooth muscle is voluntary and found adjacent to the skeleton
   (d) skeletal muscle lines the insides of vessels and organs

14. Scar tissue is generated by
   (a) fibroblasts
   (b) osteoclasts
   (c) stem cells
   (d) parenchymal cells

15. Which of the following is a type of nerve cell
   (a) neurone
   (b) neuralgia
   (c) neutron
   (d) nucleus

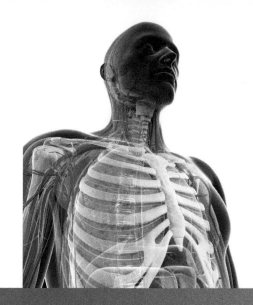

5

Embryology

Jacinta Hope Martin and Jessie Maree Sutherland

Test Your Prior Knowledge

- What are the processes which produce the gametes?
- What anatomical features develop during the embryonic period?
- At what stage is an embryo considered a foetus?
- Define the range of gestational weeks that characterise each trimester.
- List three complications of pregnancy.

Learning Outcomes

After reading this chapter you will be able to:

- Describe the maturational processes involved in making gametes fertilisation competent.
- Outline pre-implantation embryo development.
- Overview post-implantation embryogenesis.
- Discuss implantation and early placental development.
- Describe common pregnancy complications and their symptomology.

 Visit the student companion website at www.wileyfundamentalseries.com/anatomy where you can test yourself using flashcards, multiple-choice questions and more. Instructor companion site at www.wiley.com/go/instructor/anatomy where instructors will find valuable materials such as PowerPoint slides and image bank designed to enhance your teaching.

Fundamentals of Anatomy and Physiology: For Nursing and Healthcare Students, Third Edition. Edited by Ian Peate and Suzanne Evans.
© 2020 John Wiley & Sons Ltd. Published 2020 by John Wiley & Sons Ltd.
Student companion website: www.wileyfundamentalseries.com/anatomy
Instructor companion website: www.wiley.com/go/instructor/anatomy

Introduction

Embryo is derived from the Greek word 'ἔμβρυον' or 'embryon' meaning the unborn. Embryology encompasses the development of gametes (eggs and sperm), the events surrounding fertilisation of the egg by a sperm cell, as well as the subsequent development of a genetically unique embryo and later foetus (Figure 5.1). In this chapter we will investigate these processes.

A Note on Timings

When following the development of an embryo, the date of fertilisation gives us the start of embryonic development, while for clinical care purposes, gestational stage is based on a woman's last menstrual period. Since this would be approximately two weeks prior to fertilisation, there is a two-week disparity between embryonic age and gestational age. We have attempted to clarify these two scales used throughout.

Final Maturation of the Oocyte and Sperm

Oocyte Maturation and Ovulation

We will detail the process of oogenesis further in Chapter 13, but it is important to know that follicle growth occurs within the ovary and that mature follicle development is gonadotropin mediated; that is, mediated by follicle stimulating hormone (FSH) and luteinising hormone (LH).

During oogenesis, a cohort of follicles develop; however, only one is recruited to become the 'dominant follicle'. This process occurs when oestrogen levels peak towards the end of the follicular phase causing a surge in levels of LH and FSH (24–36h). A LH-induced signalling cascade results in secretion of proteolytic enzymes that degrade the follicle blister and form a hole called the stigma where the oocyte engaged in the cumulus–oocyte complex is released. This complex describes a mature oocyte surrounded by specialised somatic cells called cumulus cells. All remaining recruited yet un-ovulated follicles undergo atresia or degradation. This cumulus–oocyte complex is released from the ruptured follicle and moves out into the peritoneal cavity through the stigma, where it is caught by the fimbriae at the end of the fallopian tube/oviduct and pushed along by cilia towards the uterus, where it is then available to be fertilised. Ovulation marks the end of the follicular phase of the ovarian cycle and the start of the luteal phase (Figure 5.2).

During recruitment and ovulation, the oocyte completes meiosis I and commences meiosis II where it will arrest in the metaphase (see Chapter 13). If fertilisation does not occur, the oocyte will degenerate between 12 and 24 hours after ovulation. In the ovary, without the oocyte, the follicle will fold inward on itself, transforming into the corpus luteum (CL). The CL is responsible for the production of oestrogen and progesterone. These hormones are responsible for signalling to the endometrial glands to begin the production of the proliferative and secretory endometrium in preparation for implantation and pregnancy maintenance (Figure 5.2).

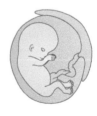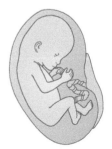

Figure 5.1 **The early embryo develops from a simple group of cells into complex shapes and structures in the early weeks.** *Source:* Webster and de Wreede (2016). Reproduced with permission of John Wiley & Sons.

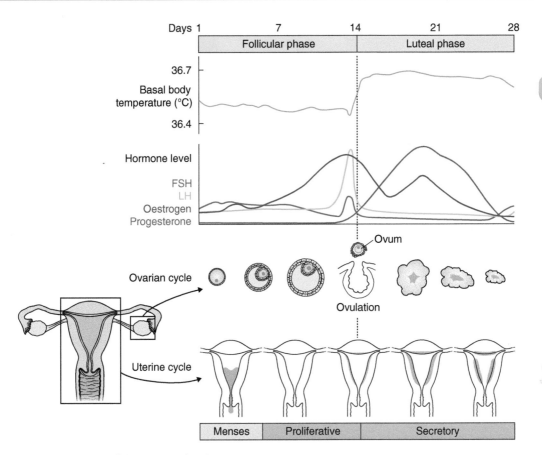

Figure 5.2 **Hormones of the menstrual cycle.** *Source:* Webster et al. (2018). Reproduced with permission of John Wiley & Sons.

Sperm Maturation

While the events of sperm and egg maturation initially occur independently, they converge and synchronise in the female reproductive tract prior to fertilisation. Chapter 13 covers the process of sperm production in the testes, but when sperm exit the testes, they still have several maturation steps to complete as they travel through the epididymis and female reproductive tract toward to site of fertilisation.

During epididymal transit the protein and lipid architecture of the sperm is altered, after which the sperm acquire the potential for forward progressive motility and zona pellucida binding. Sperm can also be stored in the epididymis. In humans, sperm may be stored in the epididymis for 2–4 days (Sullivan and Mieusset, 2016). Once sperm completely transverse the epididymis to the vas deferens in readiness for ejaculation, they are mixed with diluting fluids from the seminal vesicles and other accessory glands to form the semen (sperm and seminal plasma). At this stage, the sperm remain largely immobile until the mechanical and chemical stimulation by ejaculation and the glandular secretions stimulate the physiological activation of the sperm cells readying them for the subsequent maturational phases of capacitation, hyperactivation and acrosome reaction which occur during the accession of the female reproductive tract.

Capacitation/hyperactivation is the penultimate step in the maturation of mammalian spermatozoa required to render them competent to fertilise an oocyte. Capacitation involves the removal of steroids and non-covalently bound epididymal/seminal glycoproteins resulting in a more fluid membrane with an increased permeability to calcium (Ca^{2+}). A complementary influx of Ca^{2+} then produces increases in the intracellular cAMP levels and thus an increase in motility (Aitken and Nixon, 2013). Hyperactivation (a specialised type of motility) coincides with the onset of capacitation and is the result of the increased Ca^{2+} levels. Specifically, hyperactivation is characterised by large whipping movements of the tail together with larger sideways swinging movements of the head. The destabilisation of the acrosomal sperm head membrane by a

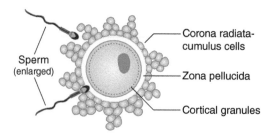

Figure 5.3 **Sperm approaching the ovum.** *Source*: Webster and de Wreede (2016). Reproduced with permission of John Wiley & Sons.

process known as the acrosome reaction is the final stages of sperm maturation (Zhou et al., 2017). The acrosome reaction allows the penetration and fusion of the sperm with the plasma membrane of the oocyte for fertilisation (Bromfield and Nixon, 2013) (Figure 5.3).

Day One: Fertilisation

Fertilisation or 'conception' involves the union of an egg and a sperm, usually occurring in the ampulla of the fallopian tube. The result of this merger is the production of a single cell zygote, or fertilised egg. Once capacitated sperm find their way to the cumulus–oocyte complex, they must penetrate through the cumulus cell mass to reach the zona pellucida; hyperactivation and the acrosome reaction aid these processes.

The zona pellucida is a specialised glycoprotein matrix which surrounds the plasma membrane of the oocytes with important roles in:

- oocyte development
- protection
- species-specific binding
- prevention of polyspermy (more than 1 sperm fertilising)
- blastocyst development and
- precluding premature implantation.

Once through the zona pellucida, the sperm must bind and fuse with the plasma membrane (or oolemma) of the oocyte. Fusion of spermatozoa with the oolemma is still poorly understood, but is believed to require the presence of membrane proteins on both the sperm and the oocyte (see Figure 5.4). Once the spermatozoon has 'docked' onto the oolemma (1), the two membranes coalesce, enabling the transfer of the paternal nucleus, centrosomes (an organelle which organises microtubules and regulates the cell division), paternal mRNA, protein and the mitochondria (which are later eliminated) (2–5).

The paternal nucleus contains highly condensed genetic material. Following fusion, the paternal nucleus is 'unpacked' (or decondensed) and reorganised into the paternal pronucleus. The maternal genome, following meiosis II, is simultaneously enclosed by its own nucleic membrane and decondensed to form the maternal pronucleus. Both pronuclei undergo DNA duplication (12–18 h) and migrate toward the cell middle and their nuclear membranes break down. The centrosome, delivered by the spermatozoa, plays an important role in the convergence of the two pronuclei for syngamy (or nuclei fusion). Syngamy enables haploid chromosomal pairing, DNA replication and the first mitotic division resulting in a 2-cell embryo.

Days 2–5: Pre-Implantation Development

While the embryo develops, it travels through the oviduct into the uterine cavity, carried by the currents created by the cilia of the epithelium lining the uterine tubes and the contractions of its muscular layer. Some 24 hours after fertilisation the zygote begins its first cell division, to produce the two-cell embryo. For the next 5 days, the cells of the embryo divide approximately every 24 hours, doubling the number of cells each time (Figure 5.5).

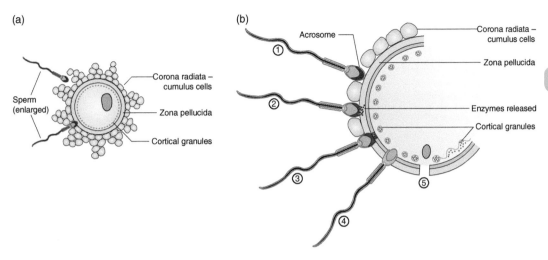

Figure 5.4 **(a) and (b): Spermatozoon passing through cumulus cells and meeting zona pellucida.** *Source:* Webster et al. (2018). Reproduced with permission of John Wiley & Sons.

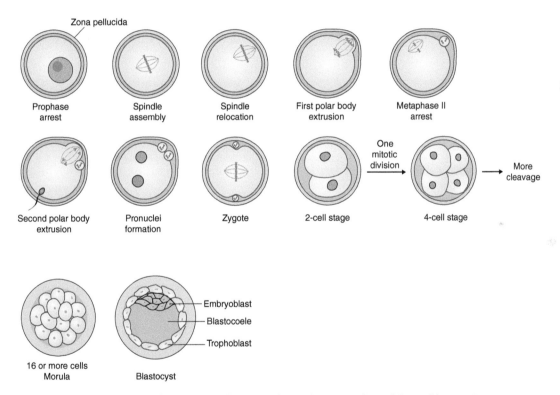

Figure 5.5 **The continuation of meiosis II and a zygote becoming a morula and then a blastocyst.** *Source:* Webster and de Wreede (2016). Reproduced with permission of John Wiley & Sons.

Approximately 3 days after fertilisation, the ball of cells reaches the uterus and begins to undergo a shape change, to produce the 'mulberry-shaped' embryo, known as a morula. The cells begin to secrete fluid into an internal cavity, around which the cells then organise themselves around a fluid filled cavity. Following this, the embryos is knowns as a blastocyst, and at this stage it contains 70–100 cells.

At the blastocyst stage, cells delineate into two distinct cell lines: one that gives rise to the extraembryonic structures, the chorionic sac and foetal portion of the placenta (trophoblast cells) and one (the inner cell mass) that constitutes the embryonic tissues (Morris et al., 2012; Niakan et al., 2012).

The trophoblast cells secrete enzymes that degrade the zona pellucida in readiness for 'hatching' required for implantation. The zona pellucida has acted as a protective immunological barrier until now, preventing premature implantation. Once hatched, the embryo is free to adhere to the uterine lining, access the uterine secretions for nutrition, and grow.

Day 6: Implantation

At the end of the 6th day of development, the embryo will embed in the endometrium of the uterus in a process known as implantation. The time during which this can occur – the 'implantation window' – is a relatively short timeframe during which the uterus is receptive to the blastocyst as a result of the action of oestrogen and progesterone on the endometrium. Implantation usually takes place in the top 1/3 of the uterus during the secretory phase of the menstrual cycle.

There are three main stages of implantation (Figure 5.6). First, the blastocyst reaches the uterus and loosely adheres to the endometrium. The trophoblast cells then interact with the endometrial cells in the adhesion stage. Finally, the blastocyst embeds itself in the uterine lining via the actions of specialised trophoblast cells which secrete enzymes and other factors to erode the endometrial cells away, allowing the embryo to penetrate down into the endometrium. These specialised trophoblasts then rapidly divide and completely surround the embryo by the time it is fully embedded in the endometrium. Implantation signals the end of the pre-embryonic stage of development and the beginning of placenta formation. A significant percentage (50–75%) of blastocysts will fail at this stage for a variety of reasons. When this occurs, the blastocyst is shed along with the endometrium during menstruation. The high rate of implantation failure explains why a pregnancy is unlikely to be achieved in a single ovulation cycle.

Week 2: Early Placental Formation

Extracellular vacuoles appear in the syncytiotrophoblasts and join together forming lacunae. These lacunae are filled with tissue fluids and uterine secretions and, following the erosion of the maternal capillaries, fill with maternal blood to establish early uteroplacental circulation. Implantation ends at the second week of development. At this stage the 'embryonic bud' consists schematically of two hemispheric cavities that lie on one above the other. These include the amniotic cavity and the umbilical vesicle (Figure 5.7).

The placenta continues to grow along with the foetus to keep pace with the increasing demand for nutrient uptake, waste elimination and gas exchange via the mother's blood supply. It also provides protection against infectious particles and produces hormones, including human chorionic gonadotropin (hCG). Specifically, hCG is secreted by the trophoblast cells and is responsible for the maintenance of the corpus luteum to ensure it continues to secrete progesterone and oestrogen to sustain pregnancy. hCG accumulates in the maternal bloodstream increasing exponentially in the first 7–10 weeks of pregnancy, peaking by 10–12 weeks (Korevaar *et al.*, 2015).The presence of hCG in the urine is used as an indicator of pregnancy.

Clinical Considerations Pregnancy Test

A pregnancy is confirmed by the presence of human chorionic gonadotropin (hCG) in the mother's urine or blood. Beginning at embryo implantation, hCG can first be detected in a blood sample approximately 11 days after conception.

Tests for blood hCG are more sensitive than those for urine levels (99.5–100%) and enable the time of pregnancy to be determined. Additionally, an hCG blood test can distinguish between normally progressing and abnormal pregnancies (e.g. molar pregnancies or ectopic pregnancies). Venous blood must be collected by a health professional and sent away for laboratory analysis.

Early diagnosis of pregnancy enables early preventative interventions to ensure maternal and foetal health (e.g. antenatal care, avoidance of alcohol and nicotine) and is also beneficial for women who do not wish to proceed with their pregnancy, as it enables the pregnancy to be terminated in the early stages.

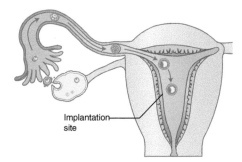

Implantation site

Normal implantation commonly occurs in the superior parts of the uterus, but can occur at a number of sites

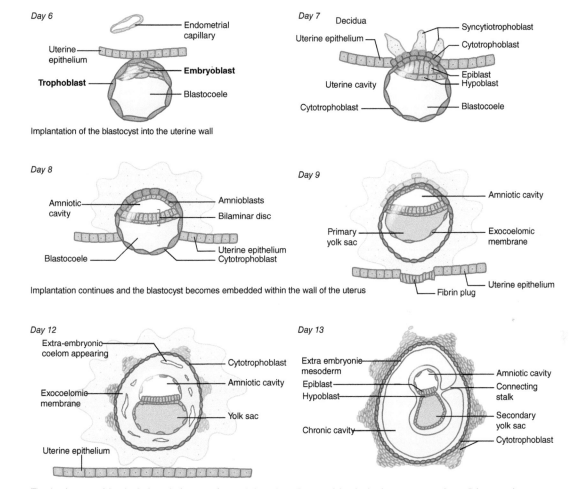

Day 6

Endometrial capillary

Uterine epithelium

Trophoblast

Embryoblast

Blastocoele

Implantation of the blastocyst into the uterine wall

Day 7

Decidua

Uterine epithelium

Syncytiotrophoblast

Cytotrophoblast

Uterine cavity

Epiblast
Hypoblast

Cytotrophoblast

Blastocoele

Day 8

Amniotic cavity

Amnioblasts

Bilaminar disc

Uterine epithelium
Cytotrophoblast

Blastocoele

Implantation continues and the blastocyst becomes embedded within the wall of the uterus

Day 9

Amniotic cavity

Primary yolk sac

Exocoelomic membrane

Uterine epithelium

Fibrin plug

Day 12

Extra-embryonic coelom appearing

Cytotrophoblast

Amniotic cavity

Exocoelomic membrane

Yolk sac

Uterine epithelium

Day 13

Extra embryonie mesoderm

Epiblast

Hypoblast

Amniotic cavity

Connecting stalk

Secondary yolk sac

Chronic cavity

Cytotrophoblast

The development of the chorionic cavity between the amniotic cavity, yolk sac and the chorion leaves a connecting stalk between the embryo and the developing placenta

Figure 5.6 **Implantation.** *Source:* Webster and de Wreede (2016). Reproduced with permission of John Wiley & Sons.

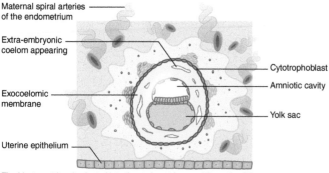

Maternal spiral arteries of the endometrium

Extra-embryonic coelom appearing

Exocoelomic membrane

Uterine epithelium

Cytotrophoblast

Amniotic cavity

Yolk sac

The blastocyst has implanted into the endometrium and the cells of the trophoblast invade the maternal tissue. (End of week 2)

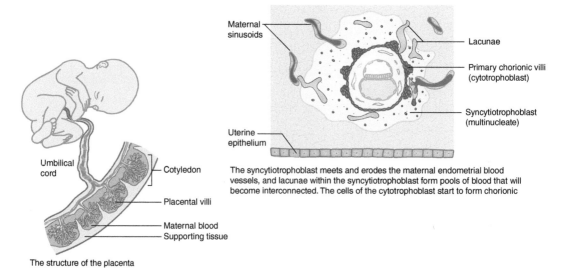

Maternal sinusoids

Lacunae

Primary chorionic villi (cytotrophoblast)

Syncytiotrophoblast (multinucleate)

Uterine epithelium

The syncytiotrophoblast meets and erodes the maternal endometrial blood vessels, and lacunae within the syncytiotrophoblast form pools of blood that will become interconnected. The cells of the cytotrophoblast start to form chorionic

Umbilical cord

Cotyledon

Placental villi

Maternal blood

Supporting tissue

The structure of the placenta

Figure 5.7 **The placenta.** *Source:* Webster and de Wreede (2016). Reproduced with permission of John Wiley & Sons.

Week 3–8: Post-Implantation Embryonic Development

The embryonic period is the developmental phase which occurs during the first eight weeks after fertilisation. The key feature of this period is the complex differentiation occurring, which establishes the basic body form.

Differentiation of Embryonic or Germ Layers

During the latter stage of embryonic development, the cells begin to form the three primary cell lineages that give rise to all adult tissues. This process is known as gastrulation and occurs shortly after implantation following the differentiation of the inner cell mass into a 2-layered plate of cells called the bilaminar embryonic disc, the 'epiblast' and the 'hypoblast' (Figure 5.8). The hypoblast forms extra-embryonic tissues while the epiblast forms the embryo proper.

Through gastrulation, the epiblast splits into the three germ layers; the ectoderm, mesoderm and endoderm. The cells of each germ layer differentiate and specialise to form tissues, organs and organ systems. Differentiation occurs when the form and function of cells changes to reflect a distinct function or developmental fate.

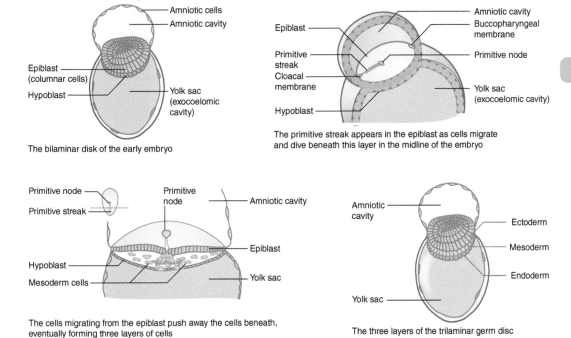

Figure 5.8 **Gastrulation.** *Source:* Webster and de Wreede (2016). Reproduced with permission of John Wiley & Sons.

The ectoderm gives rise to the skin and nervous system. The endoderm becomes the lining of digestive and respiratory tracts, parts of the liver and the pancreas, and the bladder lining. The mesoderm develops into the muscles, skeleton, circulatory system, excretory system (except the bladder lining), gonads and the inner layer of skin (dermis) (Figure 5.9).

Gastrulation is of clinical importance as it is a period highly susceptible to damaging factors such as alcohol, caffeine and tobacco – known as teratogens. Teratogens exposure during this period can result in significant developmental consequences to the embryo and may result in spontaneous abortion.

Neurulation is another critical event occurring in early embryonic development. It is the formation of the neural tube from a layer of ectoderm cells. This tube will develop into the brain, spinal cord and retina. The three-layered embryonic disc curls under with the ectoderm on the outside, resulting in the formation of the neural tube (Figure 5.10).

Week 3
During week 3, after neurulation, the brain enlarges at the site of the future head and somites develop from the mesoderm, appearing first as lumps on either side of the neural tube and developing into the vertebrae and ribs. At the same time, the epidermis is developing from the ectoderm.

Week 4
By the beginning of the fourth week, the embryo is approximately 2 mm in length. The head and tail ends begin to curl inwards, forming a C-shape. The head develops primitive eyes and the future inner ear canal. Pharyngeal arches, the future jaw and ears, develop as lumps in the neck region (Figure 5.11). The heart develops from a tube of mesoderm and begins to beat, forming the earliest functioning organ. In addition, the arm and leg buds appear arising from both the ectoderm and mesoderm.

Week 5
Rapid brain growth characterises this stage, where distinct brain areas and cranial nerves also begin to develop. The arm buds, flatten and become 'paddle-like'. Heart chambers develop, and the primitive gonads form at the genital ridge. By the end of this week the embryo is 1 cm in length.

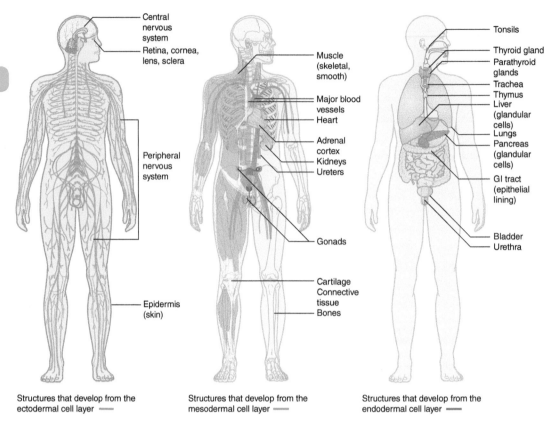

Figure 5.9 **The fate of the three germ layers.** *Source:* Webster and de Wreede (2016). Reproduced with permission of John Wiley & Sons.

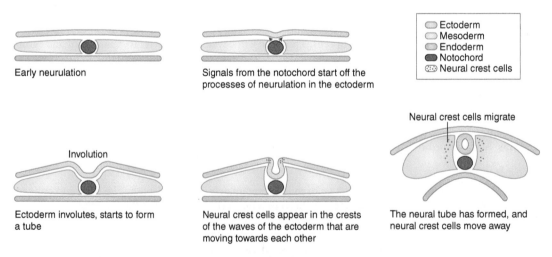

Figure 5.10 **Neurulation.** *Source:* Webster and de Wreede (2016). Reproduced with permission of John Wiley & Sons.

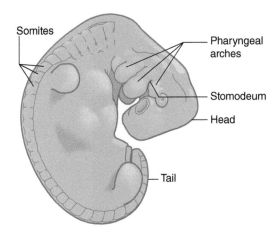

Somites

Pharyngeal
arches

Stomodeum

Head

Tail

Figure 5.11 **Fourth week embryo: lateral aspect of the fourth week embryo with visible pharyngeal arches.**
Source: Webster and de Wreede (2016). Reproduced with permission of John Wiley & Sons.

Week 6

The embryonic eyes gain pigment and the external ears form. There is also brain and head expansion, while the hand buds form finger rays. The heart further develops and circulation is established as the liver begins to produce blood cells. The primordial germ cells also complete their migration to the gonads and a distinct tail can be observed.

Weeks 7 and 8

The final two-week period of embryonic development phase is marked by distinct facial, organ system (especially the gastrointestinal tract) and neuromuscular development. The development of mouth, tongue and palate is also completed during this time. The eyelids grow and fuse together (they will not open until the 25th week) and the fingers and toes develop. The differentiation of the early gonads into testes or ovaries commences based on genetic sex and the tail bud disappears. The end of week 8 marks the end of the embryonic period and the beginning of the foetal period. Foetal movement is now visible on ultrasound.

The embryonic period is the most susceptible to major congenital complications and embryo loss or miscarriage. This is perhaps not surprising, given the extraordinary complexity of development that occurs in these first eight weeks. Embryonic loss can occur because of intrinsic errors in the developing embryo, including chromosomal anomalies and genetic defects, as well as through environmental insults, such as exposure to toxins, or uterine anomalies. Consequently, the earlier a woman is aware of a pregnancy, the sooner certain interventions, such as reducing alcohol consumption and folate and iron supplementation, can be introduced to support healthy embryo development.

Episode of Care Adult

Foetal alcohol spectrum disorder (FASD) is a disorder which includes a range of problems associated with the exposure of an unborn child to alcohol during gestation. As a spectrum disorder, FASD may affect each child differently, depending on the timing and level of alcohol consumption.

Alcohol consumed during pregnancy is able to cross the placenta into the bloodstream of the foetus. The foetus is exposed to a significantly higher alcohol level than the mother because the foetus metabolises alcohol at a much lower rate than an adult can. The risk of harm to the foetus is highest when the mother drinks a large amount of alcohol often (i.e. binge drinks).

Symptoms of FASD include:

- short stature, low body weight, small head size;
- bone and joint deformities;
- heart defects;
- miscarriage, spontaneous abortion or stillbirth;
- learning and behavioural problems (memory and coordination problems, impulsiveness and hyperactivity).

Natalie, 28, while pregnant with her first child continued to drink throughout the duration of her pregnancy. Natalie's daughter, Isabel, displays the typical characteristics of FASD. She has small eyes, a thin upper lip, a short, upturned nose and a smooth philtrum. She also displays mild behavioural problems including hyperactivity and rapidly changing moods. Isabel has been enrolled in an appropriate educational and behavioural programme following recommendation by their doctor.

Accurate diagnosis of FASD is extremely important so that the affected child receives appropriate care after birth. There is no cure for FASD, but treatment, if delivered early, may improve the long-term outcomes for the child. Treatment options can include educational and behavioural therapies or the administration of stimulant medication which may be used for the management of the associated attention-deficit/hyperactivity disorders. Importantly, treatment programmes need to be individualised to each patient and are usually coordinated by a developmental paediatrician.

Multiple Choice Questions

1. Foetal alcohol spectrum disorder (FASD) is a preventable condition:
   (a) true
   (b) false
2. Children born with FASD often exhibit characteristic facial features including:
   (a) short horizontal length from the inner corner to the outer corner of the eye
   (b) a smooth philtrum
   (c) a thin upper lip
   (d) all of the above
3. There is no known safe amount of alcohol during pregnancy:
   (a) true: there is no safe time to drink during pregnancy
   (b) false: FASD only occurs if a mother drinks during the 3rd trimester
4. It is easy to diagnose FASD:
   (a) true: all children display the same symptomology
   (b) false: the severity of foetal alcohol syndrome symptoms varies, with some children experiencing them to a greater degree than others
5. Alcohol consumed during pregnancy may lead to permanent brain damage in a child:
   (a) true
   (b) false

Late Gestation and Birth: Gestational Weeks 13–40 (Embryonic Weeks 11–38)

Human pregnancy is divided into trimesters (three-month periods). The first trimester extends from conception to about the 12th week of pregnancy (embryo week 10). The second trimester extends from weeks 13 to 27, and the third trimester from 28 weeks until birth. A typical pregnancy spans a total of 40 weeks from the first day of the last menstrual period to the birth of the baby (see Figure 5.12). Birth occurring earlier than 37 weeks is considered 'pre-term' birth and carries considerable risk for the foetus.

The First Trimester (Also See Post-Implantation Development)

During the first trimester, elevated progesterone levels and other hormonal changes can affect almost every organ in the mother's body. Women may suffer from extreme fatigue, morning sickness, food craving or aversions, mood swings and constipation, among other problems.

By the end of first trimester all major systems and organs of the baby have developed and are functioning, including the circulatory, nervous, digestive and urinary systems. The embryo is taking on a 'human shape', although the head is larger in proportion to the rest of the body. After eight weeks, the embryo is now referred to as a foetus (which means offspring). Even though the organs and body systems are fully formed by the end of 12 weeks, the foetus cannot survive independently.

The Second Trimester (13–27 Weeks Gestation)

Nausea and fatigue may be reduced or entirely eliminated, while physical signs of a baby such as the 'baby bump' will start to manifest as the women's abdomen expands to house the growing baby. During this time,

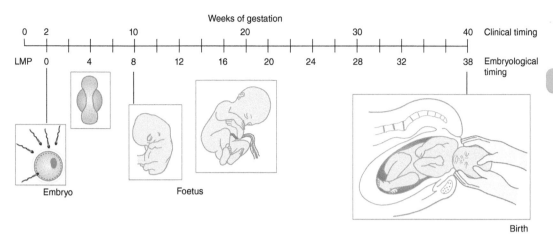

Weeks of gestation

Figure 5.12 Embryonic and foetal periods: The scale, in weeks, shows how gestation is dated clinically and embryonically. LMP refers to the date of the 'last menstrual period' from which the clinical period of gestation is determined. Embryologically, development begins with fertilisation. *Source:* Webster and de Wreede (2016). Reproduced with permission of John Wiley & Sons.

it is possible, through testing and ultrasound, to determine the baby's sex. In the later stages of this trimester, the pregnant woman may also begin to feel the foetus moving.

By week 13 the baby has begun to produce urine and release it into the amniotic sac, making amniotic fluid. Its bones are beginning to harden. By week 15 and 16 the baby's scalp pattern develops, its eyes begin to move. The baby's limb movements also become coordinated and can be detected during ultrasound exams. During weeks 17, 18 and 19 the baby's toenails develop, it gains the ability to hear, it becomes more active (rolling and flipping) and the vernix caseosa (a protective coating against abrasions, chapping and hardening that can result from exposure to amniotic fluid) begins to cover the baby. For female babies, the uterus and vaginal canal are also forming during this time.

In the final weeks of the second trimester the baby is completely covered with a fine, downy hair called 'lanugo'. The lanugo helps hold the vernix caseosa on the skin. In addition, the sucking reflex also is developing and the baby's hair becomes visible, so too are the foot and fingerprints. For males, the testes will also have begun to descend. Importantly, during week 26, the baby's lungs develop, beginning to produce surfactant, the substance that allows the air sacs in the lungs to inflate – and keeps them from collapsing and sticking together when they deflate. At week 27, the second trimester ends.

Clinical Considerations Prenatal Monitoring

Brenda, 30, is in the final trimester of her second pregnancy. During a routine antenatal visit, her midwife performs an ultrasound and measures the baby's heart rate. Brenda's baby has 130 beats per minute, within the normal range of 120–160 beats per minute.

An abnormal foetal heart rate or rhythm can indicate a problem, such as inadequate oxygen to the foetus. An abnormal foetal heart rate very late in pregnancy may indicate the need for an emergency caesarean delivery. Foetal heart rate may be monitored during labour, particularly for high-risk pregnancies. Short-lasting accelerations in the foetal heart rate during labour are a sign of a healthy foetus, and stimuli such as moving the mother's abdomen or gently pressing the baby's head as it is passing through the cervix should provoke these accelerations in heart rate.

The Third Trimester and Birth

An expectant mother may experience significant discomfort in this trimester, as the precipitous growth of the baby places more pressure on the internal organs. Upward pressure of the foetus on the diaphragm may make breathing difficult, and create gastric reflux, especially when lying down, and downward pressure on the bladder reduces its capacity and makes frequent urination a feature. Further swelling of the extremities is likely, due to the combination of an increased blood volume and compression of more veins by the foetus. Colostrum may leak from breasts, which are also likely to be tender, and uterine contractions may be felt, which can indicate real or false labour.

In readiness for birth, the baby will reposition itself in the lower abdomen/pelvis and the cervix will thin and soften in a process called 'effacement'. After week 37, the baby is considered 'full term', and at this point the baby's organs are fully functional. The average weight of a newborn ranges from 6 pounds 2 ounces (2.78 kg) to 9 pounds 2 ounces (4.13 kg) with an average length of 19 to 21 inches long (48.26–53.34 cm).

Medicines Management Pain Relief During Labour (Nitrous Oxide)

During the initial stage of labour, a woman will experience pain caused by the contraction of the uterus and dilation/stretching of the cervix. Towards the end of the first stage and into the second stage of labour, more intense pain is caused by pressure on the birth canal, vulva and perineum.

Pain perception is influenced by a variety of factors and will determine the maternal physiologic responses to the pain. If labour pain causes maternal anxiety, it is likely to manifest as muscular tension which may impair uterine contractility. There are non-medical and medical options for pain relief during labour, depending upon maternal preference, intensity of pain, and the anticipated length of labour. Non-medical methods of pain relief include relaxation, active birth, massage, heat and water, transcutaneous electrical nerve stimulation (TENS) and sterile water injections. The medical methods used most commonly are nitrous oxide gas (administered in 50/50 mix with oxygen), opioid analgesic intravenous injection, and local anaesthetic epidural administration (Table 5.1).

Table 5.1 Pharmacological methods of pain relief during labour.

DRUG	METHOD	INDICATION FOR USE	EFFECTIVENESS	SIDE EFFECTS	DURATION
Oxygen/ nitrous oxide	Inhalation 50/50 mixture of oxygen and nitrous oxide	First and second stage of labour	Mild	Faint, nausea and vomiting	Short-actin[g during inhalation
Pethidine	Intramuscular 50–150 mg	First stage	Mild – takes 'edge' off pain	Nausea and vomiting. Respiratory depression in newborn – naloxone used to reverse this effect	3–4 hours
Pudendal nerve block	Infiltration of right and left pudendal nerves (S2–S4) just below ischial spines	For operative vaginal delivery (in second-stage labour)	Moderate/good analgesia		45–90 minutes
Perineal infiltration	0.5% lidocaine at posterior fourchette	To facilitate episiotomy and/or before suturing tears/ episiotomies	Effective local analgesia within 5 minutes		45–90 minutes
Remifentanil PCA (patient-controlled analgesia)	Intravenous (powerful opiate that does not cross the placenta)	For patients in whom epidural is contraindicated or who wish a less complete analgesic block	Good		

Table 5.1 (Continued)

DRUG	METHOD	INDICATION FOR USE	EFFECTIVENESS	SIDE EFFECTS	DURATION
Epidural anaesthesia	Injection of 0.25–0.5% bupivacaine via catheter into extradural space (L3–L4)	First and second stage Caesarean section (CS)	Complete pain relief in >95% within 20 minutes	Transient hypotension (preload with i.v. fluids) Decreased mobility Dural puncture <1/100 Increased length of second-stage labour	Continuous infusion with top-ups every 3–4 hours
Spinal anaesthesia	0.5% bupivacaine into subarachnoid space	Operative delivery, e.g. forceps or CS Manual removal of placenta	Complete pain relief within few minutes	Respiratory depression	Single injection – wears off after 3–4 hours

Complications of Pregnancy

Complications of pregnancy may include 'implantation abnormalities' or problems associated with gestation. Some common pregnancy complications include the following.

Ectopic Pregnancies

Usually an embryo implants within the body of the uterus. However, in 1–2% of cases, the embryo implants outside the uterus leading to an ectopic pregnancy or an extra-uterine pregnancy. Abnormal implantation sites may include the fallopian tubes or the external surface of the uterus, ovary, bowel, gastrointestinal tract, mesentery or peritoneal wall. Almost all (99%) of ectopic pregnancies are tubal pregnancies, with all other sites combined representing only 1% of ectopic pregnancies. These pregnancies can result in haemorrhages and sterility (e.g. if the fallopian tube ruptures).

Pregnancy Loss/Miscarriage and Stillbirth

Pregnancy loss can occur at any stage of gestation. Miscarriage is the loss of a baby before 20 weeks gestation. Approximately 20% of confirmed pregnancies end in miscarriage, although it is likely that some women miscarry without knowing they are pregnant. Signs that a miscarriage has occurred include cramping, abdominal pain and vaginal spotting/bleeding.

Later term pregnancy loss, or stillbirth, occurs when a baby is lost after 20 weeks gestation or during birth. A stillbirth may occur due to congenital anomalies, chromosomal abnormalities or premature birth.

There is no evidence that exercising, stress, working or having sex causes pregnancy loss and most women who have had lost a pregnancy will go on to successfully carry a subsequent pregnancy to term. However, in rare instances, usually due to chromosomal abnormalities, some women may experience recurrent miscarriages (3 or more in a row); in these cases, assisted reproductive strategies, such as use of donor eggs or embryos, may be used to overcome infertility.

Clinical Considerations Preeclampsia

Pre-eclampsia usually affects pregnant women during the second half of pregnancy or immediately after delivery of their baby. A combination of elevated blood pressure, protein in the urine and oedema in the extremities suggest preeclampsia. Untreated, the condition can have serious complications for mother and child and can be life threatening.

During routine antenatal appointments, the mother's blood pressure will be monitored. If readings of 140 mmHg systolic and/or 90 mm Hg diastolic are observed on two occasions at least 4 hours apart the mother may have preeclampsia. To make a definitive diagnosis, protein in the urine (proteinuria) of >2+ on a dipstick test, or 300 mg/24 hours is considered indicative of preeclampsia. In more severe cases, the patient may also exhibit renal insufficiency (serum creatinine > 0.09 mmol/L), liver disease, neurological problems (including convulsions) and haematological disturbances (thrombocytopenia or placental insufficiency). While preeclampsia can be managed until the baby is mature enough to be delivered, by administration of antihypertensive medication for example, the only cure for preeclampsia is delivery of the baby.

Episode of Care Adult

Pre-term birth is defined as birth before 37 weeks gestation and is associated with an increased risk of intellectual disability. The more premature the baby, the greater the risk. Babies born between 32 and 26 weeks are more likely to have lower cognitive function, increased behavioural problems and a higher prevalence of psychiatric disorders (de Jong et al., 2012). Babies born before 28 weeks without severe disabilities still have an increased risk of autism, inattention, anxiety and obsessive-compulsive disorder (Fevang et al., 2016). Developmental delays in babies born prematurely can be an early sign of learning difficulties.

Anna Orr is 33 weeks pregnant with her second child. Anna and her partner Andy are both 38, and their first child, Kanye, was born prematurely at 35 weeks. Due to Anna's advanced maternal age and her previous pre-term birth, her pregnancy is considered high-risk and she is monitored closely by her medical team. Despite having an uncomplicated pregnancy, Anna goes into labour early and her baby, Coco, is born at 35 weeks. Coco and Anna have an extended stay in hospital before they are both cleared to return home. Coco and her brother Kanye meet their adjusted milestones and attend regular health checks and developmental checks with their family health nurse. When the children attend school, Kanye's teacher notices that he has a tendency for short periods of inattention that are impacting his learning. Anna and Andy work with Kanye to help improve his focus at school, and no further problems are noted.

Multiple Choice Questions

1. There are subcategories of pre-term birth: extremely pre-term, very pre-term and moderate to late pre-term. What weeks correspond to these categories?
   (a) less than 12 weeks, 24 weeks and 40 weeks respectively
   (b) less than 28 weeks, 28–32 weeks and 32–37 weeks respectively
2. Can induction or caesarean birth be planned before 39 completed weeks of gestation?
   (a) no
   (b) only if medically indicated
3. Pre-term birth and its associated complications are the leading cause of death among children under 5 years of age?
   (a) true
   (b) false
4. Pre-term birth may occur:
   (a) spontaneously
   (b) due to infection
   (c) due to a chronic disease (diabetes and high blood pressure)
   (d) all of the above
5. Which of the following is not a treatment for pre-term birth?
   (a) tocolytics or other medication to attempt to delay birth
   (b) antenatal steroid injections (given to pregnant women to expedite babies' lung maturation)
   (c) kangaroo mother care and frequent breastfeeding
   (d) antibiotics to treat newborn infections
   (e) administration of magnesium sulphate to prevent neurological impairment of the child
   (f) assisted reproductive technologies

Episode of Care Adult

Naomi Madden is 26 weeks pregnant with her first child. Naomi is 31 years old and obese, with a BMI of 30. Both her mother Julie and her brother Clint have type 2 diabetes. Following Naomi's oral glucose tolerance screening test, she is diagnosed with higher than normal blood sugar levels and gestational diabetes. Naomi is taught to manage her gestational diabetes through healthy eating and increased moderate physical activity, and also how to regularly monitor her blood glucose levels and give herself insulin injections (suitable for use during pregnancy) when necessary. Due to the increased risk of a larger than normal baby (macrosomia), Naomi is offered induction of labour at 38 weeks. Her baby girl Matilda is born in the normal weight range, without any further complications. Following Matilda's birth, Naomi has regular follow-up tests for diabetes and continues to maintain a healthy lifestyle which is adopted by her whole family.

Multiple Choice Questions

1. Gestational diabetes is a type of diabetes that only develops during pregnancy:
   (a) true
   (b) false
2. Development of gestational diabetes increases the risk of the expectant mother developing type 2 diabetes later in life:
   (a) true
   (b) false
3. Gestational diabetes normally occurs during the:
   (a) 6th to 12th week of pregnancy
   (b) 24th to 28th week of pregnancy
4. Which of these is not a risk factor for the development of gestational diabetes?
   (a) family history of type 2 diabetes or a first-degree relative (mother or sister) who has had gestational diabetes
   (b) obesity
   (c) history of elevated blood glucose levels
   (d) Aboriginal and Torres Strait Islander background
   (e) carrying a male baby
5. Gestational diabetes can be managed by:
   (a) healthy eating
   (b) regular physical activity
   (c) insulin injections
   (d) all of the above

Episode of Care Learning Disabilities

Down syndrome or Trisomy 21 is the most common autosomal trisomy and also the most common genetic cause of intellectual disability. Down syndrome is caused by the presence of an extra chromosome 21 or extra parts of chromosome 21. The incidence of Down syndrome is approximately 1:650 births but this increases with maternal age. Major clinical features are highlighted in Figure 5.13. Almost all babies born with Down syndrome are intellectually disabled; however, the severity of learning difficulties can vary highly between individuals and is therefore difficult to predict. It is important to note that children with Down syndrome will take longer to reach certain milestones and are likely to be delayed in cognitive development, with specific deficits in speech, language production and auditory short-term memory, and are at increased risk for depression and Alzheimer's disease (Chapman and Hesketh, 2000).

Sandra McDonald is 39 years old and pregnant with her second child. At the first trimester dating scan, the sonographer notes an above average Nuchal Translucency measurement. Follow up testing identifies that the foetus is likely to be born with Down syndrome. Sandra was aware that due to her age she was at higher risk of having a child with Trisomy 21 and together with her partner Danny, they decide to continue with the pregnancy. Sandra is monitored closely throughout the remainder of her pregnancy. The McDonald family is offered counselling and specialist services to help plan for the delivery, care and management of child who has Down syndrome. Baby Ryan is born with no further complications at 40 weeks gestation. Throughout his life, Ryan is routinely screened for Down syndrome associated complications, including those related to intellectual disability. It is identified that Ryan requires glasses and hearing aids due to vision and hearing problems. The timely implementation of these aids ensures Ryan's ability to learn and understand is not impaired.

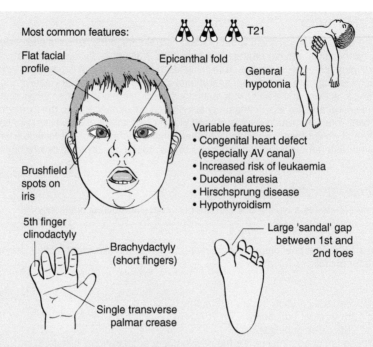

Figure 5.13 **The essential features of Down syndrome.** *Source:* Webster et al. (2018). Reproduced with permission of John Wiley & Sons.

Multiple Choice Questions

1. Down syndrome is a:
   (a) genetic condition
   (b) an illness
   (c) a disease
2. Down syndrome (DS) is a genetic condition where a person is born with an extra copy of chromosome:
   (a) 12
   (b) 21
   (c) 19
   (d) 18
3. The likelihood of giving birth to a child with Down syndrome increases with maternal age:
   (a) true
   (b) false
4. Despite abnormalities in behaviour, mental ability and physical development, individuals with Down syndrome grow up to hold jobs, live independently and enjoy normal recreational activities:
   (a) true
   (b) false
5. Pre-natal Down syndrome screening tests:
   (a) provide a definitive diagnosis of Down syndrome
   (b) identify the likelihood of a child being born with Down syndrome

Skills in Practice Ultrasound

Obstetric ultrasound is a diagnostic imaging tool used for foetal screening during pregnancy. Ultrasound uses high-frequency, non-audible, sound waves which, when reflected off internal structures, create a real-time image. It does not expose patients to ionising radiation, as occurs with X-ray imaging.

Most obstetric ultrasounds performed after 10 weeks of pregnancy are abdominal. A transducer is moved over the mother's abdomen to visualise the foetus. Ultrasound can identify severe abnormalities that may be incompatible with life or cause significant morbidity, in addition to milder anomalies amenable to antenatal intervention.

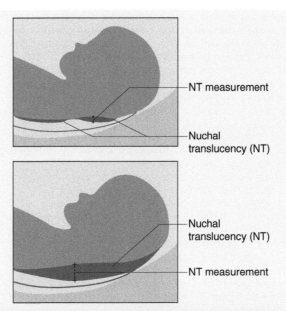

Figure 5.14 **Antenatal screening: nuchal translucency describes the space between the cervical spine and the skin that is measured during an ultrasound. The collection of fluid here increases in some developmental anomalies.** *Source:* Webster and de Wreede (2016). Reproduced with permission of John Wiley & Sons.

A routine obstetric ultrasound is recommended for all pregnant women at 18–22 weeks gestation. This scan can confirm the timing of the pregnancy by measurement of the foetus and identify any abnormalities (Salomon *et al.*, 2011). At this stage the foetus is at a size and developmental stage that allows detailed examination of the skull, central nervous system, heart, thorax, gastrointestinal tract, urogenital systems and skeleton as well as the placenta and amniotic fluid.

Additionally, when possible, it is recommended that pregnant women have an obstetric ultrasound between 11 and 13.9 weeks gestational age, known as the nuchal or dating scan. An ultrasound performed at this earlier stage provides a more accurate estimate of the timing of the pregnancy and can also identify multiple foetuses and major congenital abnormalities. Nuchal translucency (Figure 5.14) measures the space (fluid) between the cervical spine and skin and this measurement can be correlated to a number of chromosomal anomalies, e.g. Trisomy 21 or Down syndrome (see Episode of Care feature above).

The sensitivity and accuracy of ultrasound is reduced in women with a high body mass, or low amniotic fluid. Drinking a few glasses of water prior to the ultrasound may achieve a clearer image by enlarging the bladder and pushing the foetus up out of the pelvis.

Conclusion

Embryology encompasses much more than the early stages of a pregnancy; it includes all the factors responsible for a healthy and successful pregnancy. From the maturation of gametes to the birth of a healthy baby, there are numerous stages where medical monitoring and/or interventions are applicable. Consequently, there are many important roles for health professionals to play throughout this process and a robust knowledge of fertilisation, conception, embryo development, gestation and birth are essential attributes for anyone specialising in this field.

Glossary

Aneuploidy: The presence of an abnormal number of chromosomes in a cell.
Atresia: Degeneration process of the ovarian follicles that do not ovulate.
Colostrum: First secretion from the mammary glands after birth.
Conceptus: Denotes the embryo and its associated extraembryonic structures (i.e. placenta).
Corpus luteum (CL): A hormone-secreting structure that develops in an ovary at the sight of ovulation.

Ectoderm: The outermost of the three primary germ layers of an embryo.

Effacement: Process by which the cervix prepares for delivery (soften, shorten and become thinner) after the baby has repositioned itself in the lower in the abdomen/pelvis region.

Embryogenesis: The formation and development of an embryo.

Endoderm: The innermost of the three primary germ layers of an embryo.

Endometrium: The inner epithelial layer and mucous membrane of the mammalian uterus.

Epididymis: Highly convoluted which connects the testis to the vas deferens.

Fallopian tube (also known as an oviduct or uterine tube): Uterine appendages leading from the ovaries into the uterus.

Fertilisation: The union of the male and female gamete (sperm and oocyte).

Follicle stimulating hormone (FSH): Sex hormone produced by the pituitary gland.

Gametes: Haploid sex cells (eggs and called sperm).

Gastrulation: Phase of early embryonic development during which the single-layered blastula is reorganised into a multilayered structure known as the gastrula.

Gestation: The period of development between conception and birth.

Human chorionic gonadotropin (hCG): Hormone secreted by the placenta which forms the basis of pregnancy tests.

Implantation: The process of attachment and invasion of the uterus endometrium by the blastocyst.

Luteinising hormone (LH): Hormone produced in the anterior pituitary gland which triggers ovulation and corpus luteum development.

Mesoderm: The innermost layer of the three primary germ layers of an embryo.

Miscarriage: Pregnancy loss before 20 weeks of pregnancy.

Oestrogen: Steroid hormones which promote the development and maintenance of female characteristics of the body.

Ovulation: A phase of the female menstrual cycle that involves the release of an egg (ovum) from one of the ovaries.

Preeclampsia: A serious condition of pregnancy, usually characterised by high blood pressure, protein in the urine and severe swelling.

Pre-term: Labour delivery before 37 completed weeks of pregnancy.

Progesterone: Hormone released by the corpus luteum in the ovary.

Stillbirth: Loss of a foetus or baby after 20 weeks' gestation or during birth.

Zygote: Fertilised egg.

References

Aitken, R.J. and Nixon, B. (2013) Sperm capacitation: a distant landscape glimpsed but unexplored. *Molecular Human Reproduction* **19**: 785–793.

Bromfield, E.G. and Nixon, B. (2013) The function of chaperone proteins in the assemblage of protein complexes involved in gamete adhesion and fusion processes. *Reproduction* **145**: R31–42.

Korevaar, T.I., Steegers, E.A., de Rijke, Y.B., et al. (2015). Reference ranges and determinants of total hCG levels during pregnancy: the Generation R Study. *European Journal of Epidemiology* **30**: 1057–1066.

Morris, S.A., Grewal, S., Barrios, F., Patankar, S.N., Strauss, B., Buttery, L., Alexander, M., Shakesheff, K.M. and Zernicka-Goetz, M. (2012) Dynamics of anterior-posterior axis formation in the developing mouse embryo. *Nature Communications* **3**: 673.

Niakan, K.K., Han, J., Pedersen, R.A., Simon, C. and Pera, R.A. (2012) Human pre-implantation embryo development. *Development* **139**: 829–841.

Salomon, L.J., Alfirevic, Z., Berghella, V., et al. (2011) Practice guidelines for performance of the routine mid-trimester fetal ultrasound scan. *Ultrasound in Obstetrics and Gynaecology* **37**: 116–126.

Zhou, W., Anderson, A.L., Turner, A.P., De Iuliis, G.N., McCluskey, A., McLaughlin, E.A. and Nixon, B. (2017) Characterization of a novel role for the dynamin mechanoenzymes in the regulation of human sperm acrosomal exocytosis. *Molecular Human Reproduction* **23**: 657–673.

Further Reading

Australian Bureau of Statistics

https://www.abs.gov.au/ausstats%5Cabs@.nsf/0/8668A9A0D4B0156CCA25792F0016186A?Opendocument

The ABS' purpose is to inform Australia's important decisions by partnering and innovating to deliver relevant, trusted, objective data, statistics and insights. These data include usual information about births, fertility and infertility rates in Australia.

Australian Government Department of Health
https://beta.health.gov.au/resources/pregnancy-care-guidelines/part-d-clinical-assessments/risk-of-pre-eclampsia
The Australian Department of Health aims to develop and deliver policies and programs and advise the Australian
    Government on health, aged care and sport.

Diabetes UK
Diabetes UK vision is a world where diabetes can do no harm and leading the fight against the UK's biggest and growing
    health crisis, sharing knowledge and taking on diabetes together. https://www.diabetes.org.uk.

National Diabetes Services Scheme
https://pregnancyanddiabetes.com.au/
The National Diabetes Services Scheme is an initiative of the Australian Government administered with the assistance of
    Diabetes Australia. This website also provides information about pregnancy and diabetes. Fact sheet:
    http://gd.ndss.com.au/Global/GD/Understanding%20Gestational%20Diabetes%20-%20high%20res.pdf

National Institute for Health and Care Excellence
Hypertension in Pregnancy: Diagnosis and Management
https://www.nice.org.uk/guidance/cg107

Stillbirth Foundation of Australia
https://stillbirthfoundation.org.au/stillbirth/
The Stillbirth Foundation Australia's mission is to significantly reduce the incidence of stillbirth through research, educa-
    tion and advocacy.

The World Health Organisation (WHO): Sexual and Reproductive Health
https://www.who.int/reproductivehealth/en/
The WHO aims to build a better healthier future for all people over the world. Their primary role is to direct and coordinate
    international health within the United Nations system focusing on health through the life-course; non-communicable
    and communicable diseases; preparedness, surveillance and response; and corporate services. With regard to repro-
    duction, the WHO gathers information about abortion, adolescents, reproductive cancers, sexually transmitted and
    reproductive tract infections, contraception, infertility, maternal and perinatal health, sexual health, stillbirths and
    violence against women.
Martin, J.H., Bromfield, E.G., Aitken, R.J. and Nixon, B. (2017) Biochemical alterations in the oocyte in support of early
    embryonic development. *Cellular and Molecular Life Sciences* **74**: 469–485. DOI: 10.1007/s00018-016-2356-1.

Activities

Multiple Choice Questions
1. Follicular maturation is mediated by what hormones?
    (a) follicle stimulating hormone (FSH) and luteinising hormone (LH)
    (b) oestrogen
    (c) progesterone
    (d) testosterone
2. During oogenesis, a number of follicles mature but usually only 1 follicle is 'recruited' to become a
    dominant follicle in readiness for ovulation. What happens to the remaining mature follicles?
    (a) they are fertilised
    (b) they undergo atresia (or degradation)
    (c) they undergo meiosis
3. Fertilisation takes place where in the female reproductive tract?
    (a) the ampullary region of the fallopian tube
    (b) the follicle blister
    (c) the uterus
    (d) the corpus luteum
4. Sperm are considered functionally mature after:
    (a) leaving the testes. They do not need to undergo further maturation
    (b) transit of epididymis
    (c) ejaculation and activation in the female reproductive tract

5. The epidydimal maturation phase of the sperm is responsible for:
   (a) penetrate the cumulus cell layer and the zona pellucida
   (b) forward progressive motility, increased sperm concentration procurement of additional proteins required for fertilisation and development
   (c) the combination of the sperm with the diluting fluids of the seminal vesicles and other accessory glands to form semen
   (d) capacitation and hyperactivation

6. The zona pellucida is responsible for:
   (a) species-specific binding, prevention of polyspermy and precluding premature implantation.
   (b) sperm activation
   (c) decondensing the paternal (sperm) nucleus prior to the first mitotic division

7. The paternal gamete contributes what to the zygote following fertilisation?
   (a) nucleic membrane
   (b) the paternal genetics, centrosome and mRNA and protein
   (c) mitochondria

8. Five days following conception (fertilisation) the embryo is known as a
   (a) blastocyst
   (b) trophectoderm
   (c) morula
   (d) oocyte

9. Implantation is characterised by how many stages?
   (a) 1
   (b) 2
   (c) 3

10. Some of the primary roles for the placenta include
    (a) nutrient, gas and waste exchange between mother and baby
    (b) a snack for the mother post birth
    (c) thermo-regulation, hormone secretion and corpus luteum formation

11. In a process is known as gastrulation, what are the three germ layers that develop?
    (a) ectoderm, mesoderm, endoderm
    (b) endothelial, muscle, fibroblast
    (c) epidermis, dermis, hypodermis

12. Loss of a pregnancy prior to 20 weeks is classified as:
    (a) still birth
    (b) implantation failure
    (c) miscarriage

13. Loss of a pregnancy after 20 weeks is classified as:
    (a) still birth
    (b) implantation failure
    (c) miscarriage

14. Placenta previa is a condition where:
    (a) an embryo implants outside the reproductive tract on the external surface of the uterus, ovary, bowel, gastrointestinal tract, mesentery or peritoneal wall
    (b) an embryo implants in the inferior portion of the uterus and the placenta grows over the opening of the cervix
    (c) only the trophoblast cells proliferate following fertilisation

15. Preeclampsia is diagnosed on the basis of:
    (a) cramping, abdominal pain and vaginal spotting/bleeding
    (b) physical abnormalities with the uterus or cervix
    (c) hypertension following 20 weeks of gestation, end-organ dysfunction, and proteinuria
    (d) birth prior to 37 weeks of gestation

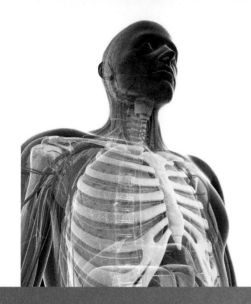

6

The Muscular System

Janet G. Migliozzi

Test Your Prior Knowledge

- List the functions of the muscular system.
- Name the different types of muscles found in the human body.
- Describe the energy sources that enable muscles to contract.
- List the stages involved in muscle contraction.
- List the different types of body movement.

Learning Outcomes

After reading this chapter you will be able to:

- Describe the structure and functions of the muscular system.
- Describe the different types of muscles in the human body.
- Name the major muscles of the body and their functions.
- Describe how a muscle contracts.
- Describe the energy sources that muscles use.

Visit the student companion website at www.wileyfundamentalseries.com/anatomy where you can test yourself using flashcards, multiple-choice questions and more. Instructor companion site at www.wiley.com/go/instructor/anatomy where instructors will find valuable materials such as PowerPoint slides and image bank designed to enhance your teaching.

Fundamentals of Anatomy and Physiology: For Nursing and Healthcare Students, Third Edition. Edited by Ian Peate and Suzanne Evans.
© 2020 John Wiley & Sons Ltd. Published 2020 by John Wiley & Sons Ltd.
Student companion website: www.wileyfundamentalseries.com/anatomy
Instructor companion website: www.wiley.com/go/instructor/anatomy

Body Map

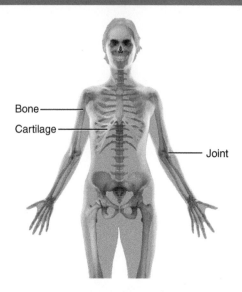

Bone

Cartilage

Joint

Introduction

All physical function of the body involves muscular activity, and as muscles are responsible for all body movement, they can be considered the 'machines' of the body (Marieb and Hoehn, 2015). This chapter will discuss the structure and function of the muscular system.

Types of Muscle Tissue

The body contains three types of muscle tissue: smooth, cardiac and skeletal. Table 6.1 provides a summary of the different types of muscle tissue.

Smooth or Visceral Muscle

Smooth or visceral muscle is located in the walls of hollow internal organs and blood vessels of the body; for example, the small intestine, blood vessels (arteries, arterioles, venules and veins), bronchioles of the respiratory tract, urinary bladder and ureters, uterus and Fallopian tubes, but not the heart. Smooth muscle fibres have a single nucleus, are usually arranged in parallel lines and are not striated. Smooth muscles are involuntary, do not fatigue easily and are controlled by the medulla oblongata in the brain, which is responsible for controlling involuntary action throughout the body. Smooth muscle is discussed in more detail in Chapter 10.

Table 6.1 **Different types of muscle tissue.**

SKELETAL MUSCLE	SMOOTH MUSCLE	CARDIAC MUSCLE
Attached to bones or the skin (facial muscles only)	Found in the walls of hollow visceral organs and blood vessels	Located in the walls of the heart
Single, long cylindrical cells	Single, narrow, rod-shaped cells	Branching chains of cells
Striated, multinucleated cells	Non-striated, uninucleated cells	Striated, uninucleated cells
Under voluntary control	Involuntary control	Involuntary control

Cardiac

Cardiac muscle, found only in the heart, is also a form of involuntary muscle and forms the walls of the heart. Its main function is to propel blood into the circulation by making the right atrium contract. Cardiac muscles also have a single nucleus, are striated, branched and tubular. Cardiac muscle is discussed in more detail in Chapter 9.

Skeletal

The skeletal muscles make up the muscular system of the body (composed of over 600 muscles) and account for 40–50% of the body weight in an adult. The skeletal muscles are the only voluntary muscles of the body (i.e. are consciously controlled) and are the muscles involved in moving bones and generating external movement. Skeletal muscle is also referred to as striped or striated muscle because of the banded patterns of the cells seen under the microscope.

The rest of this chapter will focus on skeletal muscle only as both smooth and cardiac muscle are discussed in more detail elsewhere.

Functions of the Muscular System

The muscular system plays five important roles in the body:
- maintains posture
- produces movement
- stabilises joints
- protection
- generates heat.

Maintenance of Body Posture

Despite the continuous downward pull of gravity, the body is able to maintain an erect or seated posture because of the continuous tiny adjustments that the skeletal muscles make.

Production of Movement

The body's ability to mobilise is a result of skeletal muscle activity and muscle contraction, as when muscles contract they pull on the tendons and bones of the skeleton to produce movement.

Stabilisation of Joints

Muscle tendons play a vital role in stabilising and reinforcing the joints of the body. During movement the skeletal muscles pull on bones which stabilise the joints of the skeleton.

Protection and Control of Internal Tissue Structures/Organs

Skeletal muscle plays an important role in protecting the internal organs as the visceral organs and internal tissues contained within the abdominal cavity are protected by layers of skeletal tissue within the abdominal wall and floor of the pelvic cavity. Similarly, the orifices contained within the digestive and urinary tracts are encircled by skeletal muscle, and this allows for voluntary control over swallowing, urination and defaecation (Martini and Bartholomew, 2017).

Generation of Heat

Heat generation is vital in maintaining normal body temperature, and skeletal muscles, which account for 40% of the body's mass, are the muscle type mostly responsible for the body's heat generation. During muscle contraction, adenosine triphosphate (ATP) is used to release the needed energy, with nearly three-quarters of its energy escaping as heat.

Composition of Skeletal Muscle Tissue

As muscles contain other types of tissues, such as blood vessels and connective and nervous tissue, they are considered to be organs (Logenbaker, 2017). Each cell in skeletal muscle tissue is known as a single muscle fibre, which, owing to its large size, contains hundreds of nuclei (i.e. are multinucleate). A skeletal muscle consists of individual muscle fibres that are markedly different from a 'typical' cell (not least by their size) bundled into fascicles and surrounded by three layers of connective tissue.

Clinical Consideration Rhabdomyolysis

Rhabdomyolysis is a serious syndrome that can occur following damage to a muscle. This may result in part of the muscle tissue dying and the contents entering the blood stream which can lead to complications such as renal failure.

Traumatic causes of rhabdomyolysis include:

- A crush injury such as from a road traffic collision, fall, or building collapse.
- Long-lasting muscle compression such as that caused by prolonged immobilisation after a fall or lying unconscious on a hard surface during illness or while under the influence of alcohol or medication.
- Electrical shock injury, lightning strike, or third-degree burn.
- Venom from a snake or insect bite.

Non-traumatic causes of rhabdomyolysis include:

- The use of alcohol or illegal drugs such as heroin, cocaine or amphetamines.
- Extreme muscle strain, especially in someone who is an untrained athlete; this can happen in elite athletes too, and it can be more dangerous if there is more muscle mass to break down.
- The use of medications such as antipsychotics or statins, especially when given in high doses.
- A very high body temperature (hyperthermia) or heat stroke.
- Seizures or delirium tremens.
- A metabolic disorder such as diabetic ketoacidosis.
- Diseases of the muscles (myopathy) such as congenital muscle enzyme deficiency or Duchenne's muscular dystrophy.
- Viral infections such as the flu, HIV or herpes simplex virus.
- Bacterial infections leading to toxins in tissues or the bloodstream (sepsis).

A previous history of rhabdomyolysis also increases the risk of having rhabdomyolysis again.

The 'classic triad' of rhabdomyolysis symptoms are: muscle pain in the shoulders, thighs or lower back; muscle weakness or trouble moving arms and legs; and dark red or brown urine or decreased urination. However, half of patients with the condition may have no muscle-related symptom. The presenting clinical picture and a raised level of creatinine kinase (a by-product of muscle breakdown) in the blood may assist with diagnosis. Treatment aims to support the kidneys and reverse the symptoms of renal failure; in rare cases this may require haemodialysis.

Gross Anatomy of Skeletal Muscles

Muscle is separated from skin by the hypodermis, which consists of adipose tissue (which provides insulation and protects the muscle from physical damage) and a dense, broad band of connective tissue known as fascia, which supports and surrounds muscle tissue and provides a pathway for nerves and the lymphatic and blood vessels to enter and exit a muscle. Extending from the fascia are three layers of connective tissue that also play a role in supporting and protecting the muscle and are necessary to ensure that the force of contraction from each muscle cell is transmitted to its points of attachment to the skeleton (see Figure 6.1). These include:

- the **epimysium**, which is wrapped around the entire muscle;
- the **perimysium**, which surrounds bundles of muscle fibres known as fascicles;
- the **endomysium**, which is wrapped around each individual muscle cell.

The epimysium, perimysium and endomysium blend into either strong, cord-like tendons or into sheet-like aponeuroses that attach muscles indirectly to bones, cartilages or connective tissue (Marieb and Hoehn, 2015).

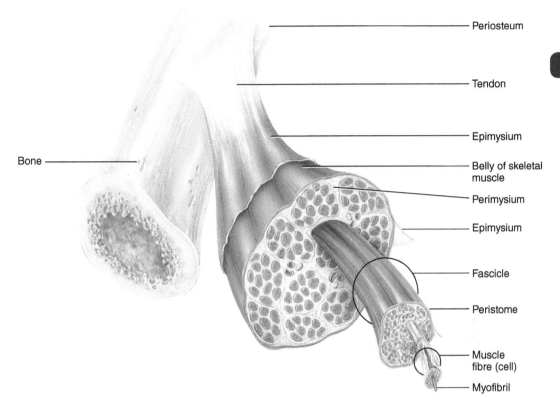

Periosteum

Tendon

Epimysium

Bone

Belly of skeletal muscle

Perimysium

Epimysium

Fascicle

Peristome

Muscle fibre (cell)

Myofibril

Figure 6.1 **Gross anatomy of a skeletal muscle.** *Source:* Tortora and Derrickson (2009). Reproduced with permission of John Wiley & Sons.

Skills in Practice Intramuscular Injection

An intramuscular (IM) injection is given directly into a selected muscle, and while there are several sites on the body that are suitable for IM injections, the most common areas used are:

- the deltoid muscle of the upper arm;
- the vastus lateralis muscle, which forms part of the quadriceps muscle group of the upper leg;
- the gluteus medius (ventrogluteal site) muscle, which runs beneath the gluteus maximus from the ilium to the femur.

IM injections are used for the delivery of certain drugs that (for various reasons) cannot be given via an oral, intravenous or subcutaneous route. The IM route enables a large amount (up to 5 mL) of drug to be introduced at one time, minimises tissue irritation and provides a faster route than subcutaneous/intradermal injections.

Microanatomy of Skeletal Muscle Fibre

When examined microscopically, skeletal muscle cells appear cylindrical in shape, have a distinctive banded appearance of alternate light and dark stripes and lie parallel to each other (see Figure 6.2). Table 6.2 provides a summary of the cellular components of a muscle fibre.

The Sarcolemma and Transverse Tubules

Each muscle fibre is covered by a plasma membrane called the sarcolemma and cylindrical structures called myofibrils that are suspended inside the muscle fibre in a matrix called the sarcoplasm (cytoplasm), which

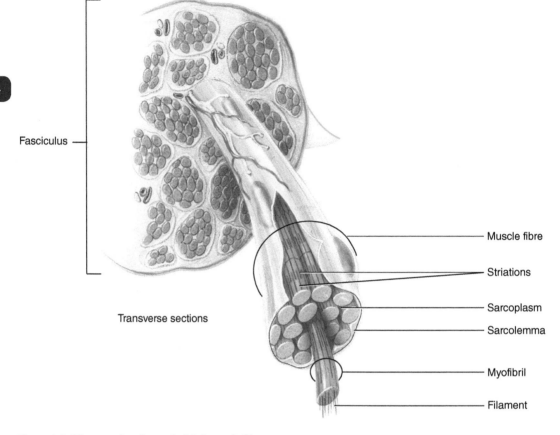

Fasciculus

Transverse sections

Muscle fibre

Striations

Sarcoplasm

Sarcolemma

Myofibril

Filament

Figure 6.2 **Diagram showing a skeletal muscle fibre.**

Table 6.2 **Cellular components of a muscle fibre.**

NAME	FUNCTION
Sarcolemma	Plasma membrane of a muscle fibre that forms T tubules
Sarcoplasm	Cytoplasm of the muscle fibre that contains myofibrils
Myofibril	Consists of bundles of myofilament and plays a key role in muscle contraction
Myofilament	Consists of thick and thin filaments that give muscle tissue its striated appearance and plays a role in muscle contraction
Myoglobin	A reddish-brown pigment (gives muscle tissue its dark-red colour) that stores oxygen for muscle contraction
T tubule	Fluid-filled tubular structure that releases calcium from the sarcoplasmic reticulum
Sarcoplasmic reticulum	Storage site for calcium ions

extends along the entire length of the muscle fibre. The surface of the sarcolemma is scattered with openings that lead into a network of narrow tubules called transverse or 'T' tubules that are filled with extracellular fluid and form passageways though the muscle fibre (Martini and Bartholomew, 2017).

The Sarcoplasm

The sarcoplasm contains multiple mitochondria, which produce large amounts of ATP during muscle contraction (Tortora and Derrickson, 2017) and it is here that the T tubules make contact with a membrane known as the sarcoplasmic reticulum (SR). The SR stores calcium ions (essential for muscle contraction) in structures called cisternae and myoglobin (a reddish-brown pigment that is similar to haemoglobin), which stores oxygen until needed to generate ATP.

The Myofibrils

Myofibrils (which are bundles of myofilaments) are thread-like structures that are found in abundance in the sarcoplasm. The myofibrils play a key role in the muscle contraction mechanism and contain two types of protein filaments: thick filaments composed of myosin and thin filaments composed of actin and two other proteins, tropomyosin and troponin. These filaments form compartments know as sarcomeres, which are the basic functional units of striated muscle fibres (Tortora and Derrickson, 2017), and each myofibril contains approximately 10,000 sarcomeres arranged end to end. The sarcomeres are separated from each other by dense zig-zagging protein-based structures called Z discs.

The Sarcomeres

Extending across each of the thick filaments found within the sarcomere is a dark area known as the A band in the centre of which is a narrow H zone. On either side of the A band there is a lighter coloured area consisting of thin filaments called the I band. The alternating A and I bands give skeletal muscles their striated (striped) appearance.

Episode of Care Child

Muscular dystrophy is a broad term applied to an inherited group of disorders that destroy the muscles by causing muscle fibres to degenerate, shrink in size and eventually die. The muscle fibres that die are replaced with fat and connective tissue.

The most common form of the disease is Duchenne's muscular dystrophy, which is inherited via a flawed gene carried by the mother and results in a lack of protein called dystrophin that plays a part in the structure and function of muscle fibres. The lack of dystrophin causes calcium to leak into muscle fibres and activate an enzyme that causes the muscle fibre to dissolve.

The condition occurs predominantly in males and manifests itself between the ages of 2 and 6 years. The disease is progressive, and most patients are wheelchair bound by the age of 12 years and do not live beyond young adulthood (Marieb and Hoehn, 2015). While treatment in the form of injections of immature muscle cells that produce dystrophin provides some relief (Longenbaker, 2013), there is no known cure.

Recent advances in medical technology have increased the number of people who can be treated at home. Community nurses offer care and support to patients and families they manage tracheostomies, ventilators, feeding tubes, intravenous therapies and many cardiac issues, as well as a range of other complex medical needs.

Siobhan

When Siobhan was born, she was floppy and very weak; she was a small baby. After her birth Siobhan was taken to the neonatal unit for care.

Siobhan was examined by numerous doctors. The medical team carried out a number of assessments and observed how she held her hands to how tall and flexible she was. A lumbar puncture was performed on Siobhan and numerous blood tests were taken.

A diagnosis was finally made by the geneticist who came to see Siobhan and after taking note of a range of symptoms, she ran them through the database of genetic disorders. Siobhan was diagnosed with congenital myotonic dystrophy.

Siobhan is now 8 years old she has mobility problems and is unable to speak as other 8 year olds do. However, she makes known her needs and plays with the other children and her sibling.

Multiple Choice Questions

1. Muscular dystrophy is
    (a) also known as cerebral palsy
    (b) a group of inherited genetic conditions
    (c) a condition that is quickly out lived
    (d) a condition that is cured by steroids

2. Muscular dystrophy is caused by:
   (a) smoking and drinking during pregnancy
   (b) syphilis
   (c) changes in the muscle fibres interfering with muscle function
   (d) a cerebral aneurysm
3. The most common form of muscular dystrophy is:
   (a) Duchenne muscular dystrophy
   (b) facioscapulohumeral muscular dystrophy
   (c) oculophrayngeal muscular dystrophy
   (d) myotonic dystrophy
4. There is no cure for muscular dystrophy:
   (a) true
   (b) false
5. Dystrophin is:
   (a) another name for muscular dystrophy in the older person
   (b) the cause of muscular dystrophy
   (c) a type of blood disease
   (d) muscle protein

Types of Muscle Fibres

Three types of muscle fibres are found in skeletal muscles and are found in varying proportions throughout the body:

- **Slow oxidative fibres** are small, dark-red fibres (due to containing large amounts of myoglobin) that generate ATP by aerobic respiration, make up approximately 50% of skeletal muscle and are capable of slow, prolonged contractions and are not easily fatigued.
- **Fast oxidative–glycolytic fibres** are medium, dark-red fibres that also generate ATP by aerobic respiration, but owing to their high glycogen content are also able to generate ATP by anaerobic glycolysis. Fast oxidative–glycolytic fibres are able to contract and relax more quickly than slow oxidative fibres.
- **Fast glycolytic fibres** are large white fibres (low myoglobin content) that generate ATP mainly by anaerobic glycolysis and provide the most rapid and powerful muscle contractions, but they fatigue easily.

Blood Supply

Skeletal muscles have a very extensive blood supply and receive a total of 1 L of blood each minute, which equates to 20% of the resting cardiac output. This increases to 15–20 L min^{-1} when exercising intensively. As a general rule, each skeletal muscle is supplied by an artery and one or two veins, and each muscle fibre is in close contact with a network of microscopic capillaries within the endomysium.

Clinical Consideration Acute Compartment Syndrome

In the limbs the connections between the muscle fibres and the skeleton are robust; consequently, muscles are commonly isolated in dense collagen-based compartments. These compartments are where the blood vessels and nerves that supply a specific muscle enter.

When an injury to a limb occurs, if the resulting oedema that normally occurs develops within a compartment where there is little room for tissue expansion, the interstitial pressure increases. As pressure within the compartment is higher than that within the capillaries, blood flow, and hence tissue perfusion, slows and may ultimately stop (Harris and Hobson, 2015). This can result in tissue ischaemia and muscle death, with the resultant contents of the affected muscle fibres potentially entering the bloodstream (rhabdomyolysis). Common causes of compartment syndrome include limb fractures, crush injuries, vascular compromise and drug overdoses involving heroin or cocaine.

Early diagnosis of compartment syndrome is essential to avoid long-term disability. Nurses and other members of the multidisciplinary team must have an awareness and understanding of the condition. They must also be aware of the signs and symptoms and initiate immediate appropriate action once compartment syndrome is suspected. Being able to identify those patients who are at greatest risk and offer appropriate analgesia while monitoring them is key element of care.

Skeletal Muscle Contraction and Relaxation

The ability of skeletal muscle to contract is controlled by the body's nervous system, and each muscle fibre is controlled by a motor neurone (nerve cell), which may stimulate a few muscle cells or several hundred depending on the particular muscle and the work it does (Marieb and Hoehn, 2015). Skeletal muscle contracts in response to stimulation by an electrical signal (muscle action potential) delivered by the motor neurone, which is found halfway along the muscle cell, where it terminates at the neuromuscular junction. Here, the muscle fibre membrane is specialised to form a motor end plate.

Although a muscle fibre normally has a single motor end plate, the densely branched motor neurone axons (see Figure 6.3) mean that one motor neurone axon can connect and control many muscle fibres. The motor neurone and the muscle fibres it controls are known as a motor unit.

When a nerve impulse reaches the axon terminals, the neurotransmitter acetylcholine (ACh) that stimulates skeletal muscle is released into the synaptic cleft, which is a small gap that separates the membrane of the nerve cell from the membrane of the muscle fibre (Shier *et al.*, 2018). The synaptic cleft and motor end plate contain acetylcholinesterase (AChE), which breaks down molecules of ACh. The release of ACh results in changes to the sarcolemma that trigger the contraction of the muscle fibre.

Clinical Consideration Botulism

Botulism can arise from the consumption of contaminated or smoked food and is caused by ingestion of spores from the bacterium *Clostridium botulinum,* which is commonly found in soil and water. One of the toxins released from the bacterium prevents the release of ACh at the synaptic terminals of muscle cells and prevents an action potential in the sarcolemma from occurring. If not treated quickly this can result in potentially fatal muscular paralysis. Treatment is with an anti-toxin and the use of mechanical ventilation if the respiratory system is affected (Public Health England, 2019).

Skeletal muscle fibres are stimulated by neurones that control the production of an action potential (electrical impulse) in the sarcolemma by:

- **The release of ACh** – an action potential travels along a motor neurone until it reaches the synaptic terminal where vesicles contained within the synaptic terminal release ACh into the synaptic cleft between the motor neurone and the motor end plate.
- **The binding of ACh at the motor end plate** – the ACh molecules diffuse across the synaptic cleft and bind to ACh receptors on the sarcolemma. This changes the permeability of the membrane and allows sodium ions (Na$^+$) into the sarcoplasm, which triggers the production of a muscle action potential in the sarcolemma.
- **The conduction of action potentials by the sarcolemma** – the action potential spreads across the entire surface of the sarcolemma and then travels down the transverse tubules to the cisternae which encircle the sarcomeres of the muscle fibre. As a result of the action potential travelling across it, the cisternae releases significant amounts of calcium ions (Ca^{2+}) which leads to the initiation of a muscle contraction. Each nerve

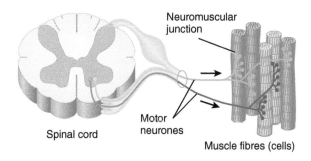

Figure 6.3 **Motor unit.** *Source:* Tortora and Derrickson (2009). Reproduced with permission of John Wiley & Sons.

impulse normally results in one muscle action potential and stages 2 and 3 are repeated if more ACh is released by another nerve impulse.

- **Muscle relaxation** – action potential generation ceases as ACh is broken down by **AChE** and the concentration of calcium ions in the sarcoplasm declines. Once calcium ions return to normal resting levels, muscle contraction will end and muscle relaxation occurs.

Figure 6.4 provides a summary of the steps involved in skeletal muscle contraction and relaxation.

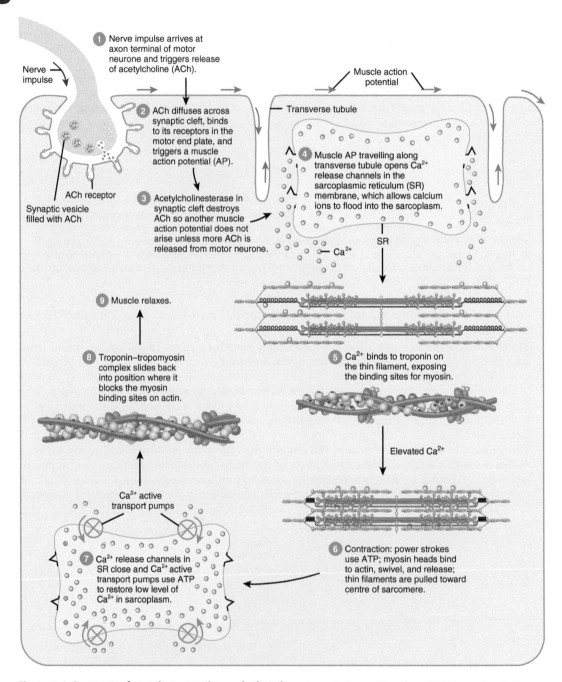

Figure 6.4 Summary of muscle contraction and relaxation. *Source:* Tortora and Derrickson (2009). Reproduced with permission of John Wiley & Sons.

Medicines Management Pyridostigmine

Pyridostigmine is an anticholinesterase agent or AChE inhibitor and is used mainly to enhance neuromuscular transmission and improve muscle strength in voluntary and involuntary muscles of patients with myasthenia gravis. AChE inhibitors inhibit AChE, raising the concentration of ACh at the neuromuscular junction. In so doing they prolong the action of ACh by inhibiting the action of the enzyme AChE (Joint Formulary Committee, 2018).

Cautions and Contraindications

The drug should be used with caution in patients who have asthma, heart disease, epilepsy, Parkinsonism, thyroid disease or stomach ulcer. AChE inhibitors should not be given to patients with intestinal or urinary obstruction.

Adverse effects of pyridostigmine include nausea, vomiting, abdominal cramps, diarrhoea, excessive salivation, sweating, bradycardia and bronchospasm. Adverse effects of the drug may be minimised by precise dosage adjustment.

129

Skills in Practice Electromyography (EMG)/Nerve Conduction Studies

This routine test is performed in specialist hospitals, patient details and consent is required before the procedure. The EMG records the electrical impulses that the muscles produce. The nerve conduction test measures the speed at which impulses travel along a nerve. These tests help to determine how well the nerves and muscles are functioning.

Before the test the patient should:

- Remove any jewellery.
- Wear clothing with short sleeves and/or loose clothing.
- Avoid using lotions and creams before the test.
- Eat and take any medication as normal.

If a patient has a pacemaker or implanted device, fitted details of the pacemaker should be discussed with the doctor or physiologist prior to the test. If the patient has a cardiac defibrillator fitted, this should be communicated with the department before the test, as the test may not be performed.

The appointment for the test is around 45 minutes. There are 3 parts to the test and these are described below. The patient may not need all three parts, this depends on the clinical problem and the findings during the test.

Part 1 Sensory Nerve Testing

The skin is cleaned with an alcohol wipe.

Then the nerves, which supply sensation, are tested using ring electrodes on the fingers or button electrodes on all other parts of the body. For a short time during the test the patient will feel a repetitive tapping/tingling sensation.

Measurements are made between the electrodes using a tape measure and a marker pen, small dots are made on the skin, but these will wash off.

Part 2 Motor Nerve Testing

This test provides a check of the nerve supply to the muscles. There is a tapping/tingling sensation similar to that felt during part 1, caused by a muscle being stimulated. Measurements are taken.

Part 3 EMG Testing

A small needle into the muscles to be tested specifically designed to carry a fine recording wire, the patient may feel a sharp scratch. Any electrical activity whilst the muscle is at rest is examined. The patient is asked to use the muscles so that they can be observed in their pattern of activity. The activity is displayed on a screen and can also be heard on a speaker as a crackling sound. The test may be repeated for different muscles.

The results are available usually within two days of the test being performed. A report is sent to the health care professional who made the referral.

The muscles tested may feel sore for a short time after the examination. The patient is able to continue their activities as normal, including driving after the test.

The nurse may be required to assist the patient before, during or after the test.

Energy Sources for Muscle Contraction

Muscle fibres require an energy source to enable them to contract as and when needed. This is provided initially in the form of ATP, which is stored in the muscle fibre. However, as only small amounts of ATP are stored in the muscle fibre, it is quickly depleted when the muscle is used and needs to be continuously available to power muscles. Therefore, working muscles require additional pathways to produce ATP, and these include:

- **Creatine phosphate:** This is broken down into creatine, phosphate and energy is the energy that is used to synthesise more ATP. Most of the creatine formed is used to resynthesise creatine phosphate and the creatine not used is converted to the waste product creatinine, which is excreted by the kidneys.
- **Anaerobic respiration:** Glycogen is the most abundant energy source found in muscle fibres and is broken down into glucose when it is needed to provide energy for muscle contraction. Glucose is initially broken down into pyruvic acid without the need for oxygen – a process known as glycolysis – and the small amounts of energy that are created by this process are captured by the bonds of ATP molecules.

During intensive muscle activity or when glucose and oxygen delivery are (temporarily) insufficient to meet the muscle requirements, the pyruvic acid generated during glycolysis converts to lactic acid. This pathway is much faster than that provided by aerobic respiration and can provide sufficient ATP for short spells of intensive exercise.

Aerobic Respiration

Approximately 95% of the ATP used at rest and during moderate exercise comes from aerobic respiration involving a series of metabolic pathways that use oxygen – collectively known as oxidative phosphorylation (Marieb and Hoehne, 2015). In order to release energy from glucose, oxygen is necessary; muscles receive this either from the haemoglobin in red blood cells or from myoglobin, a protein that stores some oxygen within the muscle cells. During aerobic respiration, glucose is broken down into carbon dioxide and water. The energy produced by the breakdown of these compounds is captured by the bonds of ATP molecules. While a rich source of ATP is obtained this way, it is a slow process that requires a continuous oxygen and fuel supply to the muscles.

Figure 6.5 provides an overview of the different ATP sources available for muscles.

Oxygen Debt

When the body is moderately active or at rest, the cardiovascular and respiratory systems of the body can usually supply sufficient oxygen to skeletal muscles to support the aerobic reactions of cellular respiration (Shier *et al.*, 2018). However, when more strenuous activity is undertaken and a muscle relies on anaerobic respiration to supply its energy needs, it incurs an oxygen debt (Longenbaker, 2013), which requires the body to dispose of lactic acid and replenish creatinine phosphate in order to repay the debt.

Medicines Management Anabolic Steroids

Anabolic steroids are synthetic substances related to testosterone and promote the growth of skeletal muscle (anabolic) by increasing protein within cells, particularly skeletal muscles and the development of male sexual characteristics (androgenic) – for example, the growth of the vocal cords, testicles (primary sexual characteristics) and body hair (secondary sexual characteristics). Anabolic steroids can be legally prescribed to treat conditions resulting from steroid hormone deficiency, such as delayed puberty, and, owing to their ability to stimulate muscle growth and appetite, diseases that result in loss of lean muscle mass, such as cancer and AIDS. But some athletes, bodybuilders and others abuse these drugs in an attempt to enhance performance and/or improve their physical appearance. Doses taken by users may be 10 to 100 times higher than doses prescribed to treat medical conditions, and the abuse of anabolic steroids may lead to aggression and other psychiatric problems, including extreme mood changes, paranoid jealousy, manic-like symptoms and anger ('roid rage') that may lead to violence. Furthermore, steroid abuse may lead to serious, even irreversible, health problems, including kidney impairment or failure, damage to the liver and cardiovascular problems, including enlargement of the heart, high blood pressure and changes in blood cholesterol leading to an increased risk of stroke and heart attack (National Institute on Drug Abuse, 2019).

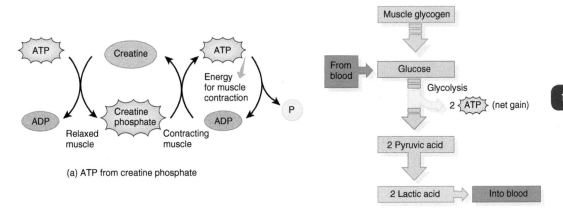

(a) ATP from creatine phosphate

(b) ATP from anaerobic glycolysis

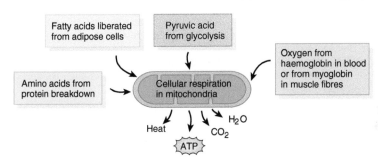

(c) ATP from aerobic cellular respiration

Figure 6.5 **(a–c) Sources of ATP for muscle energy.** *Source:* Tortora and Derrickson (2009). Reproduced with permission of John Wiley & Sons.

Muscle Fatigue

Muscle fatigue occurs when a muscle fibre can no longer contract despite continued neural stimulation and occurs as a result of the oxygen debt that occurs during prolonged muscle activity.

Episode of Care Adult

Fibromyalgia is a chronic pain condition in which people experience aches and pain throughout much of their body as well as a number of other physical and emotional complaints, including headache. Symptoms include:

- widespread body pain
- fatigue
- morning stiffness
- sleep disturbance
- numbness
- headache
- anxiety
- depression
- dry eyes
- irritable bowel syndrome (constipation and diarrhoea)
- urinary urgency
- menstrual problems
- Raynaud's syndrome (a vascular disorder in which blood circulation is restricted in the fingers and toes).

Claire is a 42-year-old mother of three and registered nurse who stopped working three years ago due to disabling pain. 'If I told you about all of my aches and pain, you'd think I was nuts,' she told her new doctor. 'I've had so many tests for my pain, fatigue, bowel problems and numbness. Everything always comes back normal and doctors always tell me I'm just stressed and I need to relax. I don't really want to talk about any of those other problems. I'm just here to get the medications for my migraines and for my depression.'

Most people with fibromyalgia experience a variety of symptoms which often causes health care providers and even patients to wonder if there really is something wrong or if the patient is exaggerating. Patients have often been told that their symptoms were make-believe, or signs of anxiety or stress. Some people, such as Claire, decide it's best to stop mentioning their problems. Unfortunately, not getting a definitive diagnosis usually results in lack of effective treatment, persistent symptoms, frustration and mental health illness. However, research studies now show that the increased pain experienced by people with fibromyalgia is not imaginary, but the result of a lower pain threshold and increased sensitivity to painful stimulation. Those with fibromyalgia feel non-painful sensations the same as other people, but they perceive painful sensations more acutely. For example, when touching a hot object, a person with fibromyalgia detects the heat as painfully hot at a temperature several degrees lower than people without fibromyalgia. Fibromyalgia affects 2% of adults. Women are more likely to have fibromyalgia than men. Some people think of fibromyalgia as a young person's disease, but fibromyalgia affects people throughout their adult years, including elderly patients. Patients with fibromyalgia typically have normal physical examinations, blood tests and x-rays. However, a number of spots on the body have been shown to be very sensitive to pressure in fibromyalgia patients. These areas are called tender points. Health care providers diagnosing fibromyalgia will typically perform a tender point examination. The possible tender points tested are shown in the figure below. With treatment, the number and pain severity of these tender points often decreases.

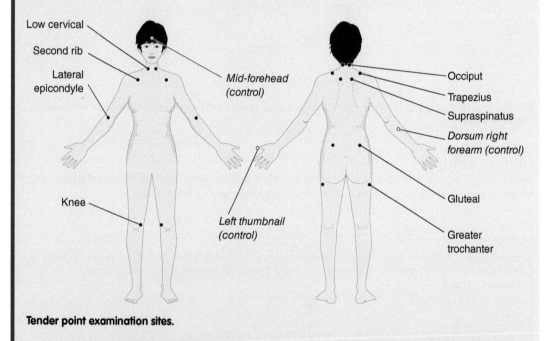

Low cervical
Second rib
Lateral epicondyle
Mid-forehead (control)
Knee
Left thumbnail (control)
Occiput
Trapezius
Supraspinatus
Dorsum right forearm (control)
Gluteal
Greater trochanter

Tender point examination sites.

Treatment for fibromyalgia attempts to ease symptoms and improve quality of life but there is no known cure at present. In Claire's case, her GP advocated the continued use of targeted pain management techniques, e.g. stress management and distraction techniques, aerobic exercise, a nutritionally dense diet and antidepressant medication. Claire's GP also reassured her that with time, her symptoms and need for medication would decrease.

Multiple Choice Questions

1. What is fibromyalgia?
   (a) small tumours in muscle tissue
   (b) a collection of painful symptoms
   (c) extra growth of fibrous tissue
   (d) tendon inflammation
2. Symptoms of fibromyalgia can include:
   (a) irritable bowel syndrome
   (b) excessive tiredness
   (c) stiffness
   (d) all of the above
3. Which of the following biological variables has been demonstrated to contribute to the development and persistence of fibromyalgia?
   (a) exposure to toxins
   (b) physical trauma
   (c) genetic inheritance
   (d) male sex
4. Which of the following is true about the treatment of fibromyalgia?
   (a) physical therapy modalities are strongly encouraged after minor trauma
   (b) first-line treatment in children suspected of having fibromyalgia is pharmacotherapy
   (c) dietary changes are essential to improving symptoms
   (d) screen all patients with fibromyalgia for Chiari malformation, and treat with skull surgery
5. Other conditions can mimic fibromyalgia. Which of these must health care providers rule out to diagnose it?
   (a) lupus
   (b) chronic fatigue syndrome
   (c) rheumatoid arthritis
   (d) all of the above

Organisation of the Skeletal Muscular System

Every one of the body's skeletal muscles is attached at a minimum of two points to bone or other connective tissue. When one part of the skeleton is moved by muscle contraction, related parts have to be steadied by other muscles for the movement to be effective. The origin of a muscle is on the stationary bone where it begins, and the muscle ends at an insertion on the bone that moves (Longenbaker, 2013).

Muscles can be named according to size, shape, location and number of origins, associated bones and the action of the muscle. Table 6.3 provides examples of the criteria used to name muscles.

The body's skeletal muscles can be divided into four areas:

- head and neck muscles
- muscles of the upper limbs (shoulder, arm, forearm)
- trunk (thorax and abdomen)
- muscles of the lower limbs (hip, pelvis/thigh, leg).

The major muscles of the body are listed according to body area in Tables 6.4, 6.5, 6.6 and 6.7 and illustrated in Figures 6.6, 6.7, 6.8 and 6.9.

Figures 6.10 and 6.11 provide an overview of the major muscles of the body.

Skeletal Muscle Movement

Skeletal muscle movement occurs as a result of more than one muscle moving, and muscles invariably move in groups. As a general rule, when a muscle contracts at a joint, one bone remains fairly stationary and the other one moves. The origin of a muscle is on the stationary bone and the insertion of a muscle is on the bone

Table 6.3 Muscle names.

CHARACTER/TERM	DEFINITION	EXAMPLE
Direction		
Transverse	Across	Transversus
Oblique	Diagonal	abdominis
Rectus	Straight	External oblique Rectus abdominis
Shape		
Trapezius	Trapezoid	Trapezius
Deltoid	Triangular	Deltoid
Obicularis	Circular	Obicularis oculi
Rhomboid	Diamond-shaped	Rhomboideus
Platys	Flat	Platysma
Size		
Major	Larger	Pectoralis major
Minor	Smaller	Pectoralis minor
Maximus	Largest	Gluteus maximus
Minimus	Smallest	Gluteus minimus
Longus	Longest	Adductor longus
Latissimus	Widest	Latissimus dorsi
Number of origins		
Biceps	Two origins	Biceps brachii
Triceps	Three origins	Triceps brachii
Quadriceps	Four origins	Quadriceps femoris

Table 6.4 Muscles of the head and neck.

MUSCLE	ORIGIN	INSERTION	FUNCTION
Frontalis	Skin and muscles around eye	Skin of eyebrow and bridge of nose	Wrinkles forehead Raises eyebrows
Occipitalis	Occipital bone	Galea aponeurotica (tendinous sheet)	Tenses and retracts scalp
Obicularis oculi	Maxillary and frontal bones	Skin around eye	Closes eye
Buccinator	Maxillary bone and mandible	Fibres of orbicularis oris	Compresses cheeks
Zygomaticus	Zygomatic bone	Obicularis oculi	Raises corner of mouth
Obicularis oris	Muscles near the mouth	Skin of central lip	Closes and protrudes lips
Masseter	Zygomatic arch/ mandible	Lateral surface of mandible	Closes jaw
Temporalis	Temporal bone		Closes jaw
Pterygoids (medial and lateral)	Sphenoid and maxillary bones	Medial and anterior surface of mandible	Elevates and depresses mandible Moves mandible from side to side
Platysma	Fascia in upper chest	Lower mandible	Draws mouth downward
Stylohyoid	Temporal bone	Hyoid bone	Depresses hyoid bone and larynx
Mylohyoid	Mandible	Hyoid bone	Depresses mandible Elevates floor of mouth
Sternocleidomastoid	Margins of sternum of clavicle	Mastoid region of skull	Flexes the neck Rotates head

Table 6.5 Muscles of the upper limbs (shoulder, arm and hand).

MUSCLE	ORIGIN	INSERTION	FUNCTION
Levator scapulae	Transverse processes of cervical vertebrae	Scapula	Elevates scapula
Trapezius	Occipital bone and cervical and thoracic vertebrae	Clavicle, spine and scapula	Help to extend the head Adduct the scapulae when shoulders are shrugged or pulled back
Rotator cuff muscles: Supraspinatus Infraspinatus Subscapularis Teres minor Teres major	Posterior surface above and below scapula	Humerus	A group of muscles that are responsible for angular and rotational movements of the arm
Pectoralis major	Clavicle, sternum and upper ribs	Humerus	Flexes and adducts the arm

Muscles that move the forearm

MUSCLE	ORIGIN	INSERTION	FUNCTION
Biceps brachii	Between the scapula and forearm	Radius	Flexes and supinates the forearm
Triceps brachii	Between the scapula and forearm	Ulna	Extends the elbow/ forearm
Brachialis	Between humerus and ulna	Ulna	Flexes forearm

Muscles that move the hand and fingers

MUSCLE	ORIGIN	INSERTION	FUNCTION
Flexor and extensor carpi	Base of second and third metacarpal bones	Base of second and third metacarpals	Flexion, extension abduction and adduction at wrist
Flexor and extensor digitorum	Posterior and distal phalanges	Base and surface of phalanges in fingers 2–5	Flexion and extension at finger joints and wrist
Palmaris longus	Distal end of humerus	Fascia of palm	Flexes the wrist

Table 6.6 Muscles of the trunk (thorax and abdomen).

MUSCLE	ORIGIN	INSERTION	FUNCTION
Internal intercostals	Superior border of each rib	Inferior border of preceding rib	Depress the rib cage and contract during forced expiration
External intercostals	Inferior border of each rib	Superior border of next rib	Elevate the ribs during inspiration
Diaphragm	Ribs 4–10, lumbar vertebrae	Tendon near to centre of diaphragm	Contracts to allow inhalation Relaxes to allow exhalation
Internal and external obliques	Between the lower ribs and pelvic girdle	Lower ribs, iliac crest and crest of pubis	Compress the abdominal cavity and protect and support the abdominal organs Rotation of the trunk
Transversus abdominis	Lower ribs, iliac crest and inguinal ligament	Extend horizontally across the abdomen from sternum to crest of pubis	Compress the abdominal cavity, protect and support the abdominal organs Rotation of the trunk
Rectus abdominis	Crest of pubic bone and symphysis pubis	Sternum and ribs	Compress the abdominal cavity, protect and support the abdominal organs Assists with flexing and rotating the lumbar spine

Table 6.7 Muscles of the lower limbs (hip, pelvis/thigh and leg).

MUSCLE	ORIGIN	INSERTION	FUNCTION
Psoas major	Lumbar vertebrae	Femur	Flexes thigh
Gluteus maximus	Sacrum, coccyx and surface of Ilium	Femur and fascia of thigh	Extends thigh at hip
Gluteus medius and minimus	Surface of Ilium	Femur	Abducts and rotates thigh
Adductor group	Pubic bone and Ischial tuberosity	Posterior surface of femur	Adducts, flexes, extends and rotates thigh
Quadriceps femoris group · Rectus femoris · Vastus lateralis · Vastus medialis · Vastus intermedius · Sartorius	Ilium, acetabulum and femur Ilium	Patella Tibia	Extends leg at knee Flexes, abducts and rotates thing to allow crossing of legs
Hamstring group · Biceps femoris · Semitendinosus · Semimembranosus	Femur, Ischial tuberosity, iliac spine	Tibia and head of fibula	Flexes and rotates leg, abducts, rotates and extends thigh
Posterior compartment · Gastrocnemius · Soleus · Tibialis posterior	Femur Fibula and tibia Tibia and fibula	Calcaneus (by means of the Achilles tendon) Second, third and fourth metatarsals	Flexes foot and leg at knee joint Flexes foot Flexes and inverts foot
Anterior compartment · Tibialis anterior · Extensor digitorum longus	Tibia Tibia and fibula	First metatarsal Middle and distal phalanges of each toe	Dorsiflexes and inverts foot Dorsiflexes and everts foot, extends toes
Lateral compartment · Fibularis longus	Fibula and tibia	First metatarsal	Flexes and everts foot

that moves. The action of each muscle is dependent upon how the muscle is attached to either side of a joint and also the kind of joint it is associated with. When a muscle contracts it produces a specific action. However, muscles can only pull; they cannot push, as when a muscle contracts it becomes shorter. Usually, there are at least two opposing muscles (agonist and antagonist) acting on a joint that bring about movement in opposite directions. An agonist or prime mover is a muscle primarily responsible for producing an action, while an antagonist of a prime mover causes muscle movement in the opposite direction; for example, an agonist may cause an arm to bend, while the antagonist will cause it to straighten.

Common types of body movements include:

- extension – a movement that increases the angle or distance between two bones or parts of the body;
- hyperextension – an extension angle greater than 180°;
- flexion – the opposite of extension, in that it is a movement that decreases the angle or distance between two bones and brings the bones closer together and is a common movement of hinge joints – for example, bending the elbow or knee;
- abduction – moving a limb away from the midline of the body;
- adduction – (the opposite of abduction) the movement of a limb towards the midline of the body;
- rotation – a movement common to ball-and-socket joints and is the movement of a bone around its longitudinal axis;
- circumduction – a combination of abduction, adduction, extension and flexion.

Table 6.8 provides a summary of the different actions of muscle movement.

(a)

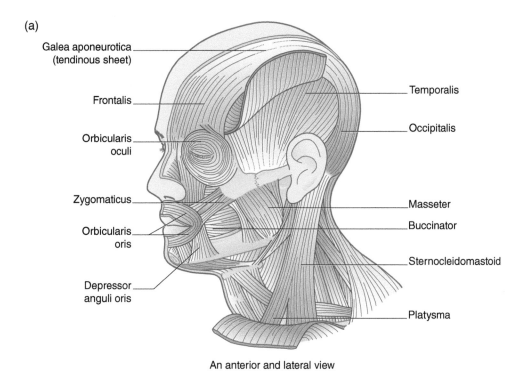

An anterior and lateral view

(b)

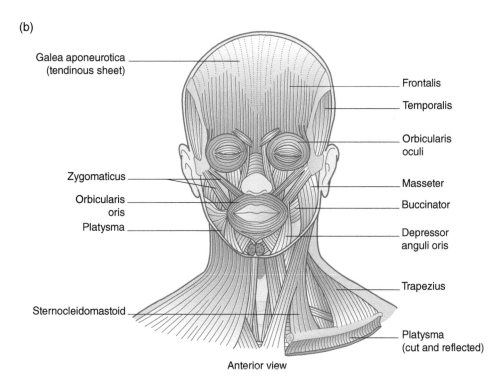

Anterior view

Figure 6.6 **(a, b) Head and neck muscles.** *Source:* Tortora and Derrickson (2009). Reproduced with permission of John Wiley & Sons.

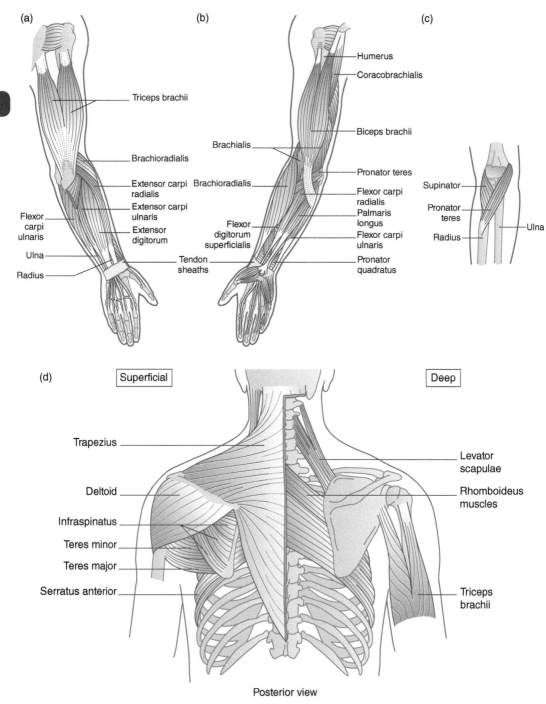

Figure 6.7 **(a–g) Muscles of the upper limbs (shoulder, arm and hand).**

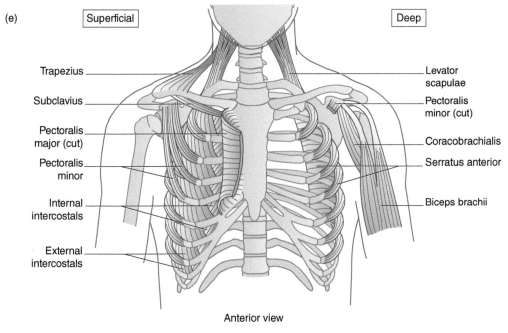

(e)

Superficial — Deep

Trapezius

Subclavius

Pectoralis major (cut)

Pectoralis minor

Internal intercostals

External intercostals

Levator scapulae

Pectoralis minor (cut)

Coracobrachialis

Serratus anterior

Biceps brachii

Anterior view

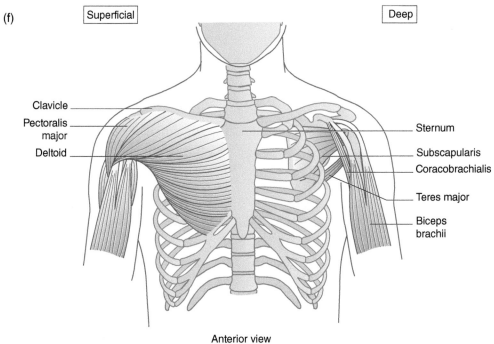

(f)

Superficial — Deep

Clavicle

Pectoralis major

Deltoid

Sternum

Subscapularis

Coracobrachialis

Teres major

Biceps brachii

Anterior view

Figure 6.7 **(Continued)**

140

(g)

Superficial

Deep

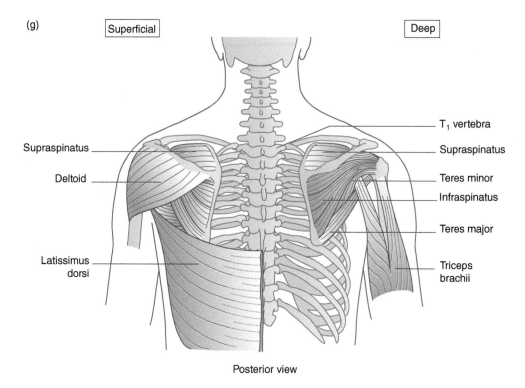

Supraspinatus

Deltoid

Latissimus dorsi

T₁ vertebra

Supraspinatus

Teres minor

Infraspinatus

Teres major

Triceps brachii

Posterior view

Figure 6.7 (Continued)

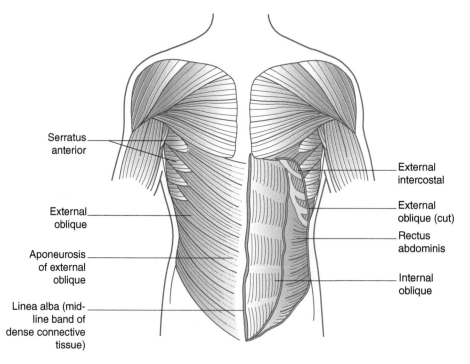

Serratus anterior

External oblique

Aponeurosis of external oblique

Linea alba (mid-line band of dense connective tissue)

External intercostal

External oblique (cut)

Rectus abdominis

Internal oblique

Figure 6.8 Trunk (thorax and abdomen).

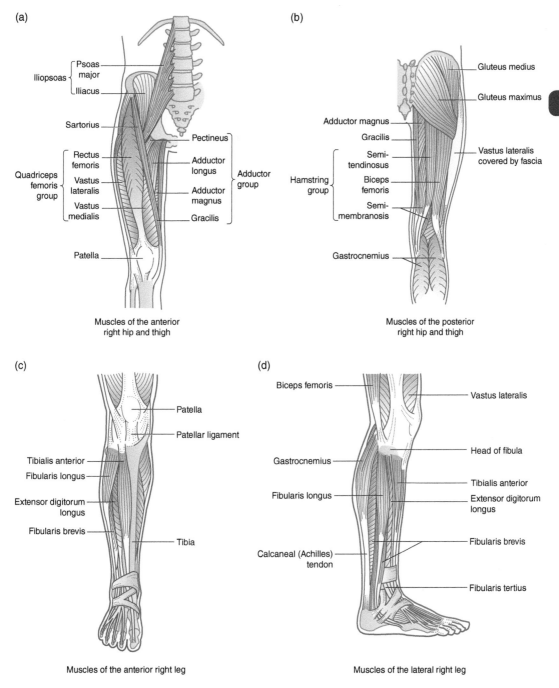

(a)

Iliopsoas { Psoas major
Iliacus

Sartorius

Quadriceps femoris group { Rectus femoris
Vastus lateralis
Vastus medialis

Patella

Pectineus
Adductor longus
Adductor magnus
Gracilis

Adductor group

Muscles of the anterior
right hip and thigh

(b)

Gluteus medius
Gluteus maximus

Adductor magnus
Gracilis

Hamstring group { Semi-tendinosus
Biceps femoris
Semi-membranosis

Gastrocnemius

Vastus lateralis
covered by fascia

Muscles of the posterior
right hip and thigh

(c)

Tibialis anterior
Fibularis longus
Extensor digitorum longus
Fibularis brevis

Patella
Patellar ligament

Tibia

Muscles of the anterior right leg

(d)

Biceps femoris
Gastrocnemius
Fibularis longus
Calcaneal (Achilles) tendon

Vastus lateralis
Head of fibula
Tibialis anterior
Extensor digitorum longus
Fibularis brevis
Fibularis tertius

Muscles of the lateral right leg

Figure 6.9 (a–f) Muscles of the lower limbs (hip, pelvis/thigh and leg).

(e)

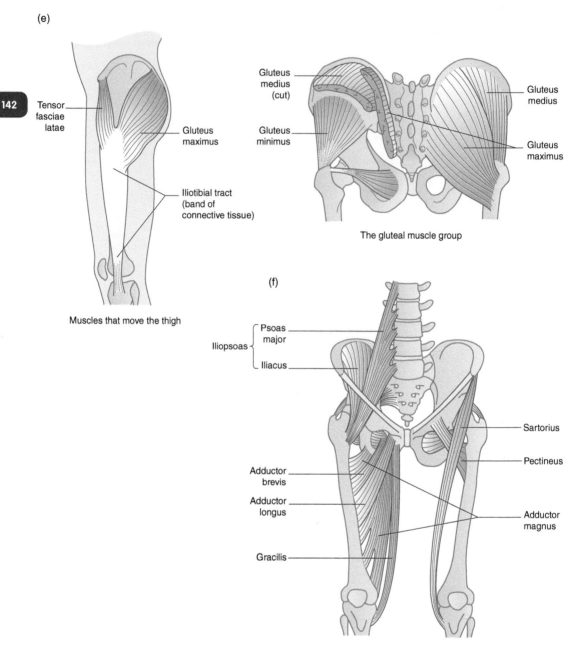

Tensor fasciae latae

Gluteus maximus

Iliotibial tract (band of connective tissue)

Muscles that move the thigh

Gluteus medius (cut)

Gluteus minimus

Gluteus medius

Gluteus maximus

The gluteal muscle group

(f)

Iliopsoas {
Psoas major
Iliacus
}

Sartorius

Pectineus

Adductor brevis

Adductor longus

Adductor magnus

Gracilis

The iliopsoas muscle and the adductor group

Figure 6.9 (Continued)

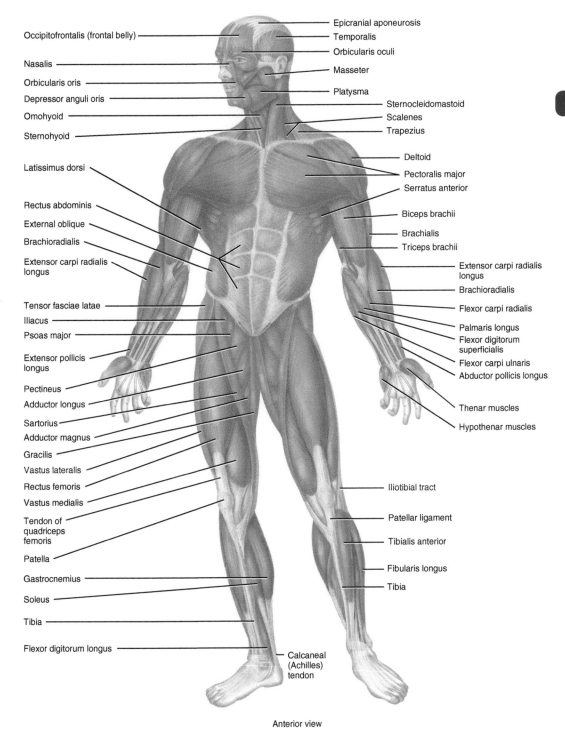

Epicranial aponeurosis
Occipitofrontalis (frontal belly)
Temporalis
Orbicularis oculi
Nasalis
Masseter
Orbicularis oris
Depressor anguli oris
Platysma
Omohyoid
Sternocleidomastoid
Scalenes
Sternohyoid
Trapezius

Deltoid
Latissimus dorsi
Pectoralis major
Serratus anterior

Rectus abdominis
Biceps brachii
External oblique
Brachialis
Brachioradialis
Triceps brachii
Extensor carpi radialis longus
Extensor carpi radialis longus
Brachioradialis
Tensor fasciae latae
Flexor carpi radialis
Iliacus
Palmaris longus
Psoas major
Flexor digitorum superficialis
Extensor pollicis longus
Flexor carpi ulnaris
Abductor pollicis longus
Pectineus
Adductor longus
Thenar muscles
Sartorius
Hypothenar muscles
Adductor magnus
Gracilis
Vastus lateralis
Rectus femoris
Iliotibial tract
Vastus medialis
Tendon of quadriceps femoris
Patellar ligament
Tibialis anterior
Patella
Gastrocnemius
Fibularis longus
Soleus
Tibia
Tibia
Flexor digitorum longus
Calcaneal (Achilles) tendon

Anterior view

Figure 6.10 **Anterior view of the major muscles of the body.** *Source:* Tortora and Derrickson (2009). Reproduced with permission of John Wiley & Sons.

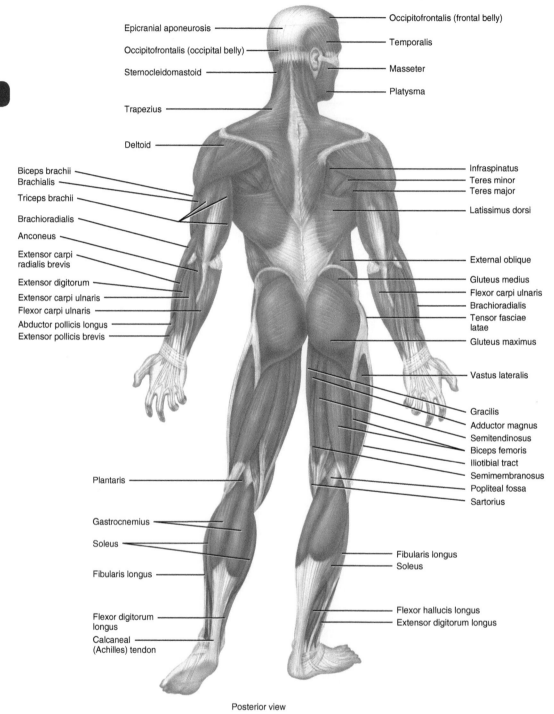

Epicranial aponeurosis

Occipitofrontalis (occipital belly)

Sternocleidomastoid

Trapezius

Deltoid

Biceps brachii
Brachialis
Triceps brachii
Brachioradialis
Anconeus
Extensor carpi
radialis brevis
Extensor digitorum
Extensor carpi ulnaris
Flexor carpi ulnaris
Abductor pollicis longus
Extensor pollicis brevis

Plantaris

Gastrocnemius

Soleus

Fibularis longus

Flexor digitorum
longus
Calcaneal
(Achilles) tendon

Occipitofrontalis (frontal belly)

Temporalis

Masseter

Platysma

Infraspinatus
Teres minor
Teres major

Latissimus dorsi

External oblique

Gluteus medius
Flexor carpi ulnaris
Brachioradialis
Tensor fasciae
latae
Gluteus maximus

Vastus lateralis

Gracilis
Adductor magnus
Semitendinosus
Biceps femoris
Iliotibial tract
Semimembranosus
Popliteal fossa
Sartorius

Fibularis longus
Soleus

Flexor hallucis longus
Extensor digitorum longus

Posterior view

Figure 6.11 Posterior view of the major muscles of the body. *Source:* Tortora and Derrickson (2009). Reproduced with permission of John Wiley & Sons.

Table 6.8 Types of muscle movement.

ACTION	DEFINITION
Extension	Increases the angle or distance between two bones or parts of the body
Flexion	Decreases the angle of a joint
Abduction	Moves away from the midline
Adduction	Moves closer to the midline
Circumduction	A combination of flexion, extension, abduction and adduction
Supination	Turns the palm up
Pronation	Turns the palm down
Plantar flexion	Lowers the foot (point the toes)
Dorsiflexion	Elevates the foot
Rotation	Moves a bone around its longitudinal axis

Episode of Care Child

The growing interest and participation in fitness and recreational events has led to an increase in soft tissue injuries. Common injuries include:

- **Sprains** – a sprain results from the twisting or wrenching of a joint that injures the surrounding tissues, ligaments and blood vessels.
- **Strains** – a strain or pulled muscle occurs from the excessive use or stretching of a muscle. This can result in the tearing of a muscle and/or its tendon.
- **Repetitive strain injury (RSI)** – this refers to a range of disorders that can develop of time and affects muscles, tendons and nerves.

Emily is an 8-year-old girl who has presented to the minor injuries department with a swollen and painful right ankle. Emily's mother reports that during her gymnastics class Emily jumped from a balance beam, landing awkwardly. On examination, Emily's ankle is swollen and discoloured, Emily is complaining of pain and is reluctant to move her ankle or allow it to be examined. A diagnosis of a sprained right ankle is made.

Ankle sprains are one of the most common injuries in children and usually happen when there is a sudden movement or twist resulting in the ligaments that surround the ankle joint to be overstretched.

The RICE principle:

R = Rest to prevent further damage
I = Ice application to reduce inflammation and pain
C = Compression to immobilise and reduce inflammation
E = Elevation above heart level reduces blood flow to the area leading to less inflammation and pain

along with physiotherapy and the use of non-steroidal anti-inflammatory drugs is a recommended conservative treatment to minimise disability and enhance full recovery of muscle functionality after injury (Dauty and Menu, 2017).

In Emily's case, she was told to rest as much as possible, prescribed an oral suspension of paracetamol to control the pain, her right ankle was firmly bandaged from just below the toes to above the ankle. Emily's mum was taught to apply an ice pack to the area every 2–4 hours using ice wrapped in a tea towel and to elevate Emily's right leg on some pillows while she was sitting or lying down. Emily and her mum were also taught some gentle exercises to stretch the ankle joint and minimise stiffness and reassured that Emily should expect to make a full recovery within 1–2 weeks.

Multiple Choice Questions

1. A soft tissue or muscle sprain:
    (a) commonly occurs in women
    (b) is most likely to occur at the wrist
    (c) is increasing in incidence
    (d) always results in loss of function to the affected area

2. RICE stands for:
   (a) relaxation, inertia, compression, elevation
   (b) rotation, ice, colour, education
   (c) rest, ice, compression, elevation
   (d) rest, inspection, colour, eradication
3. A muscle sprain usually involves damage to the muscle and:
   (a) a ligament
   (b) a nerve
   (c) a blood vessel
   (d) all of the above
4. A muscle sprain occurs as a result of:
   (a) a nearby bone fracture
   (b) stretching of adjacent ligaments
   (c) dislocation of a nearby joint
   (d) all of the above
5. Which of the following will minimise the risk of a muscle sprain?
   (a) wearing appropriate and properly fitting footwear
   (b) undertaking warming up exercises prior to commencing physical activity
   (c) building muscle strength
   (d) all of the above

The Effects of Ageing

Generally, the size and power of all muscle tissues within the body decrease as the body ages. This can be attributed to:

- Loss of elasticity to skeletal muscle – as muscles age they lose their elasticity due to a process called fibrosis (Martini and Bartholomew, 2017). Fibrosis causes ageing muscles to develop increasing amounts of fibrous connective tissue, which results in a loss of flexibility, movement and circulation.
- Decrease in size of muscle fibres – as the muscle ages, the number of myofibrils decreases and this results in a loss of muscle strength and an increased tendency for the muscle to fatigue more quickly. This tendency for rapid fatigue also means that, with age, there is a lower tolerance for exercise.
- Age-related reduction in cardiovascular performance – means that blood flow to muscles does not increase with exercise and the ability to recover from muscular injuries decreases and is likely to result in scar tissue formation.

Conclusion

Muscular tissue is either smooth, cardiac or skeletal and is a specialised tissue that is structured to contract. In so doing, it causes movement of bones at a joint or in soft tissues. Through its ability to sustain partial contraction of muscle, the muscular system also plays an important role in maintaining body posture for a long period of time. Skeletal muscle also plays an important role in heat production and is able to adjust heat production in extremes of environmental temperatures.

Glossary

Acetylcholine (ACh): Neurotransmitter responsible for the transmission of a nerve impulse across a synaptic cleft.
Acetylcholinesterase (AChE): Enzyme that breaks down acetylcholine.
Actin: One of the two major proteins of muscle that make up the myofibrils of muscle cells.
Adenosine triphosphate (ATP): Molecule used by cells when energy is needed.
Aerobic: With oxygen.
Anaerobic: Without oxygen.
Antagonist: Muscle that acts in opposition to a prime mover.

Anterior: Pertaining to the front.
Aponeurosis: Membranous sheet connecting a muscle and the part it moves.
Glycogen: A polysaccharide that stores energy for muscle contraction.
Ligament: Strong connective tissue that connects bone.
Myofibril: A bundle of myofilaments that contracts.
Myasthenia gravis: Muscle weakness due to an inability to respond to the neurotransmitter ACh.
Myofibril: Portion of a muscle fibre that contracts.
Myoglobin: A red pigment that stores oxygen for muscle contraction.
Posterior: Pertaining to the back.
Sarcolemma: Plasma membrane of a muscle fibre that forms T tubules.
Sarcoplasm: Cytoplasm of a muscle fibre that contains organelles, including myofibrils.
Tendon: Tissue that connects muscle to bone.
T tubule: Extension of the sarcolemma that extends into the muscle fibre.

References

Dauty M. and Menu, P. (2017) Therapeutic alternatives: principles and results. In Roger, B., Germazi A., Skaf, A. (eds) *Muscle Injuries in Sports Athletes. Sports and Tramatology.* Switzerland: Springer Nature

Harris, C. and Hobson, M. (2015) The management of soft tissue injuries and compartment syndrome. *Orthopaedics II: Spine and Pelvis* 33(6): 251–256.

Joint Formulary Committee (2018) *BNF 75.* London: Pharmaceutical Press.

Logenbaker, S.N. (2017) *Mader's Understanding Human Anatomy and Physiology*, 9th edn. London: McGraw-Hill.

Marieb, E.N. and Hoehn, K. (2015) *Human Anatomy and Physiology*, Global edn. San Francisco, CA: Pearson Benjamin Cummings.

Martini, F.H. and Bartholomew, E.F. (2017) *Essentials of Anatomy and Physiology*, 7th edn. Upper Saddle River, NJ: Pearson Education.

National Institute on Drug Abuse (2019) Drug Facts; Anabolic Steroids. http://www.drugabuse.gov/publications/drugfacts/anabolic-steroids (accessed May 2019).

Public Health England (2019) Botulism. https://www.gov.uk/government/publications/botulism clinical - and -public-health-management (accessed May 2019).

Shier, D., Butler, J. and Lewis, R. (2018) *Hole's Human Anatomy and Physiology*, 15th edn. Maidenhead: McGraw-Hill.

Tortora, G.J. and Derrickson, B.H. (2009) *Principles of Anatomy and Physiology*, 15th edn. Hoboken, NJ: John Wiley & Sons, Inc

Further Reading

Myaware
http://www.myaware.org
Myaware is the name for the Myasthenia Gravis Association. This association offers support to people with myasthenia and their families; they aim to increase public and medical awareness of the condition and to raise funds for research and support staff.

Talk to Frank
http://www.talktofrank.com
Provides friendly confidential information about drugs.

Activities

Multiple Choice Questions
1. How much of the average adult human body is made up of skeletal muscle?
    (a) 40–50%
    (b) 10%
    (c) 30%
    (d) 70%

2. In an isotonic muscle contraction:
   (a) movement of bones does not occur
   (b) both muscle tension and length are changed
   (c) the length of the muscle remains constant
   (d) the muscle tension remains constant
3. The innermost layer of connective tissue surrounding a skeletal muscle is:
   (a) hypodermis
   (b) perimysium
   (c) endomysium
   (d) epimysium
4. Which of the following statement is *not* true of skeletal muscle?
   (a) is under voluntary control
   (b) is not striated
   (c) can have long muscle fibres
   (d) is usually attached to the skeleton
5. The energy for muscle contraction is most *directly* obtained from:
   (a) aerobic respiration
   (b) phosphocreatinine
   (c) anaerobic respiration
   (d) ATP
6. Extension of a muscle:
   (a) decreases the angle
   (b) increases the angle
   (c) is carried out by a flexor
   (d) (b) and (c)
7. The movable attachment of muscle to bone is referred to as:
   (a) the joint
   (b) the origin
   (c) the rotator
   (d) the insertion
8. Skeletal muscles move the body by:
   (a) means of neural stimulation
   (b) pulling on the bones of the skeleton
   (c) using the energy of ATP to form ADP
   (d) activation of enzyme pathways
9. If additional ATP is required, which of the following can be used as an alternative energy source?
   (a) myosin
   (b) troponin
   (c) creatine phosphate
   (d) myoglobin
10. Relaxing and contracting the masseter muscle would mean that you were:
    (a) blinking
    (b) running
    (c) chewing
    (d) bending downwards
11. The intercostal muscles occur in:
    (a) the skull
    (b) ribs
    (c) diaphragm
    (d) pelvis
12. Sarcolemma covers:
    (a) the abdomen
    (b) nerve fibre
    (c) muscle fibre
    (d) none of the above

13. When one muscle bends one part upon the other this is known as:
    (a) abnormal
    (b) regulator
    (c) flexor
    (d) abductor

14. Red muscles are rich in:
    (a) calcium only
    (b) myosin only
    (c) myoglobin and cytochrome
    (d) haemoglobin only
15. What connect bones and muscles together:
    (a) synovial fluid
    (b) tendons
    (c) ligaments
    (d) cartilage

Find Out More

1. Name and describe the three forms of human muscle tissue and list where they are found in the body.
2. Outline how ATP is supplied to muscles.
3. Describe the processes that enable a muscle to contract.
4. Explain how ageing affects skeletal muscle.
5. Describe a neuromuscular junction.
6. Why does skeletal muscle appear striated when looked at under the microscope?
7. What role does calcium play in the muscle?
8. What do anabolic and catabolic mean?
9. What does myalgia mean?
10. What is the other name for the collarbone?

Conditions

The following is a list of conditions that are associated with the muscular system. Take some time and write notes about each of the conditions. You may make the notes taken from textbooks or other resources (e.g. people you work with in a clinical area), or you may make the notes as a result of people you have cared for. If you are making notes about people you have cared for, you must ensure that you adhere to the rules of confidentiality.

Muscular dystrophy

Myasthenia gravis

Fibromyalgia

Tetanus

Rigor mortis

Muscle cramps

Poliomyelitis

Rhabdomyolysis

Sarcoma

Fibrosis

Botulism

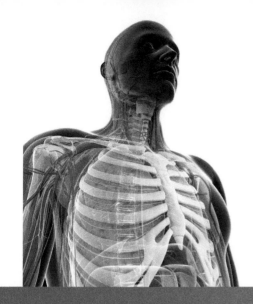

7

The Skeletal System

Suzanne Evans

Test Your Prior Knowledge

- What are the main functions of the skeletal system?
- Which minerals are particularly important with respect to bone?
- What functions does bone perform?
- What makes bones strong?
- What makes bones flexible?

Learning Outcomes

After reading this chapter you will be able to:

- Describe all the functions of the skeletal system.
- Discuss the composition and function of bone as a tissue.
- List the various types of bone and joints.
- Describe the other connective tissues associated with the skeleton and their roles.
- Outline the factors which impact bone density and explain how they do this.

Visit the student companion website at www.wileyfundamentalseries.com/anatomy where you can test yourself using flashcards, multiple-choice questions and more. Instructor companion site at www.wiley.com/go/instructor/anatomy where instructors will find valuable materials such as PowerPoint slides and image bank designed to enhance your teaching.

Fundamentals of Anatomy and Physiology: For Nursing and Healthcare Students, Third Edition. Edited by Ian Peate and Suzanne Evans.
© 2020 John Wiley & Sons Ltd. Published 2020 by John Wiley & Sons Ltd.
Student companion website: www.wileyfundamentalseries.com/anatomy
Instructor companion website: www.wiley.com/go/instructor/anatomy

Body Map

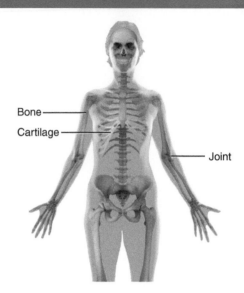

Bone

Cartilage

Joint

Introduction

Viewing a skeleton in the laboratory often creates the impression that bone is a solid, dry, inert material. In fact, in a living organism, bone is a very metabolically active tissue that has a large blood supply and is remodelled constantly. Bones are always in the process of adjusting and readjusting themselves to be able to respond optimally to the stresses placed on them, and the remodelling also plays an important role in calcium homeostasis.

The skeleton provides us with shape, protection for delicate organs, and a system of levers, which, along with muscles, give us the power of movement. This system of levers against which muscles can exert forces, includes joints, which maximise the range of movements we can make. When considering the skeleton as a whole, therefore, it is useful to consider not just the bone, but also the other connective tissues that hold the bone together, form joints and connect muscle to bone to enable movement. These tissues are the cartilage, ligaments and tendons that are found closely associated with bone, and which will also be included in this chapter.

Bone is an engineering wonder; it is a living tissue and yet it has the tensile strength of steel and the compressive strength of concrete, while being light enough to allow us to move around with ease.

While bones are strong enough to protect underlying tissue and support our bodyweight, they are not solid – only the outer edges of bones consist of dense, solid bone, known as compact bone; the interior of the bone contains lighter bone that forms a meshwork rather than a solid mass; this is known as spongy or trabecular bone. Spongy bone, while not as strong as compact bone, is much lighter, due to the many spaces in the bone, avoiding an excessively heavy skeleton. Spongy bone still adds interior strength to a bone, however; the columns of spongy bone acting as 'struts' which stabilise and strengthen the bone structure internally. In the centre of the bones there is a cavity, known as the medullary cavity, which houses the blood vessels supplying the bone, and the bone marrow, responsible for blood cell production (Figure 7.1).

In addition to these functions, bone represents a huge storage depot for minerals such as calcium and phosphate and is involved in the homeostatic regulation of these minerals in the blood. The physiological roles, therefore, that bones perform are:

- **Support and protection.** Bones are vital for providing support and form for soft tissues of the body. Since bone is an incompressible tissue, the skeleton provides the overall body shape, with soft tissues attached to the bones and around the bones.

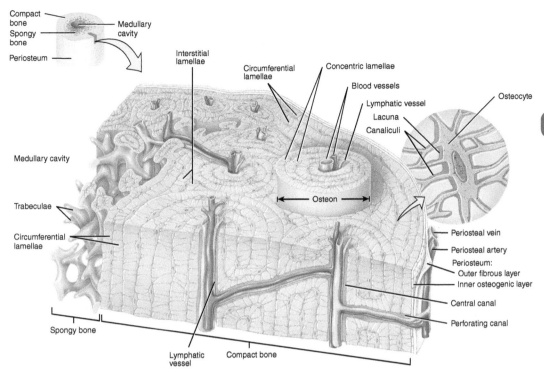

Figure 7.1 Compact and spongy bone, and their blood supply. *Source: Tortora and Derrickson (2009). Reproduced with permission of John Wiley & Sons.*

Bone also provides excellent protection for delicate organs; the skull completely encases the delicate brain, the sternum and ribs protect the lungs and heart, and the vertebrae protect the spinal cord. In the lower body, the pelvis protects the abdominal and reproductive organs. Since bone must also enable movement, some compromises have to be made in the bony protection that encases our organs. So, the organs of the chest are protected by a 'cage' formed by ribs, which allows the chest cavity to expand and contract during breathing, Similarly, the vertebral column, rather than being a rigid bony tube, consists of 26 vertebrae with movable joints between, which allow bending and stretching while still protecting the spinal cord.

- **Enabling efficient movement.** The bones enable purposeful movement, either of the whole body, or just parts of it. Bones of the limbs act as rigid levers which the muscles pull on to move. Without bone to anchor them, the movements produced by muscle would not be able to move the body very far. Other bones form the basis of supportive platforms which, when pulled on by the muscles, maintain body position and posture. Our tendency to walk on two legs instead of four creates a great deal of additional stress for the bones and muscles of the back that keep us in that upright position. The movements that are possible, from tiny, precise finger movements, to whole body movements, are enabled by the moving articulations between bones, known as joints, and the pulling action of the skeletal muscles on the bones that from the joints.

- **Haemopoiesis.** Bones also produce our blood cells – a process known as haemopoiesis. Haemopoiesis occurs only in red bone marrow (also known as myeloid tissue), which in adults fills the internal cavity of the vertebrae, pelvis, ribs, skull and the ends of the long bones. These bones are therefore the source of our red and white blood cells during adult life.

Red bone marrow contains multipotent stem cells. These are cells that are not yet committed to being a particular type of cell, and can still develop to become any of the blood cells. These stem cells give rise to the various white blood cells which are vital for our immune response, and the red blood cells, which are vital for carrying oxygen through the blood to all our tissues. The blood cells need to be regularly re-supplied, as they only last for a limited time in the circulation. Failure of the bone marrow to produce enough blood cells can result in immune deficiency and increased risk of infections if white cells are deficient, or severe anaemia if red cells are deficient. An illustration of the production of blood cells from the red bone marrow stem cells is shown in Chapter 17, the immune system, Figure 17.1.

Not all bones in the adult contain red marrow – some bones, such as the shafts of long bones, are filled with yellow marrow, which is mainly fat.

- **Calcium homeostasis.** Bone is a huge store of the minerals calcium and phosphate, and has the ability to release stored minerals in response to the body's demands. For example, when the level of calcium in the blood decreases, the bones can release calcium into the bloodstream. This release is part of the homeostatic control of plasma calcium levels, which is necessary because calcium ions are so physiologically active, and involves parathyroid hormone as the controller of this system.

A healthy skeleton is therefore vital for many aspects of our normal function.

Clinical Considerations Gout

This is an acute and very painful arthritic condition caused by a problem with uric acid metabolism, resulting in crystallisation of uric acid in the joints, which causes inflammation and pain, which can be severe. Single joints may be affected (often the metatarsophalangeal joint of the big toe), or multiple joints. The big toe is affected more often because uric acid will crystallise more readily at lower temperatures, and the joints of the toe are more likely to get cold.

The condition is related to the metabolism of compounds known as purines, which are part of the molecules that carry the genetic code, DNA and RNA. Uric acid is produced when purines are metabolised, so an abnormally high level of purine metabolism or an inadequate excretion of uric acid by the kidney can cause gout. In most sufferers, the problem is an inability to excrete adequate amounts of uric acid in the urine.

Overproduction of uric acid occurs in disorders that result in a high cell turnover, as purines are released from the dead cells. Cell death caused by chemotherapy can raise uric acid levels, as can excessive exercise and obesity.

An excessive intake of purines due to a diet rich in high-purine foods such as anchovies, sardines, sweetbreads, kidney, liver, meat extracts and alcohol is also associated with an increased risk of gout.

Bone as a Tissue

Bone is a connective tissue, and, in common with all connective tissues, consists of specialised cells embedded in an extracellular matrix. The specialised cells in bone are of three types: osteoblasts, osteoclasts and osteocytes, each performing their own specific roles. The extracellular matrix of bone consists of an organic framework made of the protein collagen, onto which an inorganic 'cement' of calcium salts is laid in successive layers. The result is a material that is hard, rigid and strong (due to the calcium salts), but also flexible (due to the collagen). These properties result in a bone which has very good tensile strength (this can be tested by trying to snap a long bone along its length), good compressive strength (this can be tested by trying to compress a bone by placing weight on top of it) and good flexibility (this can be tested by observing how much a bone will bend before it snaps). Healthy bone will contain collagen and calcium salts in the correct proportions and will display all these characteristics. Diseases which affect the production of normal collagen in the bone will result in bones which lack the normal flexibility and therefore break more easily when large forces are placed on them. An example of this is the inherited disorder brittle bone disease (osteogenesis imperfecta). A lack of calcium salts in the bone will result in bones that are softer than normal and will bend when large forces are placed on them. An example of this is childhood rickets, which occurs as a result of inadequate active vitamin D. Perhaps the most common disorder though, is one where the balance of collagen to calcium salts is normal, but the density of bone is low; the bones are not as compact and dense as they should be, a disorder known as osteoporosis. It is important to understand that in osteoporosis the bone composition is normal (unlike diseases such as brittle bone disease or rickets), but there is not enough bone present to resist all the stresses placed on the skeleton, and fractures become more of a risk.

Bone is not simply an impressively strong and flexible material – it is also a dynamic and responsive tissue, which is constantly being broken down and renewed. This turnover of bone is mainly as a result of another unique feature of bone – it's piezoelectric properties. Materials which show a piezoelectric effect can generate charge, and therefore electricity, in response to mechanical stress. When a mechanical stress is placed on a bone, therefore, the bone generates charge along the lines of greatest stress, or load. This charge stimulates the building of more bone along those stress lines. In this way, each bone strengthens itself to meet the loads that are being placed on it. This is why loading bones by taking regular weight-bearing exercise is so important for bone health – the load on the bones is what generates the signals which lead to stronger bones. Removing any kind of weight bearing exercise, by enforced bed rest for example, leads to a rapid reduction in bone density.

The functions of bone are carried out by the three bone cell types:

Osteoblasts

Osteoblasts synthesise the organic matrix of bone (the collagen) and then they control the deposition of calcium salts onto the collagen to create hardened bone. These cells are therefore responsible for the creation of new bone and the repair of fractured bone.

Osteoclasts

Osteoclasts are large cells which seal themselves onto an area of bone and secrete enzymes and acid onto the bone to dissolve it. The action of osteoclasts therefore removes bone and releases minerals from the bone into the blood stream. Osteoclast action is also the first step in bone renewal and repair; first the osteoclasts pass over the bone to be repaired and take away the surface, and then osteoblasts follow in their wake, creating new bone on the freshly cleaned surface.

The density of bone will therefore depend on the balance of osteoblast and osteoclast activity; if osteoclasts are more active than osteoblasts, there will be a loss of bone density, and if osteoblasts are more active than osteoclasts, there will be an increase in bone density. Various factors are known to influence the activity of one or other of these cells, and therefore the bone density, and more are being discovered as research on bone physiology progresses. The most important factors are shown in Table 7.1

Osteocytes

These cells start off as osteoblasts, but, during the formation of compact bone, they begin to change their form and develop long, finger-like processes. They then become sealed into the compact bone, as new bone is laid down around them, and their cell processes extend through small canals in the bone and connect with those of other osteocytes. Osteocytes can be seen in Figure 7.1, positioned along the concentric rings of the compact bone, with their cell processes extending to contact one another. Osteocytes therefore form a living network that extends throughout compact bone, capable of detecting and signalling changes in the bone. The functions of osteocytes are still not fully understood, but they are believed to be the cells which convert mechanical stress on the bone into electrical signals. The cells, sealed inside the bone matrix, are ideally positioned to detect the size and direction of the forces placed on the bone, making osteocytes the source of the piezoelectric properties of bone.

Table 7.1 **Factors affecting bone density.**

CAUSE BUILDING OF BONE, EITHER DUE TO INCREASED OSTEOBLAST OR DECREASED OSTEOCLAST ACTIVITY	CAUSE RESORPTION OF BONE, EITHER DUE TO DECREASED OSTEOBLAST OR INCREASED OSTEOCLAST ACTIVITY
Adequate oestrogen level	Decreased oestrogen level
Sufficient mechanical stress (weight-bearing activities)	Insufficient weight-bearing activities
Sufficient dietary calcium intake	Insufficient dietary calcium intake
Sufficient vitamin D	Insufficient vitamin D
Growth hormone	Parathyroid hormone

Medicines Management Bisphosphonates

 Fractures, particularly of the hip and the vertebrae, are much more common in post-menopausal women and older men with osteoporosis. The drugs known as bisphosphonates, which include alendronate and zoledronate, can reduce the occurrence of these fractures drastically. The drugs can be taken orally, or given as an infusion once a year. They act by attaching to the calcium salts in the matrix of bone tissue, and when osteoclasts start to resorb the bone, the drug is absorbed by the osteoclast, and interferes with its function by stopping it from sealing itself onto the bone, and also shortening the life of the osteoclasts. This tips the balance in favour of osteoblast activity, and helps to increase bone density. Because osteoclast activity is important in bone remodelling, there is a lower rate of remodelling in the bone when these drugs are used.

Bisphosphonates are also used in post-menopausal women who have been treated for breast cancer, as they have been found to reduce the spread of the cancer to bone.

In common with all drugs, the bisphosphonates have side effects, including osteonecrosis of the jaw, a condition in which the bone of the jaw starts to die, with the loss of teeth, and the need for dental supportive therapy. This is more likely with high dose infusion. Anyone due to start bisphosphonate therapy is advised to get any required dental work completed before starting on the drug. The most common side effect of infusion of these drugs, however, is flu-like symptoms occurring within 24 hours of the infusion and resolving after a day or two.

Other Connective Tissues Closely Associated with the Skeletal System

Connective tissues are characterised by specialised cells embedded in an extracellular matrix. The matrix gives the connective tissue its strength and resilience and the cells make and repair the matrix. Besides bone, the connective tissues that are intimately associated with the skeleton are cartilage, ligaments and tendons, and an examination of the function of the skeleton would be incomplete without these connective tissues. Collagen features strongly in the extracellular matrix of each of these tissues – closely packed collagen fibres providing the strength required for these tissues to resist the forces they are subjected to, and to provide a certain amount of elasticity too. These tissues do not have their own blood supply (they are avascular), which has implications for healing when they are damaged. They receive nutrients by diffusion from blood vessels supplying nearby structures, and from joint fluid, in the case of the cartilage found in joints.

Cartilage

This tissue forms some structures in the body (for example, the outer ear and tip of the nose), and it provides vital protection and cushioning between bones at various joints. Roughening and erosion of cartilage that occur with wear and tear in the later years of life is the first step in the joint inflammation and deterioration that we recognise as osteoarthritis.

There are three types of cartilage:

- **Hyaline cartilage**. This cartilage is adapted for protecting bones from the effects of friction as they move against each other or other structures. Hyaline cartilage has a surface that is smooth and glassy. This greatly reduces friction during movement, as it allows the cartilage-covered surfaces to slide over each other easily. Hyaline cartilage is found covering the ends of bones at each movable joint, at the tips of the ribs, the tip of the nose and forming most of the foetal skeleton.
- **Elastic cartilage**. This cartilage is similar in appearance to hyaline cartilage, but under a microscope, fibres of the protein elastin can be seen in the extracellular matrix. The elastin gives the cartilage the ability to snap back to its original position when it is pulled out of shape. This cartilage is vital to maintain the shape of structures which are regularly bent or stretched in some way as part of their function, such as the epi-glottis – a flap of cartilage located above the larynx that folds down to cover the larynx whenever swallowing occurs. This prevents food from entering and blocking the airways. The outer ear of humans and other mammals consists of elastic cartilage, maintaining the shape of the ear.
- **Fibrocartilage**. This form of cartilage forms a transition between cartilage and ligament. It contains a high proportion of collagen, which while present in many connective tissues, is at a higher concentration and in

two forms (type I and type II) in fibrocartilage. This makes this cartilage strong, reasonably elastic and resistant to compression. It is found forming the outer edge of the intervertebral discs (known as the annulus fibrosus) and the menisci in the knee joint. In these locations this cartilage forms a spongy pad, cushioning joints which take a great deal of weight. Fibrocartilage also forms the pubic symphysis – the anterior joint between the pelvic bones.

Ligaments

These are the strong 'straps' that connect bones together. They can be seen wrapping across a joint between the bones that form the joint. The number and tightness of the ligaments at a movable joint will determine both its stability and its range of motion. A more stable joint will have many ligaments holding the bones in position but will have a more limited range of motion for the same reason. People who have unusually lax, stretchable ligaments will have the ability to 'hyper-extend' their joints, a property commonly referred to as double-jointedness.

Tendons

Tendons are the dense connective tissue structures that anchor muscles to bone, enabling the contraction of a muscle to result in the movement of a bone, and the bending or straightening of a joint. Tendons are also slightly elastic, so that sudden strong muscle contractions are less likely to damage the tendon or the bone, but they are also strong enough to endure the powerful forces that muscles can generate, and transmit those forces into movement of the bones.

Episodes of Care Mental Health

Musculoskeletal disorders, particularly when they are painful and disabling, can induce or exacerbate mental health disorders. Pain always comes with an element of negative emotion as part of the experience, and this, combined with limitation of normal activities can be very depressing for the sufferer. This can feed a vicious cycle, in which lowered mood intensifies the pain, and reduces motivation for the sufferer to follow rehabilitation regimes, etc.

A musculoskeletal disorder lasting longer than 12 weeks is considered chronic. People who suffer from chronic pain symptoms often report feelings of fatigue, being 'fed up' with their symptoms, and a sense that their pain is never going to end. All of this has the potential to further exacerbate low mood and increase the risk of the injury becoming a long-term disability.

Folomi is a 36-year-old with two children under the age of 8 years. She works as a care assistant for a large residential care home. Five months ago, she sustained a back injury at work and since then has been unable to work due to the pain and restricted mobility. Folomi saw the practice nurse and told her that she feels down and tired all the time, and the pain is non-stop. She says there are days that she does not even want to get out of bed and if it was not for her children she would not bother. Folomi is tearful and tells the nurse she feels she cannot go on anymore as it is all too much.

The nurse undertakes a physical and psychological assessment of Folomi's needs, reviews her pain medication, refers her to the community mental health nursing team for an appointment that day, makes a referral to the physiotherapist, contacts the social worker (with Folomi's permission) and puts her in touch with a local support group.

Multiple Choice Questions

1. Preventing chronicity and reducing the impact of musculoskeletal disorders can:
   - (a) exacerbate the person's condition
   - (b) improve the person's mental health
   - (c) cause the person further distress
   - (d) lead to negative care outcomes
2. Exercise has been shown to:
   - (a) have a positive impact on mental health
   - (b) reduce the risk of high blood pressure
   - (c) reduce fatigue
   - (d) all of the above

3. Common signs and symptoms of depression include:
   (a) hypertension, tachycardia and palpitations
   (b) reduced urinary output and nausea
   (c) low mood, lack of interest or pleasure in activities, sleep disturbance, feelings of worthlessness or guilt
   (d) alopecia, nail biting a sense of euphoria
4. Musculoskeletal disorders:
   (a) include any injury, damage or disorder of the joints or associated tissues
   (b) is a term that is only used when the person cannot stand unaided for long periods of time
   (c) can only be diagnosed by a physiotherapist
   (d) can only be diagnosed by an occupational therapist
5. It is estimated that:
   (a) two thirds of people will experience a mental health disorder, such as anxiety and/or depression
   (b) 1 in 6 people will have experienced anxiety and/or depression in the last week
   (c) a and c
   (d) none of the above

Clinical Considerations Knee Reconstruction

The knee joint bears a lot of weight and often degenerates in the later years of life, particularly in people who have been active in sports. As a hinge joint, the knee is damaged by twisting actions such as often occur when playing football, when forcing the knee joint to twist can tear the ligaments which hold it in place and the fibrocartilage pads in the joint (the menisci). Over time and use therefore, the articular cartilage at the ends of the femur and tibia can wear away, the menisci can tear, and one or more of the ligaments that stabilise the joint (the collateral ligaments and the anterior and posterior cruciate ligaments) can tear. There are now surgical options to repair the joint, and its associated ligaments and cartilage:

- The articulating surfaces of the femur and tibia can be replaced with metal or some other hardwearing material, in a procedure known as knee replacement surgery.
- Meniscal injuries, if not too severe, may heal on their own, but bigger tears, particularly in the inner portion of the meniscus without a blood supply, can be surgically trimmed or repaired.
- Injury to the cruciate ligaments of the knee can be surgically repaired by taking a graft from the tendon of nearby muscle. These knee reconstruction procedures are performed by keyhole surgery in the joint, known as arthroscopy, and can be done quite quickly. The post-surgical recovery however, may be prolonged, due to the slow healing rate of cartilage, tendons and ligaments.

Bone Formation

The template for the bones forms *in utero*, with hyaline cartilage 'models' of the bones. By the end of the third month of pregnancy, the template for the skeleton is completely formed, but consists almost entirely of hyaline cartilage. This cartilage is gradually replaced by bone, a process known as ossification, which begins with calcification of the cartilage, followed by osteoblast invasion and bone creation to replace the cartilage. Because it occurs inside a cartilage template, this process is known as endochondral ossification (Figure 7.2) and is the way in which most of our bones are formed. During the ossification process, which starts at the centre of the cartilage and moves out, blood vessels grow into the cavity of the bone. In the case of a long bone, as shown in Figure 7.2, by the time the bone is fully developed, the only remaining cartilage is at the two bone ends, and a narrow strip between the end and the shaft of the bone. The cartilage covering the ends of the bone becomes the articular cartilage, reducing friction and protecting the bone end at the joint, and the strip of cartilage that separates the bone end from the shaft acts as a growth point, allowing the bone to elongate from this point as the person grows. This strip is called the growth plate or the epiphyseal plate.

Because the ossification of the entire skeleton is not complete by birth, infants are born with large amounts of cartilage. They also have a greater number of bones than adults, but some bones fuse together during maturation, resulting in the normal number of bones by adulthood. The bones of babies and children are softer and more porous than an adult's, but become harder and denser with age, reaching their peak density at age 20–30.

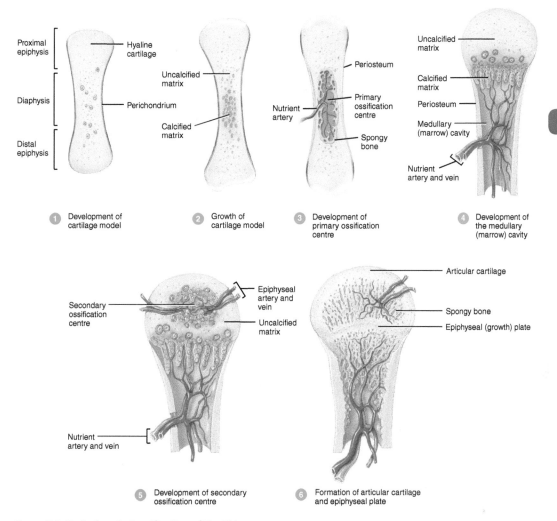

Figure 7.2 **Endochondral ossification of the tibia.** *Source:* Tortora and Derrickson (2009). Reproduced with permission of John Wiley & Sons.

Bone Growth

Growth in stature comes about because the bones of the limbs grow in length. This longitudinal growth is accompanied by an increase in the thickness of bones, so the body proportions are maintained as an individual grows.

Growth in bone length occurs at the cartilage of the epiphyseal plate. In early puberty, the chondrocytes in the cartilage divide continuously, creating new cartilage on the side of the epiphyseal plate closest to the end of the bone, while osteoblasts invade the cartilage from the shaft side of the plate, ossifying the tissue. In this way, the cartilage plate advances towards the bone end, while the bone grows in length as the trailing edge of the epiphyseal plate ossifies (Figure 7.3).

Growth of the long bones ceases when the division of chondrocytes in the leading edge of the plate slows down and eventually stops, towards the end of puberty. The ossification of the epiphyseal growth plate continues, and the plate finally becomes fully ossified when the cartilage front stops advancing. Both the growth spurt that occurs during puberty and the closure of the epiphyseal plate at the end of puberty are driven by the sex hormones; oestrogen in women and testosterone in men (Weise *et al.* 2001).

Circumferential growth of bone occurs on the outer surface of the bone. Osteoblasts lay down new bone on the outer bone surface in the concentric layers seen in compact bone. Meanwhile, osteoclast activity on the inner surface of the bone (in the bone cavity) removes bone. In this way, the size of cavity increases with the overall circumference of the bone (Figure 7.4).

(a) Radiograph showing the epiphyseal plate
of the femur of a 3-year-old

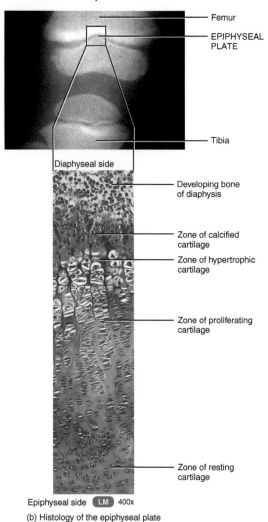

Diaphyseal side

Femur

EPIPHYSEAL
PLATE

Tibia

Developing bone
of diaphysis

Zone of calcified
cartilage

Zone of hypertrophic
cartilage

Zone of proliferating
cartilage

Zone of resting
cartilage

Epiphyseal side LM 400x

(b) Histology of the epiphyseal plate

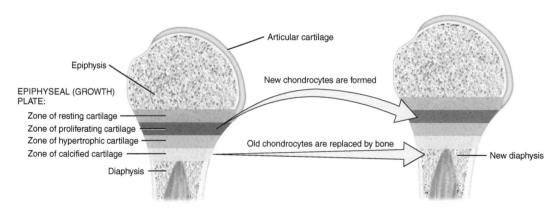

Articular cartilage

Epiphysis

New chondrocytes are formed

EPIPHYSEAL (GROWTH)
PLATE:
Zone of resting cartilage
Zone of proliferating cartilage
Zone of hypertrophic cartilage
Zone of calcified cartilage

Old chondrocytes are replaced by bone

New diaphysis

Diaphysis

(c) Lengthwise growth of bone at epiphyseal plate

Figure 7.3 **Long bones grow in length from the cartilaginous epiphyseal plates.** *Source:* Tortora and Derrickson
(2014). Reproduced with permission of John Wiley & Sons.

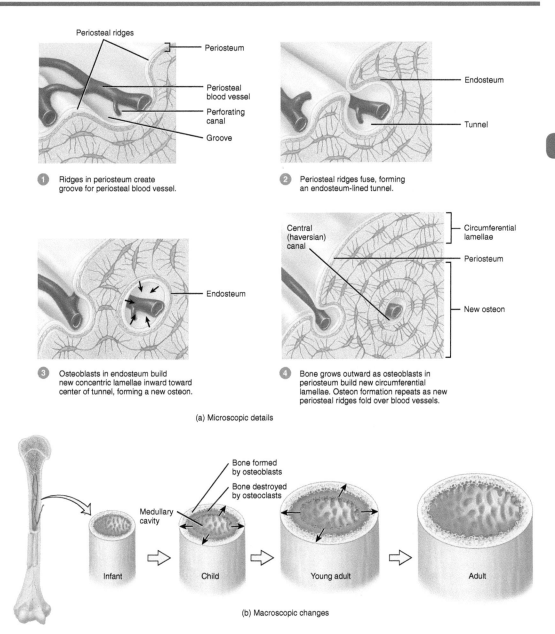

Periosteal ridges

Periosteum

Periosteal blood vessel

Perforating canal

Groove

① Ridges in periosteum create groove for periosteal blood vessel.

Endosteum

Tunnel

② Periosteal ridges fuse, forming an endosteum-lined tunnel.

Endosteum

③ Osteoblasts in endosteum build new concentric lamellae inward toward center of tunnel, forming a new osteon.

Central (haversian) canal

Circumferential lamellae

Periosteum

New osteon

④ Bone grows outward as osteoblasts in periosteum build new circumferential lamellae. Osteon formation repeats as new periosteal ridges fold over blood vessels.

(a) Microscopic details

Bone formed by osteoblasts

Bone destroyed by osteoclasts

Medullary cavity

Infant   Child   Young adult   Adult

(b) Macroscopic changes

Figure 7.4 **Bones increase in width but maintain the same proportion of compact bone to medullary cavity.**
Source: Tortora and Derrickson (2014). Reproduced with permission of John Wiley & Sons.

Bone Remodelling

The removal and renewal of the bone (remodelling), continues throughout adult life. Whether this remodelling process results in loss of bone or maintenance and strengthening of bone will be determined by the conditions the body is exposed to, many of which are within our control (Table 7.1). Lifestyle choices are important when it comes to ensuring a healthy skeleton into old age.

Episodes of Care Child

Perthes disease is a rare condition affecting the hip joint in children. Although its cause is not fully understood, it results from a temporary disruption of the blood supply to the head of one or both femurs. This loss of blood flow results in death of bone cells (osteonecrosis) and the head of the femur becomes very inflamed and painful. Over time, the dead bone is removed, and the head of the femur can become misshapen and weakened, resulting in poor articulation with the hip socket and arthritis of the hip. If allowed, the bone will regrow and the joint may recover normal function. The first sign of Perthes disease in a child is usually pain in the hip, groin or leg, often accompanied by a noticeable limp.

Kylie was 8 years of age when the school nurse contacted her parents to report that she had been consulted by Kylie's physical education teacher because Kylie had been complaining of pain in her right groin, thigh and knee during class. Kylie had a limp with a restricted range of hip movement on the right side. The nurse took a careful history and discovered that Kylie had been experiencing the pain on and off for a number of months.

Just over 60% of children with Perthes disease will recover without any treatment, but some may need additional treatment to ensure that the head of the femur is protected and kept in its correct position to allow it to regenerate. This treatment ranges from refraining from activities which stress the joint and doing regular range of motion exercises to wearing a leg brace for several weeks, keeping the hips in the ideal position for recovery.

Kylie's parents took her to see the family GP, who examined Kylie to assess whether her leg rotation was normal, and whether there was any muscle wasting on the affected side. Kylie had some restricted motion – she had difficulty rotating her right leg, and her gluteus muscles on the right side showed some wasting (they were smaller than the left side). Kylie was referred to an orthopaedic specialist for treatment.

A physiotherapy programme using muscle strengthening and stretching exercises was commenced, to improve range of motion and increase muscular strength around the affected joint.

Kylie was carefully followed up by her orthopaedic specialist, to ensure that she received prompt treatment if her condition required it. She attended the orthopaedic clinic every 4 months for examinations and x-rays. After 12 months of physiotherapy and follow up, Kylie's condition had improved and she was not suffering any pain in her hip or leg. The femoral head appeared larger and more regularly shaped on X-ray, and Kylie was discharged from specialist care.

Multiple Choice Questions

1. A condition that is said to be idiopathic means:
   (a) it is an infectious condition
   (b) it is due to an immune disorder
   (c) it only affects Caucasians
   (d) the cause is unknown
2. The head of the femur forms part of which type of joint?
   (a) hinge
   (b) ball and socket
   (c) saddle
   (d) condyloid
3. More than half of the children with Perthes disease:
   (a) will require surgical intervention
   (b) will be unable to attend school
   (c) return to normal activities within a few years
   (d) require hospitalisation for enforced bed rest
4. Diseases in the joint cause pain as a result of:
   (a) inflammation in the joint space
   (b) activation of nerves supplying nearby muscles
   (c) movement of the joints stretching ligaments
   (d) none of the above
5. Stretching exercises are likely to increase the flexibility of:
   (a) tendons
   (b) ligaments
   (c) cartilage
   (d) a and b

Episodes of Care Adult

75-year-old Deepak Singh had replacement hip surgery after suffering for years with stiffness and difficulty walking. During the surgery, the head of Deepak's femur was removed, and replaced with a metal ball that was attached by a shaft extending down into the medullary cavity of the femur. The socket of the ball and socket joint was also lined with metal.

Deepak recovered well from the surgery and was soon discharged home to the care of his wife and daughter to complete his recovery. One week after he returned home, he noticed increased pain in the hip, and was a little feverish. He returned to his GP, who called the hospital, and Deepak was readmitted to the orthopaedic ward. After a bone scan, a diagnosis of osteomyelitis (infection of the bone) was made, and aggressive antimicrobial treatment was started. The antimicrobials were chosen for their effectiveness against the bacteria most likely to be infecting the bone, such as *Staphylococcus aureus*, because identifying the infectious organism would require a bone biopsy. In the meantime, Deepak's surgeon would have to make a decision about whether to operate again and remove the prosthetic hip to ensure the infection could be completely cleared.

Osteomyelitis is a bone infection that can occur after trauma (particularly open fractures) or surgery on bones and joints. Implant-related bone infections, occurring after joint prosthesis (hip, knee, shoulder, ankle, etc.) or osteosynthesis (plates, screws, nails implant for fractures or osteotomies) are one of the most challenging complications in orthopaedic and trauma surgery. The condition often requires complex treatment in specialised centres, to reduce the risk of an infection becoming chronic. Osteomyelitis after surgery often causes no obvious signs and symptoms, making early detection and treatment a challenge, and often it will require surgery to remove the diseased or dead tissue, followed by prolonged antibiotic therapy (6 weeks or more). Fortunately, it is a relatively rare occurrence.

Multiple Choice Questions

1. Why does orthopaedic surgery increase the risk of osteomyelitis?
   (a) the anaesthetic used in the surgery slows the immune response
   (b) the bone blood flow is reduced after the surgery, making infection more likely
   (c) the surgeon's instruments often have bacteria on them, which can transfer to the bone
   (d) the opening up of the medullary cavity during surgery exposes the inner bone to possible infection
2. Why was antimicrobial treatment started before the infectious agent was identified?
   (a) antimicrobial drugs are equally effective against all bacteria
   (b) it would be impossible to get a sample of infectious tissue or fluid
   (c) treatment needed to start immediately, rather than waiting for a culture study to identify the bacteria.
   (d) the staff would have been too busy to take samples and send them to the lab
3. What advantage does bone have over cartilage when it comes to recovering from infection and healing?
   (a) a good blood supply
   (b) a rigid structure
   (c) a store of calcium
   (d) ability to move
4. What is the average life of a replacement hip?
   (a) about 15 years
   (b) about 20 years
   (c) about 40 years
   (d) none of the above
5. Where is the bacteria *Staphylococcus aureus* normally found?
   (a) mainly on undercooked meat
   (b) in poultry and eggs
   (c) on the skin of humans
   (d) mainly on instruments and surfaces

Bone Fractures

Bone is one of the few tissues with the capacity to heal completely, replacing damaged tissue with new, fully functional bone rather than with scar tissue. It is therefore able to regenerate itself after a fracture in a way similar to the initial formation of bone during development. The copious blood supply to bone is essential in fracture healing, bringing phagocytic white blood cells to the area to remove any bone fragments and dead and dying cells and to protect against infection. The regrowth of any blood vessels that were damaged is also vital for complete healing to occur (Marsell and Einhorn 2011). The steps of the healing process after a fracture of the bone are listed in Figure 7.5 below.

The broken bone ends will be stabilised somewhat by the formation of the cartilaginous callus, and fully stabilised with the formation of the hard bony callus. At this point the bone will be able to start bearing weight again. The remodelling of bone from the rather disorganised bone of the hard callus to the organised lamellar arrangement of normal compact bone with spongy bone in the interior will occur gradually, stimulated by the loading of the bone during weight-bearing activities. A completely healed fracture will show no evidence of the repair, and no scar tissue. The same is not true after injury to ligaments, cartilage or tendons, all of which lack regenerative capacity. In these tissues, an injury may be repaired, but the replacement tissue will be fibrous scar tissue rather than normally functioning tissue, and the structure will be permanently weakened unless surgical repair or replacement is carried out.

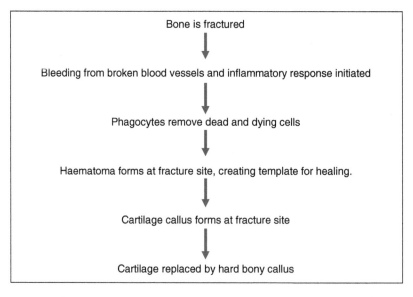

Figure 7.5 **The stages of fracture healing in bone.**

Episodes of Care Learning Disabilities

People with learning disabilities must have the same access to health care needs as everyone else, and nurses need to have a good understanding of the needs of people with learning disabilities across the life span in order to ensure that they offer the right support and make reasonable adjustments.

Bob is a 45-year-old man who has learning disabilities. He lives in supported accommodation and works in a local café for two days a week. On the way to work one morning, Bob slipped on the ice, landing on his outstretched right hand. Although it was painful, he continued his journey and went in to work.

Over the next week it was noticed that Bob was not using his right hand normally and he kept dropping items at the café. His supervisor put this down to his usual 'clumsiness'. There were episodes when Bob would cry for no apparent reason, and he would tell staff his hand was sore. He would be given two paracetamol, which seemed to help him. This went on for another week, until Bob was strongly encouraged to go and see his GP. The GP sent Bob for an X-ray, and a Colles' fracture was diagnosed. This explained Bob's pain and distress over the last two weeks.

A Colles' fracture is a fracture of the end of the radius, and is typically produced after a fall, when a person has broken their fall with their arm outstretched. The broken end of the radius is bent upwards and needs realigning (known as reducing the fracture), to prevent permanent deformation of the wrist. There is also a risk of nerve damage with this fracture, since the median nerve, which supplies the muscles of the hand, travels down the radius. This fracture can take 1–2 years to completely heal.

Bob was given pain relief while the fracture was reduced and his lower arm put in a cast. He was then sent home with pain management. This alleviated Bob's distress and he was able to go about his usual activities and return to work at the café. He became quite proud of his plaster cast after everyone at the café had signed it.

Multiple Choice Questions

1. Diagnostic overshadowing:
   (a) is associated with over-prescribing
   (b) is when signs of physical ill health are mistakenly attributed to a mental health/behavioural problem
   (c) results from a poorly developed X-ray film
2. The stages of bone healing are:
   (a) the early inflammatory stage, the repair stage, the late remodelling stage
   (b) the inflammatory stage, the repair stage, the late inflammatory stage
   (c) the early inflammatory stage, the angiogenesis stage, the late remodelling stage
   (d) the early inflammatory stage, the repair stage, the early remodelling stage
3. During the inflammatory stage:
   (a) a callus is formed
   (b) white blood cells are active in the area
   (c) the patient is highly infectious
   (d) the patient will have pyrexia
4. The complete regeneration of bone after a fracture occurs:
   (a) over hours
   (b) over days
   (c) over two weeks
   (d) over months
5. People with learning disabilities:
   (a) must have the same access to health care as everyone else
   (b) may require reasonable adjustments
   (c) may need help understanding some of the information presented to them
   (d) all of the above

The Axial and Appendicular Skeleton

There are 206 named bones in the adult human skeleton (Figure 7.6).

For classification purposes, the skeleton is divided into two parts: the axial skeleton, consisting of the skull, vertebral column, ribs and sternum, which form the central axis of the body (Table 7.2); and the appendicular skeleton, consisting of the 126 bones that form the limbs (Table 7.3).

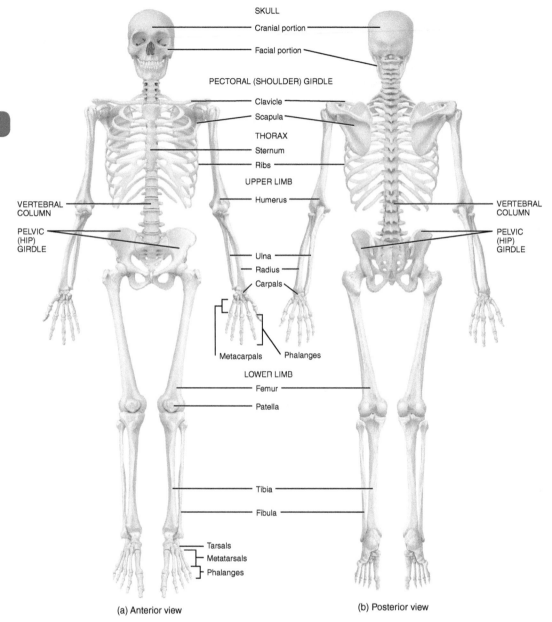

SKULL
— Cranial portion —
— Facial portion —

PECTORAL (SHOULDER) GIRDLE
— Clavicle —
— Scapula —

THORAX
— Sternum
— Ribs —

UPPER LIMB
— Humerus —

VERTEBRAL
COLUMN

PELVIC
(HIP)
GIRDLE

— Ulna —
— Radius —
— Carpals —

Metacarpals   Phalanges

LOWER LIMB
— Femur —
— Patella

— Tibia —

— Fibula —

— Tarsals
— Metatarsals
— Phalanges

VERTEBRAL
COLUMN

PELVIC
(HIP)
GIRDLE

(a) Anterior view   (b) Posterior view

Figure 7.6 **The human skeleton (a) anterior view, (b) posterior view. Axial skeleton blue and appendicular skeleton white.** *Source:* Tortora and Derrickson (2009). Reproduced with permission of John Wiley & Sons.

Bone Shapes

As can be readily seen by looking at an entire skeleton, bones can take a variety of shapes depending on their position and function. A number of bone shapes are recognised, and these bones are often collectively referred to by their shapes.

Long Bones

These bones are longer than they are wide and include the humerus, femur, radius, ulna, tibia and fibula. The clavicles, metacarpals, metatarsals and phalanges are also long bones despite their shortness. These bones allow limb movement.

Table 7.2 The bones of the axial skeleton.

STRUCTURE	NUMBER OF BONES
Skull	
Cranium	8
Face	14
Hyoid	1
Auditory ossicles	6
Vertebral column	26
This number counts the sacrum and coccyx as single vertebrae. They are actually formed from fused vertebrae (5 sacral and 4 coccygeal). Some sources give the number of vertebrae as 33 for this reason.	
Thorax	1
Sternum	24
Ribs	
Total number of bones in the axial skeleton	**80**

Table 7.3 The bones of the appendicular skeleton.

STRUCTURE	NUMBER OF BONES
Pectoral girdle	2
Clavicle	2
Scapula	
Upper limbs	2
Humerus	2
Ulna	2
Radius	16
Carpals	10
Metacarpals	28
Phalanges	
Pelvic girdle	2
Pelvic bone	
Lower limbs	2
Femur	2
Patella	2
Fibula	2
Tibia	14
Tarsals	10
Metatarsals	28
Phalanges	
Total number of bones in the appendicular skeleton	**126**
Total number of bones in the adult human skeleton	**206**

Long bones consist of a shaft (diaphysis) composed primarily of compact bone and ends (epiphyses) composed mainly of cancellous or spongy bone. Between the two is an intermediate region known as the metaphysis, also containing spongy bone.

The compact bone in the shafts forms supportive pillars of bone, which are thickest at the point where the forces applied to the bone are greatest (Figure 7.7).

Short Bones

These bones are usually roughly as wide as they are long. They tend to be found at locations in the limbs where only limited movement is required, such as the wrists and ankles. Examples include the carpals of the wrist and the tarsals of the foot (Figure 7.8). These bones have a thin layer of compact bone over predominantly spongy or cancellous bone.

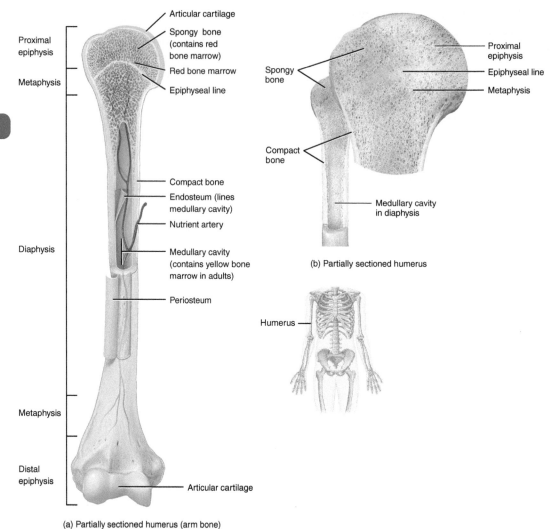

Proximal epiphysis

Metaphysis

Diaphysis

Metaphysis

Distal epiphysis

Articular cartilage

Spongy bone (contains red bone marrow)

Red bone marrow

Epiphyseal line

Compact bone

Endosteum (lines medullary cavity)

Nutrient artery

Medullary cavity (contains yellow bone marrow in adults)

Periosteum

Articular cartilage

(a) Partially sectioned humerus (arm bone)

Spongy bone

Proximal epiphysis

Epiphyseal line

Metaphysis

Compact bone

Medullary cavity in diaphysis

(b) Partially sectioned humerus

Humerus

Figure 7.7 **Parts of a long bone.** *Source:* Tortora and Derrickson (2009). Reproduced with permission of John Wiley & Sons.

Flat Bones

These are thin bones that are found encasing and protecting delicate tissue (such as the skull), or where there is a need for a broad surface for extensive muscle attachment (such as the scapula, or shoulder blade). Other examples include the sternum, ribs and some bones of the pelvis (Figure 7.9).

Irregular Bones

These are bones that, because of their irregular shapes, do not fit into any of the categories already described. They also consist of spongy bone enclosed by thin layers of compact bone. They include the vertebrae (Figure 7.10), the sphenoid and zygomatic bones of the skull and the ossicles of the ear.

Sesamoid Bones

Sesamoid bones are bones that develop within tendons at points where a tendon passes close to a joint and their role seems to be to protect the tendon from friction and rubbing at that point. They are small and round and take their name from the fact that their appearance reminded early anatomists of sesame seeds. The main example of this type of bone is the patella (Figure 7.11).

LATERAL   POSTERIOR   MEDIAL

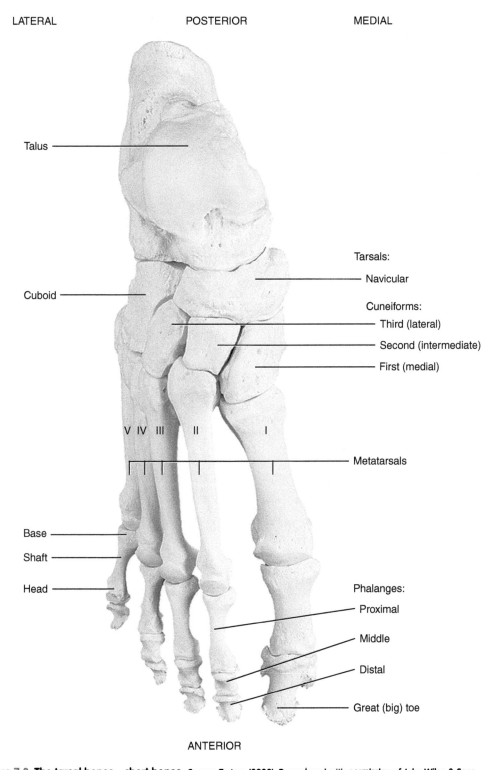

Talus

Tarsals:
Navicular

Cuboid

Cuneiforms:
Third (lateral)
Second (intermediate)
First (medial)

V IV III   II   I

Metatarsals

Base

Shaft

Head

Phalanges:
Proximal

Middle

Distal

Great (big) toe

ANTERIOR

Figure 7.8 **The tarsal bones – short bones.** *Source:* Tortora (2008). Reproduced with permission of John Wiley & Sons.

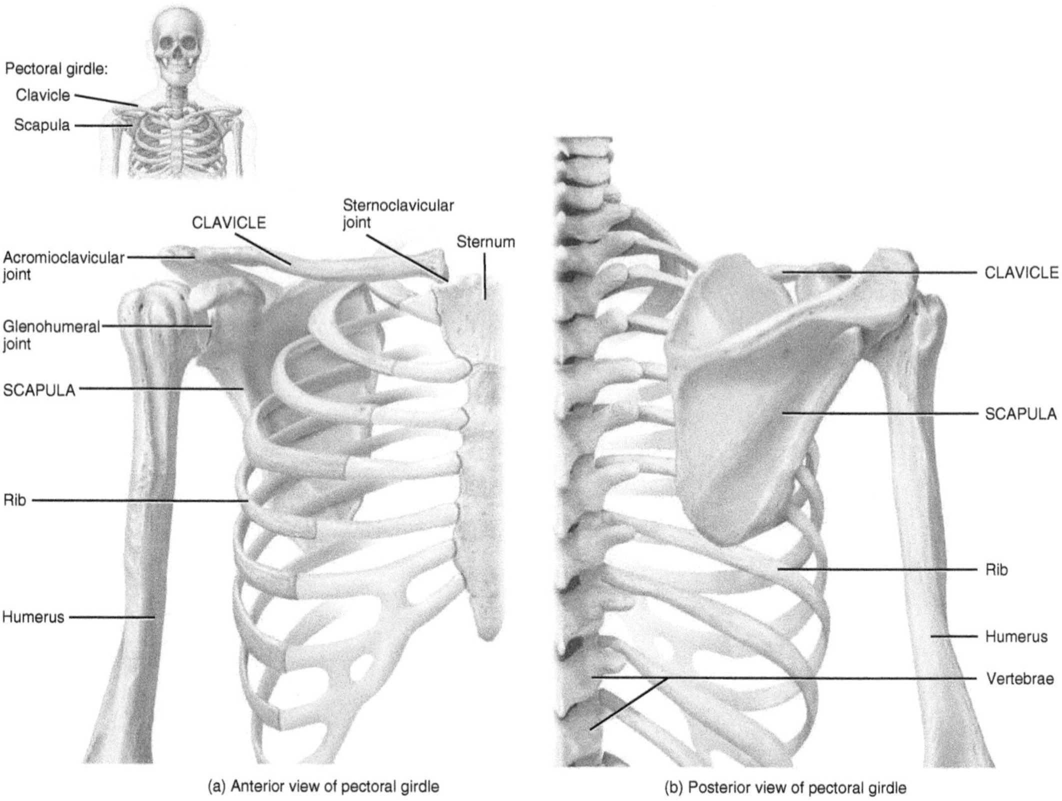

Pectoral girdle:
Clavicle
Scapula

CLAVICLE

Sternoclavicular joint

Sternum

Acromioclavicular joint

Glenohumeral joint

SCAPULA

Rib

Humerus

CLAVICLE

SCAPULA

Rib

Humerus

Vertebrae

(a) Anterior view of pectoral girdle

(b) Posterior view of pectoral girdle

Figure 7.9 **Examples of flat bones: in (a) the sternum and in (b) the scapula and ribs.** *Source:* Tortora and Derrickson (2014). Reproduced with permission of John Wiley & Sons.

Joints

A joint is the point at which two or more bones meet. There are three major types of joints: fibrous, cartilaginous and synovial.

Fibrous Joints

These joints, also called synarthrodial joints, are held together by only a ligament which fills the space between the bone ends. Examples of synarthrodial joints are the connection between the teeth and their bony sockets, the joint between the radius and the ulna, and the one between the tibia and fibula.

Cartilaginous Joints

These joints are also called symphyses (singular symphysis). They occur where the connection between the articulating bones is made up of cartilage. Examples include the intervertebral joints in the spine and the pubic symphysis, between the two halves of the pelvis.

Synovial Joints

Synovial joints, also known as diarthrodial joints, are by far the most common type of joint. They are extremely movable and adapted to allow free movement while minimising friction and the resultant heating caused by repeated movements. These joints are enclosed in a fluid-filled capsule, the lining of which produces a thick, lubricating fluid known as synovial fluid. This fluid is named after its visual similarity to the white of an egg ('*syn*' like and '*ovum*', egg), and it is similarly viscous and slippery, characteristics which reduce friction in the joint, by keeping the bone ends apart so that they do not move against one another, but against a cushion of slippery synovial fluid. The fluid also supplies nutrients to the cartilage and removes waste products. If the joint becomes immobile for a period of time the fluid becomes more gel-like, returning

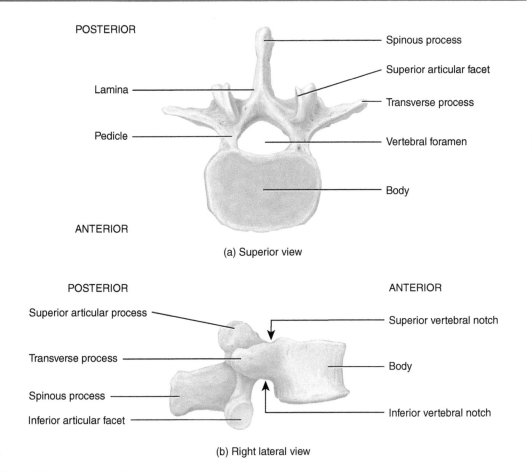

POSTERIOR

Spinous process

Superior articular facet

Lamina

Transverse process

Pedicle

Vertebral foramen

Body

ANTERIOR

(a) Superior view

POSTERIOR

ANTERIOR

Superior articular process

Superior vertebral notch

Transverse process

Body

Spinous process

Inferior articular facet

Inferior vertebral notch

(b) Right lateral view

Figure 7.10 **(a, b) The vertebrae – irregular bones.** *Source:* Tortora and Derrickson (2009). Reproduced with permission of John Wiley & Sons.

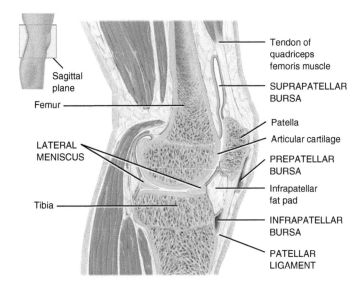

Sagittal plane

Femur

LATERAL MENISCUS

Tibia

Tendon of quadriceps femoris muscle

SUPRAPATELLAR BURSA

Patella

Articular cartilage

PREPATELLAR BURSA

Infrapatellar fat pad

INFRAPATELLAR BURSA

PATELLAR LIGAMENT

Figure 7.11 **A sesamoid bone, the patella – shown in lateral view, in the tendon of the quadriceps muscle, positioned to protect the tendon from friction when the knee joint bends.** *Source:* Tortora and Derrickson (2014). Reproduced with permission of John Wiley & Sons.

to its normal consistency when the joint begins to move again. Hyaline cartilage covers the ends of the articulating bones at the joint, and the smooth glassy surface of this cartilage further reduces friction.

There are six types of synovial joints, and these are classified by the shape of the joint and the movement available (see Table 7.4).

Table 7.4 **Six types of joint.**

TYPE OF JOINT	MOVEMENT AT JOINT	EXAMPLES	STRUCTURE
Hinge	A convex portion of one bone fits into a concave portion of another bone. The movement reflects the movement of a household hinge and bracket; movement is limited to flexion and extension as the joint opens and closes. These joints therefore move in one plane only.	Elbow, knee (shown below) 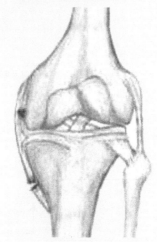	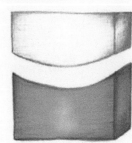
Pivot	A rounded part of one bone fits into the groove of another bone. These joints permit a rotation movement of one bone around another.	Radius and ulna, atlas and axis (shown below) 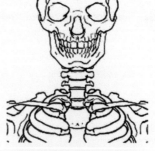	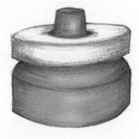
Ball and socket	The spherical end of one bone (the ball) fits into a concave socket of another bone. Movement can occur in several planes.	Hip (shown below), shoulder 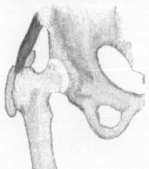	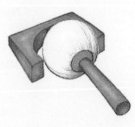

Table 7.4 (Continued)

TYPE OF JOINT	MOVEMENT AT JOINT	EXAMPLES	STRUCTURE
Condyloid	An oval surface of one bone fits into a concavity of another bone. Movement can occur in two planes.	Radiocarpal and metacarpophalangeal joints of the hand (shown below) 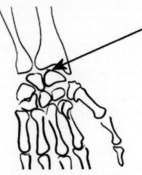	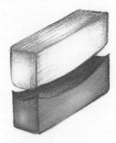
Saddle	Similar to condyloid joints, but these joints permit greater movement. Movement can occur in three planes.	Carpometacarpal joints of the thumb (shown below) 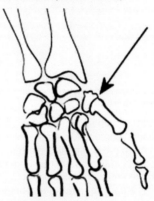	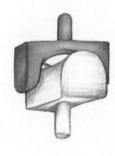
Gliding	These joints have a flat or slightly curved surface, permitting gliding movements. The joints are bound by ligaments, and movement in all directions is restricted. The joint moves back and forth and side to side.	Intertarsal and intercarpal joints of the hands (shown below) and feet 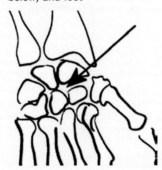	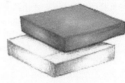

Clinical Considerations Osteoarthritis

The millions of movements that occur over a lifetime of movement inevitably result in wear and tear on the joints, particularly joints which bear a lot of weight and are involved in very basic movements like walking.

The condition osteoarthritis is a degenerative condition which occurs in most people with age. The joint damage that can be seen is a roughening of the surface of the normally smooth and glassy hyaline articular cartilage, followed by inflammation in the affected joint as a result of the increased friction on movement. This process is quite gradual and can eventually lead to the complete wearing away of the articular cartilage. If the joint is one of the major weight-bearing joints, and particularly if the person is overweight, the bones ends can be forced together until they are rubbing directly against each other when the joint moves. The result is pain and stiffness in the joint which is worse after a period of rest, but reduces after activity.

The impact of osteoarthritis will differ from person to person; the care of those with osteoarthritis will depend on the assessment of individual needs. There is no cure for osteoarthritis, but there are many interventions that can be implemented to help improve the health and well-being of the person being cared for.

A multidisciplinary approach to care is required, be this in a hospital setting or in the person's own home. Adjustments to lifestyle – for example, an increase in exercise and the modification of footwear – can help. The administration of medicines to control pain and inflammation can also help the person carry out their activities of living in a more effective way, allowing the person to remain independent and continue with their normal activities as far as possible.

For the cases in which mobility is severely affected due to pain, there is also a surgical option; hip and knee replacements are now very common – the damaged bone ends can be replaced and/or resurfaced by metal or other resistant materials. This procedure is very effective and often gives osteoarthritis sufferers a new lease of life.

Medicines Management Arthrotec

Arthrotec is a drug that contains a combination of two drugs: diclofenac, a non-steroidal anti-inflammatory drug, and misoprostol, a synthetic prostaglandin. Diclofenac has its action by reducing the production of prostaglandins that are involved in producing the inflammatory response and the associated pain. Misoprostol has a number of actions, including increasing the production of thick mucus in the stomach which protects the stomach wall, and reducing the production of stomach acid. The effects of misoprostol therefore counteract some of the side effects of the non-steroidal inflammatory drug, since these drugs are notorious for causing ulceration of the stomach as a result of the loss of the protective prostaglandins.

This drug combination is used to treat skeletal conditions such as osteoarthritis and rheumatoid arthritis, which require the long-term use of anti-inflammatory drugs, and is particularly useful for people who are at high risk for developing gastric or intestinal ulcers.

Arthrotec should not be used by pregnant women as the misoprostol may cause premature labour or uterine rupture. This is because the prostaglandin is very important in the initiation of labour, and taking a drug containing it may initiate labour early. Those who have active gastric or intestinal bleeding should not use Arthrotec. The diclofenac used in this drug can increase the risk of fatal heart attack or stroke; this risk is increased if the medication is used long term or if the person has heart disease.

Prior to administering this medicine, the nurse must determine if the person is allergic to diclofenac or misoprostol, or if there is active gastric or intestinal bleeding. The drug should not be given until after a detailed medical history has been taken as it is contraindicated in some conditions.

Conclusion

The human skeleton is a dynamic, living structure that is constantly readjusting itself to perform optimally. It provides a supportive and protective framework for our body form, with its incredible strength and flexibility, and its ability to regenerate itself after damage. The skeleton also provides the levers which can be worked by the action of muscles to produce movements, from the tiniest flick of a fingertip to the powerful impulse that propels a sprinter out of the blocks when the starting gun fires. Impressive as this is, it is not all that our skeleton does for us. The red marrow inside some of our bones is the source of all our blood cells, which provide us with immunity and with the ability to transport oxygen around the body to the tissues. And because the skeleton represents such a huge store of deposited calcium, bones are also central to the homeostatic control of plasma calcium level, and act as a source of calcium to 'top up' plasma calcium when necessary, thus ensuring that all the myriad functions that calcium ions trigger are not disrupted by abnormal calcium concentrations in the blood.

175

Glossary

Abduction: Movement away from the body's midline.

Adduction: Movement towards the body's midline.

Articulation: The meeting point for two bones at a joint.

Ball-and-socket joint: A synovial joint in which the rounded surface of one bone fits within the cup-shaped depression of the socket of the other bone.

Calcification: Deposition of mineral salts in a framework formed by collagen fibres.

Cartilage: Strong, tough material on the bone ends that helps to distribute the load within the joint; the slippery surface allows smooth movement between the bones; a type of connective tissue.

Cartilaginous joint: A joint where the bones are held together tightly by cartilage; little movement occurs in this joint. This joint does not have a synovial cavity.

Collagen: A protein that makes up most of the connective tissue.

Condyloid joint: A synovial joint that allows one oval-shaped bone to fit into an elliptical cavity of another.

Diaphysis: The shaft of a long bone.

Epiphysis: The end of long bone.

Fibrous joint: A type of joint that allows little or no movement.

Flexion: Movement at a joint which produces a decrease in the angle formed between the two bones.

Fracture: A break in a bone.

Gliding joint: A synovial joint whose articulating surfaces are usually flat, allowing only side-to-side or back-and-forth movement.

Haemopoiesis: The formation and development of blood cells in the bone marrow.

Histology: The microscopic study of tissues.

In utero: Within the uterus.

Lacuna: A small, hollow space found in any tissue.

Lamellae: Concentric rings of hard, calcified matrix found in compact bones.

Ligaments: Tough, fibrous bands of connective tissue that hold the bones together at a joint.

Macrophage: Cells that can engulf and digest cellular debris and pathogens.

Marrow: A sponge-like material found in the cavities of some bones. Red bone marrow, found in short, flat and irregular bones and the epiphyses of long bones, produces blood cells.

Mesenchyme: Embryonic connective tissue from which nearly all other connective tissue arises.

Metaphysis: The narrow transitional section of a long bone that lies between the diaphysis (bone shaft) and the epiphysis (bone end).

Ossification: The formation of bone; sometimes called osteogenesis.

Osseous: Bony.

Ossicle: A small bone of the middle ear – the malleus, the incus, the stapes.

Osteoblasts: Cells that are responsible for the formation of bone.

Osteoclasts: Large cells that are responsible for absorption and removal of bone.

Osteocytes: Cells that started as osteoblasts but become trapped within the bony matrix and serve a monitoring function.

Osteon: The basic unit of structure in adult compact bone.

Osteophytes: Overgrowth of new bone around the side of osteoarthritic joints; also known as spur growth.

Periosteum: Membrane covering bones, which consists of connective tissue, osteogenic cells and osteoblasts. This is vital for bone growth, repair and nutrition.

Pivot joint: A joint where a rounded or conical-shaped surface of a bone articulates with a ring formed partly by another bone or ligament, permitting a rotational movement, for example, shaking the head.

Remodelling: Replacement of old bone by new.

Resorption: Removal of existing tissue.

Saddle joint: A synovial joint articulates the surface of a saddle-shaped bone on the other bone that is said to be shaped like the legs of the rider.

Spongy (cancellous) bone tissue: A type of bone recognisable by its 'holey' or spongy appearance, due to the latticework of bone struts. It is found in the middle of most bones, between the outer compact bone and the inner cavity. It helps to provide some strength while keeping weight down.

Synovial cavity: The space between the articulating bones of a synovial joint, filled with synovial fluid.

Synovial fluid: A clear pale yellow, viscous fluid that lubricates and cushions joints.

References

Marsell, R and Einhorn, T.A. (2011) The biology of fracture healing. *Injury* **42**(6): 551–555.

Tortora, G.J. and Derrickson, B. (2009) *Principles of Anatomy and Physiology*, 12th edn. Hoboken, NJ: John Wiley & Sons, Inc.

Tortora, G.J. (2008) *A Brief Atlas of the Human Skeleton, Surface Anatomy and Selected Medical Images*. New York: John Wiley & Sons, Inc.

Tortora, G.J. and Derrickson, B.H. (2009) *Principles of Anatomy and Physiology*, 15th edn. Hoboken, NJ: John Wiley & Sons, Inc

Tortora, G.J. and Derrickson, B.H. (2014) *Principles of Anatomy and Physiology*, 14th edn. Hoboken, NJ: John Wiley & Sons, Inc

Weise, M., Stacy De-Levi, S., Barnes, K.M., Gafni, R.I, Abad, V., and Baron, J. (2001) Effects of estrogen on growth plate senescence and epiphyseal fusion. *Proceedings of the National Academy of Sciences* **98**(12): 6871–6876.

Further Reading

Arthritis Research UK

www.arthritisresearchuk.org

This organisation works with patients and health care professionals to take the pain away from those living with all forms of arthritis, helping them to remain active. They fund high quality research, educate health care professionals and provide information to those with arthritis and their carers.

National Osteoporosis Foundation UK

https://www.nos.org.uk

The National Osteoporosis Society is a UK-wide charity dedicated to improving the diagnosis, prevention and treatment of osteoporosis and fragility fractures. The National Osteoporosis Society UK Allied Health Professional Network has been developed to provide support and professional development to allied health professionals who are specialists working in the field of osteoporosis and/or fragility fractures in the UK.

Sarcoma UK

http://sarcoma.org.uk

Sarcoma UK is the only UK cancer charity that focuses on all types of sarcoma. Sarcomas are rare cancers developing in the muscle, bone, nerves, cartilage, tendons, blood vessels and the fatty and fibrous tissues.

Arthritis Australia

https://arthritisaustralia.com.au

A not-for-profit organisation and the peak arthritis consumer body in Australia.

Osteoporosis Australia

https://www.osteoporosis.org.au

A national not-for-profit organisation responsible for providing osteoporosis information and services to the community and health professionals.

Activities

Multiple Choice Questions

1. What is an osteophyte?
   (a) a bone cell
   (b) a small bony outgrowth
   (c) a bone cancer cell
   (d) a lymph cell

2. Where would you find the medial malleolus?
   (a) at the hip, formed by the end of the femur
   (b) in the thoracic cavity, formed by the ends of the ribs
   (c) at the ankle, formed by the lower end of tibia
   (d) in the cranium, formed by the junction between the mandible and maxilla
3. What is another name for the clavicle?
   (a) the rib
   (b) the breastbone
   (c) the collarbone
   (d) the pelvis
4. Which of the following is part of the axial skeleton?
   (a) skull
   (b) humerus
   (c) tarsal
   (d) tibia
5. A joint that allows free movement is known as:
   (a) haemathrosis
   (b) synarthrosis
   (c) diarthrosis
   (d) amphiarthroses
6. The jaw bone is:
   (a) the calcaneus
   (b) the maxilla
   (c) the ischium
   (d) the mandible
7. A joint such as the elbow joint that only moves in one plane is known as:
   (a) a hinge joint
   (b) a socket joint
   (c) an arthritic joint
   (d) a saddle joint
8. Bone is covered by a protective tissue membrane called:
   (a) the lacunae
   (b) the diaphysis
   (c) the peritoneum
   (d) the periosteum
9. The skull is part of:
   (a) the appendicular skeleton
   (b) the external skeleton
   (c) the axial skeleton
   (d) the internal skeleton
10. The ribs are attached to:
    (a) the cervical vertebrae
    (b) the thoracic vertebrae
    (c) the lumbar vertebrae
    (d) the skull

11. Why are post-menopausal women at greater risk of osteoporosis?
    (a) they have lower levels of exercise and therefore lower osteoblast activity
    (b) they have lower levels of oestrogen and therefore lower osteoblast activity
    (c) they have lower levels of calcium and therefore lower osteoclast activity
    (d) they have higher levels of progesterone and therefore higher osteoclast activity

12. Jacinta has an inherited disorder which prevents her fibroblasts from producing enough normal collagen. What effect would you predict this disorder would have on Jacinta's bones?
    (a) her bones would be brittle and fracture easily
    (b) her bones would be soft and bendy
    (c) her bones would be of low density, due to bone resorption
    (d) her bones would be of higher density, due to bone remodelling

13. George has torn one of the fibrous connective tissue straps that stabilises his knee joint. What has he torn?
    (a) cartilage
    (b) a tendon
    (c) a ligament
    (d) a muscle

14. Extended bed rest has a negative impact on the skeleton. Why is this?
    (a) reduced stress on bones in bed → reduced osteoblast activity
    (b) pressure on soft tissue in bed → calcification of soft tissue and resorption of bone.
    (c) reduced sun exposure in bed → low vitamin D → low plasma calcium levels.
    (d) lack of activity in bed → bone resorbed to replace lost proteins

15. In boys, the ossification of the growth plates in long bones is caused by testosterone increase at puberty. Boys who enter puberty at an unusually early age are therefore likely to:
    (a) be generally large-boned
    (b) have weaker bones
    (c) be taller in stature
    (d) be shorter in stature

True or False

1. The skeleton is a living organism.
2. There are more bones in adults than in babies.
3. Bone stores and releases calcium.
4. The ribs protect the pancreas.
5. Yellow bone marrow produces red blood cells.
6. There is no difference between the weight and size of male and female bones.
7. The patella is located in the humerus.
8. Osteoblasts forms new bone.
9. Replacement of old bone by new is called remodelling.
10. The axial skeleton has more bones than the appendicular skeleton.

Match Each Bone to its Correct Shape

A.

SHAPE	BONE
Irregular bone	Sternum
Long bone	Zygomatic
Flat bone	Metacarpal
Short bone	Hyoid
	Tarsal
	Femur
	Ethmoid
	Scapula

Find Out More

1. Why do healthy bones require exercise?
2. Describe the composition of bone.
3. How does the skeletal system help to maintain homeostasis?
4. In bone remodelling, how do osteoblasts and osteoclasts work together?
5. What happens to bone as we age?
6. What is synovial fluid?
7. Describe the healing that occurs after a fracture has been sustained.
8. Discuss intramembranous ossification.
9. What factors are essential for bone remodelling?
10. Where in the body are the two sesamoid bones and what are they called?

Conditions

The following is a list of conditions that are associated with the skeletal system. Take some time and write notes about each of the conditions. You may make the notes taken from textbooks or other resources, or you may make the notes from patients you have cared for. If you are doing this, you must ensure that you adhere to the rules of confidentiality.

Fractured neck of femur

Osteoarthritis

Osteoporosis

Gout

Osteomyelitis

Osteosarcoma

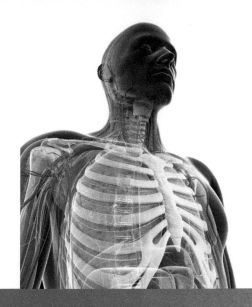

8

The Circulatory System

Noleen Jones

Test Your Prior Knowledge

- **Compare and contrast arteries and veins.**
- **List the formed elements of the blood.**
- **List the functions of the blood cells.**
- **Discuss the life cycle of a red blood cell.**
- **List the functions of the lymphatic system.**

Learning Outcomes

After reading this chapter you will be able to:

- **Discuss the normal composition of blood.**
- **List the functions of the red blood cells, white blood cells and platelets.**
- **Explain the life cycle of the red blood cells and the white blood cells.**
- **List some of the differences between an artery and a vein.**
- **Discuss the functions of the lymphatic circulation.**

 Visit the student companion website at www.wileyfundamentalseries.com/anatomy where you can test yourself using flashcards, multiple-choice questions and more. Instructor companion site at www.wiley.com/go/instructor/anatomy where instructors will find valuable materials such as PowerPoint slides and image bank designed to enhance your teaching.

Fundamentals of Anatomy and Physiology: For Nursing and Healthcare Students, Third Edition. Edited by Ian Peate and Suzanne Evans.
© 2020 John Wiley & Sons Ltd. Published 2020 by John Wiley & Sons Ltd.
Student companion website: www.wileyfundamentalseries.com/anatomy
Instructor companion website: www.wiley.com/go/instructor/anatomy

Body Map

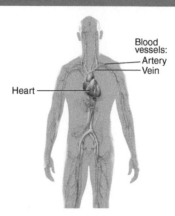

Blood vessels:
- Artery
- Vein

Heart

Introduction

The circulatory system is a complex system which deals with the distribution of nutrients, gases, electrolytes, removal of waste products of metabolism and other substances. The circulatory system includes the heart, the blood, the blood vessels and the lymphatic system. The blood vessels transport blood around the body.

Blood consists of formed elements within a fluid portion called plasma. The blood vessels form a network that allows blood to flow from the heart to all living cells and back to the heart. Blood has numerous functions including the transportation of nutrients, respiratory gases such as oxygen and carbon dioxide, metabolic wastes such as urea and uric acid, hormones, electrolytes and antibodies. As the blood is circulating throughout the body, cells are constantly exchanging nutrients, hormones, electrolytes, oxygen and other substances with it, as well as excreting unwanted wastes into the blood.

Blood is transported throughout the body by a network of blood vessels, some of which lead away and some which return to the heart. The main types of blood vessels include arteries, arterioles, capillaries, venules and veins. Another important part of the circulatory system is the lymphatic system, which drains a fluid called lymph. The lymphatic system consists of the lymph vessels, lymph nodes and lymph glands such as the spleen and the thymus gland.

This chapter will focus on the composition, structure and functions of various blood cells, discuss the structure and functions of the blood vessels, factors affecting blood pressure and the structure and functions of the lymphatic system.

Components of Blood

Blood consists of formed elements such as red blood cells (erythrocytes), leucocytes (white blood cells) and platelets. The fluid portion of blood, plasma, contains different types of proteins and other soluble molecules. When a blood sample is centrifuged, the formed elements account for 45% of the blood and plasma makes up 55% of the total blood volume. Normally, more than 99% of the formed elements are cells named for their red colour (red blood cells). White blood cells (pale in appearance) and platelets comprise less than 1% of the formed elements. Between the plasma and erythrocytes lies the buffy coat, which consists of white blood cells and platelets (Figure 8.1). The percentage of the formed elements constitutes the haematocrit or packed cell volume. Haematocrit is a blood test that measures the percentage of red blood cells in whole blood. The volume of blood is constant unless a person has physiological problems, such as haemorrhage.

Thus, blood is composed of plasma, a yellowish liquid containing nutrients, hormones, minerals and various cells, mainly red blood cells, white blood cells and platelets (Figure 8.2). Both the formed elements and the plasma play an important role in homeostasis.

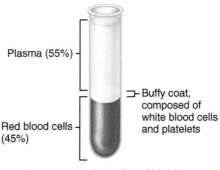

Plasma (55%)

Buffy coat,
composed of
white blood cells
and platelets

Red blood cells
(45%)

Appearance of centrifuged blood

Figure 8.1 **Components of blood.** *Source:* Tortora and Derrickson (2009). Reproduced with permission of John Wiley & Sons.

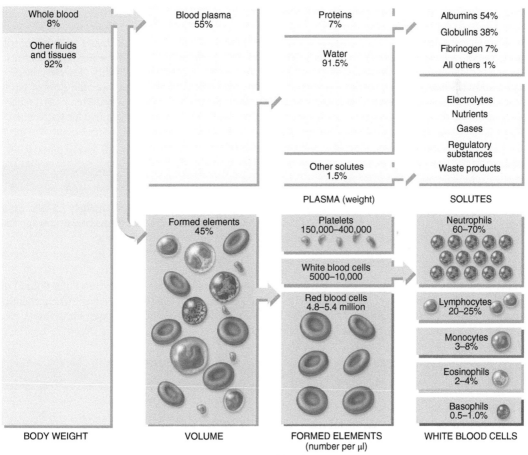

Whole blood 8%	Blood plasma 55%	Proteins 7%	Albumins 54%
Other fluids and tissues 92%			Globulins 38%
		Water 91.5%	Fibrinogen 7%
			All others 1%
			Electrolytes
			Nutrients
			Gases
			Regulatory substances
		Other solutes 1.5%	Waste products
		PLASMA (weight)	SOLUTES
	Formed elements 45%	Platelets 150,000–400,000	Neutrophils 60–70%
		White blood cells 5000–10,000	
		Red blood cells 4.8–5.4 million	Lymphocytes 20–25%
			Monocytes 3–8%
			Eosinophils 2–4%
			Basophils 0.5–1.0%
BODY WEIGHT	VOLUME	FORMED ELEMENTS (number per µl)	WHITE BLOOD CELLS

Components of blood

Figure 8.2 **Cells of the blood.** *Source:* Tortora and Derrickson (2009). Reproduced with permission of John Wiley & Sons.

Properties of Blood

The average adult has a blood volume of approximately 5 L, which accounts for 7–9% of the body's weight. Men have 5–6 L and women 4–5 L. Blood is thicker, denser and flows much slower than water due to the red blood cells and plasma proteins such as albumin and fibrinogen. Plasma proteins, including albumin, fibrinogen, prothrombin and the gamma globulins, constitute about 8% of the blood plasma in the body. These proteins help maintain water balance, and they affect osmotic pressure, increase blood viscosity and help maintain blood pressure. All the plasma proteins except the gamma globulins are synthesised in the liver.

The normal osmolality of extracellular fluid is 285–295 mosmol/kg. The osmolality of the blood is important for the cells to survive. If the osmolality is approximately 600 mosmol, the red blood cells could crenate (shrivel up) and die, and if the osmolality is below 150 mosmol, haemolysis (rupture) of the red blood cells could occur. Massive haemolysis can be fatal. Plasma osmolality is tightly controlled by homeostatic mechanisms. Changes in plasma osmolality are detected by osmoreceptors in the circulatory system. If the osmolality is too low (i.e. the blood is too dilute) the secretion of antidiuretic hormone (ADH) is switched off, and the blood slowly concentrates as water is excreted into the urine. Dehydration causes ADH to be switched on and water conserved. In order to avoid crenation or haemolysis, intravenous infusion fluids should have an osmolality as close to plasma as possible. A solution that has the same osmotic pressure as another is called isotonic. An isotonic solution generally assumes that a solution will have the same osmolality as blood.

Blood has a high viscosity, which offers resistance to blood flow. The red blood cells and proteins contribute to the viscosity of the blood, which ranges from 3.5 to 5.5 compared with 1.000 for water. Viscosity means stickiness of blood, and the normal viscosity of blood is low, allowing it to flow smoothly. However, the more red blood cells and plasma proteins in blood, the higher the viscosity and the slower the flow of blood. Normal blood varies in viscosity as it flows through the blood vessels, but the viscosity decreases as it reaches the capillaries. The specific gravity (density) of blood is 1.045–1.065 compared with 1.000 for water, and the pH of blood ranges from 7.35 to 7.45 (Nair, 2013).

Plasma

Blood plasma is a pale, yellow-coloured fluid and its total volume in an adult is approximately 2.5–3 L. Blood plasma is approximately 91% water and 10% solutes, most of which are proteins. Plasma constitutes approximately 55% of blood's volume (Figure 8.2). See Table 8.1 for the composition of plasma.

Water in Plasma

Water constitutes approximately 91% of plasma and is available to cells, tissues and extracellular fluid of the body to maintain homeostasis. It is considered the liquid portion of the blood. It is a solvent where chemical reactions between intracellular and extracellular reactions occur. Water contains solutes; for example, electrolytes whose concentrations change to meet body needs.

Functions of Blood

The functions of the blood are:
- **Transportation:** The blood is the means whereby all nourishment and respiratory gases are transported into and out of the cells.
- **Maintaining body temperature:** Blood helps to maintain the body temperature by distributing the heat produced by the chemical activity of the cells evenly, throughout the body.
- **Maintaining the acid-base balance:** Blood pH is maintained by the excretion or reabsorption of hydrogen ions and bicarbonate ions.
- **Regulation of fluid balance:** When the blood reaches the kidneys, excess fluid is excreted or reabsorbed to maintain fluid balance.

Table 8.1 **Compositions of plasma and their functions.**

SUBSTANCES	FUNCTIONS
Water 91%	Lubricates, transports, heat distribution and a solvent
Plasma protein • Albumin • Globulin • Prothrombin • Fibrinogen	Responsible for colloid osmosis, provides blood viscosity, transports hormones, fatty acids and calcium. Protection from infections. Transport of insoluble substances by allowing them to bind to protein molecules. Regulates pH of blood. An imbalance of plasma proteins can lead a patient to experience symptoms ranging from abnormally dilated blood vessels to a weakened immune system.
Electrolytes • Sodium • Potassium • Calcium • Bicarbonate • Phosphate • Chloride	Help maintain osmotic pressure and cell functions
Nutrients • Amino acids • Fatty acids • Glucose • Glycerol • Vitamins • Minerals	Cell function growth and development
Gases	Cellular function and regulation of blood pH
Enzymes, hormones and vitamins	Chemical reactions, regulate growth and development and cofactors for enzymatic reaction
Waste products • Urea • Uric acid • Creatinine • Bilirubin • Ammonia	Broken down and transported by blood to organs of excretion

Source: Adapted from Jenkins and Tortora (2013).

185

- **Removal of waste products:** The blood removes all waste products from the tissues and cells. These waste products are transported to the appropriate organs for excretion – lungs, kidneys, intestine, skin and so on.
- **Blood clotting:** By the mechanism of clotting, loss of blood cells and body fluids is prevented.
- **Defence action:** The blood aids in the defence of the body against the invasion of microorganisms and their toxins due to:
  - the phagocyte action of neutrophils and monocytes;
  - the presence of antibodies and antitoxins.

Clinical Considerations Intravenous Fluid Therapy

Intravenous (IV) fluid replacement is a common treatment used in hospitals and community settings to restore blood circulating volume, vital electrolytes and glucose.

Acute fluid losses, which can occur from prolonged episodes of vomiting and diarrhoea, or dehydration in the very young or elderly populations, can lead to hypovolaemia and is potentially fatal. Vital signs like low blood pressure and a high pulse and respirations are indicators of the body's attempt to compensate for intravascular fluid deficit. The severity of the fluid deficit is displayed through how much a vital sign deviates from the normal. Another condition for which patients may require fluid replacement is sepsis, a life-threatening infection which causes circulatory collapse.

The aim of fluid replacement is to re-establish homeostatic fluid balance. The monitoring of patients during fluid therapy must be carefully managed.

Common conditions that require fluid replacement include:
- prolonged or severe vomiting
- prolonged or severe diarrhea
- infection
- gastrointestinal (GI) suctioning
- heart failure
- septic shock
- respiratory failure
- haemorrhage
- cardiovascular collapse.

An accurate fluid balance chart must be maintained to track the intake and output of fluids in the body. Patients receiving IV fluids should also be observed for the normalisation of vital signs, a good indicator of how adequately volume is being replaced.

IV fluids are replaced cautiously in patients with chronic heart failure (CHF). This is because supplemental IV fluids may cause additional stress to an already weak heart and lead to fluid overload (Pellicori et al., 2015). Patients with CHF may be on restricted IV fluid regimens and need to be weighed daily to observe for signs of fluid retention.

Formation of Blood Cells

Red blood cells and most white blood cells and platelets are produced in the bone marrow. The red blood and white blood cells and the platelets are the formed elements of blood (Figure 8.3). The bone marrow is the soft fatty substance found in bone cavities. Within the bone marrow, all blood cells originate from a single type of unspecialised cell called a stem cell. When a stem cell divides, it first becomes an immature red blood cell, white blood cell or platelet-producing cell. The immature cell then divides, matures further and ultimately becomes a mature red blood cell, white blood cell or platelet (Figure 8.1).

In order to produce blood cells, multipotent (also called pluripotent) stem cells divide into myeloid and lymphoid stem cells in the bone marrow. The myeloid stem cells further subdivide in the bone marrow to produce red blood cells, platelets (thrombocytes), basophils, eosinophils, neutrophils and monocytes. The lymphoid stem cells begin the development in the bone marrow as B- and T-lymphocytes. B-lymphocytes continue development in bone marrow, before migrating to other lymph organs such as lymph nodes, spleen or tonsils. T-lymphocytes continue their development in the thymus, and may then migrate to other lymph tissues.

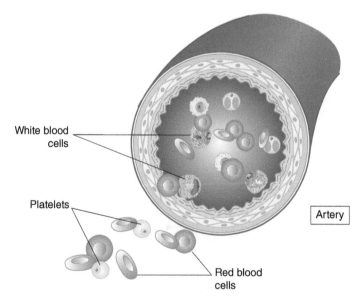

White blood cells

Platelets

Artery

Red blood cells

Figure 8.3 **Formed elements of blood.**

Red Blood Cells

Red blood cells (also known as erythrocytes) are the most abundant blood cells. They are biconcave discs (Figure 8.4) and contain oxygen-carrying protein called haemoglobin. The biconcave shape is maintained by a network of proteins called spectrin. This network of protein allows the red blood cells to change shape as they are transported through the blood vessel. The plasma membrane of a red blood cell is strong and flexible. There are approximately 4 million to 5.5 million red blood cells in each cubic millimetre of blood. They are a pale buff colour that appears lighter in the centre. Young red blood cells contain a nucleus; however, the nucleus is absent in a mature red blood cell and without any organelles such as mitochondria, thus increasing the oxygen-carrying capacity of the red blood cell.

The main function of haemoglobin in the red blood cell is to transport oxygen and carbon dioxide (approximately 20%). As the blood flows through the capillaries in the tissues, carbon dioxide is picked up by the haemoglobin and oxygen is released. As the blood reaches the lungs, carbon dioxide is released and oxygen is picked up by the haemoglobin molecules. As red blood cells lack mitochondria to produce energy (adenosine triphosphate), they utilise anaerobic respiration to produce energy and do not use any of the oxygen they are transporting. Apart from transporting oxygen and carbon dioxide, the haemoglobin plays an important role in maintaining blood pressure and blood flow.

8 µm

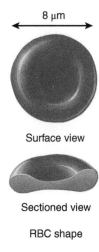

Surface view

Sectioned view

RBC shape

Figure 8.4 **Red blood cells.** *Source:* Tortora and Derrickson (2009). Reproduced with permission of John Wiley & Sons.

Medicines Management Iron Deficiency Anaemia

Anaemia occurs when the body does not have enough red, oxygen-carrying blood cells, which means the body's tissues and cells are not getting enough oxygen. Treatment for iron deficiency anaemia usually involves taking iron supplements and changing the diet to increase the iron levels, as well as treating the underlying cause. Iron supplements may be prescribed to restore the iron missing from the body. The most commonly prescribed supplement is ferrous sulphate which is taken as a tablet two or three times a day. Nurses need to be aware that patients receiving iron tablets may experience:

- abdominal pain
- constipation or diarrhoea
- heartburn
- feeling sick
- black stools (faeces).

Black stools may also result from an upper gastrointestinal bleed. If these symptoms persist, advise the patient to see their GP so that prompt action can be taken to alleviate the side effects.
See NHS Choices (2018a).

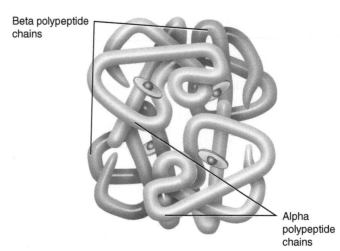

Beta polypeptide chains

Alpha polypeptide chains

Haemoglobin molecule

Figure 8.5 **Haemoglobin molecule.** *Source:* Tortora and Derrickson (2009). Reproduced with permission of John Wiley & Sons.

Haemoglobin

Haemoglobin is composed of a protein called globin bound to the iron-containing pigments called haem. Each globin molecule has four polypeptide chains consisting of two alpha and two beta chains (Figure 8.5). Each haemoglobin molecule has four atoms of iron, and each atom of iron transports one molecule of oxygen; therefore, one molecule of haemoglobin transports four molecules of oxygen. There are approximately 250 million haemoglobin molecules in one red blood cell; therefore, one red blood cell transports 1 billion molecules of oxygen. At the capillary end the haemoglobin releases the oxygen molecule into the interstitial fluid, which is then transported into the cells.

Formation of Red Blood Cells

Erythroblasts undergo development in the red bone marrow to form red blood cells (Figure 16.1). During maturation, red blood cells lose their nucleus and organelles and gain more haemoglobin molecules, thus increasing the amount of oxygen they transport. Mature red blood cells do not have a nucleus; their life span is approximately 120 days. It is estimated that approximately 2 million red blood cells are destroyed per second; however, an equal number are replaced each time to maintain the balance. The production of red blood cells is controlled by the hormone erythropoietin. Other essential components for the synthesis of red blood cells include:

- iron
- folic acid
- vitamin B_{12}.

Episodes of Care Child

Cristiana is 5 years old and the only child to her parents, Samara and Leo. Cristiana's mother is of Maltese descent. She has reached the expected development goals for a child of her age, although she has always been in the lower percentile for growth. She has had no major childhood illnesses but seems to take a little longer than other children to get over colds and minor infections. Lately, Cristiana has been under the weather and her mother is concerned that she is sleeping more than normal and appears a little short of breath after activities. She books an appointment for Cristiana to be seen at her family health practice.

When she arrives at the surgery, the practice nurse performs an assessment and collects information from Cristiana and Samara. She notes that the child looks pale, has slightly yellow corneas and is a little underweight for her age. She books the child in for a blood test and records the information in her notes.

Blood tests reveal a low haemoglobin (Hb) count and smaller than normal red blood cells. Cristiana is diagnosed with the condition Thalassaemia minor.

Thalassaemia is a genetically inherited anaemia caused by the abnormal formation of haemoglobin (Sharma et al., 2017). It is prevalent among Mediterranean cultures and ranges in severity. In its major form, people with the condition require regular blood transfusions and may have a limited life expectancy. It can cause symptoms such as shortness of breath, growth retardation and skeletal deformities.

During her follow-up appointment, the nurse explains that Cristiana will need to take the vitamin B supplement, Folic Acid, to help her body to produce more effective red blood cells. She also refers Cristiana to a nutritionist so that her mother can get advice on the best diet to help her with her anaemia.

At her review three months later, Cristiana's blood tests show an improved haemoglobin count and Samara reports that Cristiana's energy levels have increased.

Multiple Choice Questions

1. The following are types of thalassaemia:
   (a) beta thalassemia minor, beta thalassemia intermedia and beta thalassemia major
   (b) beta thalassemia majora, beta thalassemia intermedia and beta thalassemia major
   (c) beta thalassemia minor, beta thalassemia media and beta thalassemia major
   (d) beta thalassemia minor, beta thalassemia intermedia and beta thalassemia majora
2. In beta thalassemia:
   (a) there is a deficit of chromosomes
   (b) the gene change causes an imbalance of haemoglobin proteins
   (c) the person will have to undergo blood transfusion every other week
   (d) treatment always begins *in utero*
3. Children with beta thalassemia intermedia or major:
   (a) will not survive longer than 10 years of age
   (b) need lifelong medical care
   (c) will need a splenectomy
   (d) should avoid places where large group of people congregate such as schools
4. Beta thalassemia minor is also called:
   (a) Cooley's disease
   (b) beta thalassaemia trait
   (c) beta haemolytic streptococcus
   (d) beta minora
5. If a woman is pregnant and both parents have beta thalassaemia trait, doctors can check the foetus by:
   (a) ultrasound scan
   (b) MRI
   (c) chorionic villus sampling
   (d) none of the above

Erythropoietin is a hormone produced by the kidneys, which is then transported by the blood to the bone marrow. In the bone marrow erythropoietin stimulates the production of red blood cells, which then enter the bloodstream. The production and release of erythropoietin is through a negative feedback system (Figure 8.6).

Life Cycle of the Red Blood Cell

Without a nucleus and other organelles, the red blood cell cannot synthesise new structures to replace the ones that are damaged. The breakdown (haemolysis) of the red blood cell is carried out by macrophages in the spleen, liver and the bone marrow (Figure 8.7). The globin is broken down into amino acids and reused for protein synthesis. Iron is separated from haem and is stored in the muscles and the liver and reused in the bone marrow to manufacture new red blood cells. Haem is the portion of the haemoglobin that is converted to bilirubin and is transported by plasma albumin to the liver and eventually secreted in bile. In the large intestine, bacteria convert bilirubin into urobilinogen, some of which is reabsorbed into the bloodstream where it is converted into a yellow pigment called urobilin, which is excreted in urine, giving the urine a yellowish colour. The remainder of the urobilinogen is eliminated in faeces as a brown pigment called stercobilin.

190

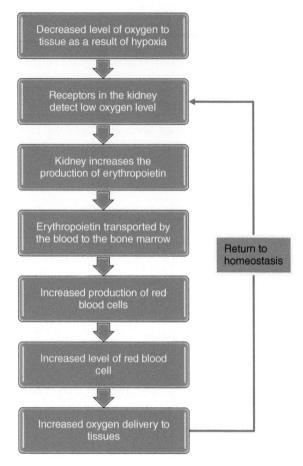

Figure 8.6 **Negative feedback for erythropoiesis.**

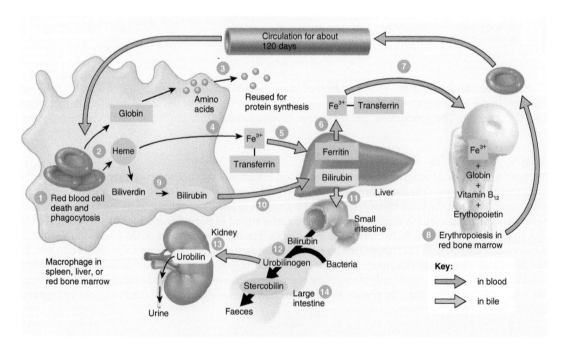

Figure 8.7 **Destruction of the red blood cell.** *Source:* Tortora and Derrickson (2009). Reproduced with permission of John Wiley & Sons.

Transport of Respiratory Gases

The major role of red blood cells is to transport oxygen from the lungs to the tissues. The oxygen in the alveoli (air sac) of the lungs combines with iron molecules in the haemoglobin to form oxyhaemoglobin. This is then transported by the blood to the tissues. As the oxygen level in the red blood cell increases it becomes bright red, and when the level of oxygen content drops the colour changes to dark bluish-red.

In addition to transporting oxygen from the lungs to the body tissues, red blood cells transport carbon dioxide from the tissues to the lungs. Carbon dioxide is transported in three ways:

- 10% of the carbon dioxide is dissolved in the plasma;
- 20% of the carbon dioxide combines with haemoglobin of the red blood cell to form carbaminohaemoglobin;
- 70% of the carbon dioxide reacts with water to form carbonic acid, which is converted to bicarbonate and hydrogen ions:

$$CO_2 + H_2O \overset{\text{carbonic anhydrase}}{\longleftrightarrow} \underset{\text{carbonic acid}}{H_2CO_3} \longleftrightarrow \underset{\text{bicarbonate ion}}{HCO_3^-} + \underset{\text{hydrogen ion}}{H^+}$$

The reaction occurs primarily in red blood cells, which contain large amounts of carbonic anhydrase (an enzyme that facilitates the reaction). Once the bicarbonate ions are formed, they move out of the red blood cells into the plasma.

White Blood Cells

White blood cells are also known as leucocytes. There are approximately 5000–10,000 white blood cells in every cubic millimetre of blood. The number may increase in infections to approximately 25,000 per cubic millimetre of blood. An increase in white blood cells is called leucocytosis, and an abnormally low level of white blood cell is called leucopenia. Unlike red blood cells, white blood cells have nuclei and they are able to move out of blood vessel walls into the tissues. White blood cells are able to produce a continuous supply of energy, unlike the red blood cells. They are able to synthesise proteins, and thus their life span can be from a few days to years. There are two main types of white blood cells:

- granulocytes (contain granules in the cytoplasm)
  - neutrophils
  - eosinophils
  - basophils
- agranulocytes (despite the name contain a few granules in the cytoplasm)
  - monocytes
  - lymphocytes.

Neutrophils

Neutrophils are the most abundant white blood cells and play an important role in the immune system. They form approximately 60–65% of granulocytes and are phagocytes. They are approximately 10–12 µm in diameter and capable of ingesting microorganisms. They contain lysozymes; therefore, their main function is to protect the body from any foreign material. They are capable of moving out of blood vessel walls by a process called diapedesis and are actively phagocytic. A non-active neutrophil lasts approximately 12 h, while an active neutrophil may last 1–2 days. Neutrophils are the first immune cells to arrive at a site of infection, through a process known as **chemotaxis**. A deficiency of neutrophils is called **neutropenia**, which may be congenital or acquired; for example, in certain kinds of anaemia and leukaemia, or as a side effect of chemotherapy. Since neutrophils are such an important part of the immune response, a lowered neutrophil count results in a compromised immune system.

The nuclei of the neutrophils are multi-lobed (Figure 8.8). The number of neutrophils increases in:

- pregnancy
- infection

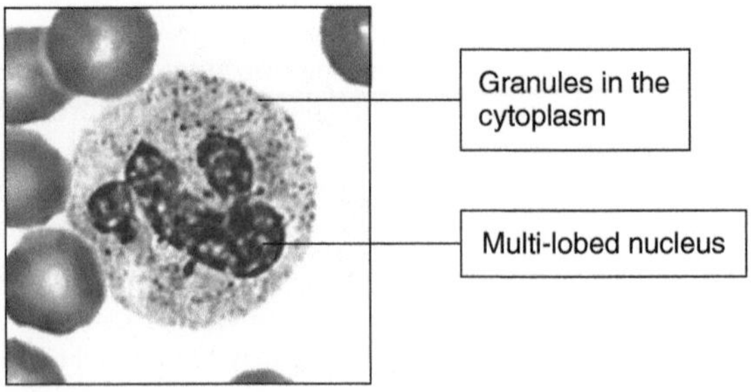

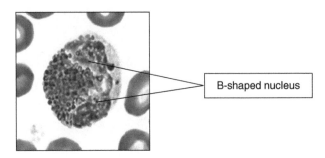

Figure 8.8 **Neutrophil.** *Source:* Tortora and Derrickson (2009). Reproduced with permission of John Wiley & Sons.

Figure 8.9 **Eosinophil.** *Source:* Tortora and Derrickson (2009). Reproduced with permission of John Wiley & Sons.

- leukaemia
- metabolic disorders such as acute gout
- inflammation
- myocardial infarction.

Eosinophils

These form approximately 2–4% of granulocytes and have B-shaped nuclei (see Figure 8.9). Like neutrophils, they too migrate from blood vessels and they are 10–12 μm in diameter. They are phagocytes; however, they are not as active as neutrophils. They contain lysosomal enzymes and peroxidase in their granules, which are toxic to parasites, resulting in the destruction of the organism. Numbers increase in allergy (e.g. hay fever and asthma) and parasitic infection (e.g. tapeworm infection).

Basophils

Basophils are least abundant, accounting for approximately 1% of granulocytes, and contain elongated lobed nuclei (Figure 8.10). Basophils are 8–10 μm in diameter. In inflamed tissue they become mast cells and secrete granules containing heparin, histamine and other proteins that promote inflammation. They also secrete lipid mediators such as leukotrienes and several cytokines. Basophils play an important role in providing immunity against parasites and also in the allergic response, as they have immunoglobulin E (IgE) on their surface and release chemical mediators that cause allergic symptoms when the IgE binds to its specific allergen.

Monocytes

Monocytes account for 5% of the agranulocytes and are circulating leucocytes (Figure 8.11). Monocytes develop in the bone marrow and spread through the body in 1–3 days. They are approximately 12–20 μm in diameter. The nucleus of the monocyte is kidney- or horseshoe-shaped. Some of the monocytes migrate into the tissue, where they develop into macrophages and engulf pathogens or foreign proteins. Macrophages play a vital role in immunity and inflammation by destroying specific antigens.

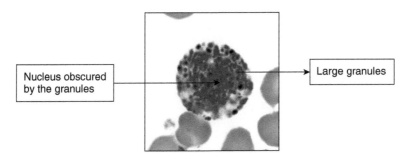

Figure 8.10 **Basophil.** *Source:* Tortora and Derrickson (2009). Reproduced with permission of John Wiley & Sons.

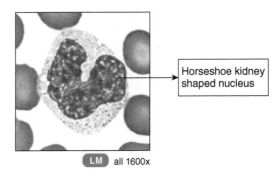

Figure 8.11 **Monocytes.** *Source:* Tortora and Derrickson (2009). Reproduced with permission of John Wiley & Sons.

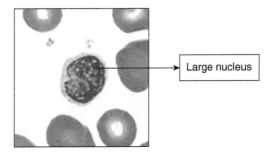

Figure 8.12 **Lymphocyte.** *Source:* Tortora and Derrickson (2009). Reproduced with permission of John Wiley & Sons.

Lymphocytes

Lymphocytes account for 25% of the leucocytes, and most are found in the lymphatic tissue such as the lymph nodes and the spleen (Figure 8.12). Small lymphocytes are approximately 6–9 μm in diameter, while the larger ones are 10–14 μm in diameter. They get their name from the lymph, the fluid that transports them. They can leave and re-enter the circulatory system, and their life span ranges from a few hours to years. The main difference between lymphocytes and other white blood cells is that lymphocytes are not phagocytes. Two types of lymphocytes are identified, and they are T- and B-lymphocytes. T-lymphocytes originate from the thymus gland (hence the name), while B-lymphocytes originate in the bone marrow. T-lymphocytes mediate cellular immune response, which is part of the body's own defence. The B-lymphocytes, on the other hand, become large plasma cells and produce antibodies that attach to antigens.

Platelets

Platelets are small blood cells consisting of some cytoplasm surrounded by a plasma membrane. They are produced in the bone marrow from megakaryocytes and fragments of megakaryocytes break off to form platelets. They are approximately 2–4 μm in diameter but have no nucleus and the life span is approximately 5–9 days. Old and dead platelets are removed by macrophages in the spleen and the Kupffer cells in the liver. The surface of platelets contains proteins and glycoproteins that allow them to adhere to other proteins such as collagen in the connective tissues. Platelets play a vital role in blood loss by the formation of platelet plugs, which seal the holes in the blood vessels and release chemicals that aid blood clotting. If the platelet number is low, excessive bleeding can occur; however, if the number increases, blood clots (thrombosis) can form, leading to cerebrovascular accident, deep vein thrombosis, heart attack or pulmonary embolism.

Haemostasis

Haemostasis is a sequence of responses that stops bleeding and can prevent haemorrhage from smaller blood vessels. Haemostasis plays an important part in maintaining homeostasis, and it consists of three main components:

- vasoconstriction
- platelet aggregation
- coagulation.

Vasoconstriction

- Results from contraction of the smooth muscle of the vessel wall, a reaction called vascular spasm.
- Constriction blocks small blood vessels, thus preventing blood flow through them.
- The action of the sympathetic nervous system is to cause vasoconstriction, which restricts blood flow for several minutes or several hours.
- Platelets release thromboxanes, which belong to the lipid group eicosanoids. Thromboxanes are vasoconstrictors and potent hypertensive agents; they facilitate platelet aggregation.

Platelet Aggregation

- Platelets adhere to the exposed collagen fibres of the connective tissue of the damaged blood vessels.
- Platelets release adenosine diphosphate, thromboxane and other chemicals that make other platelets in the area stick, and they all clump together to form a platelet plug. Platelet plugs are very effective in preventing blood loss in small blood vessels, and with fibrin threads form tight plugs.

Coagulation

Blood coagulation is an important process to maintain homeostasis. If blood vessel damage is so extensive that platelet aggregation and vasoconstriction cannot stop the bleeding, the complicated process of coagulation (blood clotting) will begin to take place with the aid of clotting factors (Table 8.2). Coagulation factors are a group of proteins essential for clotting, and most of the clotting factors are synthesised in the liver and some are obtained from our diet.

The simplified clotting stages involve the following:

1. Thromboplastinogenase is an enzyme released by the blood platelets and combines with antihaemophilic factor to convert the plasma protein thromboplastinogen into thromboplastin.
2. Thromboplastin combines with calcium ions to convert the inactive plasma protein prothrombin into thrombin.

Table 8.2 **Blood clotting factors.**

FACTOR	COMMON NAME
I	Fibrinogen
II	Prothrombin
V	Proaccelerin, labile factor
VII	Proconvertin
VIII	Antihaemophilic factor A
IX	Antihaemophilic factor B
X	Thrombokinase, Stuart-Prower factor
XI	Antihaemophilic factor C
XII	Hageman factor
XIII	Fibrin stabilising factor

3. Thrombin acts as a catalyst to convert the soluble plasma protein fibrinogen into insoluble plasma protein fibrin.
4. The fibrin threads trap blood cells to form a clot.
5. Once the clot is formed, the healing of the damaged blood vessel takes place, which restores the integrity of the blood vessel.

Two pathways are responsible for triggering a blood clot, known as intrinsic and extrinsic pathways. The extrinsic pathway is a rapid clotting system activated when the blood vessels are ruptured and tissue damage takes place. The intrinsic pathway is slower than the extrinsic pathway and is activated when the inner walls of the blood vessels are damaged.

Clinical Considerations Clotting Disorders

Sometimes a blood clot forms within a blood vessel that has not been injured or cut. For example:

- A blood clot that forms within an artery supplying blood to the heart or brain is a common cause of heart attack and stroke. The platelets become sticky and clump next to patches of atheroma (fatty material) in blood vessels and activate the clotting mechanism.
- Sluggish blood flow can make the blood clot more readily than usual. This is a factor in deep vein thrombosis, which is a blood clot that sometimes forms in a leg vein.
- Certain genetic conditions can make the blood clot more easily than usual.
- Certain medicines can affect the blood clotting mechanism, or increase the amount of some clotting factors, which may result in the blood clotting more readily.
- Liver disorders can sometimes cause clotting problems, as the liver makes some of the chemicals involved in preventing and dissolving clots.

There are a number of different blood tests which can identify clotting problems. The ones chosen depend on the circumstances and the suspected problem. Some of them include:

- Blood count – full blood count is a routine blood test that can count the number of red cells, white cells and platelets per millilitre of blood. It will detect a low level of platelets.
- Bleeding time – in this test, a tiny cut is made in the earlobe or forearm and the time taken for the bleeding to stop is measured. It is normally 3–8 minutes.
- Blood clotting tests – there are a number of tests that may be done. For example, the 'prothrombin time' and the 'activated partial thromboplastin time' are commonly done. These tests measure the time it takes for a blood clot to form after certain activating chemicals are added to the blood sample.
- Platelet aggregation test – this measures the rate at which, and the extent to which, platelets form clumps (aggregate) after a chemical is added that stimulates aggregation. It tests the function of the platelets.

See Knott (2017).

Medicines Management Anticoagulants

 Anticoagulant medicines reduce the ability of the blood to clot. This is necessary if the blood clots too much, as blood clots can block blood vessels and lead to conditions such as a stroke or a heart attack. The two most common anticoagulant medicines are:

- heparin
- warfarin.

Rixaroxaban, dabigatran and apixaban are newer anticoagulants that may be used as an alternative to warfarin for certain conditions. Some of the side effects for these medications include:

- passing blood in the urine or stool
- severe bruising
- excessive bleeding (haemorrhage)
- bleeding gums
- prolonged nose bleeds
- passing black faeces
- difficulty in breathing/chest pain
- in women, heavy or increased bleeding during a period, or any other bleeding from the vagina.

Patients taking anticoagulant medicines should be monitored closely to check that they are on the correct dose and not at risk of excessive bleeding (haemorrhage). The most common test for this is the international normalisation ratio.

See NHS Choices (2018b).

Episode of Care Learning Disabilities

Jonathan Gray is a 25-year-old student nurse in his first year of college. He loves playing rugby during the weekend, an outlet for the pent up energy build-up of his Attention Deficit Disorder (ADD). Jonathan employs prescribed strategies given to him by a neurologist to concentrate hard at college during the week. One Saturday when playing rugby, Jonathan received a blow to his face during a rugby tackle. His nose started to bleed heavily and did not stop. He was rushed to the local Emergency Department with a severe nose bleed.

He was seen by the triage nurse and during the assessment Jonathan informed the nurse that he has haemophilia, inherited from his mother. This genetic condition is normally carried asymptomatically by women, but it is men who usually display the symptoms of the disorder. People with haemophilia have impaired clotting mechanisms and bleed more easily, meaning that major injuries could cause life-threatening haemorrhages. The nurse recorded his vital signs as temperature 37 °C, pulse 68 beats per minute, respiration 16 breaths per minute and blood pressure 116/60 mmHg. He informed the nurse that he was told to avoid contact sports, but confessed that 'Rugby is my stress-relief. Without it, I don't think I'd be able to carry on at college.' The nurse makes a note that his ADD has not impeded Jonathan's capacity to understand the possible consequences of continuing to engage in a contact sport.

He was also seen by the duty doctor, who carried out some blood tests. The result of the test indicated that his activated partial thromboplastin time (APTT) was slightly delayed and his bleeding times were abnormal.

Jonathan was treated with desmopressin, a synthetic hormone. Hormones are powerful chemicals that can have a wide range of effects on the body. Desmopressin works by stimulating the production of clotting factor VIII (8) and is usually given by injection.

He was admitted for overnight observations and to assess the effect of the treatment.

Multiple Choice Questions

1. Haemophilia is:
   - (a) a condition affecting the lymph glands
   - (b) only found in women and children
   - (c) always associated with the white blood cells
   - (d) none of the above
2. Haemophilia:
   - (a) is always inherited, all people who have it are male
   - (b) is usually inherited, most people who have it are male
   - (c) can be transmitted during close sexual relationships
   - (d) is cured with radiotherapy and chemotherapy

3. With regards to haemophilia:
    (a) there is a cure, treatment allows a person with the condition to enjoy a good quality of life
    (b) the person requires high levels of Vitamin C
    (c) there is no cure, treatment can help a person enjoy a good quality of life
    (d) a blood transfusion of red blood cells is required every month
4. If a person with haemophilia gets a cut:
    (a) they will bleed to death
    (b) they will always be prone to infection
    (c) they always bleed into the knee joint
    (d) none of the above
5. Haemophilia:
    (a) results from a missing or deficient protein needed for blood clotting
    (b) is due to anaemia
    (c) can be outgrown
    (d) can cause HIV

Blood Groups

It is the red blood cells that define which blood group an individual belongs to. On the surface of the red cells there are markers called antigens, which are so small they cannot even be seen under a microscope. Apart from identical twins, each person has different antigens, and these antigens are the key to identifying blood types and must be matched in transfusions to avoid serious complications. The structure for defining blood groups is known as the ABO system. If an individual has blood group A, then they have A antigens covering their red cells. Group B has B antigens on their red blood cell, while group O has neither antigens and group AB has both antigens (Tortora and Derrickson, 2011).

The ABO system also covers antibodies in the plasma that are the body's natural defence against foreign antigens. So, for example, blood group A has anti-B in their plasma, B has anti-A, and so on. However, group AB has no antibodies and group O has both (see Figure 8.13). If these antibodies find the wrong red blood cells, they will attack them and destroy them. That is why transfusing the wrong blood to a patient can be fatal.

There is also another factor (factor D) to be considered – the rhesus factor (Rh) system. Rh antigens can be present in each of the blood groups. Not everyone has the Rh antigen on the red blood cell; however, if a person has Rh antigen on their red blood cells then they are Rh positive and if they do not have the Rh antigen then they are Rh negative. A person with blood group A and Rh positive is known as A+, while if the Rh is negative they are A–. The same applies for B, AB and O. In the UK, approximately 85% of the population are rhesus positive; that is, they possess factor D on their red blood cells. The remaining 15% of the

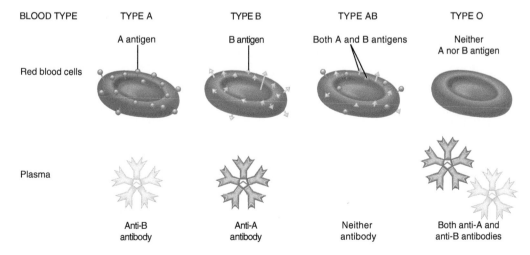

Figure 8.13 **ABO blood groups.** *Source:* Tortora and Derrickson (2009). Reproduced with permission of John Wiley & Sons.

Table 8.3 **Blood groups.**

BLOOD TYPE	ANTIGENS	ANTIBODIES	CAN DONATE BLOOD TO	CAN RECEIVE BLOOD FROM
A	Antigen A	Anti-B	A, AB	A, O
B	Antigen B	Anti-A	B, AB	B, O
AB	Antigen A Antigen B	None	AB	A, B, AB, O
O	None	Anti-A Anti-B	A, B, AB, O	O

population are rhesus negative as their red blood cells do not have factor D. It is important to consider the rhesus factor when cross-matching and transfusing blood to patients to avoid unnecessary complications such as agglutination (Table 8.3).

Skills in Practice Blood Transfusion

Blood transfusion is the common term employed in medicine for the delivery of blood components directly (intravenously) into a person's circulation. Blood is usually administered through a plastic tube inserted into a vein in the arm. It can take between 30 minutes and 4 hours, depending on how much blood is needed.

The components may be administered as a whole or individually. For example, a patient may need a replacement of red and white cells, as well as platelets and plasma, and receive a whole unit of blood. On the other hand, the patient may only require a platelet or plasma transfusion and the other components of the blood will not be given.

There are strict regulations regarding blood donations and blood transfusions. The aim of the regulations is to minimise the risk of a person being given blood contaminated with a virus, such as hepatitis C, or receiving blood from a blood group that is unsuitable for them.

Before the procedure, rigorous checks must be undertaken to ensure that the correct product and blood type is given to the correct patient. This includes careful confirmation of the patient's identity, their specific transfusion requirements, that the transfusion bag matches the details and blood typing on the patient's prescription and laboratory form, and that the product is in date and appears healthy and intact (Cowan and Davies, 2018).

A patient receiving a blood transfusion will be placed under close observation during and after the procedure. Adverse reactions to a blood transfusion can be hazardous and potentially life-threatening.

Patients undertaking blood transfusions will have their vital signs, including respiration rate, pulse, blood pressure and temperature monitored carefully. Initial symptoms of a reaction may include shortness of breath and a fast pulse (Jones, 2018). Any sign of a reaction requires that the transfusion is stopped immediately and that the patient is reviewed quickly by a doctor.

Blood Vessels

Blood vessels are part of the circulatory system that transports blood throughout the body. There are three major types of blood vessels: the arteries, which carry the blood away from the heart; the capillaries, which enable the actual exchange of water, nutrients and chemicals between the blood and the tissues; and the veins, which carry blood from the capillaries back towards the heart (Figure 8.14). All arteries, with the exception of the pulmonary and umbilical arteries, carry oxygenated blood, while most veins carry deoxygenated blood from the tissues back to the heart; exceptions are the pulmonary and umbilical veins, both of which carry oxygenated blood. The capillaries form the microcirculatory system, and it is at this point that nutrients, gases, water and electrolytes are exchanged between the blood and the tissue fluid. Capillaries are tiny, extremely thin-walled vessels and act as a bridge between arteries and veins. The thin walls of the capillaries allow oxygen and nutrients to pass from the blood into tissue fluid and allow waste products to pass from tissue fluid into the blood.

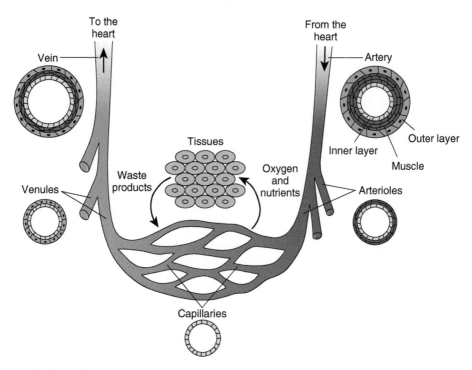

Figure 8.14 **Blood vessels.**

Structure and Function of Arteries and Veins

For most of the blood vessels, the walls consist of three layers:

- the tunica interna
- the tunica media
- the tunica externa (adventia) (Figure 8.15).

The **tunica interna** is a thin layer (only a few cells thick) of a vein and artery. It is sometimes referred to as the intima membrane. It is this layer that gives smoothness to the lining of the vessel, enhancing blood flow. It is lined by endothelial cells and elastic tissues; however, it varies in thickness between the blood vessels:

- arteries – most elastic tissue;
- veins – very little tissue;
- capillaries – no elastic layer.

The **tunica media** consists of elastic fibres and smooth muscle that allow for vasoconstriction, changing blood flow and pressure. The tunica media is supplied by the sympathetic branch of the autonomic nervous system. When stimulated, the walls contract, narrowing the lumen and increasing pressure within the blood vessel:

- arteries – varies by the size of the artery;
- veins – thin layer;
- capillaries – do not have tunica media.

The **tunica externa** (adventia) consists of collagen fibres and varies in thickness between the vessels. The collagen serves to anchor the blood vessel to nearby organs, giving it support and stability:

- arteries – relatively thick;
- veins – relatively thick;
- capillaries – very delicate.

Although the arteries and veins have similar layers, there are some clear differences between these two vessels. For a summary, see Table 8.4 and Figure 8.16.

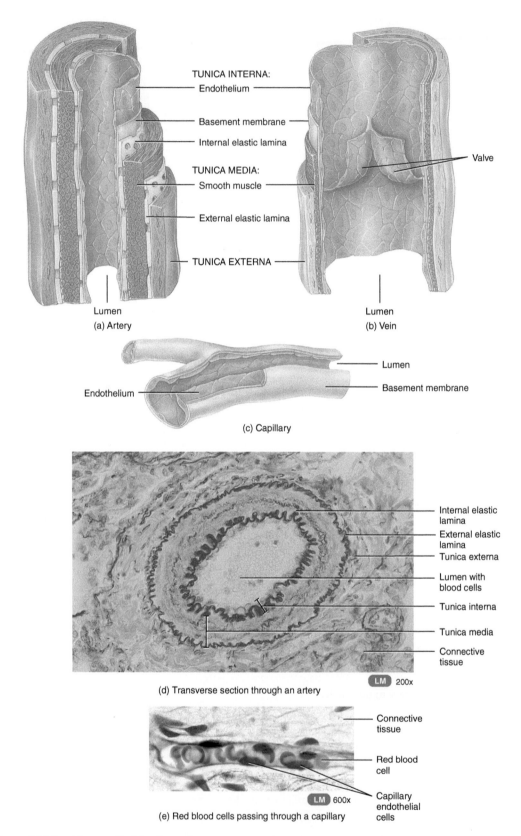

Figure 8.15 (a–e) Layers of a blood vessel. *Source:* Tortora and Derrickson (2009). Reproduced with permission of John Wiley & Sons.

Table 8.4 **Differences between arteries and veins.**

ARTERIES	VEINS
Transport blood away from the heart	Transport blood to the heart
Carry oxygenated blood, except the pulmonary and umbilical arteries	Carry deoxygenated blood, except the pulmonary and umbilical veins
Have a narrow lumen	Have a wider lumen
Have more elastic tissue	Have less elastic tissue
Do not have valves	Do have valves
Transport blood under pressure	Transport blood under low pressure

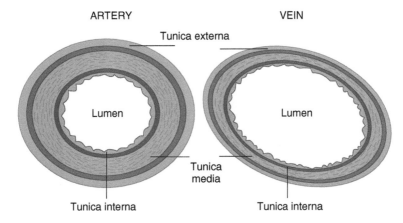

Figure 8.16 **Artery and vein.**

Capillaries

Capillaries are tiny blood vessels, approximately 5–20 µm in diameter. There are networks of capillaries (see Figure 8.17) in most of the organs and tissues of the body. Capillary walls are only one cell thick, which allows exchange of material between the contents of the capillary and the surrounding tissue fluid. The walls of capillaries are composed of a single layer of cells, the endothelium. This layer is so thin that molecules such as oxygen, water and lipids can pass through them by diffusion and enter the tissues. Waste products such as carbon dioxide and urea can diffuse back into the blood to be carried away for removal. Capillaries are so small that the red blood cells need to change shape in order to pass through them in single file.

Skills in Practice Caring for a Patient with an Intravenous Cannula

A cannula is a narrow tube which is inserted in a blood vessel or body cavity. It is a common procedure carried out in most health care facilities and the device may be kept in for a number of hours or days, depending on what it is needed for.

A peripheral intravenous cannula, also known as an intravenous catheter, is placed in a vein, usually in the lower arm. Its main purpose is to facilitate the administration of fluids or medications straight into the circulation. However, infections of the skin surrounding the device, or of the blood, can occur if they are not cared for properly.

Catheter-related blood stream infections are a dangerous complication which can develop into the life-threatening condition, sepsis. Once the cannula is in place, it must be monitored carefully in order to prevent sepsis and other complications associated with an indwelling intravenous device. These include irritation of the site, phlebitis and blood or air emboli (Barton et al., 2017).

An assessment tool, such as the Visual Infusion Phlebitis score (Jackson, 1999), is implemented to allow the catheter site to be monitored and maintained safely. The patient with an intravenous device is also advised to report symptoms such as pain, redness or swelling of the site so that any developing problems can be identified and treated quickly.

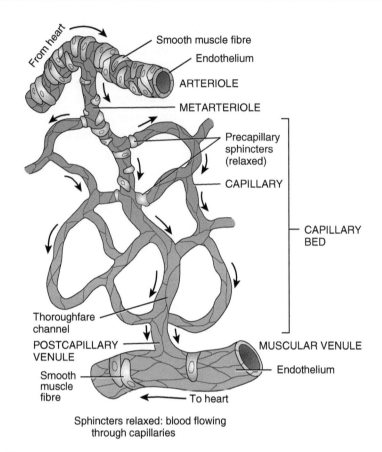

Figure 8.17 **Capillary.** *Source:* Tortora and Derrickson (2009). Reproduced with permission of John Wiley & Sons.

Blood Pressure

Blood pressure is the pressure exerted by blood within the blood vessel. The pressure is at its greatest near the heart and decreases as the blood moves further from the heart. Three factors regulate blood pressure. They are:

- neuronal regulation – through the autonomic nervous system
- hormonal regulation – adrenaline, noradrenaline, renin and others
- autoregulation – through the renin-angiotensin system.

Physiological Factors Regulating Blood Pressure

Several factors affect blood pressure, including:

- Cardiac output, the volume of blood pumped out by the heart in 1 minute. Cardiac output is a function of heart rate and stroke volume. The heart rate is simply the number of heart beats per minute. The stroke volume is the volume of blood, in millilitres, pumped out of the heart with each beat.
- Circulating volume, the volume of circulating blood perfusing tissues.
- Peripheral resistance, the resistance provided by the blood vessels.
- Blood viscosity, the measure of the resistance of blood flow. The resistance is provided by plasma proteins and other substances in the blood.
- Hydrostatic pressure, the pressure exerted by the blood on the vessel wall.

Control of Arterial Blood Pressure

Blood pressure within the large systemic arteries must be maintained to ensure adequate blood flow to the tissues. This is maintained by:

- Baroreceptors situated in the arch of the aorta and the carotid sinus, which are sensitive to pressure changes within the blood vessel. When blood pressure increases, signals are sent to the cardio-regulatory centre (CRC) in the brainstem (medulla oblongata). The CRC increases the parasympathetic activity to the heart, reducing heart rate and inhibiting sympathetic activity to the blood vessels, causing vasodilatation. This reduces blood pressure. On the other hand, if the blood pressure falls, the CRC increases the sympathetic activity to the heart and the blood vessels, thus increasing heart rate and vasoconstriction, resulting in increased blood pressure.
- Chemoreceptors situated in carotid and aortic bodies help to regulate blood pressure by detecting changes in the levels of oxygen, carbon dioxide and hydrogen ions. Changes in the levels of carbon dioxide, oxygen and hydrogen ions can affect heart and respiration rates.
- Circulating hormones, such as antidiuretic and atrial natriuretic peptide hormones, help to regulate circulating blood volume, thus affecting blood pressure.
- The renin–angiotensin system helps to maintain blood pressure through its action on vasoconstriction.
- The hypothalamus responds to stimuli such as emotion, pain and anger and stimulates sympathetic nervous activity, affecting blood pressure.

Lymphatic System

The lymphatic system (Figure 8.18) is part of the circulatory system and it transports a clear fluid called lymph. The lymphatic system begins with very small, closed-end vessels called lymphatic capillaries (Figure 8.19), which are in contact with the surrounding tissues and the interstitial fluid. The lymphatic system consists of:

- lymph
- lymph vessels
- lymph nodes
- lymphatic organs such as spleen and the thymus.

Lymph

Lymph is a clear fluid found inside the lymphatic capillaries and has a similar composition to plasma. Lymph is the ultrafiltrate of the blood, which occurs at the capillary ends of the blood vessels. Blood pressure in the blood vessel forces fluid and other substances such as small protein (albumin) from the capillaries into the tissue space as interstitial fluid, which then enters the lymphatic capillaries as lymph. The body contains approximately 1–2 L of lymph, which forms about 1–3% of body weight. Lymph transports plasma proteins, bacteria, fat from the small intestine and damaged tissues to the lymph nodes for destruction. The lymph contains lymphocytes and macrophages, which play an important role in the immune system.

Lymph Capillaries and Large Lymph Vessels

Both the blood and the lymphatic capillaries have a similar structure, in that they both consist of a single-layered endothelial cell that allows movement of substances from the interstitial space into the lymphatic capillaries (Figure 8.19). However, lymphatic capillaries are one-way vessels with a blind end (Figure 8.20) in the interstitial space. Lymphatic vessels resemble veins in structure; however, the lymphatic vessels have thinner walls and more valves in them. The larger lymphatic vessels have numerous valves to prevent backflow of lymph. The lymphatic vessels combine to form two large ducts, the right lymphatic and thoracic ducts, which then empty into the subclavian veins.

Lymph Nodes

Lymph nodes are bean-shaped organs located along the lymphatic vessels. These nodes are found in the largest concentrations in the neck, armpit, thorax, abdomen and the groin; lesser concentrations are found behind the elbows and knees. The lymphocytes in the lymph nodes filter out harmful substances from the

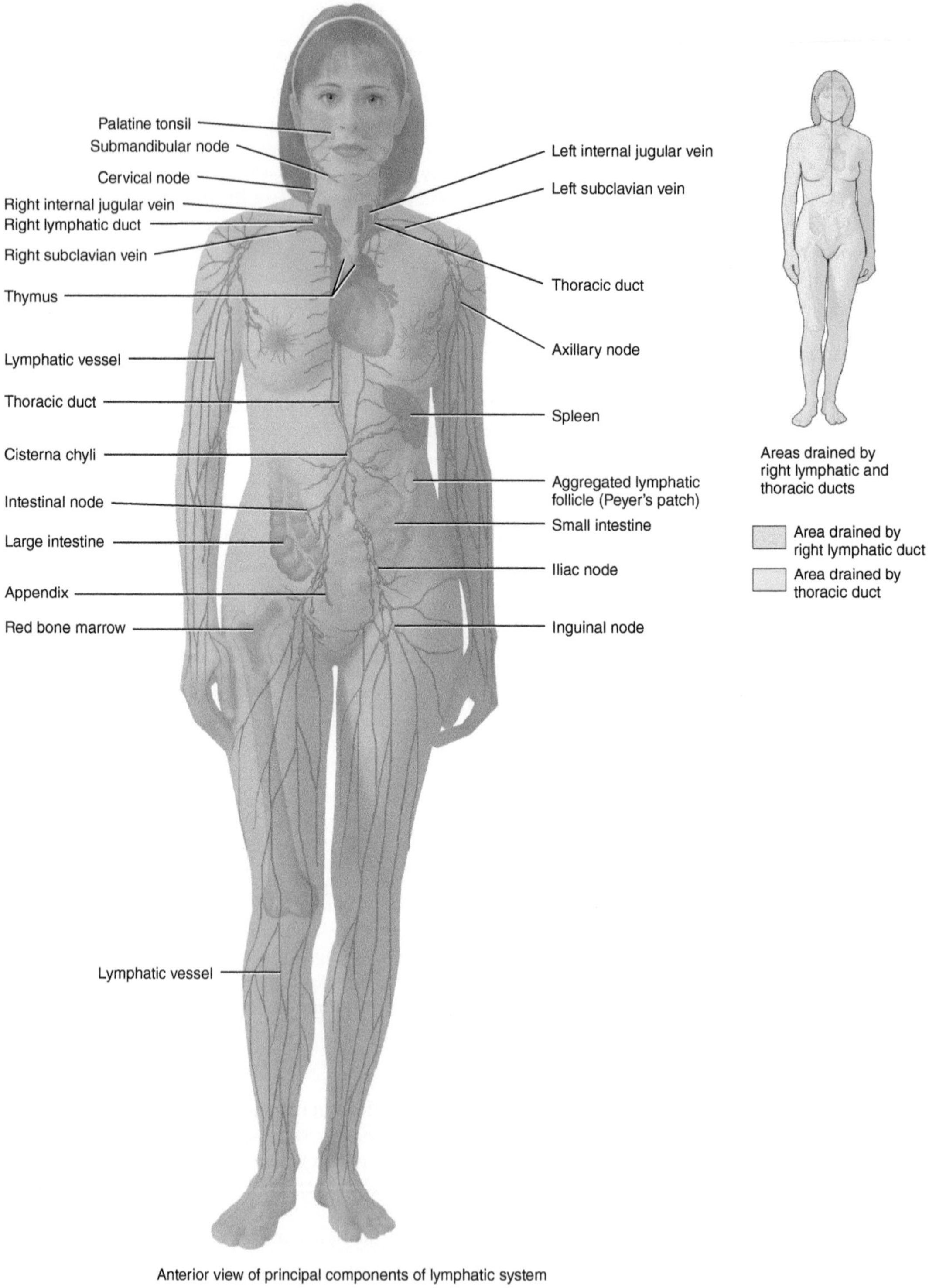

Anterior view of principal components of lymphatic system

Figure 8.18 **Lymphatic system.** *Source:* Tortora and Derrickson (2009). Reproduced with permission of John Wiley & Sons.

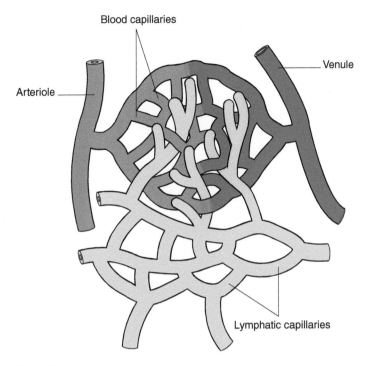

Figure 8.19 **Lymphatic capillaries.**

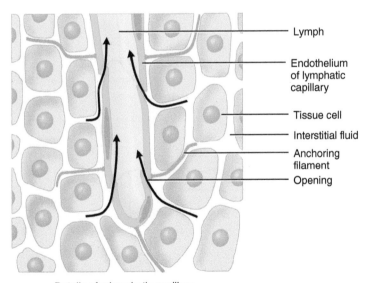

Details of a lymphatic capillary

Figure 8.20 **Lymphatic circulation.** *Source:* Tortora and Derrickson (2009). Reproduced with permission of John Wiley & Sons.

lymph and are sites for specific defences of the immune system. The lymph node is made up of an outer fibrous capsule that dips down into the node to form partitions (trabeculae), thus dividing the node into compartments (Figure 8.21). Approximately four or five afferent vessels may enter a lymph node; however, only one efferent vessel will transport the lymph out of the node.

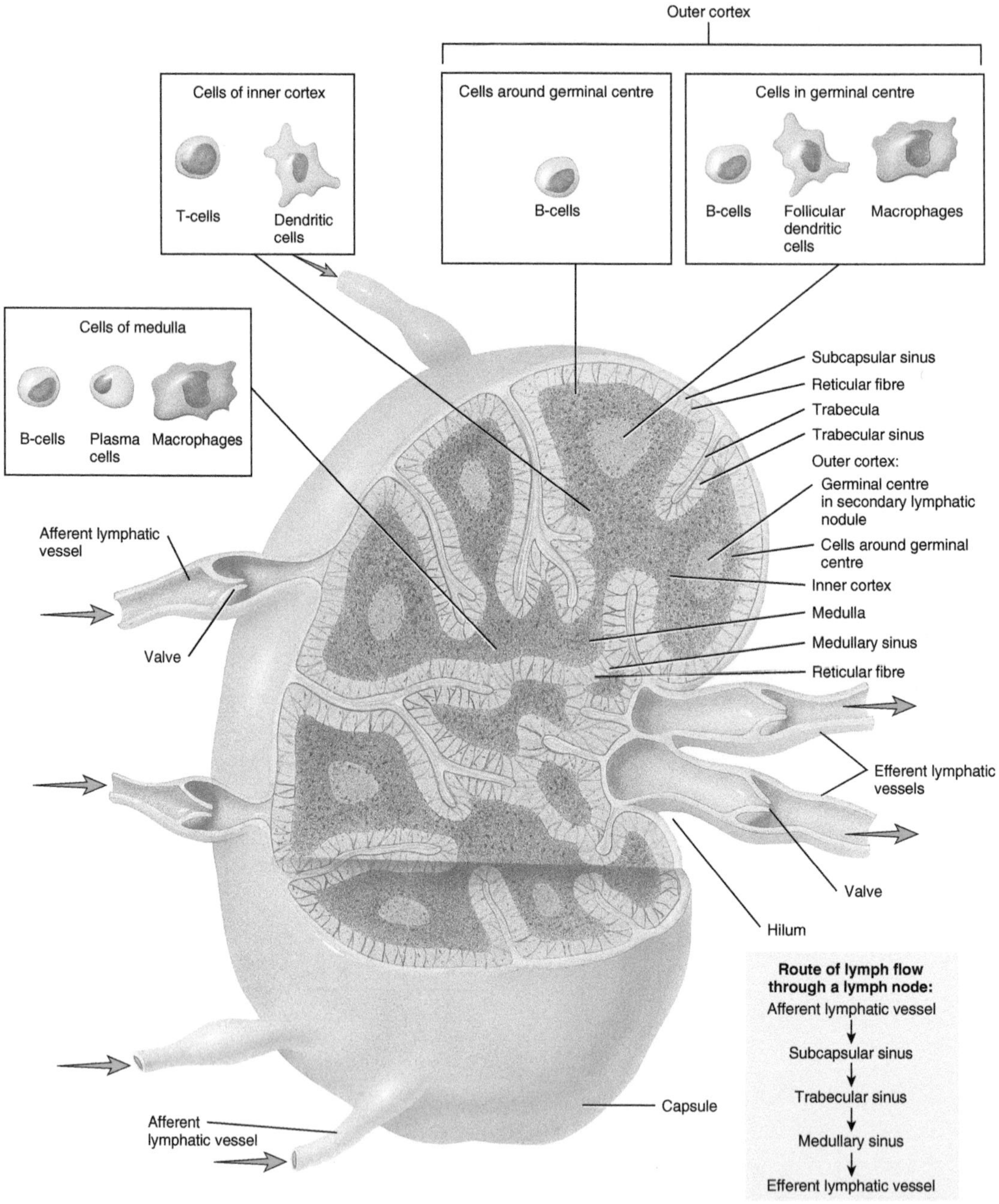

Outer cortex

Cells of inner cortex

T-cells | Dendritic cells

Cells around germinal centre

B-cells

Cells in germinal centre

B-cells | Follicular dendritic cells | Macrophages

Cells of medulla

B-cells | Plasma cells | Macrophages

Afferent lymphatic vessel

Valve

Subcapsular sinus
Reticular fibre
Trabecula
Trabecular sinus
Outer cortex:
Germinal centre in secondary lymphatic nodule
Cells around germinal centre
Inner cortex
Medulla
Medullary sinus
Reticular fibre

Efferent lymphatic vessels

Valve

Hilum

Route of lymph flow through a lymph node:
Afferent lymphatic vessel
↓
Subcapsular sinus
↓
Trabecular sinus
↓
Medullary sinus
↓
Efferent lymphatic vessel

Capsule

Afferent lymphatic vessel

Figure 8.21 **A lymph node.** *Source:* Tortora and Derrickson (2009). Reproduced with permission of John Wiley & Sons.

Clinical Considerations Oedema

Oedema, also known as dropsy, is the medical term for fluid retention in the body. The build-up of fluid causes affected tissue to become swollen. The swelling can occur in one particular part of the body – for example, as the result of an injury – or it can be more general.

The latter is usually the case with oedema that occurs as a result of certain health conditions, such as heart failure or kidney failure. Some of the possible symptoms include:

- skin discolouration
- areas of skin that temporarily hold the imprint of the finger when pressed (known as pitting oedema)
- aching, tender limbs
- stiff joints
- weight gain or weight loss
- raised blood pressure and pulse rate.

The treatment includes treating the underlying cause, including losing weight, exercise and diuretics to get rid of excess body water.

207

See Robinson (2015).

Medicines Management ABVD and Chemotherapy Treatments for Hodgkin Lymphoma

Hodgkin lymphoma is a blood cancer. Hodgkin lymphoma is a cancer that develops in the lymph nodes of the lymphatic system. It is the most common form of blood cancer in teenagers and young adults. It appears as a solid tumour in the glands in the neck, chest, armpit or groin.

Chemotherapy for Hodgkin lymphoma uses combinations of different anticancer drugs rather than just one drug. This reduces the chances of the patient developing resistance to any one of the drugs. It also reduces the side effects, because lower doses of individual drugs are used. The drug combination most widely used for Hodgkin lymphoma is called ABVD (adriamycin, bleomycin, vinblastine and dacarbazine). This regimen is usually given in 4-week cycles by administering the drugs into the vein on days 1 and 15 of each cycle. Patients with late-stage Hodgkin lymphoma are given more cycles of treatment.

Side effects of chemotherapy:

- nausea, which can be relieved using other medication;
- hair loss;
- low white blood cell count.

Side effects of ABVD include:

- heart problems caused by adriamycin;
- fever or rash caused by bleomycin;
- lung condition called fibrosis caused by bleomycin;
- ulcers or blisters caused by vinblastine;
- headaches, fatigue or diarrhoea caused by dacarbazine.

 Link To/Go To

See Blood Wise home page at:
https://bloodwise.org.uk/info-support/hodgkin-lymphoma/what.

Lymphatic Organs

Spleen

The two main organs of the lymphatic system are the spleen and the thymus gland. The spleen is the largest lymphoid organ and is approximately 12 cm in length, 7 cm wide and 2.5 cm thick. It weighs about 200 g and is purplish in colour. The main functions of the spleen are:

- filtering the blood – the destruction of old red blood cells and the remnants of manufacturing phagocytic lymphocytes and monocytes;
- storage of blood – approximately 350 mL.

The structure of the spleen is similar to the lymph node. The spleen is surrounded by a capsule of connective tissue and, like the lymph nodes, it is divided into compartments by trabeculae. The two main functional sections of the spleen are the red and the white pulp. It is in contact with the stomach, the left kidney and the diaphragm. The blood supply to the spleen derives from the splenic artery, and the splenic vein transports the blood out of the spleen.

The Thymus Gland

The thymus gland is a ductless, pinkish-grey mass of lymphoid tissue located in the thorax. At birth it is about 5 cm in length, 4 cm in breadth and about 6 mm in thickness. The organ enlarges during childhood and atrophies at puberty. The thymus gland consists of two lobes joined by connective tissue, and each lobe is covered by an outer cortex and an inner portion called the medulla. Each lobe is divided into lobules by trabeculae, and each lobule has an outer cortex and inner medulla. The cortex contains many immature lymphocytes, which migrate from the bone marrow to the thymus gland to become specialised T-lymphocytes (T-cells). Mature T-cells then migrate to the medulla and it is from the medulla the mature T-cells enter the general circulation, where they are transported by the blood to the spleen and the lymph nodes.

Functions of the lymphatic system

- The lymphatic system aids the immune system in destroying pathogens and filtering waste so that the lymph can be safely returned to the circulatory system.
- The lymphatic system removes excess fluid, waste, debris, dead blood cells, pathogens, cancer cells and toxins from these cells and the tissue spaces between them.
- The lymphatic system also works with the circulatory system to deliver nutrients, oxygen and hormones from the blood to the cells that make up the tissues of the body.
- Important protein molecules are created by cells in the tissues. These molecules are too large to enter the capillaries of the circulatory system; thus, these protein molecules are transported by the lymph to the bloodstream.

Episode of Care Mental Health

Molly Hopkins, a 62-year-old, is a retired nurse who has been living with anxiety for some years. She is married to Percy and they have two grown-up children who live abroad. Lately, Molly has been feeling more tired than usual and is waking up at night covered with sweats. She put this down to her anxiety, which has been worse of late after a minor car accident.

One evening, while having a shower, she felt a large swollen lump on the left side of her neck. Encouraged by her husband, she makes an appointment to see her GP. During the conversation, Molly informs her GP that she has lost an unplanned 4 kg over a 2-month period, which she has attributed to her 'nerves'. Concerned, her GP refers Molly to hospital for tests.

Molly is seen in the haematology clinic. After taking a medical history, the haematologist carries out some blood tests and a biopsy of the lump in the neck. In order to help Molly manage her increased anxiety while awaiting her results, the haematologist also refers her to a counselor. When Molly returns to the hospital after a couple of weeks for her results with her husband, she is informed that blood tests have revealed mild anaemia and an increased neutrophil count. The lymph node biopsy showed Reed-Sternberg cells, abnormally large lymph cells. A diagnosis of Hodgkin disease, described as cancer of the lymphatic system, is given, but the prognosis is good.

The haematologist takes his time to explain the recommended treatments to Molly so that she can ask questions and discuss her worries and fears. Molly continues to see the counselor during and after a short course of chemotherapy, followed by radiotherapy to the affected site. After these treatments, Molly returns under the care of her GP and community mental health team.

Multiple Choice Questions

1. Hodgkin disease is type of cancer of the:
   (a) endocrine system
   (b) lymphatic system
   (c) gastrointestinal system
   (d) the lymphatic and endocrine systems
2. The causes of Hodgkin disease is:
   (a) due to poor standards of living
   (b) unknown
   (c) due to hepatitis C
   (d) only found in adolescents
3. Hodgkin disease:
   (a) begins when a lymphocyte develops a genetic mutation
   (b) is always associated with TB
   (c) is identified on chest X-ray
   (d) can be transmitted via fomites

4. Factors that can increase the risk of Hodgkin disease include:
   (a) being female, obese and an elderly primigravida
   (b) being male and age
   (c) living in overcrowded accommodation
   (d) having recurrent bouts of flu and cold
5. The goal of treatment for Hodgkin disease is:
   (a) to offer palliation
   (b) to reduce the amount of red blood cells bringing the disease into remission
   (c) to destroy as many cancer cells as possible bringing the disease into remission
   (d) all of the above

Conclusion

The circulatory system is a very efficient and complex system. It ensures that all the cells and tissues of the body receive all they need, including oxygen, nutrients and electrolytes to ensure that all systems are functioning efficiently. The blood transports many substances, such as red blood cells, white blood cells, hormones and electrolytes essential for cellular function. It also plays a major role in the body's defence against bacteria and other organisms through the action of the white blood cells. The blood also transports waste products of metabolism; for example, urea, carbon dioxide and uric acid.

Blood that is pumped out of the left ventricle of the heart is transported by a network of vessels called arteries and the blood is returned to the heart by the veins. There are three types of blood vessels: arteries, veins and capillaries. Arteries carry blood away from the heart, while the veins transport blood to the heart. The blood vessels of the circulatory system are a closed system, in that blood does not leave or leak out of the blood vessels unless they are damaged. It is at the capillary end that nutrients and other products essential for cellular function leave the blood vessels. White blood cells may also leave the blood vessels at the capillary end; however, red blood cells are contained within the circulatory system.

The lymphatic system is also known as the secondary circulation. It transports fluid called lymph, which is an ultrafiltrate of the blood. It plays an important part in the immune system. The fluid lymph is transported by the lymphatic system from all parts of the body and returned to the circulatory system via the right lymphatic and thoracic ducts, which then empty into the subclavian veins.

Glossary

Active transport: The process by which substances move against a concentration gradient by utilising cellular energy.

Adenosine diphosphate: The end product that results when adenosine triphosphate loses one of its phosphate groups located at the end of the molecule.

Adenosine triphosphate: Compound that is necessary for cellular energy.

Chemical reactions: Reactions that involve molecules, in which they are formed, changed or broken down.

Compartments: Spaces.

Cytoplasm: Fluid found inside the cell.

Diffusion: The most common form of passive transport of materials; it is the means by which gases, liquids and solutes disperse randomly and occupy any space available so that there is an equal distribution.

Electrolytes: Substances that dissociate in water to form ions.

Embolus (plural: emboli): A mass that travels through the bloodstream, with the potential to clog up a blood vessel.

Endocytosis: Processes by which cells ingest foodstuffs and infectious microorganisms.

Extracellular: Space found outside the cell.

Exocytosis: The system of transporting material out of cells.

Facilitated diffusion: Diffusion with the aid of a transport protein.

Hydrophilic: Water loving.

Hydrophobic: Water hating.

Hypertonic: Solution that has a large amount of solutes dissolved in it.

Hypotonic: Solution that has a low concentration of solutes.

Hypovolaemia: Decreased volume of circulating blood.

Interstitial: Space between cells.

Intracellular: Space inside the cell.

Organelles: Structural and functional parts of a cell.

Osmosis: Movement of water through a selectively permeable membrane so that concentrations of substances in water are the same on either side of the membrane.

Osmotic pressure: The pressure that must be exerted on a solution.

Passive transport: The process by which substances move on their own down a concentration gradient without utilising cellular energy.

Phlebitis: Inflammation of a vein.

Plasma membrane: Outer layer of the cell.

Transport protein: Small molecules that help in the movement of ions across a cell membrane.

References

Barton, A., Ventura, R., **and** Vavrick, B. (2017) Peripheral intravenous cannulation: protecting patients and nurses. *British Journal of Nursing* **26**(8): 28–33.

Cowan, K. and Davies, A. (2018) How to undertake a blood component transfusion. *Nursing Standard* doi: 10.7748/ns.2018.e11196.

Jackson, A. (1999) Infection control: a battle in vein infusion phlebitis. *Nursing Times* **94**(4): 68–71.

Jenkins, G. and Tortora, G.J. (2013) *Anatomy and Physiology: From Science to Life,* vol. **2**, 3rd edn. Hoboken, NJ: John Wiley & Sons, Inc.

Jones, A. (2018) Safe transfusion of blood components. *Nursing Standard* **32**(25): 50–63.

Knott, L. (2017) Blood Clotting Tests. http://www.patient.co.uk/health/blood-clotting-tests (accessed 10 December 2018).

Nair, M. (2013) The blood and associated disorders. In Nair, M. and Peate, I. (eds), *Fundamentals of Applied Pathophysiology – An Essential Guide for Nursing and Healthcare Students*, 2nd edn. Chichester: John Wiley & Sons, Ltd.

NHS Choices (2018a) Iron Deficiency Anaemia – Treatment. http://www.nhs.uk/Conditions/Anaemia-iron-deficiency-/Pages/Treatment.aspx (accessed 9 December 2018).

NHS Choices (2018b) Anticoagulant Medicines. http://www.nhs.uk/conditions/anticoagulant-medicines/Pages/Introduction.aspx (accessed 10 December 2018).

Pellicori, P., Kaur, K. and Clark, A.L. (2015) Fluid management in patients with chronic heart failure. *Cardiac Failure Review* **1**(2): 90–95.

Robinson, A. (2015) Oedema (Swelling). http://www.patient.co.uk/health/oedema-swelling (accessed 10 December 2018).

Sharma, D. C., Arya, A., Kishor, P. and Woike, P. (2017) Overview on Thalassemias: a review article. *Medical Research Chronicles* **4**(3): 325–327.

Tortora, G.J. and Derrickson, B.H. (2009) *Principles of Anatomy and Physiology*, 12th edn. Hoboken, NJ: John Wiley & Sons, Inc.

Tortora, G.J. and Derrickson, B.H. (2011) *Principles of Anatomy and Physiology*, 13th edn. Hoboken, NJ: John Wiley & Sons, Inc.

Further Reading

Anaemia – iron deficiency

http://cks.nice.org.uk/anaemia-iron-deficiency#!scenariorecommendation:6

In this link you will find National Institute for Health and Care Excellence recommendation in the treatment and management of iron deficiency anaemia.

Blood clotting disorders

http://www.patient.co.uk/doctor/bleeding-disorders

Use this link to find out more about clotting disorders. It provides information on investigation and diagnosis, treatment and management.

Non-Hodgkin lymphoma – rituximab

http://guidance.nice.org.uk/TA65

Use this to find out National Institute for Health and Care Excellence (NICE) guidance on the use of rituximab (Mab Thera) to treat aggressive non-Hodgkin lymphoma.

210

Activities

Multiple Choice Questions

1. The first immune cells to arrive at a site of infection are:
   (a) basophils
   (b) monocytes
   (c) neutrophils
   (d) lymphocytes

2. Which of the options given below is correct?
   (a) blood is composed of plasma, red cells, white cells and platelets
   (b) lymph is composed of plasma, white cells and platelets
   (c) lymph is composed of plasma, red and white cells
   (d) plasma is composed of red cells, platelets and no white cells
3. Platelets release which chemicals to repair blood vessels?
   (a) fibrinogen
   (b) prothrombin
   (c) Factor VIII
   (d) thromboplastin
4. Which of the statements provided are incorrect?
   (a) monocytes circulate the bloodstream for many weeks
   (b) monocytes account for 5% of circulating white cells
   (c) monocytes are produced by the thymus gland
   (d) monocytes are the largest of the white cells
5. A person of blood O type:
   (a) has no antigens on their red cells
   (b) has antigens on their red cells
   (c) have parents who both have type O blood group
   (d) may receive blood from the A and B groups
6. Heparin is:
   (a) an antihistamine
   (b) an antibiotic
   (c) an anticoagulant
   (d) an antibody
7. When compared to blood, lymph:
   (a) contains more red than white cells
   (b) has no serum
   (c) has no white cells
   (d) has no red cells
8. Which of the organs below disposes of red blood cells?
   (a) the lymph glands
   (b) the spleen
   (c) the kidneys
   (d) the stomach
9. A person with the blood group A- can receive blood from:
   (a) group A+, A-, B+, B-
   (b) group O-, B-, O+, AB+
   (c) AB-, A-, B-, O-
   (d) A-, B-, O+, O-
10. Some of the checks performed prior to a blood transfusion include:
    (a) identity check and the taking of vital signs
    (b) blood typing and urine test
    (c) haemoglobin check and liver enzyme check
    (d) identity check and blood glucose check

11. Anticoagulants:
    (a) dissolve clots
    (b) reduce the ability for blood to clot
    (c) increase platelet production
    (d) increase blood clotting
12. Where are the chemoreceptors which detect blood pressure changes located?
    (a) between the left atria and left ventricle of the heart
    (b) in the carotid and aortic arch
    (c) in the medulla oblongata
    (d) in the jugular vein

13. Vital signs which indicate hypovolaemia:
    (a) high blood pressure, high pulse, high respirations
    (b) low blood pressure, low pulse, low respirations
    (c) low blood pressure, low pulse, high respirations
    (d) low blood pressure, high pulse, high respirations
14. Anaemia can result from a lack of vitamin:
    (a) A
    (b) B1
    (c) B12
    (d) D
15. The lining of large blood vessels consists of:
    (a) epithelial cells
    (b) endothelial cells
    (c) endometrial cells
    (d) smooth cells

Find Out More

1. Explain why blood is called connective tissue.
2. Within the classification of white blood cells there are some grouped under the term granulocytes. List these white blood cells and their functions.
3. What is acute myeloid leukaemia?
4. List the checks you would make to ensure that the patient is receiving the correct blood transfusion.
5. Describe the forces that move fluid across capillary walls.
6. Describe the physiological factors affecting blood pressure.
7. Explain the term 'essential hypertension'.
8. Describe the flow of lymphatic fluid through the lymphatic.
9. In our body there are MALT tissues. Explain the term MALT and its function.
10. How does the structure of a lymph node aid lymphocytes and macrophages in their protective function?

Conditions

Below is a list of conditions that are associated with the circulatory system. Take some time and write notes about each of the conditions. You may make the notes taken from textbooks or other resources (e.g. people you work with in a clinical area) or you may make the notes as a result of people you have cared for. If you are making notes about people you have cared for, you must ensure that you adhere to the rules of confidentiality.

Thrombocyte disorders

Aplastic anaemia

Deep vein thrombosis

Peripheral vascular disease

Non-Hodgkin's lymphoma

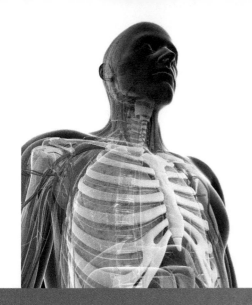

9

The Cardiac System

Carl Clare

Test Your Prior Knowledge

- Name the chambers of the heart.
- Describe blood flow through the heart.
- Name one of the valves in the heart.
- Describe the position of the heart in the body.
- Describe the factors that affect heart rate.

Learning Outcomes

After reading this chapter you will be able to:

- Describe the structure of the heart.
- List the arteries that supply blood to the heart muscle.
- Describe the electrical excitation of the heart.
- Describe the cardiac action potential.
- Discuss the cardiac cycle.

Visit the student companion website at www.wileyfundamentalseries.com/anatomy where you can test yourself using flashcards, multiple-choice questions and more. Instructor companion site at www.wiley.com/go/instructor/anatomy where instructors will find valuable materials such as PowerPoint slides and image bank designed to enhance your teaching.

Fundamentals of Anatomy and Physiology: For Nursing and Healthcare Students, Third Edition. Edited by Ian Peate and Suzanne Evans.
© 2020 John Wiley & Sons Ltd. Published 2020 by John Wiley & Sons Ltd.
Student companion website: www.wileyfundamentalseries.com/anatomy
Instructor companion website: www.wiley.com/go/instructor/anatomy

Body Map

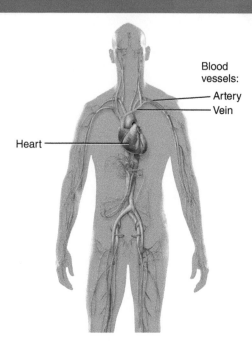

Blood
vessels:

— Artery

— Vein

Heart ————

Introduction

The heart is a muscular organ containing four chambers. Its main function is to pump blood around the circulatory system of the lungs and the systemic circulation of the rest of the body. In the average day the heart beats about 100,000 times and never rests. It must continue its cycle of contraction and relaxation in order to provide a continuous blood supply to the tissues and ensure the delivery of nutrients and oxygen and the removal of waste products. The purpose of this chapter is to review the structure and function of the heart, including:

- the size and location of the heart;
- the overall structure of the heart;
- the heart muscle and the cells of the heart;
- the blood supply to the heart muscle;
- the flow of blood through the heart;
- the electrical pathways of the heart;
- the cardiac cycle;
- factors affecting cardiac output.

Size and Location of the Heart

The heart weighs 250–390 g in men and 200–275 g in women and is a little larger than the owner's closed fist, being approximately 12 cm long and 9 cm wide (Jenkins and Tortora, 2013). It is located in the thoracic cavity (chest) in the mediastinum (between the lungs), behind and to the left of the sternum (breastbone) (see Figure 9.1).

As can be seen, the apex of the heart (the pointed end) is below the base of the heart and lies on the diaphragm. The base of the heart is itself made up of two of the chambers of the heart known as the atria (atrium is the singular of atria).

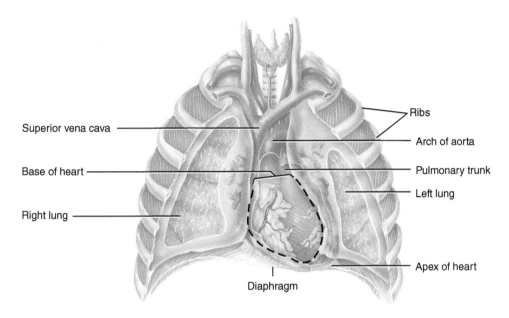

Figure 9.1 **Location of the heart.** *Source:* Tortora and Derrickson (2009). Reproduced with permission of John Wiley & Sons.

The Structures of the Heart

Heart Wall

Pericardium

The heart is surrounded by a membrane called the pericardium (peri = around). This is often referred to as a single sac surrounding the heart but is in fact made up of two sacs (the fibrous pericardium and the serous pericardium) that are closely connected to each other (see Figure 9.2). These two sacs have very different structures (Jenkins and Tortora, 2013):

- The fibrous pericardium, a tough, inelastic layer made up of dense, irregular, connective tissue. The role of this layer is to prevent the overstretching of the heart. It also provides protection to the heart and anchors it in place.
- The serous pericardium, a thinner, more delicate, layer that forms a double layer around the heart:
  - the parietal pericardium, the outer layer fused to the fibrous pericardium;
  - the visceral pericardium (otherwise known as the epicardium) adheres tightly to the surface of the heart.

Between the parietal and visceral pericardium is a thin film of fluid (pericardial fluid) that reduces the friction between the membranes as the heart moves during its cycle of contraction and relaxation. The space containing the pericardial fluid is known as the pericardial cavity; however, it must be noted that this 'space' is so small it is normally considered to be a 'virtual' space.

Myocardium

Underlying the pericardium is the heart muscle known as the myocardium (myo = muscle). The myocardium makes up the majority of the bulk of the heart. It is a type of muscle only found within the heart and is specialised in its structure and function. The myocardium can be divided into two categories: the majority is specialised to perform mechanical work (contraction); the remainder is specialised to the task of initiating and conducting electrical impulses (this second type of cardiac muscle cell will be reviewed later in the chapter). The cardiac muscle cells (myocytes) are held together in interlacing bundles of fibres that are arranged in a spiral or circular bundles. Compared with skeletal muscle fibres, cardiac muscle fibres are shorter in length and have branches (see Figure 9.3). The ends of the cardiac myocytes are attached to the adjacent cells

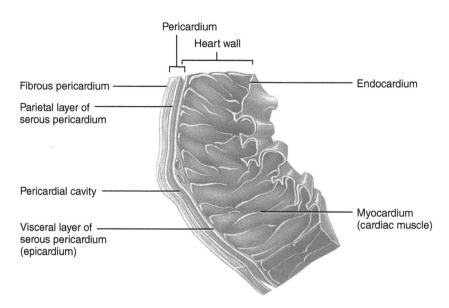

Figure 9.2 **Heart wall.** *Source:* Tortora and Derrickson (2009). Reproduced with permission of John Wiley & Sons.

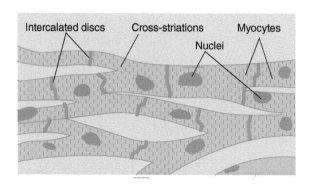

Figure 9.3 **Cardiac muscle cells (cardiac myocytes).**

in an end-to-end fashion. At this point there is a thickening of the sarcolemma (plasma membrane) known as intercalated discs. These discs contain two types of junction:

- desmosomes hold the cells together so that the fibres do not pull apart;
- gap junctions allow the rapid passage of action potentials (electrical current) between cells.

Compared with skeletal muscle cells, the cardiac myocyte contains one nucleus (or occasionally two nuclei) and the mitochondria are larger and more numerous, making cardiac muscle cells less prone to fatigue. However, cardiac muscle requires a large supply of oxygen and is less able to cope with reductions in the amount of available oxygen.

The cardiac muscle cells are divided into two discrete networks separated by a fibrous layer, the atria and the ventricles, and these two networks contract as separate units. Thus, the atria contract separately from the ventricles (see later). Within each myocyte are long contractile bundles of myofibrils. Myofibrils are in turn made up of smaller units known as sarcomeres. Contraction of the cardiac muscle is by the shortening of its sarcomeres.

Episode of Care Child

Stephen is a 14-year-old boy who is reporting increasing shortness of breath when playing sports at school. Knowing that Stephen's mother has hypertrophic cardiomyopathy, the GP refers Stephen for an echocardiogram. Echocardiographic testing shows the development of hypertrophy of the ventricular septum (the wall between the ventricles) which causes some obstruction of blood flow into the aorta. This obstruction does not cause problems in everyday life but when exercising the reduction in blood flow out of the heart leads to a reduction of blood flow to the tissues and the shortness of breath Stephen has been experiencing when playing sports. Further testing (such as 24-hour ECG monitoring) shows no evidence of cardiac arrythmias, echocardiography whilst exercising (stress echo) makes it clear that whilst Stephen has shortness of breath when exercising there is no need for surgical intervention. The cardiologist prescribes Stephen beta blockers and regularly reviews Stephen in clinic.

Hypertrophic cardiomyopathy (HCM) is the most common inherited cardiac condition (about 1:500 live births) and in many causes no symptoms. HCM is a condition that leads to the muscles of the heart (the myocardium) becoming thickened and stiff. In cases like Stephen's, the thickening of the muscles of the septum between the ventricles can lead to the obstruction of blood flow out of the heart into the aorta: this is known as hypertrophic obstructive cardiomyopathy (HOCM). HCM nearly always affects the left ventricle, occasionally it will affect the right ventricle as well.

The treatment of HCM depends on the severity of the disease. In mild cases (such as Stephen's) medication will be used. Commonly used medications are beta blockers and calcium channel blockers. If there is evidence of arrhythmias (disturbance of the heart rhythm) then anti-arrhythmic medications (such as amiodarone) will be prescribed. In severe cases an implantable cardioverter-defibrillator (ICD) will be implanted into the patient's chest. Severe cases of HCM may require surgical reduction of the heart muscle thickness or in very severe cases heart transplant.

As well as medical treatment patients with HCM should be counselled regarding lifestyle changes to reduce the impact of HCM on their life. Recommendations include: minimising alcohol, stopping smoking, reducing salt intake, maintaining a healthy weight and reducing caffeine intake. Whilst patients with HCM can (and should) exercise, the levels of exercise recommended differ from patient to patient and should be discussed with a doctor before a new exercise regimen is started.

For more information on HCM (and other cardiomyopathies) go to Cardiomyopathy UK at: https://www.cardiomyopathy.org/.

Multiple Choice Questions

1. Hypertrophic cardiomyopathy normally affects:
   (a) the right ventricle
   (b) the left ventricle
   (c) the left atrium
   (d) the right atrium
2. Echocardiography carried out whilst exercising is known as a:
   (a) treadmill test
   (b) stress echo
   (c) exercise echo
   (d) exercise test
3. Common medications used in the treatment of hypertrophic cardiomyopathy are:
   (a) beta blockers
   (b) calcium channel blockers
   (c) amiodarone
   (d) all of the above
4. Patients with hypertrophic cardiomyopathy should exercise:
   (a) following discussion with their doctor
   (b) following discussion with their physiotherapist
   (c) following discussion with their occupational therapist
   (d) following discussion with the nurse
5. Implantable cardioverter-defibrillators are implanted into patients to treat:
   (a) shortness of breath
   (b) arrhythmias
   (c) pain
   (d) dizziness

The Cardiac Action Potential

Unlike the normal skeletal muscle, in response to a single action potential a cardiac muscle fibre develops a prolonged contraction that is approximately 10–15 times longer in duration than a skeletal muscle contraction due to a plateau phase. Cardiac muscle fibres also have a longer refractory period, and thus a new contraction cannot be initiated until muscle relaxation is well advanced. Thus, a maintained contraction (tetany) cannot occur in cardiac muscle (Figure 9.4).

Endocardium

The endocardium (endo = within) is a layer of smooth simple epithelium lining the inside of the heart muscle (see Figure 9.2) and the heart valves. It is connected seamlessly with the lining of the large blood vessels that are connected to the heart.

The Heart Chambers

The heart is divided into four chambers (see Figure 9.5): the atria (entry halls or chambers) and the ventricles (little bellies). Even though the heart is referred to as a pump, it is better to think of it as two pumps:

- The right heart pump receives deoxygenated blood (blood that has given up some of its oxygen to the cells) from the tissues and pumps it out into the pulmonary circulation (the lungs).
- The left heart pump receives oxygenated blood from the pulmonary circulation and pumps it out to the rest of the body (the systemic circulation).

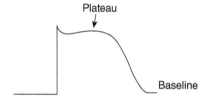

Figure 9.4 **Cardiac action potential.**

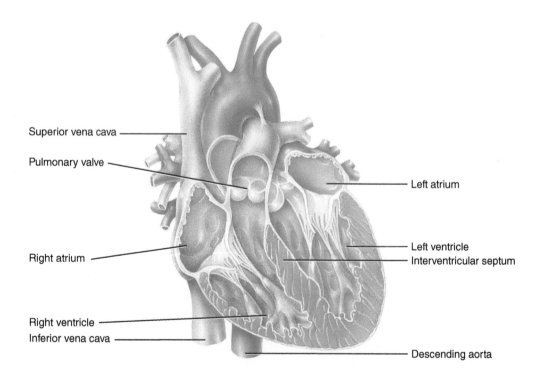

Figure 9.5 **The chambers of the heart.** *Source:* Tortora and Derrickson (2009). Reproduced with permission of John Wiley & Sons.

Atria

The atria are the smaller chambers of the heart and lie superior to (above) the ventricles. There are two atria:

- The right atrium receives blood from three veins: the superior vena cava, the inferior vena cava and the coronary sinus. The superior vena cava drains blood from the upper parts of the body, the inferior vena cava drains blood from the lower parts of the body and the coronary sinus drains blood from the circulation of the heart itself.
- The left atrium forms most of the base of the heart and receives blood from the lungs through four pulmonary veins.

Between the atria is a thin dividing wall, the interatrial septum (inter = between, septum = dividing wall).

The thickness of a chamber's wall varies according to the work the chamber has to perform. As the atria are only pumping blood into the ventricles they have much thinner walls than the ventricles, which have to pump blood around the pulmonary and systemic circulation.

Between the atria and the ventricles are two valves (the atrioventricular (AV) valves):

- the tricuspid valve is made up of three cusps (leaflets) and lies between the right atrium and the right ventricle;
- the bicuspid (mitral) valve is made up of two cusps and lies between the left atrium and the left ventricle.

The purpose of the AV valves is to prevent the backward flow of blood from the ventricles into the atria.

Ventricles

There are two ventricles: the right ventricle and the left ventricle. Each ventricle pumps the same amount of blood per beat but they have very different pressures.

- The right ventricle receives blood from the right atrium and pumps this blood out into the pulmonary circulation (the lungs). As the pressure in the pulmonary circulation is quite low the right ventricle has a thinner wall than the left ventricle.
- The left ventricle receives blood from the left atrium and pumps this blood out into the systemic circulation (the rest of the body) via the aorta. As the left ventricle has to pump against a higher pressure and over a greater distance it has a much thicker (more muscular) wall.

Between the ventricles is a dividing wall, the interventicular septum. Thus, with the septum between the atria and the septum between the ventricles there is no mixing of blood between the two sides.

At the outlet of each ventricle is a valve. Both of these valves are made up of three semilunar (half-moon-shaped) cusps (leaflets):

- the pulmonary valve lies between the right ventricle and the pulmonary arteries and prevents the backward flow of blood into the right ventricle from the pulmonary arteries;
- the aortic valve lies between the left ventricle and the aorta (the main artery leading to the systemic circulation) and prevents the backward flow of blood into the left ventricle from the systemic circulation.

Episode of Care Learning Disabilities

Daisy is a 43-year-old lady with Down syndrome (Trisomy 21) living in residential care, she has been reporting increasing shortness of breath on exertion and regular chest pain. Daisy has difficulty describing her symptoms and this has led to her reports often being ignored. The GP is suspicious of Daisy's shortness of breath and auscultates her lungs and heart. Though her lungs are clear, the GP hears a murmur when listening to Daisy's heart sounds.

The cardiologist refers Daisy for an electrocardiogram and an echocardiogram. The echocardiogram shows mild regurgitation of the aortic valve with a normal heart size. As Daisy's valve disease is relatively minor (not requiring surgery) he suggests the GP commences ACE inhibitor therapy (Baumgartner et al, 2017). Daisy will then be followed up yearly by the cardiologist to monitor the progression of the valve disease. Eventually Daisy may require valve replacement surgery.

Any of the four valves of the heart can become disordered in their functioning. There are two main processes that can affect the valves (Clare, 2007):

- **Valvular incompetence (regurgitation).** The valve becomes unable to close properly and thus there is backward flow of blood into the heart chamber behind the valve. Incompetence is most common in the mitral and aortic valves; it is very rare in both the tricuspid and pulmonary valves. Common causes of incompetence include age-related degeneration of the valve, infection of the valve and coronary heart disease.

- **Valve stenosis.** The valve becomes stiff and the leaflets of the valve may fuse together, thus narrowing the opening that blood can pass through. Stenosis is rare in the pulmonary valve and is usually only found in the tricuspid valve in conjunction with aortic and/or mitral valve stenosis. Common causes of stenosis are rheumatic fever, and age-related changes in the case of aortic valve stenosis.

Congenital heart defects are common in people with Down syndrome (Pfitzer et al., 2018), as screening programmes improve the rates of diagnosed congenital heart disease in those with Down syndrome are likely to increase. However, undiagnosed congenital heart disease remains common in the adult Down population (Vis et al., 2010). Adults with Down syndrome are entitled to free annual health checks with their GP and ideally this should include a cardiovascular examination.

Obesity is more prevalent in adults with Down syndrome than in the general population (Wong et al., 2014) and obesity predisposes patients to diabetes and coronary heart disease and exacerbates any congenital heart problems already present. As with many aspects of the care of patients with learning disabilities, a multidisciplinary approach is recommended for addressing obesity in those with Down syndrome. Approaches include, education, carer involvement, diet plans and regular health checks.

Multiple Choice Questions

1. Valve stenosis is a condition that causes:
   (a) stiffening of the valve
   (b) floppiness of the valve
   (c) the valve to collapse
   (d) the valve to stop working
2. Obesity is common in Down syndrome and predisposes the patient to:
   (a) diabetes
   (b) coronary heart disease
   (c) exacerbation of congenital heart disease
   (d) all of the above
3. A common cause of valve disease is:
   (a) infection
   (b) dehydration
   (c) age
   (d) smoking
4. Congenital heart disease can be missed in patients with Down syndrome due to:
   (a) a lack of concern from their carers
   (b) communication difficulties
   (c) different presentation of congenital heart disease in Down syndrome
   (d) it only develops later in life.
5. Patients with Down syndrome are entitled to a free health check:
   (a) every 6 months
   (b) every year
   (c) every 2 years
   (d) every 5 years

Skills in Practice Auscultation of Heart Sounds

The auscultation of heart sounds requires a stethoscope and good hearing (amplified stethoscopes are available for nurses with hearing impairments). A normal heart will have two sounds: 'lub' (known as S1) which is the closing of the atrioventricular valves and 'dub' (S2) which is caused by the closing of the semilunar valves (between atrium and ventricle). Other sounds that may be heard (adventitious sounds) include:

- Murmurs. These are caused by turbulent blood flow. The most common murmurs are related to heart valve disease.
- Rubs. A rub will almost always be a pericardial friction rub that is almost diagnostic of pericarditis (inflammation of the pericardium).
- Clicks. Clicks are difficult to hear, the aid of modern imaging technology has helped with the appreciation of these sounds.

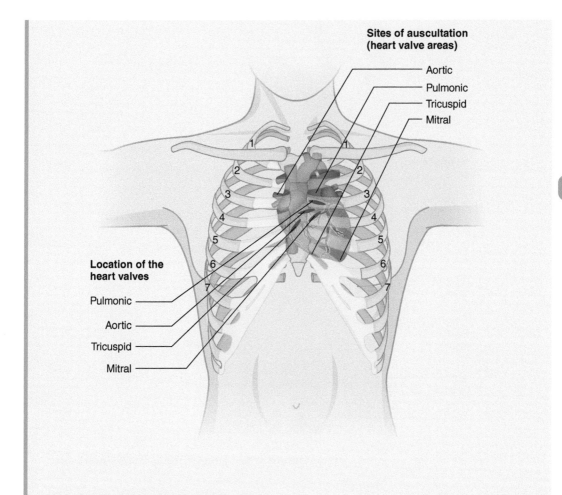

Figure 9.6 Auscultation sites for heart sounds.

Listening to heart sounds requires the placement of the stethoscope in four positions that correspond to different parts of the heart (see Figure 9.6)

Identifying abnormal heart sounds requires the ability to be able to recognise normal heart sounds and, as such, until a nurse is proficient in listening to heart sounds any suspected abnormalities should be reported to medical staff.

The recording of heart sounds in the notes requires the use of specific notation and the ability to grade murmurs according to their intensity and is a skill that can be learned after the nurse is able to identify the sounds to be recorded.

The Blood Supply to the Heart

Although small, the heart receives about 5% of the body's blood supply. Ensuring that the heart receives a plentiful supply of blood is essential to ensure the constant supply of oxygen and nutrients and the efficient removal of waste products required by the myocardium.

Only the inner part of the endocardium (about 2 mm in thickness) is supplied with blood directly from the inside of the heart chambers. The rest of the heart is supplied by the coronary arteries. The coronary arteries come directly off the aorta just after the aortic valve. They continuously divide into smaller branches, forming a web of blood vessels to supply the heart muscle. Figure 9.7 shows the main coronary arteries.

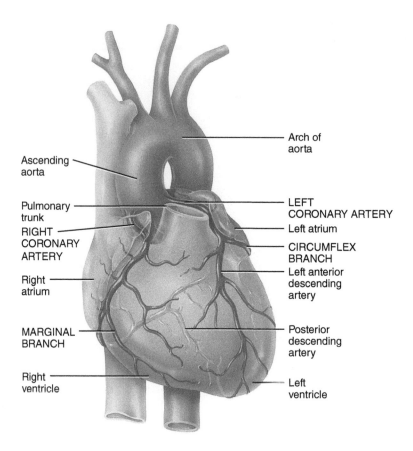

Figure 9.7 **Coronary arteries.** *Source:* Tortora and Derrickson (2009). Reproduced with permission of John Wiley & Sons.

Table 9.1 **Names of the coronary arteries, their major branches and the areas of the heart they supply.**

ARTERY	AREA OF THE HEART SUPPLIED	MAJOR BRANCHES
Left anterior descending (LAD)	Front and side of the left ventricle, apex of the heart	Diagonals Septals
Circumflex artery	Back and side of the left ventricle	Oblique marginal
Right coronary artery (RCA)	Right ventricle, base of the heart and interventricular septum	Posterior descending artery

Each artery (and its branches) supplies different areas of the heart muscle; Table 9.1 gives a summary of the main arteries, their branches and the areas of the heart they supply. It is important to note that Table 9.1 gives the anatomy as it pertains to most people, but there are normal variations in this pattern of blood supply in as much as 30% of the population. These variations have no significance in the normal, healthy person but can be important in the treatment of cardiac patients.

As the coronary arteries are compressed during each heart beat, blood does not flow through the coronary arteries at this time. Thus, blood flow to the myocardium occurs during the relaxation phase; this is the opposite of every other part of the body.

Episode of Care Mental Health

George is a 45-year-old gentleman who has been complaining of recurrent chest pain for the last few weeks. His GP has referred him to the local hospital for investigation and the cardiologist has decided that, given George's test results and his risk factors for coronary heart disease, George should undergo an angiogram (cardiac catheter).

George was diagnosed with schizophrenia at the age of 21 and after trying other antipsychotics over several years he has been taking clozapine (a second generation or atypical antipsychotic) for 15 years. The side effects of clozapine include weight gain, raised blood sugar, hypertension and raised cholesterol levels. George is a known smoker and has a poor diet. The increased risk of heart disease in patients with mental ill health have traditionally been associated with poor lifestyle choices (smoking, a lack of exercise and poor diet) and the side effects of medications used to treat conditions. In recent years there has been a growing evidence base to suggest that the increased risk may also be a direct result of the mental illness itself. Proposed mechanisms include increased platelet activity, increased cortisol levels and increased inflammatory markers (De Hert et al., 2018).

Cardiac catheterisation is the insertion of a catheter through a large artery (normally in the groin or the arm) to the heart where X-ray dye (contrast) can be injected into the coronary arteries in order to obtain an image of any narrowing of the lumen that may be reducing blood flow to the cardiac muscle (Figure 9.8).

The procedure is safe and is usually carried out as a day-case procedure under local anaesthetic. As with all procedures there is some risk, but the patient should be reassured that complications are rare and usually minor.

George undergoes cardiac catheterisation through the femoral artery. After the procedure George will be required to remain on flat bed rest and then bed rest sat up at a 30° angle before he can be allowed to mobilise. The insertion site should be monitored for active bleeding or the development of a haematoma, and regular blood pressure, pulse and pedal pulse monitoring should take place according to local practice.

The patient should be encouraged to drink to help the kidneys excrete the radio-opaque dye that has been injected into the blood (see O'Grady, 2007).

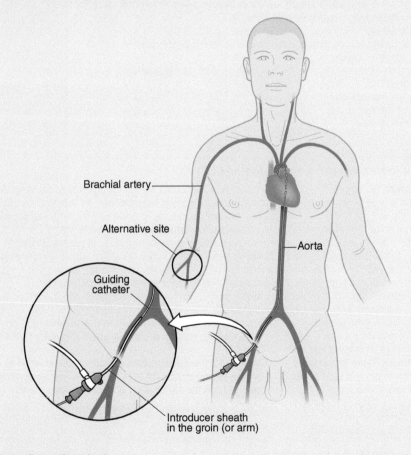

Brachial artery

Alternative site

Aorta

Guiding catheter

Introducer sheath in the groin (or arm)

Figure 9.8 **Cardiac catheterisation.**

During the bed rest after an angiogram is a good time to discuss cardiac health promotion with George. Health promotion delivered at the point the patient is attending for diagnosis or investigation is known as opportunistic health promotion. Though there is little George can do about the physiological effects of his mental illness and some of the side effects of the antipsychotic he is taking, he is able to modify some of his cardiovascular risk factors, for instance losing weight, stopping smoking and exercising. In this instance George may be responsive to a discussion about his risk factors but it is still recommended that written materials are supplied and he is signposted to resources that may be available for him (for instance the British Heart Foundation, MIND and his GP).

Multiple Choice Questions

1. Which side effects of clozapine can predispose the patient to heart disease?
   (a) weight gain
   (b) raised blood sugar
   (c) high cholesterol
   (d) all the above
2. Hypertension means:
   (a) raised blood pressure
   (b) raised cholesterol level
   (c) raised blood sugar
   (d) raised inflammatory markers
3. Opportunistic health promotion occurs:
   (a) in a formal teaching programme
   (b) online (via the internet)
   (c) when the patient is attending for other reasons (such as an angiogram)
   (d) when the patient asks for it.
4. Following the cardiac catheterisation, why is George advised to drink plenty of water?
   (a) because his blood pressure will be low
   (b) to encourage him to mobilise to the toilet
   (c) to encourage the excretion of the dye used in the procedure
   (d) to stop his blood clotting
5. What should the nurse observe for following cardiac catheterisation?
   (a) bleeding
   (b) haematoma formation
   (c) loss of the foot pulse
   (d) all of the above

Medicines Management Cardiac Medication

Following his angiogram, George is informed that he has narrowing in some of his coronary arteries and the pain he is experiencing is angina due to an imbalance between the heart muscles' need for oxygen and the ability of blood to flow through the narrowed arteries. The cardiologist prescribed George a drug called dilitiazem to help stop the pain from affecting his day-to-day life.

Diltiazem is one of a class of drugs known as calcium channel blockers. In angina they work by reducing the force of contraction of the heart by reducing the influx of calcium into the myocytes. This reduction in the force of contraction reduces the work of the heart, and therefore the need for oxygen.

Calcium channel blockers are also commonly used in the treatment of hypertension.

The side effects of calcium channel blockers include swollen ankles, ankle or foot pain, constipation, skin rashes, a flushed face, headaches, dizziness or tiredness (National Institute for Health and Care Excellence, 2013). Both diltiazem and clozapine are known to increase the risk of low blood pressure (hypotension) and thus it is recommended that George reports any episodes of dizziness to his GP and his blood pressure is monitored regularly (BNF, 2019b).

While diltiazem is not known to be affected, many of the calcium channel blockers are affected by grapefruit, and thus patients are generally advised not to drink grapefruit juice or eat grapefruit when taking calcium channel blockers. Other citrus fruits do not seem to have the same effect and can be eaten as normal.

 Link To/Go To

A list of medications that can interact with grapefruit can be found at
http://www.evidence.nhs.uk/formulary/bnf/current/a1-interactions/list-of-drug-interactions/grapefruit-juice.

Clinical Considerations Myocardial Infarction

 When one of the arteries supplying the heart muscle with blood becomes blocked by a thrombus (blood clot), the patient needs rapid treatment in order to try to limit the damage to the heart muscle. There are two main treatment options available:

- **Thrombolysis** – the administration of a thrombolytic drug in order to try to break up the clot and return blood flow through the artery. This form of treatment is very common and requires no specialist equipment to administer. However, patients are closely monitored for side effects, including haemorrhage, hypotension and disturbances in the heart rhythm.
- **Percutaneous coronary intervention (PCI)** – this is a specialist procedure requiring a dedicated cardiac catheterisation suite (a form of operating theatre with special imaging equipment), trained staff and various cardiac catheters, balloons and stents (Figure 9.9). The patient has a catheter inserted through a hole made in the femoral artery and the catheter is manoeuvred to the artery where the blockage is situated. A balloon is then passed through and inflated to push the thrombus into the walls of the artery and if necessary a metal cage (a stent) is inserted into the artery to keep the artery open. Though a specialist procedure, PCI is becoming more common in the UK.

See University of Michigan Health System (2014) for diagrams on coronary stent placement.

227

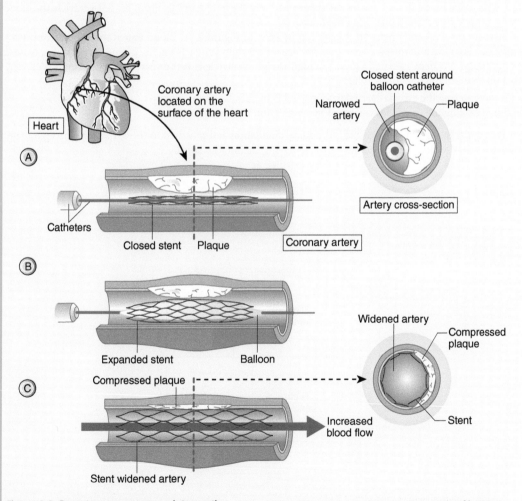

Figure 9.9 **Percutaneous coronary intervention.** *Source:* National Heart, Lung, and Blood Institute, National Institutes of Health.

Blood Flow Through the Heart

As noted earlier in the chapter, though the heart is a single organ it is best to think of it as two pumps, the right and the left heart pumps. Each pump is made up of two chambers (atrium and ventricle) and their associated valves.

- The right heart pump receives blood from the systemic circulation (the body) and pumps it through the pulmonary circulation (the lungs).
- The left heart pump receives blood from the pulmonary circulation and pumps it out around the systemic circulation.

Figure 9.10 gives a simplified explanation of the flow of blood through the heart. In this diagram, deoxygenated blood is in blue and oxygenated blood is in red. It is important to note that 'deoxygenated blood' does not refer to blood that has no oxygen in it but to blood that has given up some of its oxygen to the tissues. Typically, deoxygenated blood contains 75% of the oxygen that oxygenated blood carries.

So, as can be seen, deoxygenated blood returns from the body to the right atrium and then into the right ventricle, from where it is pumped out to the lungs. In the lungs the waste gases are exchanged for oxygen and the oxygenated blood flows into the left atrium and into the left ventricle. From the left ventricle the blood is then pumped into the circulation of the body.

A more detailed and anatomical view can be seen in Figure 9.11. Blood enters the right atrium via the superior vena cava and inferior vena cava and leaves the right ventricle via the pulmonary arteries. Note that even though it is deoxygenated blood leaving the right ventricle it is the vessels that the blood is carried in that make it arterial or venous. Thus:

- blood entering the atria is carried in veins and is therefore venous blood;
- blood leaving the ventricles is carried in arteries and is arterial blood.

Blood is transported through the pulmonary circulation and returned to the left atrium through the pulmonary veins; it is then pumped out by the left ventricle into the aorta.

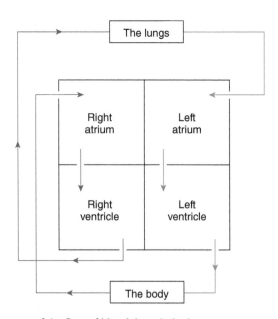

Figure 9.10 **A simplified diagram of the flow of blood though the heart.**

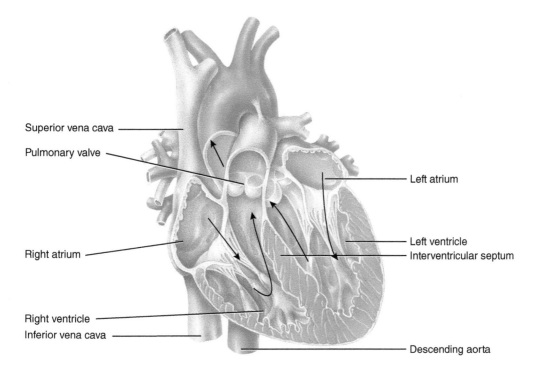

Figure 9.11 Anatomical view of the blood flow through the heart. *Source:* Tortora and Derrickson (2009). Reproduced with permission of John Wiley & Sons.

The Electrical Pathways of the Heart

Within the heart there is a specialised network of electrical pathways dedicated to ensuring the rapid transmission of electrical impulses. This ensures that the myocardium is excited rapidly in response to an initiating impulse so that the chambers contract and relax in the right order and the different pairs of chambers (atria and ventricles) contract at the same time. So, for instance, the left and right ventricles will contract simultaneously in response to an impulse (but after the atria). Also, the way in which the conduction system is organised means that the ventricles contract in a certain way to ensure they eject blood effectively. For example, if you wanted to empty out a tube of toothpaste you would squeeze from the base to ensure maximum effect. Likewise, the ventricles contract in such a way as to push blood towards and through the semilunar valves.

The cardiac muscles have a specialised property not seen in any other part of the body. All cells within the myocardium have the ability to create their own action potential without external excitation from another cell or a hormone. This is known as automaticity (or auto-rhythmicity). The problem with this is that, uncontrolled, the cells would all act independently and the heart would not beat effectively as there would be no coordination of the electrical activity and the subsequent muscle contractions. This is overcome by the use of the specialised cells in the conduction system. These cells create and distribute an electrical current that leads to a controlled and effective heart contraction. An overview of the anatomy of the conduction system can be seen in Figure 9.12.

Normal electrical excitation/distribution begins in the sinoatrial (SA) node, which is located in the right atrium, and is rapidly transmitted across the atria by fast pathways. This ensures that the right and left atria are excited together and beat as one unit. The impulse is transmitted to the AV node, where further transmission is delayed for approximately 0.1 s (Martini *et al.*, 2014). This ensures that the atria have completely

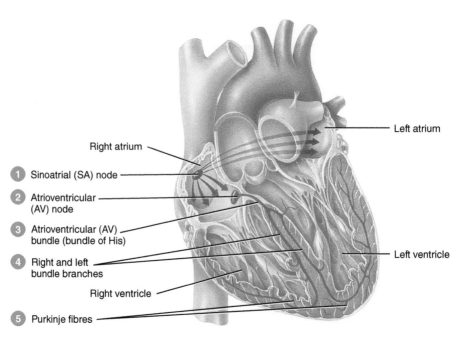

Right atrium

Left atrium

1 Sinoatrial (SA) node

2 Atrioventricular (AV) node

3 Atrioventricular (AV) bundle (bundle of His)

4 Right and left bundle branches

Left ventricle

Right ventricle

5 Purkinje fibres

Figure 9.12 **Conduction system of the heart.** *Source:* Tortora and Derrickson (2009). Reproduced with permission of John Wiley & Sons.

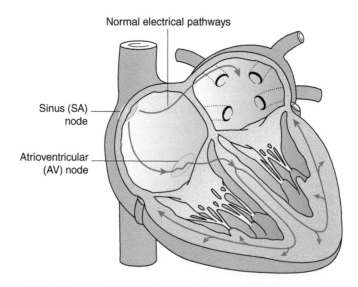

Normal electrical pathways

Sinus (SA) node

Atrioventricular (AV) node

Figure 9.13 **Normal electrical conduction.** *Source:* Tortora and Derrickson (2009). Reproduced with permission of John Wiley & Sons.

contracted before ventricular contraction is initiated. It should be noted that the atria and the ventricles are electrically isolated from each other by a band of non-conducting fibrous tissue, and thus the only electrical connection between the two is the bundle of His (AV bundle) (Figure 9.13).

Once the impulse has been 'held' in the AV node it is then transmitted down the bundle of His (AV bundle) to the fast pathways of the two bundle branches (one bundle branch per ventricle). The bundles then divide into the smaller and smaller branches of the Purkinje system, which transmits the impulses to the muscles of the ventricles.

Medicines Management Digoxin

Pauline is a 72-year-old lady admitted to the coronary care unit with a heart rate of 35 and a blood pressure of 90/40 mmHg. She is feeling very unwell and is restless, confused and agitated. The ECG recording of her heart shows signs of digoxin toxicity and on questioning Pauline's daughter it appears Pauline had been prescribed digoxin a few months ago.

Digoxin is a cardiac glycoside used in the treatment of heart failure and arrhythmias of the atria. Once a very popular drug, its use has reduced, but it is still prescribed. Digoxin slows and strengthens the heart beat (decreasing heart rate and increasing force of contraction). Owing to these effects, an excess of digoxin in the blood can lead to a slow heart rate, leading to dizziness. In the elderly, excretion of digoxin is reduced and thus digoxin levels can rise above the therapeutic threshold even on normal doses.

The signs of digoxin toxicity include nausea, vomiting, confusion, delirium and headache. It can also lead to very high levels of blood potassium. In life-threatening cases the digoxin can be counteracted by the use of digoxin-specific antibodies (digibind) infused into the blood. Otherwise supportive treatment and monitoring may be instituted and the digoxin withheld.

When administering digoxin, the nurse is required to take the pulse of the patient and, if it is below 60 beats per minute, the drug should be withheld and medical advice sought. The actions the nurse has taken must also be documented.

See British National Formulary (2019a).

Clinical Considerations Nodal Cells

Otherwise known as pacemaker cells, these are specialised cells that not only create electrical impulses but also create them at regular intervals.

Nodal cells are divided into two groups:

1. The SA node located in the right atrium, which generates electrical impulses at approximately 70–80 impulses per minute.
2. The AV node, located just above the point where the atria and ventricles meet. This node generates impulses at 40–60 impulses per minute.

The difference in the rate of impulse creation is important in the normal functioning of the heart as every time an impulse is transmitted down the electrical system it 'resets' the cells 'lower down'. Hence, the SA node is the normal pacemaker of the heart as it creates impulses faster than the AV node.

Thus, like a military command structure, the SA node could be seen to be a general who commands the captain (AV node), but if the general no longer issues commands then the captain will take over command.

Even with the 'command structure' created by the nodal cells the conduction system of the heart can slow considerably and the patient can become very unwell. For instance, if the AV node no longer transmits impulses into the bundle of His, the cells in the lower parts of the conduction system can produce action potentials of their own, but this will be at a very slow rate (between 20 and 35 impulses per minute). In order to deal with this problem the patient would need to have a permanent pacemaker fitted (Figure 9.14).

The 'generator' (battery and circuitry) is contained in a small box that is buried beneath the skin of the chest wall. Wires lead from the generator through a vein into the patient's heart. Depending on the type of pacemaker fitted, there may be one or two wires. So, for instance, in the case of a failed AV node the pacemaker would have two wires: one in the right atrium and one in the right ventricle. The pacemaker would sense the atrial action potential and then (after a short delay to mimic the action of the AV node) the ventricle would receive an electrical impulse, causing it to contract. Thus, the pacemaker acts as a replacement AV node (O'Grady, 2007).

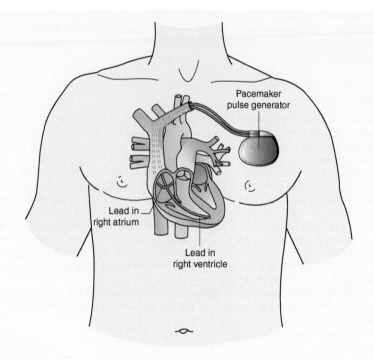

Figure 9.14 **Pacemaker.**

Skills in Practice ECG

 On admission to the coronary care unit, Pauline required a 12-lead ECG and cardiac monitoring. While they both record the electrical activity of the heart, 3-lead monitoring and a 12-lead ECG have different purposes.

Three-lead cardiac monitoring is used for the continuous monitoring of the heart rhythm in patients thought to be at risk of a heart rhythm disturbance. The lead placement is as follows:

Red lead	Right arm
Yellow lead	Left arm
Green lead	Left leg
Or	
Black lead	Right leg

It should be noted that the leads of a monitoring system are normally attached to the relevant shoulder for the arm leads and the lower chest for the leg leads, thus leaving the patient freedom of movement and leaving the chest clear for resuscitation (if required).

For a 12-lead ECG, the limb leads are placed as noted above but at the wrists and ankles; the chest leads are then attached. Many nurses use mnemonics to remember limb lead placement such as: 'Ride Your Green Bike'; others will think of *red for right* and *lemon for left*.

Twelve-lead ECGs are used for diagnostic purposes, and correct lead placement is essential.

Chest lead placement for a 12-lead ECG is a skill that should be practised under supervision until competent. Figure 9.15 shows the lead placement.

- V1: fourth intercostal space, right sternal border.
- V2: fourth intercostal space, left sternal border.
- V3: midway between V2 and V4.
- V4: fifth intercostal space, left midclavicular line.
- V5: level with V4, left anterior axillary line.
- V6: level with V4, left mid axillary line.

In female patients, electrodes are never placed on top of the breast unless you cannot gain access to the normal position. If you do have to move onto the breast, document this on the recording.

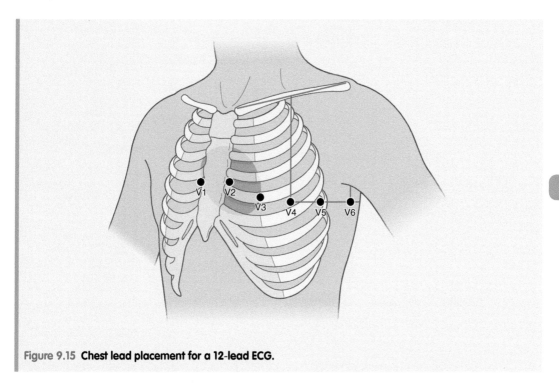

Figure 9.15 **Chest lead placement for a 12-lead ECG.**

The Cardiac Cycle

The cardiac cycle is the name given to the mechanical activity of the heart and is best understood by looking at the pressure changes in the heart chambers and the aorta and relating these to the mechanical activity of the heart and its chambers.

Systole and Diastole

These are two terms that require definition as they are unique in anatomy and physiology to the functioning of the heart.
- Systole: the contraction of a heart chamber (atrium or ventricle).
- Diastole: the relaxation of a heart chamber (atrium or ventricle).

The cardiac cycle can be seen in Figure 9.16. Note, the diagram refers to the pressures in the left side of the heart (atrium and ventricle); the cardiac cycle is the same on the right side but the pressures are lower. The cardiac cycle can be broken down into a series of steps that are detailed below. The flow of blood in the heart and the circulatory system is always from a point of higher pressure to a point of lower pressure.

The cardiac cycle is usually divided into five phases:

1. A period of ventricular filling in mid to late relaxation (ventricular diastole). Pressure in the ventricle is low. Blood that is returning to the heart through the vena cava is flowing passively through the atria and the open AV valves into the ventricle. The pressure in the atria is higher than that in the ventricles and this forces the bicuspid and tricuspid valves open. As the pressure in the ventricles rises due to the increased amount of blood in the ventricles, the leaflets of the AV valves begin to drift upwards to their closed positions. The semilunar valves (the aortic and the pulmonary valves) are closed; the pressure in the aorta and the pulmonary arteries is greater than that in the ventricles, thus forcing these valves shut. About 70% of ventricular filling happens during this phase.

2. Late in this phase the atria begin to contract (atrial systole) in response to excitation by an action potential from the SA node; this compresses the blood in the atria, leading to a slight rise in the pressure in the atria. This rise in pressure leads to a greater flow of blood into the ventricles from the atria.

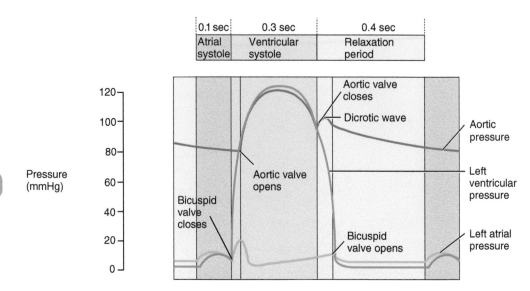

Figure 9.16 **The cardiac cycle.** *Source:* Tortora and Derrickson (2009). Reproduced with permission of John Wiley & Sons.

The ventricles remain in diastole as the electrical excitation that led to atrial contraction is delayed in the AV node. By the end of this point in time the ventricles are in the last part of their relaxation phase and contain the largest amount of blood they will contain during the cardiac cycle. This is known as the end diastolic volume (EDV) and is about 130 mL of blood (Jenkins and Tortora, 2013); that is, the volume of blood contained in the ventricles at the end of their relaxation phase (diastole). The EDV is the main factor in the creation of the end diastolic pressure, as the pressure is directly related to the amount of blood within the ventricle when the ventricle is relaxed.

3. Ventricular contraction (systole). The atria relax, leading to a drop in atrial pressure. The ventricles begin to contract as the electrical excitation is transmitted from the AV node to the ventricles through the bundle of His, then the bundle branches and finally the Purkinje fibres; this leads to a sharp rise in ventricular pressure without any change in ventricular volume (i.e. the amount of blood in the ventricles does not change). Once this pressure rises above the pressure in the atria, the AV valves are forced closed. As the semilunar valves remain closed at this point (the ventricular pressure is still lower than the pressure in the aorta and the pulmonary arteries), the ventricles are completely closed off and blood volume in the ventricles remains the same while pressure rises. This is known as the isovolumetric contraction phase ('iso' means remaining the same). Eventually, the pressure in the ventricles becomes greater than the pressure in the aorta and the pulmonary arteries. At this point, the semilunar valves are forced open and blood is ejected from the ventricles.

4. Early ventricular diastole (relaxation). The ventricles begin to relax. The blood in the ventricles is no longer compressed by the action of the heart muscle, and the pressure within the ventricles drops rapidly. As the blood volume in the ventricles remains constant (the AV valves are closed), the pressure in the aorta and the pulmonary arteries becomes greater than the pressure in the ventricles, and the semilunar valves are forced closed. This is the ventricular isovolumetric relaxation phase. Closure of the semilunar valves causes a brief rise in the pressure in the aorta as backflowing blood rebounds off the closed aortic valve; this can be seen as a slight 'bump' in the pressure tracing known as the 'dicrotic notch'.

5. During the period of ventricular systole the atria have been in diastole and filling with blood from the veins. When the pressure in the atria is greater than the pressure in the ventricles, the AV valves are forced open and blood begins to flow into the ventricles again.

Clinical Considerations Electrocardiogram and the Cardiac Cycle

Though the cardiac cycle refers to the mechanical action of the heart, the electrical activity that stimulates this mechanical action can be seen by the use of an ECG, an electrical tracing produced by attaching electrodes to the patient's skin and generated by an ECG machine. However, it is possible for the electrical tracing to be present without mechanical activity in certain types of cardiac arrest.

The normal ECG of one cycle of the heart is shown in Figure 9.17 (adapted from Jenkins and Tortora, 2013).

The changes from the baseline on the ECG are labelled by letters of the alphabet:

P – atrial depolarisation; corresponds to atrial contraction.

QRS – ventricular depolarisation; corresponds approximately to ventricular contraction (though this happens just after the peak of the R wave).

T – ventricular repolarisation; corresponds to the relaxation phase of the ventricle; atrial repolarisation cannot be seen as it is hidden by the greater electrical activity of ventricular depolarisation.

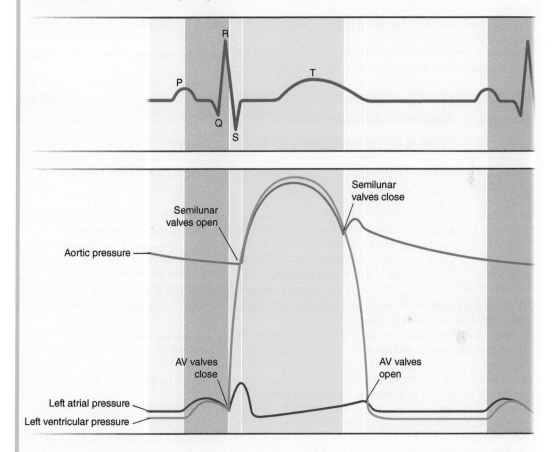

Figure 9.17 **Normal ECG of one cycle of the heart.** *Source:* Adapted from Jenkins and Tortora (2013). Reproduced with permission of John Wiley & Sons.

Despite this appearing to be a long process, if we assume a heart rate of 75 beats per minute then the average cardiac cycle would take approximately 0.8 s. The atria are in systole for 0.1 s and then in diastole for 0.7 s, while the ventricles are in systole for 0.3 s and diastole for 0.5 s. As heart rate increases, the cardiac cycle becomes shorter due to the shortening of the diastolic phase; the systolic phase remains the same. As already noted, the heart muscle is supplied with blood during the diastolic (relaxation) phase, as blood cannot flow in the coronary arteries when the heart is contracting; thus, as heart rate increases, blood flow in the coronary arteries (and blood supply to the heart muscle) is reduced.

Factors Affecting Cardiac Output

This section gives an overview of the factors affecting the cardiac output. 'Cardiac output' is a term relating to the amount of blood the heart pumps out in 1 minute and is defined by

$$\text{Cardiac Output}(CO) = \text{Stroke Volume}(SV) \times \text{Heart Rate}(HR)$$

Thus, the amount of blood the heart pumps out in a minute is made up of the amount of blood ejected from the ventricle in one beat (SV) times the heart rate (HR) in beats per minute. This gives a total volume. Thus, if we said that SV is 70 mL and the heart rate is 75, then cardiac output is 70 × 75 = 5250 mL (or 5.25 L) per minute.

To review the factors affecting cardiac output, the following sections will look at the factors regulating stroke volume and the factors regulating heart rate separately.

Regulation of Stroke Volume

Stroke volume is effectively the difference between the EDV (i.e. the amount of blood in the ventricle at the end of relaxation) and the end systolic volume (ESV – i.e. the amount of blood in the ventricle at the end of systole). The factors that affect stroke volume are preload, force of contraction and afterload.

Preload

The force the cardiac muscle fibres contract with during systole is affected by the amount of stretch they are subjected to (the greater the stretch, the greater the force). This is known as the Frank–Starling law.

The stretch of the cardiac muscle is directly related to the amount of blood in the ventricle at the end of diastole (EDV), which is, in turn, dependent on the volume of blood returned to the heart via the veins (venous return). Thus, venous return is related to the force of contraction of the ventricles. Anything that affects the speed or volume of venous return affects EDV, and therefore force of contraction. So, for instance:

- A slower heart rate allows for more time for blood to fill the ventricle, increasing the volume of blood in the ventricle at the end of diastole.
- Exercise increases venous return, as the increase in heart rate increases the pressure in the veins and the speed of venous return and the effect of skeletal muscle activity squeezes the veins 'pushing' blood back to the heart (skeletal muscle pumps). Conversely, standing still means that venous return is reduced. Thus, the guardsmen who have to stand still outside Buckingham Palace are taught to discretely contract and relax their feet to aid venous return and prevent fainting.
- Hormonal and nervous influences. The release of adrenaline or the excitation of the sympathetic nervous system leads to the contraction of the veins and the 'squeezing' of blood back to the heart.
- Very fast heart rates reduce the diastolic filling time, and thus there is less time for the ventricle to receive blood before systole starts.
- Certain heart arrhythmias stop the atria contracting effectively, and thus atrial systole is no longer effective at 'pushing' the last bit of blood into the ventricles.
- A reduced blood volume (for instance, due to a haemorrhage) reduces venous return.

Force of Contraction

Though EDV is a major component of the force of contraction (because of the Frank-Starling law), force of contraction can also be affected by other factors. The contractility of the heart can be affected by several factors:

- Hormones, such as adrenaline, glucagon and thyroxine, all increase the force of contraction.
- Sympathetic nervous system activity increases the force of contraction through the action of noradrenaline.
- Contractility can be reduced by acidaemia (excess hydrogen ions in the blood) and high potassium levels in the blood.

Afterload

Afterload refers to the pressure in the arteries leading from the ventricles (aorta or pulmonary arteries) that the ventricle must overcome in order to eject blood. In the normal adult the pressure is 80 mmHg in the aorta and 8 mmHg in the pulmonary arteries. This difference in the pressure to be overcome is reflected in the relative thickness of the ventricular walls, with the left ventricular wall being thicker (more muscular) than the right (see previous discussion on the structure of the heart).

In the average adult, aortic and pulmonary pressure is not an important factor in determining afterload as it is constant, but changes in anatomy and/or physiology, such as hypertension or aortic valve disease, can increase afterload. Increased afterload increases the amount of blood left in the ventricle after each systole, and thus also has an effect in increasing the preload (by increasing ventricular ESV and therefore pressure).

Medicines Management Hypercholesterolemia (High Cholesterol Levels)

Dave is a 45-year-old office worker who has recently returned to work after a myocardial infarction (MI). The rehabilitation nurse has given Dave a lot of information on healthy eating and exercise, but she notes his blood cholesterol test result is significantly higher than is advisable for someone who has had an MI. The nurse consults with the medical team and Dave is prescribed 80 mg atorvastatin once a day.

Atorvastatin is a cholesterol-lowering medication that lowers the amount of cholesterol produced in the body. It is commonly used in patients who have had an MI and have high cholesterol as it has been shown to reduce the chance of another MI. The patient is still required to maintain a healthy diet as atorvastatin will not treat the dietary intake of cholesterol and fat by the patient.

The nurse advises Dave to take the atorvastatin at night as one of the more common side effects is muscle pain and the patient is less likely to notice this when asleep. Dave is also advised not to eat grapefruit or drink grapefruit juice while taking atorvastatin as it can interact.

See National Institute for Health and Care Excellence (2014).

Regulation of Heart Rate

Heart rate is controlled by two main mechanisms:

- autononomic nervous system activity;
- hormone activity.

Resting heart rate is also affected by factors such as age, gender, temperature and physical fitness (Jenkins and Tortora, 2013).

Autonomic Nervous System Activity

When activated by a stimulus, such as exercise or stress, the sympathetic nerve fibres release the neurotransmitter noradrenaline at their cardiac endings. This leads to the excitation of the SA node and an increase in its production of action potentials and thus an increase in heart rate.

Alternatively, when the parasympathetic nervous system is stimulated, this results in the release of acetylcholine at the parasympathetic cardiac nerve endings, which has the effect of reducing the rate of action potential generation in the SA node and thus reducing heart rate.

Both the sympathetic and parasympathetic nervous systems are active at all times, but the parasympathetic nervous system is normally the dominant influence. This can be seen if the vagus nerve (cranial nerve X) is cut, for instance in heart transplant patients. In these situations the SA node will normally produce action potentials at a rate of 100 a minute and therefore the heart rate increases to 100 beats per minute. The removal of the influence of the parasympathetic nervous system (by the disconnection of the vagus nerve) removes the heart rate reducing effect of this system.

Baroreceptors and the Cardiovascular Centre

Baroreceptors are specialised mechanical receptors located in the carotid sinus and the aortic arch. They are sensitive to the amount of stretch in these blood vessels and have direct outflow via the autonomic nervous system to the cardiovascular centre in the medulla oblongata.

The cardiovascular centre of the medulla oblongata is the main centre for the control of autonomic nervous activity that affects the heart. As can be seen in Figure 9.18, the cardiovascular centre is made up of two sub-centres:

- The cardioinhibitory centre directly controls parasympathetic outflow to the heart (especially the SA node); thus, increased outflow from this centre has the effect of reducing heart rate.
- The vasomotor centre is further divided into the pressor area and the depressor area. The pressor area has a relatively constant outflow of action potentials to the heart via the sympathetic nervous system. This has a direct effect on both heart rate and the force of ventricular contraction (and therefore stroke volume) as

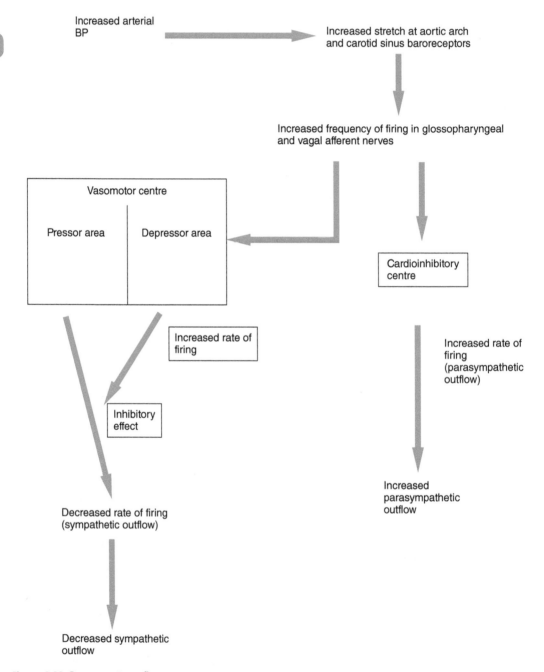

Figure 9.18 **Baroreceptor reflex.**

well as effects on the vasculature, which subsequently will affect heart function by changing preload and afterload. Outflow from the pressor area is moderated by nerves transmitting impulses from the depressor area that have a directly inhibiting effect on the transmission of impulses from the pressor area. Thus, it can be thought that the nerve impulses of the depressor area act like a 'collar' or tap: the greater the number of impulses from the depressor area the tighter the collar or tap is made, reducing the number of impulses from the pressor area to the heart, and thus the effect on heart rate and force of contraction.

Hormone Activity
Two hormones are normally associated with the control of heart rate:
- Adrenaline – from the adrenal medulla. Adrenaline has the same effect as noradrenaline released by the sympathetic nervous system.
- Thyroxine – from the thyroid gland. Released in large quantities, thyroxine has the effect of increasing the heart rate.

Conclusion

The heart is a single organ situated in the thoracic cavity between the lungs. Though a single organ, the heart is effectively two separate pumps made up of four chambers:
- The right heart pump, comprised of the right atrium and right ventricle, pumps blood through the pulmonary circulation.
- The left heart pump, comprised of the left atrium and the left ventricle, pumps blood through the systemic circulation.

Surrounding the heart is a double protective sac called the pericardium. Underlying the pericardium is the heart muscle (myocardium), which is a specialised type of muscle that is branched in its structure and is laid down in spiral bundles to make up the walls of the various heart chambers.

Control of the heart muscle is achieved by the use of a specialised series of nerve cells that make up the conduction system of the heart, including:
- the SA node, the pacemaker of the heart;
- the AV node, an area of the heart's conduction system that controls the delivery of the action potential to the ventricles;
- Purkinje fibres, conductive fibres that aid rapid distribution of the action potential throughout the ventricles.

Blood flow through the heart is based on changes of pressure in the cardiac cycle. These pressure changes also lead to the opening and closing of the cardiac valves, thus further controlling blood flow.

Regulation of the heart's activity is based on the actions of:
- hormones, especially adrenaline;
- autonomic nervous system activity, for instance via the cardiovascular centres.

Glossary

Action potential: Momentary change in the electrical status of a cell wall.
Afterload: The 'load' that the heart has to pump against, mostly created by the blood pressure in the arteries.
Aorta: Main artery leading from the left ventricle.
Aortic valve: Semilunar valve that lies between the left ventricle and the aorta.
Arterial: Pertaining to the arteries.
Arterial blood: Blood carried in the arteries.
Atria: Upper chambers of the heart (singular = atrium).
Atrioventricular bundle: Bundle of conductive nerve fibres that transmit action potentials from the AV node to the ventricular conduction system. Otherwise known as the bundle of His.
Atrioventricular node: Otherwise known as the AV node. Specialised area of cardiac cells located just above the point where the right atrium and right ventricle meet.

Atrioventricular valve: Collective name for the two valves that lie between the atria and the ventricles (bicuspid and tricuspid).

Automaticity: The ability of certain cells to generate their own action potential without an external stimulus.

Baroreceptors: Specialised mechanical receptors located in the aortic arch and the carotid sinus.

Bicuspid valve: The AV valve that lies between the left atrium and the left ventricle. Also known as the mitral valve.

Bundle of His: See **atrioventricular bundle**.

Cardiac action potential: Specialised action potential of the heart muscle cells, it is of longer duration than normal cellular action potentials.

Cardiac cycle: The sequence of events that occurs when the heart beats.

Cardiac output: The amount of blood pumped out by a ventricle in millilitres per minute.

Cardioinhibitory centre: Part of the cardiovascular centre; when stimulated, the major effect is to slow down the heart rate.

Cardiovascular centre: Located in the medulla oblongata, this centre controls most of the nervous activity that affects the heart.

Coronary arteries: Arteries that supply the myocardium with oxygenated blood.

Coronary sinus: Collection of veins that come together to form a single large vessel that returns blood from the myocardium to the right atrium.

Depolarisation: Change in the electrical potential of a cell membrane to a more positive charge.

Desmosomes: A specialised cell structure whose function is to hold cells together.

Diastole: The relaxation of a heart chamber (atrium or ventricle).

Dicrotic notch: A small bump in the pressure tracing of the arteries created by a backflow of blood after the closure of the aortic valve.

End diastolic pressure: The pressure created by the blood in a named chamber (usually the left ventricle) at the end of diastole.

End diastolic volume: The volume of blood in a named chamber (usually the left ventricle) at the end of diastole.

Endocardium: Innermost layer that lines the chambers of the heart and also lines the cardiac valves.

Epithelium: Layer of body tissue that lines the inside of cavities and the surface of many structures.

Fibrous pericardium: The outer, tough layer of the pericardium that provides protection to the heart, prevents overstretching of the heart and helps to anchor the heart in place.

Gap junction: A specialised connection between cell membranes that allows the passage of ions and molecules.

Hormone: Chemical substance that is released into the blood by the endocrine system and has a physiological control over the function of cells or organs other than those that created it.

Inferior vena cava: Large vein that returns blood to the right atrium from the lower parts of the body.

Interatrial septum: Dividing wall between the atria.

Interventricular septum: Dividing wall between the ventricles.

Ion: An electrically charged atom or molecule.

Isovolumetric: No change in volume (amount).

Medulla oblongata: The lower half of the brainstem.

Mitral valve: See bicuspid valve.

Myocardium: Muscle layer of the heart.

Myocyte: Cardiac muscle cell.

Nodal cells: Otherwise known as pacemaker cells, these are specialised cells that not only create electrical impulses but create them at regular intervals. The two main groupings of these cells are located in the SA node and the AV node.

Parietal pericardium: The outer layer of the serous pericardium, it is fused to the fibrous pericardium.

Pericardial fluid: A thin film of fluid that reduces the friction between the pericardial membranes as the heart moves during its cycle of contraction and relaxation.

Pericardium: Double-layered sac that surrounds the heart.

Pulmonary circulation: Circulatory system of the lungs.

Pulmonary valve: Semilunar valve that lies between the right ventricle and the pulmonary circulation.

Pulmonary veins: Veins of the pulmonary circulation that return blood from the lungs to the left atrium.

Purkinje fibres (system): Specialised conductive fibres that rapidly transport action potentials through the ventricle walls.

Repolarisation: Return of the electrical potential of a cell membrane to a negative resting state.

Sarcolemma: Cell membrane of a muscle cell.

Semilunar valves: The valves that lie between the ventricles and the pulmonary or systemic circulation (aortic valve and pulmonary valve).

Septum: A dividing wall.

Serous pericardium: Inner (double) layer of the pericardium comprised of the parietal and visceral pericardial layers.

Sinoatrial node: Otherwise known as the SA node. Specialised area of cardiac cells located in the upper part of the right atrium. Usually referred to as the pacemaker of the heart.

Stroke volume: The amount of blood ejected by a ventricle in one beat.

Superior vena cava: The large vein that returns blood to the right atrium from the upper part of the body.

Systemic circulation: The circulatory system of the body (excluding the lungs).

Systole: The contraction of a heart chamber (atrium or ventricle).

Tetany: Sustained involuntary contraction of a muscle.

Tricuspid valve: The AV valve that lies between the right atrium and ventricle.

Vasomotor centre: Part of the cardiovascular centre; has effects on heart rate and the force of contraction of the heart.

Venous: Pertaining to the veins.

Venous blood: Blood carried in the veins.

Ventricles: The large lower chambers of the heart.

Visceral pericardium: The inner layer of the serous pericardium (otherwise known as the epicardium); adheres tightly to the surface of the heart.

241

References

Baumgartner, H., Falk, V., Ruschitza, F. and Windecker, S. (2017) 2017 ESC/EACTS Guidelines for the management of valvular heart disease. *European Heart Journal.* **38**(36): 739–2791.

British National Formulary (2019a) Cardiac Glycosides. https://bnf.nice.org.uk/treatment-summary/cardiac-glycosides.html (accessed 5 June 2019).

British National Formulary (2019b) Interactions – Clozapine. https://bnf.nice.org.uk/interaction/clozapine-2.html (accessed 5 June 2019).

Clare, C. (2007) Valve disorders. In Hatchett, R. and Thompson, D.R. (eds), *Cardiac Nursing: A Comprehensive Guide.* London: Churchill Livingstone Elsevier; pp. 357–382.

De Hert, M., Detraux, J and Vancampfort, D. (2018) The intriguing relationship between coronary heart disease and mental disorders. *Dialogues in Clinical Neuroscience.* **20**(1): 31–40.

Jenkins, G.W. and Tortora, G.J. (2013) *Anatomy and Physiology: From Science to Life*, 3rd edn. Hoboken, NJ: John Wiley & Sons, Inc.

Martini, F.H., Nath, J.L. and Bartholemew, E.F. (2014) *Fundamentals of Anatomy and Physiology*, 10th edn. San Francisco, CA: Pearson Benjamin Cummings.

National Institute for Health and Care Excellence (2013) Myocardial Infarction: Cardiac Rehabilitation and Prevention of Further MI. NICE guidelines [CG172]. https://www.nice.org.uk/guidance/cg172 (accessed 5 June 2019).

National Institute for Health and Care Excellence (2014) Lipid Modification Therapy for Preventing Cardiovascular Disease: Secondary Prevention. NICE Pathways. http://pathways.nice.org.uk/pathways/cardiovascular-disease-prevention#path=view%3A/pathways/cardiovascular-disease-prevention/lipid-modification-therapy-for-preventing-cardiovascular-disease.xml:S_P_I_A_M_Pcontent=view-node%3Anodes-secondary-prevention (accessed 5 June 2019).

O'Grady, E. (2007) *A Nurse's Guide to Caring for Cardiac Intervention Patients.* Chichester: John Wiley & Sons, Ltd.

Pfitzer, C., Helm, P.C., Rosenthal, L.M., Berger, F., Bauer, U.M.M. and Schmitt, K.R. (2018) Dynamics in prevalence of Down Syndrome in children with congenital heart disease. *European Journal of Pediatrics* **177**(1): 107–115.

Tortora, G.J. and Derrickson, B.H. (2009) *Principles of Anatomy and Physiology*, 12th edn. Hoboken, NJ: John Wiley & Sons, Inc.

University of Michigan Health System (2014) Coronary Angioplasty and Stenting. http://www.med.umich.edu/cardiac-surgery/patient/adult/adultcandt/coronary_angioplasty.shtml (accessed 5 June 2019).

Vis, J.C., de Bruin-Bon, R.H., Bouma, B.J., Huisman, S.A., Imschoot, L., van den Brink, K. and Mulder, B.J. (2010) Congenital heart defects are under-recognised in adult patients with Down's syndrome. *Heart* **96**:1480–1484.

Wong, C., Dwyer, J. and Holland, M. (2014) Overcoming weight problems in adults with Down Syndrome. *Nutrition Today* **49**(3): 109–119.

Further Reading

British Heart Foundation

https://www.bhf.org.uk/

The British Heart Foundation is the UK's largest charity for heart disease. The website has many useful resources for patients and professionals.

Arrhythmia Alliance

http://www.heartrhythmcharity.org.uk/www/436/0/About/

The Arrhythmia Alliance is an alliance of several independent charities devoted to raising awareness of heart arrhythmias, improving diagnosis and improving the life of people with arrhythmias.

Resuscitation Council (UK)

https://www.resus.org.uk/index.html

The Resuscitation Council (UK) is an organisation devoted to promoting evidence-based resuscitation guidelines and contributing to saving lives through training and education.

Activities

Multiple Choice Questions

1. The double sac surrounding the heart is:
   (a) the myocardium
   (b) the pericardium
   (c) the endocardium
   (d) the epicardium

2. Which heart chamber has the thickest muscle wall?
   (a) right ventricle
   (b) right atrium
   (c) left ventricle
   (d) left atrium

3. Blood flowing into the right atrium comes from:
   (a) the lungs
   (b) the body (systemic circulation)
   (c) the left heart
   (d) the right heart

4. Blood pumped out from the left heart is carried by:
   (a) the vena cava
   (b) the pulmonary arteries
   (c) the aorta
   (d) the coronary arteries

5. The contraction of a heart chamber is known as:
   (a) automaticity
   (b) diastole
   (c) isovulmetric
   (d) systole

6. The blood flow through the heart is caused by changes in:
   (a) pressure
   (b) electricity
   (c) transport molecules
   (d) oxygen

7. The artery supplying blood to the front of the left ventricle is:
   (a) the posterior descending artery
   (b) the circumflex artery
   (c) the right coronary artery
   (d) the left anterior descending artery

8. Normal electrical excitation of the heart begins in:
   (a) the bundle of His
   (b) the Purkinje fibres
   (c) the AV node
   (d) the SA node
9. The effect of increased parasympathetic nervous system activity is to:
   (a) increase heart rate
   (b) decrease heart rate
   (c) increase force of contraction
   (d) decrease force of contraction
10. Preload is mostly a factor of:
    (a) ESV
    (b) EDV
    (c) the Frank–Starling law
    (d) adrenaline release

11. Typically, deoxygenated blood contains what percentage of the oxygen that oxygenated blood carries.
    (a) 70%
    (b) 75%
    (c) 80%
    (d) 85%
12. Digoxin toxicity can lead to very high blood levels of:
    (a) potassium
    (b) sodium
    (c) calcium
    (d) magnesium
13. The condition that leads to the muscles of the heart (the myocardium) to become thickened and stiff is:
    (a) dilated cardiomyopathy
    (b) restrictive cardiomyopathy
    (c) hypertrophic cardiomyopathy
    (d) constrictive cardiomyopathy
14. 'Statin' drugs, such as Atorvastatin, are used to:
    (a) stop heart arrhythmias
    (b) reduce blood cholesterol levels
    (c) reduce blood clotting
    (d) reduce pressure in the heart
15. The vagus nerve is also known as:
    (a) cranial nerve VIII
    (b) cranial nerve IX
    (c) cranial nerve X
    (d) cranial nerve XI

Conditions

The following is a list of conditions that are associated with the cardiac system. Take some time and write notes about each of the conditions. You may make the notes taken from textbooks or other resources (e.g. people you work with in a clinical area), or you may make the notes as a result of people you have cared for. If you are making notes about people you have cared for, you must ensure that you adhere to the rules of confidentiality.

Heart failure

Myocardial infarction	
Aortic stenosis	
Mitral regurgitation	
Pericarditis	

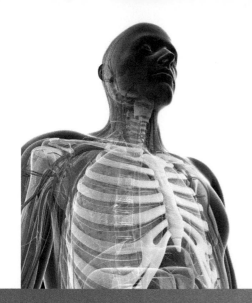

10

The Digestive System

Louise McErlean

Test Your Prior Knowledge

- What is the main function of the digestive system?
- List the structures that form the digestive system.
- List the hormones and enzymes involved in the digestive system.
- Name the main food groups.
- Differentiate between macronutrients and micronutrients.

Learning Outcomes

After reading this chapter you will be able to:

- Identify the organs of the digestive system, including the accessory organs of the digestive system and describe the functions of each of these organs, as well as the overall function of the digestive system.
- Explain the action of the enzymes and hormones associated with the digestion of proteins, carbohydrates and fats.
- Describe what proteins, carbohydrates and fats are broken down into and how the body uses these constituent parts.
- Describe the structure and function of the accessory organs of the digestive system.
- List the common vitamins and minerals and the problems associated with a deficit or excess.

Visit the student companion website at www.wileyfundamentalseries.com/anatomy where you can test yourself using flashcards, multiple-choice questions and more. Instructor companion site at www.wiley.com/go/instructor/anatomy where instructors will find valuable materials such as PowerPoint slides and image bank designed to enhance your teaching.

Fundamentals of Anatomy and Physiology: For Nursing and Healthcare Students, Third Edition. Edited by Ian Peate and Suzanne Evans.
© 2020 John Wiley & Sons Ltd. Published 2020 by John Wiley & Sons Ltd.
Student companion website: www.wileyfundamentalseries.com/anatomy
Instructor companion website: www.wiley.com/go/instructor/anatomy

Body Map

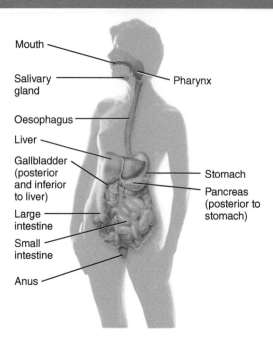

Mouth

Salivary gland

Pharynx

Oesophagus

Liver

Gallbladder (posterior and inferior to liver)

Stomach

Pancreas (posterior to stomach)

Large intestine

Small intestine

Anus

Introduction

The digestive system is also known as the gastrointestinal system or the alimentary canal. This vast system is approximately 10 m long. It travels the length of the body from the mouth through the thoracic, abdominal and pelvic cavities, where it ends at the anus (see Figure 10.1). The digestive system has one major function: to convert food from the diet into a form that can be utilised by the cells of the body in order to carry out their specific functions. This chapter discusses the structure and function of the digestive system and explains how dietary nutrients are broken down and used by the body for cell metabolism and for growth and repair.

The Activity of the Digestive System

The activity of the digestive system can be categorised into five processes:
- **Ingestion:** taking food into the digestive system.
- **Propulsion:** moving the food along the length of the digestive system.
- **Digestion:** breaking down food. This can be achieved *mechanically* as food is chewed or moved through the digestive system, or *chemically* by the action of *enzymes* mixed with the food as it moves through the digestive system.
- **Absorption:** the products of digestion exit the digestive system and enter the blood or lymph capillaries for distribution to where they are required.
- **Elimination:** the waste products of digestion are excreted from the body as faeces.

The Organisation of the Digestive System

The digestive system consists of the main digestive system structures and the accessory organs. The main digestive system structures include the mouth, pharynx, oesophagus, stomach, small intestine and large intestine. Accessory organs also contribute to the function of the digestive system. The accessory organs are the salivary glands, the liver, the gallbladder and the pancreas.

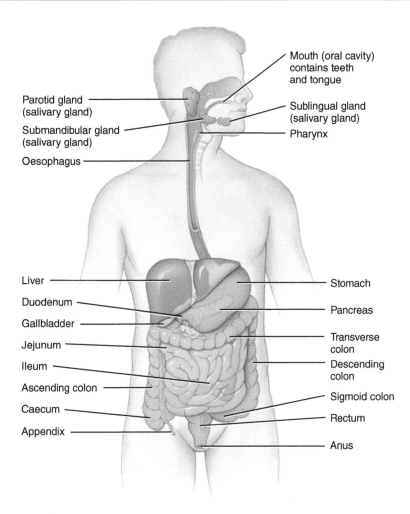

Mouth (oral cavity)
contains teeth
and tongue

Parotid gland
(salivary gland)

Sublingual gland
(salivary gland)

Submandibular gland
(salivary gland)

Pharynx

Oesophagus

Liver

Stomach

Duodenum

Pancreas

Gallbladder

Jejunum

Transverse
colon

Ileum

Descending
colon

Ascending colon

Sigmoid colon

Caecum

Rectum

Appendix

Anus

Figure 10.1 **The digestive system.** *Source:* Tortora and Derrickson (2009). Reproduced with permission of John Wiley & Sons.

The Digestive System Organs

The Mouth (Oral Cavity)

Food enters the mouth or oral cavity, and this is where the process of digestion begins. The oral cavity consists of several structures (see Figure 10.2). Food enters the oral cavity in a process called ingestion. The food mixes with saliva.

The lips and cheeks are formed of muscle and connective tissue. This allows the lips and cheeks to move food mixed with saliva around the mouth and begin mechanical digestion. The teeth contribute to mechanical digestion by grinding and tearing food. This process of chewing and mixing food with saliva is called mastication. The oral cavity can be exposed to very hot and very cold food as well as rough food particles. It is lined with mucus-secreting, stratified squamous epithelial cells. This layer provides some protection against abrasion, the effects of heat and continuous wear and tear.

The lips and cheeks are also involved in speech and facial expression.

Tongue

The tongue is a large, voluntary muscular structure that occupies much of the oral cavity. It is attached posteriorly to the hyoid bone and inferiorly by the lingual frenulum (see Figure 10.2).

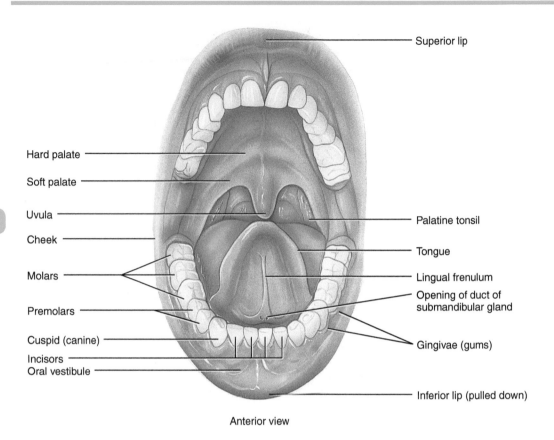

Anterior view

Figure 10.2 **The oral cavity.** *Source:* Tortora and Derrickson (2009). Reproduced with permission of John Wiley & Sons.

The superior surface of the tongue is covered in stratified squamous epithelium for protection against wear and tear. This surface also contains many little projections called papillae. The papillae (or taste buds) contain the nerve endings responsible for the sense of taste (Tortora and Derrickson, 2012). The taste buds contribute to our enjoyment of food. As well as taste, other functions of the tongue include swallowing (deglutition), holding and moving food around the oral cavity and speech.

Palate
The palate forms the roof of the mouth and consists of two parts: the hard palate and the soft palate. The hard palate is located anteriorly and is bony. The soft palate lies posteriorly and consists of skeletal muscle and connective tissue (see Figure 10.2). The palate plays a part in swallowing. The palatine tonsils lie laterally and are lymphoid tissue. The uvula is a fold of tissue that hangs down from the centre of the soft palate.

Teeth
Temporary teeth are also known as deciduous teeth or milk teeth. Temporary teeth begin to appear at about 6 months old. There are 20 temporary teeth, and these are replaced by permanent teeth from about the age of 6 years (Nair and Peate, 2018). There are 32 permanent teeth. Sixteen are located in the maxilla arch (upper) and 16 are located in the mandible (lower) (see Figure 10.3).

Canines and incisors are cutting and tearing teeth. Premolars and molars are used for the grinding and chewing of food. Despite their different functions and shape, the structure of each tooth is the same. The visible part of the tooth is called the crown. The crown sits above the gum or gingiva. The centre of the tooth is called the pulp cavity. Blood and lymph vessels as well as nerves enter and leave the tooth here. The tooth receives nutrients and sensations via the pulp. Surrounding this is a calcified matrix, not unlike bone, called the dentine. Surrounding the dentine is a very hard, protective material called enamel. The neck of the tooth is where the crown meets the root. The teeth are anchored in a socket with a bone-like material called cementum, and the function of the teeth is to chew (masticate) food.

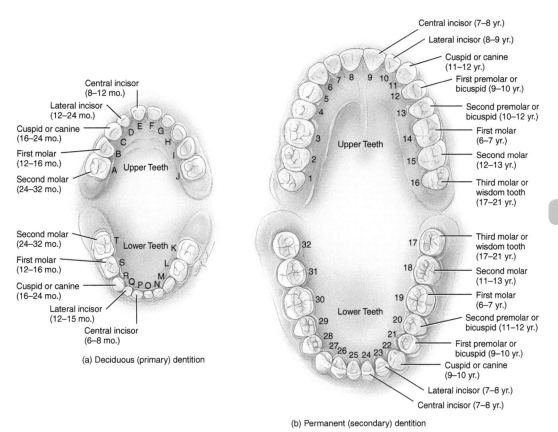

Central incisor (7–8 yr.)

Lateral incisor (8–9 yr.)

Cuspid or canine (11–12 yr.)

First premolar or bicuspid (9–10 yr.)

Second premolar or bicuspid (10–12 yr.)

First molar (6–7 yr.)

Second molar (12–13 yr.)

Third molar or wisdom tooth (17–21 yr.)

Upper Teeth

Central incisor (8–12 mo.)

Lateral incisor (12–24 mo.)

Cuspid or canine (16–24 mo.)

First molar (12–16 mo.)

Second molar (24–32 mo.)

Upper Teeth

Second molar (24–32 mo.)

First molar (12–16 mo.)

Cuspid or canine (16–24 mo.)

Lateral incisor (12–15 mo.)

Central incisor (6–8 mo.)

Lower Teeth

(a) Deciduous (primary) dentition

Third molar or wisdom tooth (17–21 yr.)

Second molar (11–13 yr.)

First molar (6–7 yr.)

Second premolar or bicuspid (11–12 yr.)

First premolar or bicuspid (9–10 yr.)

Cuspid or canine (9–10 yr.)

Lateral incisor (7–8 yr.)

Central incisor (7–8 yr.)

Lower Teeth

(b) Permanent (secondary) dentition

Figure 10.3 **(a, b) Teeth.** *Source: Tortora and Derrickson (2009). Reproduced with permission of John Wiley & Sons.*

Salivary Glands

There are three pairs of salivary glands (see Figure 10.4). The parotid glands are the largest and they are located anterior to the ears. Saliva from the parotid glands enters the oral cavity close to the level of the second upper molar tooth. The submandibular glands are located below the jaw on each side of the face. Saliva from these glands enters the oral cavity from beside the lingual frenulum of the tongue. The sublingual glands are the smallest. They are located in the floor of the mouth.

Although saliva is continuously secreted in order to keep the oral cavity moist, the activity of the parasympathetic fibres that innervate the salivary glands will lead to an increased production of saliva in response to the sight, smell or taste of food. The action of sympathetic fibres leads to a decreased secretion of saliva.

In health, approximately 1–1.5 L of saliva are secreted daily. Saliva consists of:

- water
- salivary amylase
- mucus
- mineral salts
- lysozyme
- immunoglobulins
- blood clotting factors.

Saliva has several important functions:

- Salivary amylase is a digestive enzyme responsible for beginning the breakdown of carbohydrate molecules from complex polysaccharides to the disaccharide maltase.
- The fluid nature of saliva helps to moisten and lubricate food that enters the mouth. This makes it easier to hold the food in the mouth and also assists in forming the food into a bolus in preparation for swallowing.

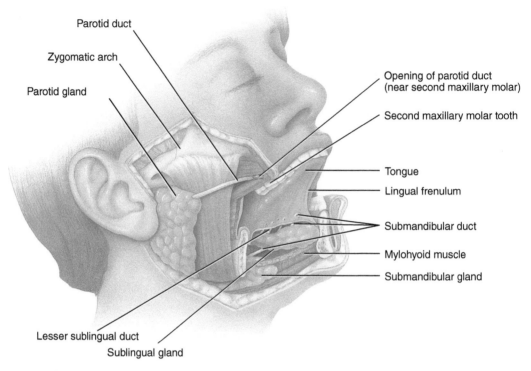

Figure 10.4 **Salivary glands.**

- The continuous secretion of saliva is cleansing and helps to maintain moisture in the oral cavity. A lack of moisture can lead to oral mucosal infections and formation of mouth ulcers.
- The oral cavity is an entry route for pathogens from the external environment. Lysozyme, a constituent of saliva, has an antibacterial action. Immunoglobulin and clotting factors also contribute to the prevention of infection.
- Taste is only possible when food substances are moist. Saliva is required to moisten food.

Skills in Practice Mouth care

Patients who are ill can also be dehydrated and therefore their production of saliva is reduced. This can lead to an increased risk of oral infections, as wear and tear within the oral cavity increases.

Reduced amounts of saliva lead to less washing away of pathogens to the acid environment of the stomach where they may be destroyed. The oral cavity provides a route for pathogens to enter the respiratory tract, and therefore good oral hygiene practices may help prevent respiratory infections, particularly in patients who are vulnerable because of acute illness, cancer treatments or immobility.

When patients are ill, diet is essential for tissue repair and healing; however, a lack of saliva will lead to the food not tasting as it should. The food will not easily form into the required bolus size for ease of swallowing. This may put the patient off eating and drinking and may lead to the patient losing their appetite and potentially delayed healing.

Ill health can lead to neglect of hygiene standards for individuals. Mouth care is easy for patients to ignore when they are feeling poorly. However, it is an essential consideration for nursing.

Pharynx

The pharynx consists of three parts: the oropharynx, the nasopharynx and the laryngopharynx. The naso-pharynx is considered a structure of the respiratory system. The oropharynx and the laryngopharynx are passages for both food and respiratory gases (see Figure 10.5). The epiglottis is responsible for closing the entrance to the larynx during swallowing, and this essential action prevents food from entering the larynx and obstructing the respiratory passages.

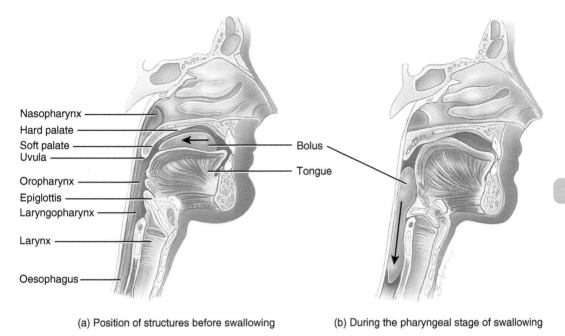

Nasopharynx
Hard palate
Soft palate
Uvula
Oropharynx
Epiglottis
Laryngopharynx
Larynx
Oesophagus

Bolus
Tongue

251

(a) Position of structures before swallowing

(b) During the pharyngeal stage of swallowing

Figure 10.5 **(a, b) Swallowing.** *Source:* Tortora and Derrickson (2009). Reproduced with permission of John Wiley & Sons.

Swallowing (Deglutition)

Once ingested food has been adequately chewed and formed into a bolus, it is ready to be swallowed. Swallowing (deglutition) occurs in three phases.

1. The voluntary phase: During this phase the action of the voluntary muscles serving the oral cavity manipulates the food bolus into the oropharynx. The tongue is pressed against the palate and this prevents the food from moving forward again.
2. The pharyngeal phase: During this phase a reflex action is initiated in response to the sensation of the food bolus in the oropharynx. This reflex is coordinated by the swallowing centre in the medulla oblongata, and the motor response is contraction of the muscles of the pharynx. The soft palate elevates, closing off the nasopharynx and preventing the food bolus from using this route. The larynx moves up and moves forward, allowing the epiglottis to cover the entrance to the larynx so the food bolus cannot move into the respiratory passages.
3. The oesophageal phase: The food bolus moves from the pharynx into the oesophagus. Waves of oesophageal muscle contractions move the food bolus down the length of the oesophagus and into the stomach. This wave of muscle contraction is known as **peristalsis** (see Figure 10.6).

Episode of Care Learning Disabilities

Dysphagia is the medical term used to describe swallowing difficulties. There are four stages to deglutition (swallowing) and problems in any of the stages can lead to dysphagia.

People can describe problems with choking while eating or drinking, coughing while eating or drinking, a feeling of food being 'stuck', problems with chewing, issues with controlling and swallowing liquids and foods.

Some people with learning disabilities are more likely to have dysphagia and issues associated with eating too fast. There can also be issues around eating inappropriate or items not usually considered as food (pica).

Dysphagia increases the risk of dehydration, undernutrition, frequent upper respiratory tract infections, aspiration pneumonia and choking.

Asif is a 34-year-old man with moderate learning disabilities. He lives in a community care home. The staff note that Asif has had two upper respiratory tract infections, coughs frequently at mealtimes and is losing weight. Asif's situation appears to have changed and they are concerned about his dysphagia.

Asif is referred to his doctor as the dysphagia is new and while the dysphagia may be due to eating and drinking difficulties, the care team are conscious that there could be other pathologies associated with dysphagia and further investigation may be required.

Asif's medications are reviewed. He is not on any medications that can affect his alertness (for example, antipsychotic medication) or medicines that increase salivation (for example, cholinergic medications). Medications are eliminated from the potential cause of Asif's current dysphagia.

Asif is referred to the speech and language therapy team who conduct a thorough examination to include:

- examination of the inside of the mouth and tongue movements;
- assessment while eating different types of food;
- swallow test;
- breathing assessment;
- ordering video fluoroscopy.

Following the assessment, the speech and language therapists advise the following for Asif:

- Ensure Asif is upright during meal or snack times and for 30 minutes after eating.
- Supervise Asif during eating and drinking and allow time for him to eat
- Reduce distractions during meal times to allow Asif to focus on swallowing.
- Cut Asif's food into small manageable portions, large enough to stimulate chewing but small enough to prevent choking.
- Check on oral hygiene following meals to ensure no food is left in the oral cavity
- Use a food chart to monitor how much Asif is eating and ensure he is weighed weekly.

One month later, Asif has not had any further upper respiratory tract infections and is back to his original weight.

Multiple Choice Questions

1. Which of these risk assessment tools can inform the health care practitioner that there is an issue around eating and drinking:
   (a) the Falls Risk Assessment Tool
   (b) the Malnutrition Universal Screening Tool
   (c) the PQTSR Tool
   (d) the Waterlow Score
2. Which statement with regard aspiration pneumonia is true?
   (a) it often occurs as a result of dysphagia
   (b) weight loss and reduced appetite could be an indicator of aspiration pneumonia
   (c) coughing up purulent sputum could be an indication of aspiration pneumonia
   (d) all of the above
3. Which of the following is not a phase associated with swallow?
   (a) the voluntary phase
   (b) the cardiac phase
   (c) the pharyngeal phase
   (d) the oesophageal phase
4. Which of the following medicines are associated with an overproduction of saliva?
   (a) Risperidone
   (b) Paracetamol
   (c) Glycopyrrolate
   (d) Amitriptyline
5. Where is saliva produced?
   (a) the sublingual glands
   (b) the parotid glands
   (c) the submandibular glands
   (d) all of the above

Oesophagus

The food bolus leaves the oropharynx and enters the oesophagus. The oesophagus extends from the laryngopharynx to the stomach. It is a thick-walled structure, measuring about 25 cm in length, and lies in the thoracic cavity, posterior to the trachea. The function of the oesophagus is to transport

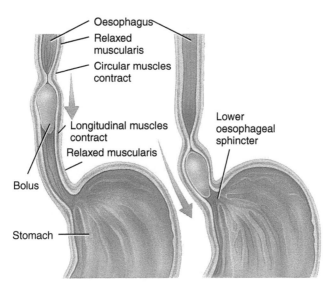

Anterior view of frontal sections of peristalsis in oesophagus

Figure 10.6 **Peristalsis in the oesophagus.** *Source:* Tortora and Derrickson (2009). Reproduced with permission of John Wiley & Sons.

substances (the food bolus) from the mouth to the stomach. Thick mucus is secreted by the mucosa of the oesophagus, and this aids the passage of the food bolus and also protects the oesophagus from abrasion.

The upper oesophageal sphincter regulates the movement of substances into the oesophagus, and the lower oesophageal sphincter (also known as the cardiac sphincter) regulates the movement of substances from the oesophagus to the stomach. The muscle layer of the oesophagus differs from the rest of the digestive tract, as the superior portion consists of skeletal (voluntary) muscle and the inferior portion consists of smooth (involuntary) muscle. Breathing and swallowing cannot occur at the same time (Nair and Peate, 2018).

Medicines Management Omeprazole

Omeprazole is a medicine used to treat a number of digestive system conditions, including dyspepsia, acid reflux, oesophagitis and peptic ulcer disease. It belongs to a group of medicines known as proton pump inhibitors (Galbraith *et al.*, 2007). Hydrochloric acid produced in the stomach can escape into the oesophagus or the duodenum of the small intestine and irritate the delicate epithelium in these areas. Omeprazole works on the parietal cells in the stomach, inhibiting the production of hydrochloric acid.

Omeprazole is usually prescribed as 20–40 mg once daily.

The common side effects for patients taking omeprazole are:

- vomiting
- diarrhoea
- constipation
- pain (stomach)
- headaches
- increased flatulence
- nausea.

NICE (2014) produced guidance on the investigation and management of dyspepsia.

The Structure of the Digestive System

There are four layers of tissue or tunicas that exist throughout the length of the digestive tract from oesophagus to anus (see Figure 10.7).

The mucosa is the innermost layer. The products of digestion are in contact with this layer as they pass through the digestive tract. The mucosa consists of three layers: the mucous epithelium (mucous membrane), which is involved in the secretion of mucus and other digestive system secretions such as saliva or gastric juice. This layer helps to protect the digestive system from the continuous wear and tear it endures. In the small intestine this layer is involved in absorption of the products of digestion. The next layer is the lamina propria, which consists of loose connective tissue that has a role in supporting the blood vessels and lymphatic tissue of the mucosa. The outermost layer is called the muscularis mucosa and consists of a thin smooth muscle layer that helps to form the gastric pits or the microvilli of the digestive system.

The submucosa is a thick layer of connective tissue. It contains blood and lymphatic vessels and some small glands. It also contains Meissner's plexus – nerves that stimulate the intestinal glands to secrete their products.

The muscularis consists of an inner layer of circular smooth muscle and an outer layer of longitudinal smooth muscle. The stomach has three layers of smooth muscle, and the upper oesophagus has skeletal muscle. Blood and lymph vessels and the myenteric plexus (a network of sympathetic and parasympathetic nerves) are located between the two layers of smooth muscle. The wave-like contraction and relaxation of this muscle layer are responsible for moving food along the digestive tract – a process known as peristalsis (see Figure 10.7). Peristalsis helps to churn and mechanically digest food.

The outer layer of the digestive tract is the serosa (adventitia). The largest area of serosa is found in the abdominal and pelvic cavities and is known as the peritoneum. The peritoneum is a closed sac. The visceral peritoneum covers the organs of the abdominal and pelvic cavity, and the parietal peritoneum lines the

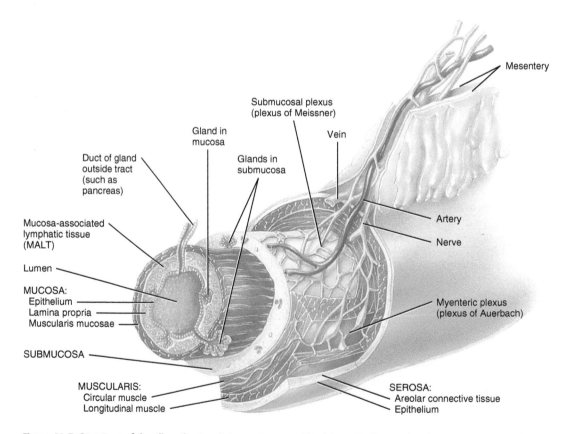

Figure 10.7 **Structure of the digestive tract.** *Source:* Tortora and Derrickson (2009). Reproduced with permission of John Wiley & Sons.

abdominal wall. A small amount of serous fluid lies between the two layers. The peritoneum has a good blood supply and contains many lymph nodes and lymphatic vessels. It acts as a barrier, protecting the structures it encloses, and can act to isolate areas of infection to prevent damage to neighbouring structures.

Stomach

The stomach lies in the abdominal cavity. It lies between the oesophagus superiorly and the duodenum of the small intestine inferiorly. It is divided into regions (see Figure 10.8).

The entrance to the stomach from the oesophagus is via the lower oesophageal sphincter or cardiac sphincter. This leads to a small area within the stomach called the cardiac region or cardia. The fundus is the dome-shaped region in the superior part of the stomach. The body region occupies the space between the lesser and greater curvature of the stomach, and the pyloric region narrows into the pyloric canal. The pyloric sphincter controls the exit of chyme from the stomach into the small intestine. Chyme is the name given to the food bolus as it leaves the stomach.

The stomach is supplied with arterial blood from a branch of the celiac artery, and venous blood leaves the stomach via the hepatic vein. The vagus nerve innervates the stomach with parasympathetic fibres that stimulate gastric motility and the secretion of gastric juice. Sympathetic fibres from the celiac plexus reduce gastric activity.

The stomach has the same four layers of tissue as the digestive tract, but with some differences. The muscularis contains three layers of smooth muscle instead of two. It has longitudinal, circular and oblique muscle fibres. The extra muscle layer facilitates the churning, mixing and mechanical digestion of food that occurs within the stomach, as well as supporting the onward journey of the food by peristalsis.

The mucosa within the stomach is also different from the rest of the digestive tract. When the stomach is empty, the mucosal epithelia falls into long folds known as rugae. The rugae fill out when the stomach is full. A very full stomach can contain approximately 4 L, while an empty stomach contains only about 50 mL (Marieb and Hoehn, 2010). The shape and size of the stomach vary from person to person and depending on the quantity of food stored within it.

255

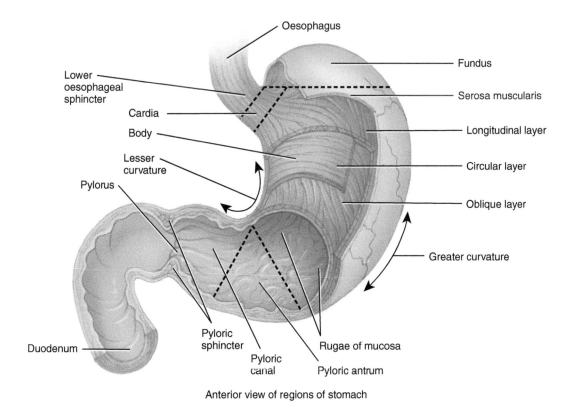

Anterior view of regions of stomach

Figure 10.8 **The stomach.** *Source:* Tortora and Derrickson (2009). Reproduced with permission of John Wiley & Sons.

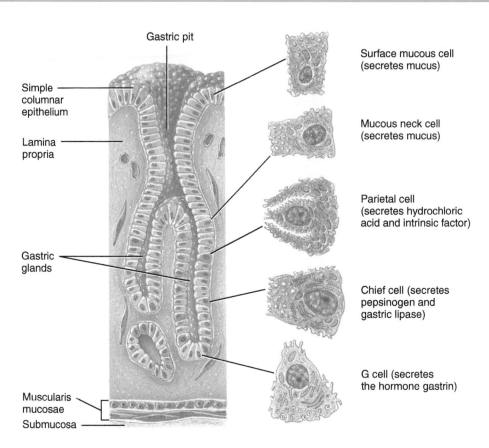

Figure 10.9 **Gastric glands and cells.** *Source:* Tortora and Derrickson (2009). Reproduced with permission of John Wiley & Sons.

The mucosa contains many gastric glands that secrete many different substances (see Figure 10.9).

- Surface mucous cells produce thick bicarbonate-coated mucus. This thick layer of mucus protects the stomach mucosal epithelia from corrosion by acidic gastric juice. When these cells become damaged, they are quickly shed and replaced.
- Mucous neck cells also secrete mucus – this mucus is different from surface cell mucus.
- Parietal cells produce hydrochloric acid and intrinsic factor. Intrinsic factor is necessary for the absorption of vitamin B_{12}. This vitamin is essential for the production of mature erythrocytes. Hydrochloric acid creates the acidic environment of the stomach (pH 1–3) and begins denaturing dietary protein in preparation for the action of pepsin.
- Chief cells produce pepsinogen, which is converted to pepsin in the presence of hydrochloric acid. Pepsin is necessary for the breakdown of protein into smaller peptide chains.
- Enteroendocrine cells, such as g cells, produce a variety of hormones, including gastrin. These hormones help regulate gastric motility.

This concoction of secretions plus water and mineral salts is more commonly called gastric juice. About 2 L of gastric juice is produced daily.

Clinical Considerations Enteral Feeding

Enteral feeding is the ingestion of food via the digestive tract.

Food is mainly ingested via the oral cavity but there are times when this route is not possible; for example, during critical illness, when consciousness is affected or when swallow is affected. Other methods of providing enteral nutrition include via the following:

- Nasogastric tube – a thin tube inserted via the nose, down the oesophagus and into the stomach.
- Nasojejunal tube – a tube inserted as per the nasogastric tube. However, it passes the stomach and enters the jejunum of the small intestine. It is useful when people have conditions that affect the function of the stomach or the duodenum and may be placed after pancreatic surgery.

- Percutaneous Endoscopic Gastrostomy (PEG) tube – this tube is placed where longer term enteral feeding is required. The tube is inserted via the abdominal wall into the stomach. This procedure requires the appropriate health care practitioner to use endoscopy to place the tube in the correct position. Sedation is administered for this procedure.
- Percutaneous Endoscopic Jejunostomy (PEJ) tube – this tube is placed in the same way as a PEG tube; however, it bypasses the stomach and is placed beyond the duodenum in the jejunum. PEJ may be chosen over PEG if the patient has a condition affecting the stomach.
- Enteral tubes are often required in clinical practice. They can be placed for short term use – for example for aspirating the gastric contents – or more longer term for enteral nutrition including the administration of medicines.

The health care worker must ensure that they understand the care required for each tube including the risks associated with misplacement, the tube blocking and pressure where the tubes are in contact with the skin.

257

Regulation of gastric juice secretion is divided into three phases (see Figure 10.10).

1. The cephalic phase: The sight, taste or smell of food stimulates the secretion of gastric juice.
2. The gastric phase: When food enters the stomach, the hormone gastrin is secreted into the bloodstream, and this stimulates the secretion of gastric juice. The secretion of hydrochloric acid reduces the pH of the stomach contents, and when the pH drops below 2 the secretion of gastrin is inhibited.
3. The intestinal phase: As the acidic contents of the stomach enter the duodenum of the small intestine, the hormones secretin and cholecystokinin (CCK) are secreted. These hormones also act to reduce the secretion of gastric juice and gastric motility.

The rate of gastric emptying depends on the size and content of the meal. A large meal takes longer than a small meal. Liquids quickly pass through the stomach, while solids require longer to be thoroughly mixed with gastric juice. Most meals will have left the stomach 4 h after ingestion.

The functions of the stomach are:

- to act as a store for food;
- production of mucus to protect the stomach;
- mechanical digestion, by the churning action facilitated by an additional layer of smooth muscle;
- mixing food with hydrochloric acid to help eradicate pathogens and denature proteins in preparation for the action of pepsin;
- production of chyme;
- production of intrinsic factor.

Medicines Management Ondansetron

Nausea and vomiting are the most common digestive system symptoms. Vomiting (emesis) occurs when the emetic or vomiting centre in the brain is activated. It can be activated as a result of irritation in the stomach. The irritation could be due to bacteria or often medication. Some medications cross the blood–brain barrier and stimulate the vomiting centre. When stimulated, the abdominal muscles and diaphragm are activated and a reverse peristalsis occurs in the stomach, leading to the ejection of the stomach contents (Marieb, 2017).

This unpleasant reaction can be treated with medications such as ondansetron. Ondansetron belongs to a group of medications known as anti-emetics. It acts by blocking serotonin, which promotes vomiting.

The usual adult dose is 8 mg twice daily. This can be adjusted according to need. Ondansetron is often prescribed during chemotherapy, and the dose required may be increased if this is prescribed. Ondansetron may also be prescribed intravenously if the patient is too nauseous to tolerate oral medication.

The most common side effects associated with Ondansetron are:

- constipation
- headaches
- flushing.

The side effects associated with this medication are minimal, and allergy reactions are sometimes seen when given intravenously (Galbraith et al., 2007).

258

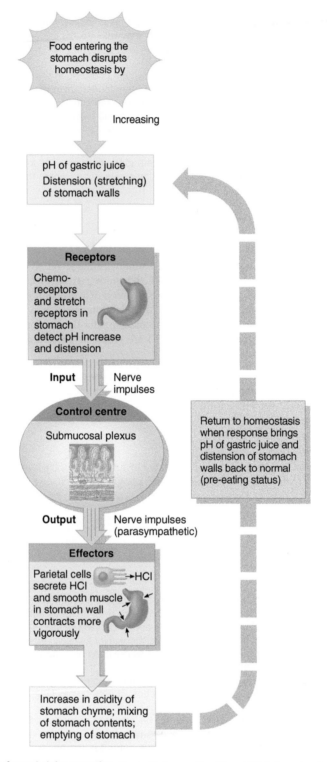

Figure 10.10 **Phases of gastric juice secretion.** *Source:* Tortora and Derrickson (2009). Reproduced with permission of John Wiley & Sons.

Episode of Care Mental Health

There are a range of anxiety disorders that affect the mental well-being of people. These include:

- generalised anxiety disorder
- social anxiety disorder
- panic disorders
- phobias
- post-traumatic stress disorder (PTSD)
- obsessive compulsive disorders (OCD)
- health anxiety
- body dysmorphic disorder (BDD)
- perinatal anxiety or perinatal OCD.

An increase in anxiety can lead to the following changes in the digestive system:

- An increase in the amount of hydrochloric acid produced by the stomach. This leads to symptoms associated with heart burn and acid reflux.
- Anxiety leads to an increase in the sympathetic nervous system's activity and a decrease in the parasympathetic nervous system's activity. Long-term anxiety can affect the body's ability to rest and digest.
- Parasympathetic activity occurs most when people are asleep. Insomnia is a symptom common for those who have an anxiety disorder.
- Anxiety disorders can affect the bacterial flora within the digestive system, and this can affect the digestive system and the gut–brain axis.

Mannir is 27 years old and has been diagnosed with generalised anxiety disorder.

He has described symptoms to his GP of severe heartburn, despite increased use of Gaviscon, and insomnia. Mannir has tried several self-help options but his GP has referred Mannir for cognitive behavioural therapy which should help.

For the increased heart burn, the doctor has prescribed omeprazole 40 mg once a day. Mannir reports that this has helped, and his symptoms have greatly improved. The reduction in the heartburn is now helping Mannir to sleep as the symptoms were worse when he was lying down and trying to sleep.

Multiple Choice Questions

1. Where is hydrochloric acid produced in the body?
   (a) the oral cavity
   (b) the oesophagus
   (c) the stomach
   (d) the small intestine
2. Hydrochloric acid is necessary for the digestion of which type of food?
   (a) carbohydrates
   (b) proteins
   (c) fats
   (d) water
3. Which part of the nervous system promotes digestive activities?
   (a) the limbic system
   (b) the somatic nervous system
   (c) the sympathetic nervous system
   (d) the parasympathetic nervous system
4. What protects the stomach from the effects of hydrochloric acid?
   (a) secretion of pepsin
   (b) secretions of bicarbonate rich mucous
   (c) secretion of lipase
   (d) secretion of intrinsic factor
5. Which of the following would you recommend for you patient with acid reflux?
   (a) head slightly elevated
   (b) lying on the left-hand side
   (c) not eating before going to bed
   (d) all of the above

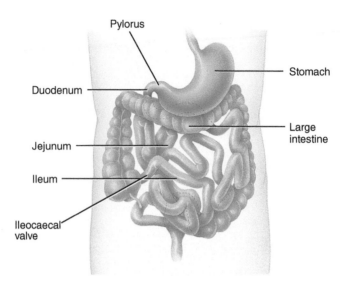

Figure 10.11 **The small intestine.** *Source:* Tortora and Derrickson (2009). Reproduced with permission of John Wiley & Sons.

Small Intestine

The small intestine is approximately 6 m long. In the small intestine food is further broken down by mechanical and chemical digestion, and absorption of the products of digestion takes place. The small intestine is divided into three parts (see Figure 10.11):

1. The duodenum is approximately 25 cm long. It is the entrance to the small intestine.
2. The jejunum measures 2.5 m and is the middle part of the small intestine.
3. The ileum measures 3.5 m. It meets the large intestine at the ileocaecal valve. This valve prevents the backflow of the products of digestion from the large intestine back into the small intestine.

The small intestine is innervated with both parasympathetic and sympathetic nerves. It receives its arterial blood supply from the superior mesenteric artery and nutrient-rich venous blood drains into the superior mesenteric vein and eventually into the hepatic portal vein towards the liver.

There are four types of cell present in the mucosa of the small intestine (see Figure 10.12):

- The absorptive cell produces digestive enzymes and absorbs digested foods.
- Goblet cells secrete mucus to protect the intestine from abrasion and from the acidic chyme entering the small intestine.
- Enteroendocrine cells produce regulatory hormones such as secretin and CCK. These hormones are secreted into the bloodstream and act on their target organs to release pancreatic juice and bile.
- Paneth cells produce lysozyme, which protects the small intestine from pathogens that have survived the acid conditions of the stomach. Peyer's patches (lymphatic tissue of the small intestine) also protect the small intestine.

Partially digested food enters the small intestine and spends from 3–6 h moving through its 6 m length. The smooth muscle activity within the small intestine continues the process of mechanical digestion. There are two types of mechanical digestion in the small intestine: segmental contractions, which help to mix the various enzymes in the small intestine with the contents of the chyme; and peristalsis, which propels the food down the length of the small intestine as well as facilitating mixing.

Chemical digestion completes the breakdown of the carbohydrates, fats and proteins. Pancreatic juice from the pancreas, bile from the gallbladder and intestinal juice contribute to this.

Chemical Digestion

Within the small intestine, any carbohydrates that have not been broken down by the action of salivary amylase will be broken down by pancreatic amylase.

Bile will emulsify fat and fatty acids, making it easier for lipase (also from the pancreatic juice) to break the fats into fatty acids and glycerol. Proteins are denatured by hydrochloric acid in the stomach. In the small

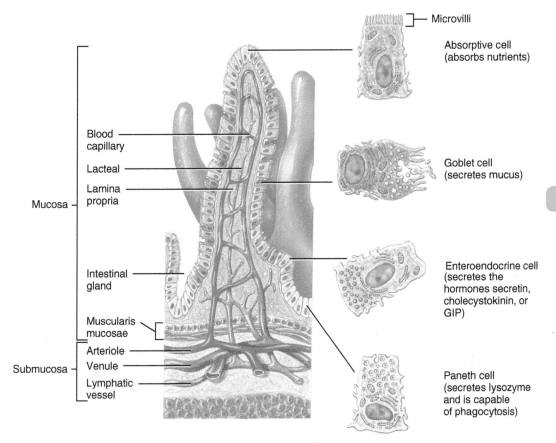

Microvilli

Absorptive cell
(absorbs nutrients)

Goblet cell
(secretes mucus)

Blood
capillary

Lacteal

Lamina
propria

Mucosa

261

Enteroendocrine cell
(secretes the
hormones secretin,
cholecystokinin, or
GIP)

Intestinal
gland

Muscularis
mucosae

Arteriole

Venule

Submucosa

Lymphatic
vessel

Paneth cell
(secretes lysozyme
and is capable
of phagocytosis)

Enlarged villus showing lacteal, capillaries, intestinal glands and cell types

Figure 10.12 **The cells within the villi of the small intestine.** *Source:* Tortora and Derrickson (2009). Reproduced with permission of John Wiley & Sons.

intestine they are further acted upon by the enzymes trypsin, chymotrypsin and carboxypeptidase. The end product of protein digestion are tripeptidases, dipeptidases and amino acids.

The small intestine produce 1–2 L of intestinal juice daily. It is secreted from the cells of the crypts of Lieberkühn (located between the villi) in response to either acidic chyme irritating the intestinal mucosa or distension from the presence of chyme in the small intestine. Intestinal juice is slightly alkaline (pH 7.4–8.4) and watery. Intestinal juice and pancreatic juice from the pancreas mix with the acidic chyme as it enters the duodenum and increase the pH, thus preventing the corrosive action of chyme on the mucosa of the duodenum. Intestinal juice contains mucus, which helps protect the intestinal mucosa, mineral salts and enterokinase.

The primary function of the small intestine is absorption of water and nutrients, and it has several anatomical adaptations to facilitate this:

- Permanent circular folds, called plicae circulars, within the mucosa and submucosa slow down the movement of the products of digestion, allowing time for absorption of nutrients to occur.
- On the surface of the mucosa are tiny, finger-like projections called villi. At the centre of the villi is a capillary bed and a lacteal (lymph capillary). This allows nutrients to be absorbed directly into the blood or the lymph.
- On the surface of the villi are cytoplasmic extensions called microvilli. The presence of the microvilli greatly increases the surface area available for absorption. The appearance of the microvilli resembles the surface of a brush; hence it is called the brush border. The brush border produces some enzymes used to

further break down carbohydrates such as lactase, maltase, dextrinase and sucrase. It also produces enzymes to further break down proteins: aminopeptidase, carboxypeptidase and dipeptidase.

The absorption of nutrients occurs by diffusion or active transport. Some nutrients will be absorbed into the blood capillary and some will be absorbed into the lacteal.

Function of the small intestine

- Production of mucus to protect the duodenum from the effects of the acidic chyme.
- Secretion of intestinal juice and pancreatic juice from the pancreas increase the pH of the chyme to facilitate the action of the enzymes.
- Bile enters the small intestine to emulsify fat so that it can be further broken down by the action of lipase.
- Many enzymes are secreted to complete the chemical digestion of carbohydrates, proteins and fats.
- Mechanical digestion is by peristalsis and segmentation and slows down to allow adequate mixing and maximum absorption.
- The small intestine is structurally designed with a large surface area for maximum absorption of the products of digestion.
- The small intestine is where the majority of nutrients, electrolytes and water are absorbed.

The Pancreas

The pancreas is composed of exocrine and endocrine tissue. It consists of a head, body and tail (see Figure 10.13). The cells of the pancreas are responsible for making the endocrine and exocrine products.

- The islet cells of the islets of Langerhans produce the endocrine hormones insulin and glucagon. These hormones control carbohydrate metabolism.
- The acini glands of the exocrine pancreas produce 1.2–1.5 L of pancreatic juice daily. Pancreatic juice travels from the pancreas via the pancreatic duct into the duodenum at the hepatopancreatic ampulla.

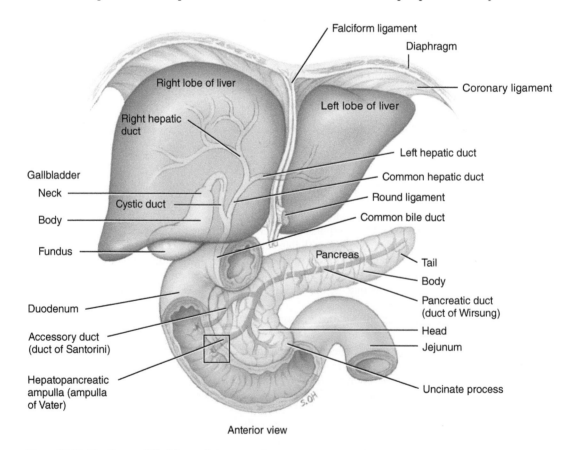

Anterior view

Figure 10.13 **The liver, gallbladder and pancreas.** *Source:* Tortora and Derrickson (2009). Reproduced with permission of John Wiley & Sons.

262

- The cells of the pancreatic ducts secrete bicarbonate ions, which gives pancreatic juice its high pH (pH 8). This helps to neutralise acidic chyme from the stomach, thus protecting the small intestine from damage by the acidity. Additionally, the actions of amylase and lipase are most effective at the higher pH (pH 6–8).

Pancreatic juice consists of:

- water;
- mineral salts;
- pancreatic amylase, which completes the digestion of carbohydrates;
- lipase, used in the digestion of fat;
- trypsinogen, chymotrypsinogen and procarboxypeptidase, which are released in an inactive form to protect the digestive system structures from the protein-digesting enzymes that they become – once they enter the duodenum they are activated by enterokinase from intestinal juice and become trypsin, chymotrypsin and carboxypeptidase respectively and are then used in the digestion of protein.

Two hormones regulate the secretion of pancreatic juice. Secretin, produced in response to the presence of hydrochloric acid in the duodenum, promotes the secretion of bicarbonate ions. CCK, secreted in response to the intake of protein and fat, promotes the secretion of the enzymes present in pancreatic juice. Parasympathetic vagus nerve stimulation also promotes the release of pancreatic juice.

In summary, the exocrine function of the pancreas is to secrete pancreatic juice into the duodenum. The actions of pancreatic juice lead to the further breakdown of carbohydrate, fat and protein.

Medicines Management Creon

Creon is a medication prescribed for patients who have cystic fibrosis or pancreatic insufficiency. It contains the following enzymes:

- amylase – for the breakdown of carbohydrate;
- lipase – for the breakdown of fats;
- proteases – for the breakdown of protein.

Pancreatic insufficiency can occur as a result of pancreatic cancer, pancreatic surgery and acute or chronic pancreatitis. In cystic fibrosis the ducts that transport the pancreatic enzymes become obstructed with the increased mucus production associated with this disease pathway.

The dosage of creon required will depend on the diet of the patient. If the symptoms of loose stool and weight loss persist, then the dose of creon may be increased. Creon is usually taken for life. There are some side effects associated with creon, and these include:

- abdominal distension
- nausea
- vomiting
- diarrhoea
- constipation.

The tablets are enteric coated to protect them from inactivation in the stomach (Galbraith *et al.*, 2007). NICE (2016) produced a Clinical Knowledge Summary on managing chronic pancreatitis.

Episode of Care Child

Crohn's disease is an inflammatory bowel disease. While the symptoms of Crohn's disease can occur at any time, they often begin in childhood. The causes of Crohn's disease are unknown but are thought to be linked to a number of things including the immune system, genetic makeup, following from a viral illness and abnormal gut flora.

The inflammation in Crohn's disease may occur anywhere in the digestive tract. It may be patchy covering small areas, or it may extend further and deeper into the tissue. It is a chronic condition.

Zoe is 10 years old. She complains constantly to her mum that she is so tired all the time and does not want to go to school. Her teachers have reported lethargy and an inability to join in with the other children for any length of time.

Zoe attends the dentist for her routine 6 monthly check up and the dentist reports mouth ulcers. Zoe's is mum is concerned as all of the symptoms, including a failure to gain weight and develop, are starting to mount up. Zoe visits the GP with her mum. The GP asks for a stool sample. There is no evidence of any obvious blood in the sample, but it is sent off for analysis.

The GP is concerned and refers Zoe to paediatric services for further investigation. Zoe's stool test does reveal blood in the stool and her blood tests show anaemia. When talking to the consultant, Zoe discusses her symptoms which include:

- diarrhoea
- crampy tummy pain
- mouth ulcers
- tiredness
- weight loss.

Following some additional tests including an MRI scan, the consultant diagnoses Crohn's disease and prescribes some anti-inflammatory medication for Zoe.

Multiple Choice Questions

1. Which of the following is not an inflammatory bowel disease?
   (a) ulcerative colitis
   (b) Crohn's disease
   (c) irritable bowel syndrome
   (d) all of the above
2. Which of the following describes normal protection within the gastro-intestinal system?
   (a) secretion of hydrochloric acid
   (b) mucosa associated lymphatic tissue (MALT)
   (c) the secretion of saliva
   (d) all of the above
3. Which of the following is a symptom of Crohn's disease?
   (a) diarrhoea that lasts for longer than 7 days
   (b) the presence of blood in the faeces
   (c) fatigue
   (d) all of the above
4. A narrowed area of the bowel caused by recurrent inflammation and healing is called:
   (a) stricture
   (b) fistula
   (c) stoma
   (d) fissure
5. Which area of the intestine is most commonly affected by Crohn's disease?
   (a) duodenum
   (b) jejunum
   (c) pylorus
   (d) ileum

The Liver and Production of Bile

The liver is the body's largest gland. It weighs between 1 and 2 kg. It lies under the diaphragm partly protected by the ribs. The liver occupies most of the right hypochondriac region and extends through part of the epigastric region into the left hypochondriac region. The right lobe is the largest of the four liver lobes. On the posterior surface of the liver there is an entry and exit to the organ called the portal fissure. Blood, lymph vessels, nerves and bile ducts enter and leave the liver through the portal fissure.

The liver is composed of tiny hexagonal-shaped lobules that contain hepatocytes (see Figure 10.14). The hepatocytes are protected by Kupffer cells (hepatic macrophages). The Kupffer cells deal with any foreign particles and worn-out blood cells.

Each corner of the hexagonal-shaped lobule has a portal triad. A branch of the hepatic artery, a branch of hepatic portal vein and a bile duct are present here. The hepatic artery supplies the hepatocytes with oxygenated arterial blood. The hepatic portal vein delivers nutrient-rich deoxygenated blood from the digestive tract to the hepatocytes. The hepatocytes' function is to filter, detoxify and process the nutrients from the digestive tract. Nutrients can be used for energy, stored or used to make new molecules. The liver sinusoids are large, leaky capillaries that drain the blood from the hepatic artery and hepatic portal vein into the central vein. This processed blood is then drained into the hepatic vein and on to the inferior vena cava.

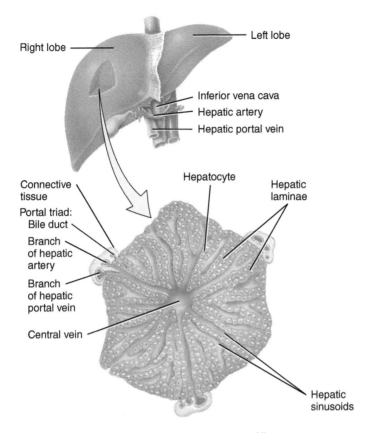

Overview of histological components of liver

Figure 10.14 **Liver lobule.** *Source:* Tortora and Derrickson (2009). Reproduced with permission of John Wiley & Sons.

As the blood flows towards the centre of the triad to exit at the central vein, the bile produced by the hepato-cyte as a metabolic by-product moves in the opposite direction towards the bile canaliculi and on to the bile ducts. Bile then leaves the liver via the common hepatic duct towards the duodenum of the small intestine.

The liver produces and secretes up to 1 L of yellow/green alkaline bile per day. Bile is composed of:

- bile salts, such as bilirubin from the breakdown of haemoglobin;
- cholesterol;
- fat-soluble hormones;
- fat;
- mineral salts;
- mucus.

The function of bile is to emulsify fats, giving the fat-digesting enzyme, lipase a larger surface area to work on.

Bile is stored and concentrated in the gallbladder.

The Functions of the Liver

Apart from the production of bile and the metabolism of carbohydrate, fat and protein (discussed further on in this chapter), the liver has many additional functions:

- detoxification of drugs – the liver deals with medication, alcohol, ingested toxins and the toxins produced by the action of microbes;
- recycling of erythrocytes;
- deactivation of many hormones, including the sex hormones, thyroxine, insulin, glucagon, cortisol and aldosterone;
- production of clotting proteins;

- storage of vitamins, minerals and glycogen;
- synthesis of vitamin A;
- heat production.

The Gallbladder

The gallbladder is a small, green, muscular sac that lies posterior to the liver. It functions as a reservoir for bile. It also concentrates bile by absorbing water. The mucosa of the gallbladder, like the rugae of the stomach, contains folds that allow the gallbladder to stretch in order to accommodate varying volumes of bile. When the smooth muscle walls of the gallbladder contract, bile is expelled into the cystic duct and down into the common bile duct before entering the duodenum via the hepatopancreatic ampulla.

The stimulus for gallbladder contraction is the hormone CCK. This enteroendocrine hormone, secreted from the small intestine into the blood, is produced in response to the presence of fatty chyme in the duodenum. CCK stimulates the secretion of pancreatic juice and the relaxation of the hepatopancreatic sphincter. When the sphincter is relaxed, both bile and pancreatic juice can enter the duodenum.

The Large Intestine

The contents of the small intestine move slowly through it by a process called segmentation. This allows time to complete digestion and absorption. Entry to the large intestine is controlled by the ileocaecal sphincter. The sphincter opens in response to the increased activity of the stomach and the action of the hormone gastrin. Once food residue has reached the large intestine it cannot backflow into the ileum (see Figure 10.15).

The large intestine measures 1.5 m in length and 7 cm in diameter. It is continuous with the small intestine from the ileocaecal valve and ends at the anus.

Food residue enters the caecum and has to pass up the ascending colon along the transverse colon, down the descending colon and out of the body via the rectum, anal canal and anus. The caecum is a descending,

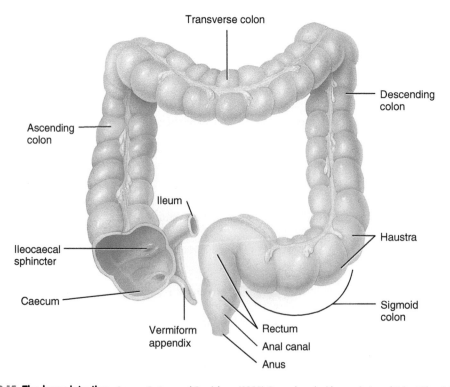

Figure 10.15 **The large intestine.** *Source:* Tortora and Derrickson (2009). Reproduced with permission of John Wiley & Sons.

sac-like opening into the large intestine. The vermiform appendix is a narrow, tube-like structure that leaves the caecum but is closed at its distal end. It is composed of lymphoid tissue and has a role in immunity. Two sphincter muscles control exit from the anus. The internal anal sphincter is smooth muscle and is under the control of the parasympathetic nervous system, whereas the external anal sphincter is composed of skeletal muscle and is under voluntary control.

Clinical Considerations Appendicitis

The narrow lumen of the appendix does not allow much room for inflammation. If it becomes blocked by faecoliths (hard faecal material) or becomes twisted and kinked, this results in inflammation of the appendix. The swelling associated with this can lead to ulceration of the mucosal lining. This presents initially as central abdominal pain that eventually localises at the region of the appendix. Appendicitis can subside, but it can result in abscess formation and even rupture.

267

The large intestine mucosa contains large numbers of goblet cells that secrete mucus to ease the passage of faeces and protect the walls of the large intestine. The simple columnar epithelium changes to stratified squamous epithelium at the anal canal. Anal sinuses secrete mucus in response to faecal compression. This protects the anal canal from the abrasion associated with defaecation.

The longitudinal muscle layer of the large intestine is formed into bands called the taeniae coli. These give the large intestine its gathered appearance. The sac created by this gathering is called a haustrum.

The food residue from the ileum is fluid when it enters the caecum and contains few nutrients. The small intestine is responsible for some of the absorption of water, but the primary function of the large intestine is to absorb water and turn the food residue into semi-solid faeces. The large intestine also absorbs some vitamins, minerals, electrolytes and drugs. Food residue usually takes 24–48 h to pass through the large intestine; 500 mL of food residue enters the large intestine daily and approximately 150 mL leaves as faeces.

As faeces enters the rectum, the stretching of the walls of the rectum initiates the defaecation reflex. Acquired, voluntary control of the defaecation reflex occurs between the ages of 2 and 3 years. The external anal sphincter is under voluntary control, and, if it is appropriate to do so, defaecation can occur. Contraction of the abdominal muscles and diaphragm (the Valsalva manoeuvre) creates intra-abdominal pressure and assists in the process of defaecation. If it is not appropriate to defaecate, as it is under voluntary control, it can be postponed. After a few minutes the urge to go will subside and will only be felt again when the next mass movement through the large intestine occurs.

Faeces is a brown, semi-solid material. It contains fibre, stercobilin (from the breakdown of bilirubin), water, fatty acids, shed epithelial cells and microbes. Stercobilin gives faeces its brown colour. An excess of water in faeces results in diarrhoea. This occurs when food residue passes too quickly through the large intestine, so that the absorption of water cannot occur. Conversely, constipation occurs if food residue spends too long in the large intestine.

Medicines Management Lactulose

Lactulose belongs to a group of medications called laxatives or aperients. It is used to treat constipation. Constipation occurs as a result of a lack of fluid intake or dehydration, a lack of exercise or immobility, during pregnancy or due to a lack of dietary fibre.

People who experience constipation should try to increase their mobility and fluid intake. They should examine their diet to see whether additional fibre can be taken. Lactulose may also be prescribed.

The usual adult dose for lactulose is 15 mL three times a day. Lactulose acts in the large intestine and can take 48 h to have an effect. Increasing fluid intake to 2 L will also help.

Lactulose is an osmotic laxative (Galbraith et al., 2007), and leads to a change in the osmotic pressure in the bowel, and therefore more water is available in the intestine. This leads to the stool having more water content, making it pass through the intestine easier.

The side effects of taking lactulose include:

- nausea
- diarrhoea
- flatulence
- abdominal discomfort.

NICE (2017) produced a Clinical Knowledge Summary on constipation.

Digestive Tract Hormones

Many hormones are responsible for the activity of the digestive system. A summary of their role is contained in Table 10.1.

Nutrition, Chemical Digestion and Metabolism

This chapter has hitherto concentrated on how the digestive tract deals with food ingested in order to break it down into its constituent parts for use by the cells of the body. This section will consider nutrition and the role of a balanced diet in health.

An adequate intake of nutrients is essential for health. Nutrition also has an important role in social and psychological well-being. If managed inappropriately, nutrition can lead to many physical and psychological illnesses. Therefore, it is important to have an understanding of the role of nutrients within the body in order to understand how a lack or excess of nutrients will lead to ill health.

The remainder of this chapter will identify the macro-and micronutrients and the food groups that provide the source of macro-and micronutrients. It will examine what the nutrients are broken down into and how the body uses these constituent parts.

Nutrients

A nutrient is a substance that is ingested and processed by the gastrointestinal system. It is digested and absorbed and can be used by the body to produce energy or become the building block for a new molecule or to participate in essential chemical reactions. Nutrients are required for body growth, repair and maintenance of cell function. Not all of the food ingested can be classed as nutrients. Some non-digestible plant fibres are not nutrients but are required for healthy functioning of the digestive system.

Balanced Diet

The body has the ability to break down some nutrients in order to create new molecules, but this ability is finite and there remains a group of essential nutrients that the body cannot make but are required to be ingested in the diet for homeostasis to be maintained. A balanced diet is therefore essential for health (Public Health England, 2018). The daily recommended portions of food groups required for a balanced diet are shown in the food pyramid (see Figure 10.16). Lack of a balanced diet can lead to malnourishment, and overindulgence can lead to obesity.

Table 10.1 **Summary of the role of the digestive system hormones.**

HORMONE	ORIGIN	TARGET	ACTION	STIMULUS
Gastrin	Stomach	Stomach	Increases gastric gland secretion of hydrochloric acid Gastric emptying	Presence of protein in the stomach
Secretin	Duodenum	Stomach	Inhibits gastric gland secretion Inhibits gastric motility	Acidic and fatty chyme in the duodenum
		Pancreas	Increases pancreatic juice secretion Promotes cholecystokinin action	
		Liver	Increases bile secretion	
Cholecystokinin	Duodenum	Pancreas	Increases pancreatic juice secretion	Chyme in the duodenum
		Gallbladder	Stimulates contraction	
		Hepatopancreatic sphincter	Relaxes – entry to duodenum open	

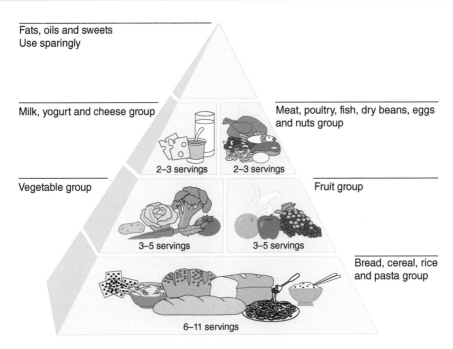

Fats, oils and sweets
Use sparingly

Milk, yogurt and cheese group

Meat, poultry, fish, dry beans, eggs
and nuts group

2–3 servings   2–3 servings

Vegetable group

Fruit group

3–5 servings   3–5 servings

Bread, cereal, rice
and pasta group

6–11 servings

Figure 10.16 **The food pyramid.** *Source:* Tortora and Derrickson (2009). Reproduced with permission of John Wiley & Sons.

Clinical Considerations Bariatric Surgery

Bariatric surgery is used as a last resort to treat those who are severely obese. The procedure works by reducing intake or the absorption of calories and is used to treat people with potentially life-threatening obesity if other treatments (e.g. lifestyle changes) have not worked. Indications include:

- a body mass index (BMI) greater than 40;
- a BMI of 35 or above and having another serious health condition that may be improved if weight is lost (e.g. type 2 diabetes or hypertension);
- other non-surgical methods have failed to maintain weight loss for at least 6 months;
- the person commits to long-term follow-up.

Weight loss surgery can help to significantly and quickly reduce excess body fat for those who meet the criteria. Bariatric surgery has to be undertaken in a specialist centre with long-term follow-up of patients. National guidelines are available concerning bariatric surgery. Contraindications include those who are unfit for surgery and those people with an uncontrolled alcohol or drug dependency.

Dietary nutrients begin life as large food molecules. They enter the digestive tract and are broken down into smaller molecules. This process is called catabolism. Digestive enzymes facilitate the breakdown of foods by a process called hydrolysis. Hydrolysis is the addition of water to break down the chemical bonds of the food molecules. Each of the three different types of food is broken down (lysed) by different enzymes.

Nutrient Groups

Carbohydrates, proteins and lipids are known as the major nutrients or macronutrients. They are required in quite large quantities. Vitamins and minerals are required in much smaller quantities, but they also are crucial for the maintenance of health, they are also known as the micronutrients. There are therefore six classes of nutrients:

- water
- carbohydrates
- proteins
- lipids (fats)
- vitamins
- minerals.

Water

Water is essential for the action of many digestive system functions. It is required to produce the many different juices of the digestive system. As the enzymes act on the different food molecules within the diet, water is added. This process is known as hydrolysis (Cohen and Hull, 2018).

Carbohydrates

Monosaccharides, disaccharides and polysaccharides are all carbohydrates. The dietary source of carbohydrates is plants. However, the milk sugar lactose is a form of carbohydrate found in cow and human milk. Carbohydrates are found in many foods, such as bread, pasta, cereal, biscuits, vegetables and fruit.

Carbohydrates consist of carbon, hydrogen and oxygen. They can be complex, such as the polysaccharides starch and glycogen, or simple, such as the disaccharides sucrose (table sugar) and lactose (milk sugar) and the monosaccharides glucose, fructose and galactose.

Digestion of carbohydrates supplies the body with fructose, galactose and glucose. The liver converts fructose and galactose to glucose as glucose is the molecule used by the body's cells.

Digested carbohydrates are absorbed into the blood via the villi of the small intestine. They enter the hepatic portal circulation and are transported to the liver for processing. The liver is a highly metabolic organ that requires a plentiful supply of glucose to carry out its metabolic activity.

Glucose is used by the cells to produce adenosine triphosphate (ATP). Glucose plus oxygen makes ATP, carbon dioxide and water. The process of breaking down glucose is called glycolysis.

Insufficient carbohydrate intake will lead to an inability to meet the cells' energy demands. If this happens, the body will break down amino acids and lipids to create new glucose, a process called gluconeogenesis.

Excess glucose is converted to glycogen and stored in the liver. It can also be converted to fat and stored.

Fats

Dietary sources of fat include butter, eggs, cheese, milk, oily fish and the fatty part of meat. These contain saturated fat, which is mainly saturated fatty acids and glycerol. Vegetable oils and margarine are sources of unsaturated fats. The body can also create fat from excess carbohydrate and protein intake.

Fat also contains carbon, hydrogen and oxygen, but in a different combination from carbohydrates.

When fat enters the small intestine it mixes and is emulsified by bile. The action of pancreatic lipase completes the digestion of fat and it is broken down into monoglycerides, glycerol and fatty acids. The monoglycerides and some of the fatty acids enter the lacteals of the villi and are transported via the lymph to the thoracic duct and into the circulation, where they eventually reach the liver. Glycerol and the remaining fatty acids are absorbed more directly into the capillary blood and reach the liver via the hepatic portal vein.

The liver uses some of the fatty acids and glycerol to provide energy and heat. In fact, hepatocytes and skeletal muscle use triglycerides as their major energy source. Excessive triglycerides can also be stored as adipose tissue, and this can also be used as an energy store when glucose is not available to body cells.

Dietary fats make food seem tender and lead to a feeling of satisfaction with food. They are necessary for the absorption of fat-soluble vitamins. Adipose tissue protects, cushions and insulates vital organs in the body. Phospholipids are required to form the myelin sheath and cell membranes. Cholesterol is obtained from egg yolk and dairy produce but is also synthesised in the body to form steroid hormones and bile salts.

Excess fat in the diet can lead to obesity and cardiovascular disease. A lack of fat in the diet can lead to weight loss, poor growth and skin lesions.

Proteins

Dietary sources of protein include meat, eggs and milk. Beans and peas (legumes), nuts, cereals and leafy green vegetables are also sources of amino acids.

Protein digestion begins in the stomach and is completed in the small intestine. Proteins are broken down into amino acids. They are absorbed via the villi of the small intestine, where they reach the capillaries and then the hepatic portal circulation to the liver or general circulation.

Proteins are used by the body for many purposes. They are used to form muscle, collagen and elastin, necessary for body structure and tissue repair. The hormones insulin and growth hormone are required for this. Amino acids are also used to form hormones and enzymes within the body. All of the amino acids required to form a required protein must be available within the cell in order for that protein to be made. This is called the all or nothing rule. Protein can also be used as a source of energy for the body. The amino acid is broken down mainly at the liver, where the nitrogenous part of the amino acid is removed and converted first to ammonia and then to urea. Urea is excreted as a waste product in urine. The remainder of the amino acid is used to produce energy. Protein cannot be stored by the body. Any excess amino acids are converted to carbohydrate or fat to be stored as adipose tissue.

Too much protein in the diet can lead to obesity. A lack of dietary protein can lead to muscle/tissue wasting and weight loss. A lack of plasma proteins can lead to oedema.

Vitamins

Vitamins are organic molecules that are required in small amounts for healthy metabolism. Essential vitamins cannot be manufactured by the body and must come from the diet, highlighting again the importance of a balanced diet. Some vitamins can be manufactured. Vitamin K is synthesised by intestinal bacteria; the skin makes vitamin D; and vitamin A is made from beta-carotene, found for example in carrots.

Many vitamins act as *coenzymes* (Seeley *et al.*, 2008). These vitamins combine with enzymes to make them functional. For example, the formation of clotting proteins requires the presence of vitamin K.

Vitamins are either fat soluble or water soluble. The fat-soluble vitamins combine with lipids from the diet and are absorbed in this way. Apart from vitamin K, the fat-soluble vitamins can be stored in the body; therefore, there can be problems associated with toxicity when these vitamins accumulate.

The water-soluble vitamins are absorbed with water along the digestive tract. They cannot be stored, and any excess ingested will be excreted in urine. A summary of vitamins and their functions is given in Table 10.2.

Table 10.2 **Vitamins summary.**

VITAMIN	SOURCE	FUNCTION	DEFICIENCY
Fat soluble			
A, retinol	Manufactured from beta-carotene. Egg yolk, cream, fish oil, cheese, liver	Skin, mucosa integrity; bone and tooth development during growth; photoreceptor pigment synthesis in the retina, normal reproduction, antioxidant	Night blindness, dry skin and hair, loss of skin integrity, increased infection particularly respiratory, gastrointestinal and urinary
D	Manufactured by the skin. Cheese, eggs, fish oil, liver	Regulates calcium and phosphate metabolism	Rickets in children, osteomalacia in adults
E	Egg yolk, wheat germ, whole cereals, milk and butter	Antioxidant	In severe deficiency, ataxia and visual disturbances, decreased life span of red blood cells
K	Synthesised by bacteria in the large intestine. Liver, fish, fruit and leafy green vegetables	Formation of clotting proteins at the liver	Prolonged clotting times, bruising, bleeding
Water soluble			
B_1, thiamine	Egg yolk, liver, nuts, meat, legumes cereal germ	Coenzyme required for carbohydrate metabolism	Beriberi – muscle wasting, stunted growth polyneuritis and infection. Vision disturbances, confusion, unsteadiness, memory loss, fatigue, tachycardia, heart enlargement
B_2, riboflavin	Milk, green vegetables, yeast, cheese, fish roe, liver	Coenzyme required for carbohydrate and protein metabolism	Skin-cracking, particularly around the corners of the mouth, blurred vision, corneal ulcers, intestinal mucosa lesions

(Continued)

Table 10.2 (Continued)

VITAMIN	SOURCE	FUNCTION	DEFICIENCY
Folic acid	Liver, kidney, yeast, fresh leafy vegetables, eggs, whole grains	Coenzyme essential for DNA synthesis, red blood cell formation	Anaemia, spina bifida in newborn, increased risk of heart attack and stroke
Niacin, nicotinic acid	Liver, cheese, yeast, eggs, cereals, nuts, fish	Coenzyme involved in glycolysis, fat breakdown – assists with breakdown and inhibits cholesterol production	Pellagra – skin reddening to light, anorexia, nausea and dysphagia, delirium and dementia
B_6, pyridoxine	Meat, liver, fish, grains, bananas, yeast	Coenzyme involved in amino acid metabolism	Increased risk of heart disease, eye and mouth lesions. In children, nervous irritability, convulsions, abdominal pain and vomiting
B_{12} cyanocobalamin	Meat, fish, liver, eggs, milk	Coenzyme in all cells, involved in DNA synthesis. Formation and maintenance of myelin around nerves	Pernicious anaemia, peripheral neuropathy
B_5 pantothenic acid	Meat, grains, legumes, yeast, egg yolk	Coenzyme associated with amino acid metabolism and formation of steroids	Non-specific symptoms
Biotin	Egg yolk, liver, legumes, tomatoes	Coenzyme in carbohydrate metabolism	Pallor, anorexia, nausea, fatigue
C, ascorbic acid	Fruit, particularly citrus fruit, vegetables	Antioxidant, enhances iron absorption and use, maturation of red blood cells	Poor wound healing, joint pain, anaemia, scurvy

Minerals

Small quantities of inorganic compounds called minerals are required by the body for many purposes. For example, calcium gives structure and strength to tissues, and sodium forms ions essential for maintaining osmotic pressure. They also form approximately 5% of the body weight (Nair and Peate, 2018).

There are minerals that are required in moderate amounts, such as calcium and magnesium, and many others known where trace amounts are required, such as cobalt and copper. A summary of some of the minerals and their function is given in Table 10.3.

Clinical Considerations Obesity

Obesity is on the increase in Western society. Obesity occurs when more calories are taken in than are used by the body. Lack of exercise, a sedentary lifestyle and generous diet all contribute to weight gain. Obesity has serious health consequences as it predisposes people to indigestion, gallstones, hernias, cardiovascular disease, varicose veins, osteoarthritis and type 2 diabetes mellitus.

Conclusion

Digestion and nutrition play a vital role in the maintenance of health. The digestive tract processes ingested nutrients by breaking them down chemically and mechanically. Accessory structures – such as the pancreas, liver and gallbladder – have an essential role in providing the digestive tract with bile and pancreatic juice to

Table 10.3 **Minerals summary.**

MINERAL	SOURCE	FUNCTION	DEFICIENCY(D)/EXCESS(E)
Calcium	Milk, egg yolk, shellfish, cheese, green vegetables	Bones and teeth, cell membrane permeability, nerve impulse transmission, muscle contraction, heart rhythm, blood clotting	D: osteomalacia, osteoporosis, muscle tetany. In children – rickets and retarded growth E: lethargy and confusion, kidney stones
Chloride	Table salt	Works with sodium to maintain osmotic pressure of extracellular fluid	D: alkalosis, muscle cramps E: vomiting
Magnesium	Nuts, milk, legumes, cereal	Constituent of coenzymes. Muscle and nerve irritability	D: neuromuscular problems, irregular heartbeat E: diarrhoea
Sodium	Table salt	Extracellular cation. Works with chloride to maintain osmotic pressure of extracellular fluid. Muscle contraction, nerve impulse transmission, electrolyte balance	D: rare – nausea E: hypertension, oedema
Potassium	Fruit and vegetables and many foods	Intracellular cation. Muscle contraction, nerve impulse transmission electrolyte balance	D: Rare – muscle weakness, nausea, tachycardia E: cardiac abnormalities, muscular weakness
Iron	Liver, kidney, beef, green vegetables	Constituent of haemoglobin	D: anaemia E: haemochromatosis, liver damage
Iodine	Saltwater fish, vegetables	Constituent of thyroid hormones	D: hypothyroidism E: thyroid hormone synthesis depressed

facilitate the digestion of the macronutrients protein, carbohydrate and fat. The small intestine provides the large surface area available for the absorption of nutrients, and the liver processes the products of digestion. The large intestine plays an excretory role, ridding the body of the waste products from digestion and absorbing any remaining water back into the body.

The maintenance of homeostasis is achieved through the ingestion of a balanced diet, containing a variety of elements from each of the food groups.

Without all of this activity, normal cell functioning would be at risk and this would lead to ill health. Digestive health contributes greatly to physical, psychological and social well-being.

Glossary

Absorption: Process whereby the products of digestion move into the blood or lymph fluid.
Acini glands: Produce pancreatic juice.
Amylase: Carbohydrate-digesting enzyme.
Anus: End of the digestive tract.
Bile: Fluid produced by the liver and required for the digestion of fat.
Bile duct: Tube that carries bile from the liver.
Body region: Region of the stomach.
Caecum: Beginning of the large intestine.
Canine: Type of tooth.
Carbohydrate: One of the major food groups.

Cardiac region: Region of the stomach closest to the oesophagus.
Catabolism: Process of breaking down substances into simpler substances.
Chief cells: Pepsinogen-producing cells.
Cholecystokinin: Digestive system hormone.
Chyme: Creamy, semi-fluid mass of partially digested food mixed with gastric secretions.
Deglutition: Swallowing.
Digestion: The chemical and mechanical breakdown of food for absorption.
Duodenum: First part of the small intestine.
Enamel: Covering of the tooth.
Epiglottis: Cartilage that covers the larynx during swallowing.
Faeces: Brown, semi-solid digestive system waste.
Fats: One of the major food groups.
Frenulum: Fold between the lip and gum.
Fundus: Anatomical base region of the stomach.
Gluconeogenesis: The creation of glucose from non-carbohydrate molecules.
Glycolysis: The anaerobic breakdown of glucose to form pyruvic acid.
Goblet cell: Mucus-producing cell.
Haustrum: Sac-like section of the large intestine.
Hepatocyte: Liver cell.
Hepatic portal vein: Vein that delivers dissolved nutrients to the liver.
Hepatopancreatic ampulla: The site where the bile duct and pancreatic duct meet.
Hepatopancreatic sphincter: Muscular valve that controls the entrance of pancreatic juice and bile to the duodenum.
Hyoid bone: Bone that acts as the base of the tongue.
Hydrochloric acid: Acid produced by the parietal cells of the stomach.
Hydrolysis: Addition of water to breakdown food molecules.
Hypochondriac region: Upper lateral divisions of the abdominopelvic cavity.
Ileum: The end part of the small intestine.
Ileocaecal valve: Site where the small and large intestine meet.
Ingestion: The process of taking food into the body via the mouth.
Incisors: Type of tooth.
Intestinal crypts: Also known as the crypts of Lieberkuhn – glands found in the villi of the small intestine.
Intrinsic factor: Substance required for the absorption of vitamin B$_{12}$.
Jejunum: The middle part of the small intestine between the duodenum and the ileum.
Kupffer cell: Hepatic macrophage.
Lacteal: Lymphatic capillary of the small intestine.
Lamina propria: Loose connective tissue layer of the digestive tract.
Laryngopharynx: Where the larynx and pharynx meet.
Lipase: Fat-digesting enzyme.
Liver: Accessory organ located in the abdominal cavity that has many metabolic and regulatory functions.
Liver sinusoid: Liver capillary.
Lower oesophageal sphincter: Valve between the oesophagus and stomach.
Lysozyme: Bactericidal enzyme.
Macronutrient: Food consumed in large quantities.
Mastication: Chewing.
Metabolism: Sum total of the chemical reactions occurring in the body.
Meissner's plexus: Nerves of the small intestine.
Mesenteric plexus: Digestive tract innervation.
Micronutrient: Nutrient required in small quantities.
Microvilli: Cytoplasmic extensions of the villi.
Minerals: Salts – inorganic compounds.
Molars: Type of tooth.
Mucosa: Layer of the digestive tract.
Mucous neck cells: Mucous-secreting cells of the stomach.
Muscularis mucosa: Muscular layer of the digestive tract.
Nutrient: Product obtained from the digestion of food and used by the body.
Oesophagus: Muscular tube from laryngopharynx to stomach.
Oral cavity: The first part of the digestive system.
Oropharynx: Part of the pharynx closest to the oral cavity.
Palate: Roof of the mouth.

Pancreatic duct: Duct that links the pancreas and common bile duct.
Paneth cell: Cell that produces lysozyme.
Papillae: Small mucosal projections.
Parasympathetic fibres: Autonomic nervous system nerve fibres.
Parietal cells: Hydrochloric acid-producing cell of the stomach.
Parotid glands: Salivary glands located close to the ears.
Pepsin: Enzyme required for the breakdown of protein.
Pepsinogen: Enzyme precursor of pepsin.
Peristalsis: Wave-like contractions that move food through the digestive tract.
Peritoneum: Serous membrane that lines the abdominal cavity.
Peyer's patches: Lymphatic tissue of the small intestine.
Pharyngeal phase: Second phase of swallowing.
Pharynx: Tube between the mouth and the oesophagus.
Plicae circulars: Permanent circular folds in the small intestine.
Portal fissure: Area where blood vessels and nerves enter and leave the liver.
Portal triad: Corner of liver lobule.
Premolars: Type of tooth located between the canine and molar teeth.
Propulsion: The process of moving the food along the length of the digestive system.
Proteins: Substance that contains carbon, hydrogen, oxygen and nitrogen.
Pulp cavity: Centre of the tooth.
Pyloric canal: Area where the stomach opens into the small intestine.
Pyloric region: Area of the stomach that occurs where the stomach meets the small intestine.
Pyloric sphincter: Valve that controls food movement from the stomach to the small intestine.
Rectum: Final portion of the large intestine.
Rugae: Folds or ridges found in the digestive tract.
Salivary amylase: Carbohydrate-digesting enzyme found in saliva.
Secretin: Hormone that regulates secretion of pancreatic juice.
Segmentation: Movement of chyme in the small intestine.
Serosa: Outer layer of the digestive tract.
Sphincter of Oddi: Valve that controls the movement of bile and pancreatic juice into the small intestine.
Splanchnic circulation: Blood vessels of the digestive system.
Stercobilin: Waste product of bilirubin breakdown.
Stomach: Food reservoir where the digestion of protein begins.
Sublingual glands: Salivary gland located on the floor of the mouth.
Submandibular glands: Salivary glands located below the jaw bilaterally.
Submucosa: Thick connective tissue layer of the digestive tract.
Superior mesenteric artery: Vessel that supplies the small intestine with arterial blood.
Superior mesenteric vein: Blood vessel that drains venous blood from the small intestine.
Surface mucous cells: Mucus-secreting cells of the stomach.
Stomach: Reservoir for food involved in both chemical and mechanical digestion.
Taeniae coli: Muscle bands in the large intestine.
Upper oesophageal sphincter: Controls the movement of food into the oesophagus from the oropharynx.
Uvula: Small piece of tissue that protrudes from the soft palate.
Vermiform appendix: Blind-ended tube connected to the caecum and composed of lymphatic tissue.
Villi: Tiny, finger-like projections found on the surface of the mucosa of the small intestine.
Visceral peritoneum: The innermost part of the peritoneum that is in contact with the abdominal organs.
Vitamins: Essential organic compounds require in small amounts.
Voluntary phase: The first phase of swallowing.

References

Cohen, B.J. and Hull, K.L. (2018) *Memmlers's The Human Body in Health and Disease*, 14th edn. Philadelphia, PA: Wolters Kluwer.

Public Health England (2018) *A Quick Guide to the Governments Healthy Eating Recommendations*. London: Public Health England.

Galbraith, A., Bullock, S., Manias, E., Hunt, B. and Richards, A. (2007) *Fundamentals of Pharmacology. An Applied Approach for Nursing and Health*, 2nd edn. Abingdon: Routledge.

Marieb E.N. (2017) *Essentials of Human Anatomy & Physiology*, 12th edn. San Francisco, CA: Pearson Benjamin Cummings.

Marieb, E.N. and Hoehn K. (2010) *Human Anatomy and Physiology*, 8th edn. San Francisco, CA: Pearson Benjamin Cummings.

Nair, M. and Peate, I. (2018) *Fundamentals of Applied Pathophysiology. An Essential Guide for Nursing and Healthcare Students*, 3rd edn. Chichester: John Wiley & Sons, Ltd.

NICE (2014) Gastro-oesophageal Reflux and Dyspepsia in Adults: Investigation and Management. NICE guidelines [CG184]. http://www.nice.org.uk/guidance/cg184 ().

NICE (2016) Pancreatitis – Chronic. https://cks.nice.org.uk/pancreatitis-chronic ().

NICE (2017) Constipation. https://cks.nice.org.uk/constipation (accessed 18th June 2019).

Seeley, R.R., Stephens, T.D. and Tate, P. (2008) *Anatomy and Physiology*, 8th edn. New York: McGraw-Hill.

Tortora, G.J. and Derrickson, B.H. (2009) *Principles of Anatomy and Physiology*, 12th edn. Hoboken, NJ: John Wiley & Sons, Inc.

Tortora, G.J. and Derrickson, B.H. (2012) *Essentials of Anatomy and Physiology*, 9th edn. New York: John Wiley & Sons, Inc.

Further Reading

Crohn's & Colitis UK
A charity for those affected by inflammatory bowel disease.
http://www.crohnsandcolitis.org.uk/
Link to clinical guidelines on Crohn's disease: management in adults, children and young people https://www.nice.org.uk/guidance/cg152.

Colostomy Association
A charity for people with colostomy.
http://www.colostomyassociation.org.uk/

National Smile Month
An initiative to improve oral health and hygiene. It is organised by a charity called the British Dental Health Foundation.
http://www.nationalsmilemonth.org/

Activities

Multiple Choice Questions

1. Which of these vitamins is essential for blood clotting?
   (a) vitamin A
   (b) vitamin B_{12}
   (c) vitamin E
   (d) vitamin K

2. Which mineral found in broccoli provides the body with an essential constituent of the thyroid hormone thyroxine?
   (a) iron
   (b) iodine
   (c) calcium
   (d) potassium

3. Which of these is true of fat?
   (a) it is used for the growth and repair of body cells
   (b) it is a constituent of myelin sheaths
   (c) it is essential for the transport of the water-soluble vitamins
   (d) all of the above

4. Which layer of the digestive tract is responsible for peristalsis?
   (a) mucosa
   (b) submucosa
   (c) muscularis
   (d) peritoneum

5. Which of these structures is considered an accessory organ?
   (a) salivary gland
   (b) pancreas
   (c) liver
   (d) all of them
6. Where does most of the absorption of nutrients occur?
   (a) small intestine
   (b) large intestine
   (c) stomach
   (d) oesophagus
7. Which of these is *not* a constituent of gastric juice?
   (a) hydrochloric acid
   (b) mucus
   (c) intrinsic factor
   (d) trypsinogen

8. Which enzyme is involved in the breakdown of protein?
   (a) chymotrypsin
   (b) lipase
   (c) amylase
   (d) bile
9. Where is bile produced?
   (a) the small intestine
   (b) the gallbladder
   (c) the pancreas
   (d) the liver
10. Which part of the large intestine is lymphoid tissue?
    (a) the appendix
    (b) the caecum
    (c) the ascending loop
    (d) the sigmoid colon
11. Chyle is:
    (a) a gastric hormone
    (b) a milky type of fluid consisting of a mixture of lymphatic fluid and chylomicrons
    (c) a protein rich fluid that has a very high acid content and is only produced when the stomach is empty
    (d) all of the above
12. Achlorhydria refers to:
    (a) the absence of hydrochloric acid in the gastric secretions
    (b) excessive production of hydrochloric acid
    (c) is a type of peptic ulcer
    (d) is a type of gastric cancer
13. The pancreas is:
    (a) a non-essential organ
    (b) considered an accessory organ to the gastrointestinal system
    (c) an organ that is essential in the production of red blood cell
    (d) only fully functional after the person reaches the age of 18 years
14. The Peyer's patches are:
    (a) small in number and are located in the areas of lymphoid tissue in the wall of the large intestine
    (b) numerous in number and are located in the wall of the oesophagus, they are involved in the development of immunity to antigens present there
    (c) large areas of lymphoid tissue that are found only in the sigmoid colon
    (d) numerous areas of lymphoid tissue found in the wall of the small intestine; they are involved in the development of immunity to antigens present there.

15. Motility of the gut is known as:
    (a) paralysis
    (b) peristalsis
    (c) periosteum
    (d) peritoneum

True or False

1. The large intestine is colonised with bacteria.
2. The first section of small intestine is called the jejunum.
3. Pancreatic juice reaches the duodenum through the cystic duct.
4. The function of bile is to emulsify fats.
5. There are 20 milk teeth.
6. The enzyme that acts on carbohydrate is lipase.
7. The sense of taste is improved when food is not dry.
8. The oesophagus contains only smooth muscle.
9. Intrinsic factor is produced by enteroendocrine cells.
10. The secretion of gastric juice is increased during the intestinal phase.

Find Out More

1. What is gingivitis and what advice would you give to help prevent this condition?
2. Oral candidiasis (oral thrush) affects many hospital in-patients. Can you suggest why this might be and discuss the treatment available?
3. What is the role of the nurse in caring for a patient with dysphagia?
4. Discuss the conditions that may lead to a patient requiring an ileostomy.
5. Differentiate between colostomy and ileostomy.
6. A 28-year-old woman has had a colostomy formed. She asks you how the colostomy would be affected should she become pregnant. How would you advise this patient?
7. Discuss how the digestive system would respond to starvation.
8. Investigate the services available to patients who have irritable bowel syndrome to help them manage everyday life.
9. A range of medications is available to minimise or eliminate digestive system conditions associated with the acid environment of the stomach. Research these medications and consider when they may be used.
10. Constipation is a very common digestive system condition. What is the role of the nurse in relation to prevention of constipation?

Test Your Learning

1. Where does bile and pancreatic juice enter the duodenum?
2. Which teeth are used for grinding of food?
3. What is the exocrine pancreatic product essential for?
4. What are carbohydrates broken down into?
5. List the enzymes involved in the breakdown of protein.

Conditions

The following is a list of conditions that are associated with the digestive system. Take some time and write notes about each of the conditions. You may make the notes taken from textbooks or other resources (e.g. people you work with in a clinical area), or you may make the notes as a result of people you have cared for. If you are making notes about people you have cared for, you must ensure that you adhere to the rules of confidentiality.

Peptic ulcer

Peritonitis

Ulcerative colitis

Paralytic ileus

Obesity

Malnutrition

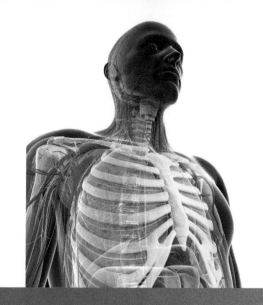

11

The Renal System

Karen Nagalingam

Test Your Prior Knowledge

- **Name the functions of the kidneys.**
- **List the organs of the renal system.**
- **Describe the components of a nephron.**
- **List the composition of urine.**
- **Describe the structure and function of the bladder.**

Learning Outcomes

After reading this chapter you will be able to:

- **Describe the structure and functions of the kidney.**
- **Describe the microscopic structures of the kidney.**
- **Explain glomerular filtration.**
- **List the chemical compositions of urine.**
- **Discuss the production of urine.**

Visit the student companion website at www.wileyfundamentalseries.com/anatomy where you can test yourself using flashcards, multiple-choice questions and more. Instructor companion site at www.wiley.com/go/instructor/anatomy where instructors will find valuable materials such as PowerPoint slides and image bank designed to enhance your teaching.

Fundamentals of Anatomy and Physiology: For Nursing and Healthcare Students, Third Edition. Edited by Ian Peate and Suzanne Evans.
© 2020 John Wiley & Sons Ltd. Published 2020 by John Wiley & Sons Ltd.
Student companion website: www.wileyfundamentalseries.com/anatomy
Instructor companion website: www.wiley.com/go/instructor/anatomy

Body Map

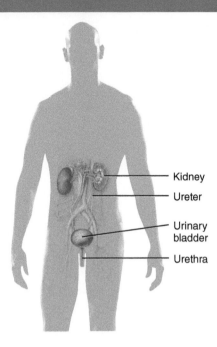

Kidney

Ureter

Urinary bladder

Urethra

Introduction

The kidneys play an important role in maintaining homeostasis. They remove waste products through the production and excretion of urine and regulate fluid balance in the body. As part of their function, the kidneys filter essential substances from the blood, such as sodium and potassium, and selectively reabsorb substances essential to maintain homeostasis. Any substances not essential are excreted in the urine. The formation of urine is achieved through the processes of filtration, selective reabsorption and excretion. The kidneys also have an endocrine function, secreting hormones such as renin and erythropoietin. This chapter will discuss the structure and functions of the renal system. It will also include some common disorders and their related nursing management and treatment.

Renal System

The renal system, also known as the urinary system, consists of:
- kidneys, which filter the blood to produce urine;
- ureters, which convey urine to the bladder;
- urinary bladder, a storage organ for urine until it is eliminated;
- urethra, which conveys urine to the exterior.

See Figure 11.1 for the organs of the renal system.

The organs of the renal system ensure that a stable internal environment is maintained for the survival of cells and tissues in the body – homeostasis.

Kidneys: External Structures

There are two kidneys, one on each side of the spinal column. They are approximately 11 cm long, 5–6 cm wide and 3–4 cm thick. They are said to be bean-shaped organs, where the outer border is convex; the inner border is known as the hilum (also known as hilus), and it is here that the renal arteries, renal veins, nerves and the ureters enter and leave the kidneys. The renal artery carries blood to the kidneys; and once the blood is filtered, the renal vein takes the blood away. The right kidney is in contact with the liver's large right lobe, and hence the right kidney is approximately 2–4 cm lower than the left kidney.

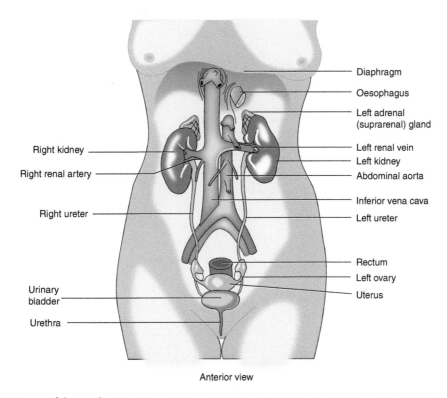

Anterior view

Figure 11.1 **Organs of the renal system.** *Source:* Tortora and Derrickson (2009). Reproduced with permission of John Wiley & Sons.

Covering and supporting the kidneys are three layers:

- renal fascia
- adipose tissue
- renal capsule.

The renal fascia is the outer layer and consists of a thin layer of connective tissue that anchors the kidneys to the abdominal wall and the surrounding tissues. The middle layer is called the adipose tissue and surrounds the capsule. It cushions the kidneys from trauma. The inner layer is called the renal capsule. It consists of a layer of smooth connective tissue that is continuous with the outer layer of the ureter. The renal capsule protects the kidneys from trauma and maintains their shape. See Figure 11.2 for the external layers.

Clinical Considerations Acute Kidney Injury

When the kidneys suddenly stop working this is known as acute kidney injury. It occurs for many reasons with the most common reason being a reduction in fluid volume or pressure. This can be caused by a reduction in blood volume from loss of blood or fluid or from a reduction in pressure caused by sepsis or reduced cardiac output.

There are two ways to determine if the kidneys are working effectively. The first is with blood tests to measure changes in creatinine and the other is to measure urine output.

Clinical assessment of hydration status can be difficult to determine. However, some signs and symptoms can help you to decide if a patient has too little fluid as well as too much.

- A visual inspection of the skin and mucus membranes: consider temperature, colour and dryness of the skin, lips and mouth (should be moist and pink).
- Assessment of peripheral circulation can be undertaken by measuring the capillary refill time (CRT): apply enough pressure to the fingernail bed to cause blanching (up to 5 seconds). Measure the time until the skin returns to normal. This should be less than 2 seconds in a well hydrated person.
- A useful indicator of reduced blood volume is the body's compensatory mechanisms. A raised NEWS2 score including reduced blood pressure, raised heart rate and breathing rate can all be a sign.
- A variation in lying and standing blood pressure.
- Visible signs of oedema usually found in the peripheries or occasionally the lungs (frothy sputum).

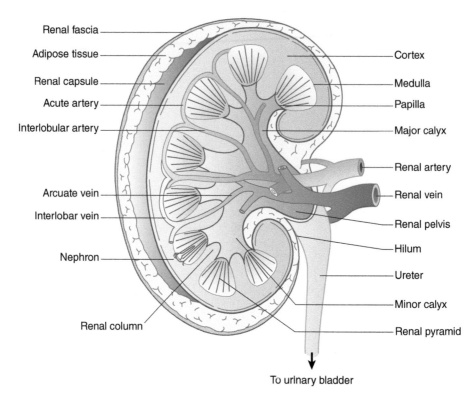

Renal fascia

Adipose tissue

Renal capsule

Acute artery

Interlobular artery

Arcuate vein

Interlobar vein

Nephron

Renal column

Cortex

Medulla

Papilla

Major calyx

Renal artery

Renal vein

Renal pelvis

Hilum

Ureter

Minor calyx

Renal pyramid

To urinary bladder

Figure 11.2 **External layers of the kidney.**

Kidneys: Internal Structures

There are three distinct regions inside the kidney:

• renal cortex
• renal medulla
• renal pelvis.

The renal cortex is the outermost part of the kidney. In adults, it forms a continuous, smooth outer portion of the kidney with a number of projections (renal columns) that extend down between the pyramids. The renal column is the medullary extension of the renal cortex. The renal cortex is reddish in colour and has a granular appearance, which is due to the capillaries and the structures of the nephron. The medulla is lighter in colour and has an abundance of blood vessels and tubules of the nephrons (see Figure 11.3). The medulla consists of approximately 8–12 renal pyramids (see Figure 11.3). The renal pyramids, also called malpighian pyramids, are cone-shaped sections of the kidneys. The wider portion of the cone faces the renal cortex, while the narrow end points internally, and this section is called the renal papilla. Urine formed by the nephrons flows into cup-like structures, called calyces, via papillary ducts. Each kidney contains approximately 8–18 minor calyces and two or three major calyces. The minor calyces receive urine from the renal papilla, which conveys the urine to the major calyces. The major calyces unite to form the renal pelvis, which then conveys urine to the bladder (see Figure 11.4). The renal pelvis forms the expanded upper portion of the ureter, which is funnel-shaped and it is the region where two or three calyces converge.

Skills in Practice Undertaking a Fluid Balance

A fluid balance chart is designed to identify fluid intake and fluid output to determine what the balance of fluid is. An accurate fluid balance chart is essential for managing an unwell patient and it can be a key sign in identifying when the kidneys are not working correctly. When calculating fluid balance, it is important to consider all types of fluid that will influence hydration status. Any drinks, soups, gravy and custard need to be accounted for. As well as accurately documenting input, output needs to be accounted for. This includes all urine, any drains, vomiting and diarrhoea. Other considerations include fluid loss that cannot be measured. This is known as insensible loss; when the environment is hot or when a person has an elevated temperature or a high respiratory rate, more fluid will be lost.

To accurately measure fluid intake, make sure you are aware of the volumes contained in cups, mugs, soup bowls and so on so that the correct volume can be recorded. Ask the patient to keep a note if appropriate of what they have drunk and when. Measure all urine output, by asking the patient to use a urinal or a measuring device that can be placed in the toilet. Or weighing pads to determine the fluid volume. Fluid balance is a team effort and requires teamwork.

Daily fluid balance total and daily weights can supplement any clinical assessment regarding fluid status and can be a useful indicator when determining how to manage a patient.

1 kg increase in weight = 1 litre of fluid.

Any short-term elevation in weight could indicate that the patient is retaining fluid.

285

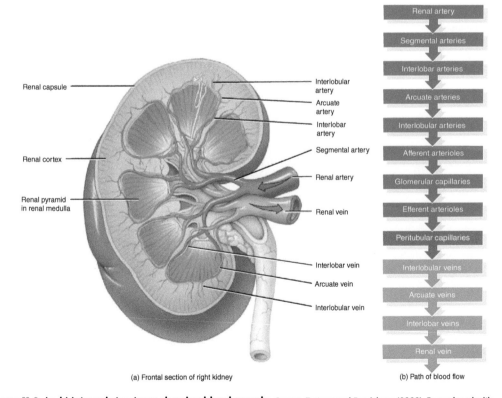

(a) Frontal section of right kidney

(b) Path of blood flow

Figure 11.3 (a, b) Internal structures showing blood vessels. *Source:* Tortora and Derrickson (2009). Reproduced with permission of John Wiley & Sons.

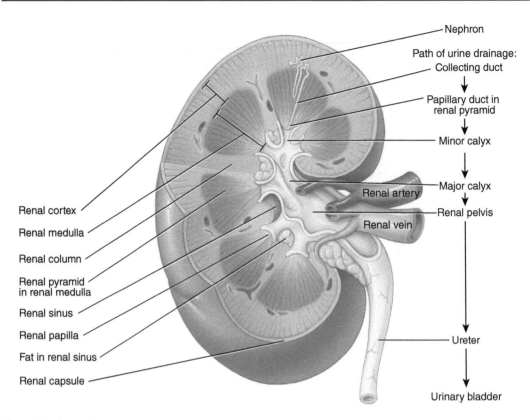

Figure 11.4 **Internal structures.** *Source:* Tortora and Derrickson (2009). Reproduced with permission of John Wiley & Sons.

Medicines Management Blood Pressure Management

 High blood pressure (hypertension) is a common comorbidity and is regularly managed using blood pressure medication and lifestyle changes. Elevated blood pressure can have a direct effect on the heart and vascular system meaning that patients are at increased risk of coronary heart disease and stroke.

There are many different types of blood pressure medications and patients may be on combinations of medications in order to achieve the desired effect.

Angiotensin-converting enzyme inhibitors, such as ramipril and lisinopril, are known as ACE inhibitors. They work by interrupting the renin angiotensin cycle instigated by the juxtaglomerular cells located near the glomerulus of the nephron. Angiotensin II has powerful vasoconstriction properties which cause a rise in blood pressure. ACE inhibitors work by stopping the conversion of Angiotensin I to Angiotensin II. Whilst on this medication, patients must drink plenty of fluids and avoid dehydration.

Episodes of Care Learning Disabilities

Jamie has come into the emergency department with his carer with weakness and fatigue. He is 47 years old with Down syndrome and multiple comorbidities, including raised blood pressure, Type 2 diabetes and chronic back pain. As a result of this he is taking multiple medications.

Jamie has had diarrhoea and vomiting for the last 3 days and although this has subsided Jamie's carer is concerned for him. On assessment Jamie is alert and orientated. His mouth and skin are dry, and his lips are cracked. His blood pressure is also low for him (105/65mm/Hg) and he is complaining of feeling dizzy. Jamie cannot remember when he last went to the toilet to pass urine. Blood tests confirm that Jamie has acute kidney injury (AKI).

Multiple Choice Questions

1. What tests are undertaken to identify AKI?
   (a) blood tests
   (b) urine tests
   (c) blood cultures
   (d) sputum cultures
2. How much urine should a patient produce?
   (a) 30 mL an hour
   (b) 1.5 litres in a day
   (c) 0.5 mL/kg/hr
   (d) 1 litre in 6 hours
3. Jamie weighs 96 kg, how much urine will he be expected to produce an hour?
   (a) 30 mL/hr
   (b) 60 mL/hr
   (c) 48 mL/hr
   (d) 15 mL/hr
4. If the kidneys suddenly stopped working, which electrolytes would be affected (identify all that apply)?
   (a) vitamin D
   (b) sodium
   (c) potassium
   (d) bilirubin
5. Why might Jamie's mouth be dry and lips cracked?
   (a) he has a mouth ulcer
   (b) he is dehydrated
   (c) he is too cold
   (d) he is too hot

Nephrons

These are small structures and they form the functional units of the kidney. The nephron consists of a glomerulus and a renal tubule (see Figure 11.5). There are approximately 1 million nephrons per kidney, and it is in these structures where urine is formed. The nephrons:

- filter blood;
- perform selective reabsorption;
- excrete unwanted waste products from the filtered blood.

The nephron is part of the homeostatic mechanism of the body. This system helps regulate the amount of water, salts, glucose, urea and other minerals in the body. The nephron is a filtration system located in the kidney and is responsible for the reabsorption of water and salts. The nephron is divided into several sections:

- Bowman's capsule
- proximal convoluted tubule
- loop of Henle
- distal convoluted tubule (DCT)
- the collecting ducts.

Each section performs a different function; these will be discussed in the following sections.

Bowman's Capsule

Also known as the glomerular capsule (see Figure 11.6), Bowman's capsule is a cup-like sac and is the first portion of the nephron. Bowman's capsule is part of the filtration system in the kidneys. When blood reaches the kidneys for filtration, it enters Bowman's capsule first, with the capsule separating the blood into two components: a filtrated blood product and a filtrate that is moved through the nephron, another structure in the kidneys. The glomerular capsule consists of visceral and parietal layers (see Figure 11.6). The visceral layer is lined with epithelial cells called podocytes, while the parietal layer is lined with simple squamous epithelium and it is in Bowman's capsule that the network of capillaries called the glomerulus (Marieb, 2016) is found. Filtration of blood takes place in this portion of the nephron.

288

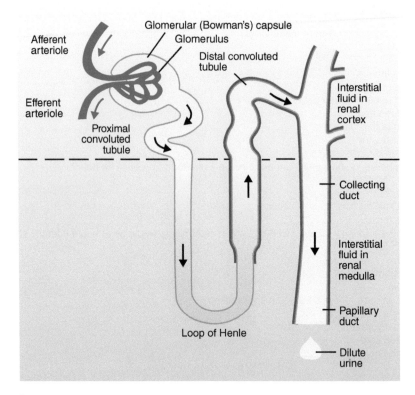

Figure 11.5 **Nephron.** *Source:* Tortora and Derrickson (2009). Reproduced with permission of John Wiley & Sons.

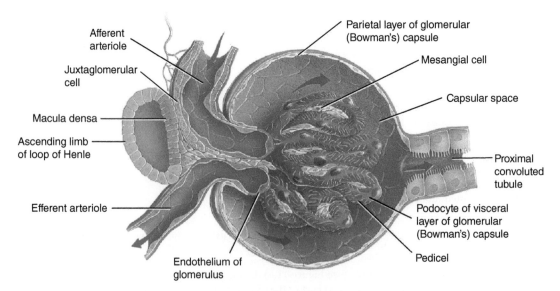

Figure 11.6 **Bowman's capsule.** *Source:* Tortora and Derrickson (2009). Reproduced with permission of John Wiley & Sons.

Proximal Convoluted Tubule

From Bowman's capsule, the filtrate drains into the proximal convoluted tubule (see Figure 11.6). The surface of the epithelial cells of this segment of the nephron is covered with densely packed microvilli. The microvilli increase the surface area of the cells, thus facilitating their resorptive function. The infolded membranes forming the microvilli are the site of numerous sodium pumps. Resorption of salt, water and glucose from the glomerular filtrate occurs in this section of the tubule; at the same time, certain substances, including uric acid and drug metabolites, are actively transferred from the blood capillaries into the tubule for excretion.

Loop of Henle

The proximal convoluted tubule then bends into a loop called the loop of Henle (see Figure 11.6). The loop of Henle is the part of the tubule that dips or 'loops' from the cortex into the medulla (descending limb), and then returns to the cortex (ascending limb). The loop of Henle is divided into the descending and ascending loops. The ascending loop of Henle is much thicker than the descending portion. The main function of the loop of Henle is to generate a concentration gradient that creates a region of a high concentration of sodium in the medulla of the kidney. The descending portion of the loop of Henle is highly permeable to water and has low permeability to ions and urea. The ascending loop of Henle is permeable to ions but not to water. When required, urine is concentrated in this portion of the nephron. This is possible because of the high concentration of solute in the substance or interstitium of the medulla. Different parts of the loop of Henle have different actions:

- The descending loop of Henle is relatively impermeable to solute but permeable to water, so that water moves out by osmosis and the fluid in the tubule becomes hypertonic.
- The thin section of the ascending loop of Henle is virtually impermeable to water, but permeable to solute, especially sodium and chloride ions. Thus, sodium and chloride ions move out down the concentration gradient; the fluid within the tubule first becomes isotonic and then hypotonic as more ions leave. Urea, which was absorbed into the medullary interstitium from the collecting duct, diffuses into the ascending limb. This keeps the urea within the interstitium of the medulla, where it also has a role in concentrating urine.
- The thick section of the ascending loop of Henle and early distal tubule are virtually impermeable to water. However, sodium and chloride ions are actively transported out of the tubule, making the tubular fluid very hypotonic.

Distal Convoluted Tubule

The thick ascending portion of the loop of Henle leads into the distal convoluted tubule (DCT) (see Figure 11.6). The DCT is lined with simple cuboidal cells, and the lumen of the DCT is larger than the proximal convoluted tubule lumen because the proximal convoluted tubule has a brush border (microvilli). The DCT is an important site:

- it actively secretes ions and acids;
- it plays a part in the regulation of calcium ions by excreting excess calcium ions in response to calcitonin hormone;
- it selectively reabsorbs water;
- arginine vasopressin receptor 2 proteins are also located there;
- it plays a role in regulating pH by absorbing bicarbonate and secreting protons (H^+) into the filtrate.

The final concentration of urine, in this section, is dependent on a hormone called antidiuretic hormone (ADH). If ADH is present, the distal tubule and the collecting duct become permeable to water. As the collecting duct passes through the medulla with a high solute concentration in the interstitium, the water moves out of the lumen of the duct and concentrated urine is formed. In the absence of ADH the tubule is minimally permeable to water, so a large volume of dilute urine is formed.

Collecting Ducts

The DCT then drains into the collecting ducts (see Figure 11.6). Several collecting ducts converge and drain into a larger system called the papillary ducts, which in turn empty into the minor calyx (plural: calices). From here the filtrate, now called urine, drains into the renal pelvis. This is the final stage where sodium and water are reabsorbed. When a person is dehydrated, approximately 25% of the water filtered is reabsorbed in the collecting duct. The cells of the collecting ducts are impermeable to water, but with the aid of the ADH and aquaporins water is reabsorbed from the collecting ducts. Aquaporins are proteins embedded in the cell membrane that regulate the flow of water. Aquaporins selectively transport water molecules in and out of the cell, while preventing the passage of ions and other solutes. Aquaporin 1 is abundant in the proximal convoluted tubule and the descending thin limb of the loop of Henle, and aquaporins 2, 3 and 4 are present in the collecting ducts; however, aquaporin 4 is predominantly found in the brain.

Clinical Considerations Chronic Kidney Disease and Contrast Procedures

Chronic kidney disease is the progressive and irreversible loss of functioning nephrons. This damage to the nephrons in the kidney can be caused by multiple factors including hypertension, diabetes and heart disease. Urea and creatinine in the blood can be used to identify how well the kidneys are working. Glomerular filtration rate is an estimated measurement of how well the kidneys are working, it represents the amount of blood filtering through the glomeruli each minute.

When a patient requires an MRI, CT scan or angiogram procedure, a contrast dye may be used to help enhance the tests. This dye can cause problems with the kidney and patients with reduced renal function have an increased risk of developing contrast-induced acute kidney injury. Therefore, the patient may require increased monitoring of their renal function, extra fluid and, in some rare cases, haemodialysis or peritoneal dialysis may be instigated straight after the procedure.

Functions of the Kidney

The kidneys maintain fluid balance, electrolyte balance and the acid–base balance of the blood.

- The kidneys remove waste products and excess water (fluid) collected by, and carried in, the blood as it flows through the body. Approximately 190 L of blood enter the kidneys every day via the renal arteries. Millions of tiny filters, called glomeruli, inside the kidneys separate waste products and water from the blood. Most of these unwanted substances come from what we eat and drink. The kidneys automatically remove the right amount of salt and other minerals from the blood to leave just the quantities the body needs.
- By removing just the right amount of excess fluid, healthy kidneys maintain what is called the body's fluid balance. In women, fluid content stays at about 55% of total weight. In men, it stays at about 60% of total weight. The kidneys maintain these proportions by balancing the amount of fluid that leaves the body against the amount entering the body. When a large volume of fluid is drunk, healthy kidneys remove the excess fluid and produce a lot of urine. On the other hand, if fluid intake is low, the kidneys retain fluid and the patient does not pass much urine. Fluid also leaves the body through sweat, breath and faeces. If the weather is hot and we lose a lot of fluid by sweating, then the kidneys will not produce much urine.
- Kidneys synthesise hormones such as renin and angiotensin. These hormones regulate how much sodium (salt) and fluid the body keeps, and how well the blood vessels can expand and contract. This, in turn, helps control blood pressure.
- Kidneys produce a hormone known as erythropoietin, which is carried in the blood to the bone marrow where it stimulates the production of red blood cells. These cells carry oxygen throughout the body. Without enough healthy red blood cells anaemia develops, a condition that causes weakness, cold, tiredness and shortness of breath.
- Healthy kidneys keep bones strong by producing the hormone calcitriol. Calcitriol maintains the right levels of calcium and phosphate in the blood and bones. Calcium and phosphate balance are important to keep bones healthy. When the kidneys fail they may not produce enough calcitriol. This leads to abnormal levels of phosphate, calcium and vitamin D, causing renal bone disease. For a summary of the functions of the kidney, see Table 11.1.

Table 11.1 **Summary of the functions of the kidneys.**

Regulation of electrolytes – help to regulate ions such as sodium, potassium, calcium, chloride and phosphate ions

Regulation of blood pH – excrete hydrogen ions into the urine and conserve bicarbonate ions, thus helping to regulate pH of blood

Regulation of blood volume – by conserving or eliminating water in the urine

Secretes renin (regulates blood pressure) and erythropoietin (production of red blood cells)

Production of calcitriol for the regulation of calcium level

Aids in regulation of blood glucose level by gluconeogenesis

Detoxification of free radicals and drugs

Excretion of waste products, such as urea, uric acid and creatinine

Medicines Management Nephrotoxic Drugs

Renal impairment may be acute or chronic – both of which can result in problems with medications. Renal impairment may be the result of a variety of renal or systemic diseases, such as diabetic nephropathy or systemic lupus erythematosus. Normal ageing results in a decline in renal function due to loss of nephrons. When prescribing for elderly patients, it should therefore be assumed that some degree of renal impairment exists.

Reasons for problems with medications in renal failure include:

- failure to excrete a drug or its metabolites;
- many side effects being poorly tolerated by patients in renal failure;
- some drugs ceasing to be effective when renal function is reduced.

For example, prescribing any drug that increases potassium level is potentially very dangerous – for example, potassium supplements and potassium-sparing diuretics. Other products that contain potassium include ispaghula husk laxatives. Non-steroidal anti-inflammatory drugs (NSAIDs), such as ibuprofen and diclofenac, given over a short period of time can cause acute kidney injury as a result of renal under-perfusion. ACE inhibitors can also cause a deterioration in renal function. However, this is a problem only in patients with compromised renal perfusion, particularly those with renal artery stenosis. Care should be taken when an ACE inhibitor and NSAID are prescribed together, as this combination may precipitate an acute deterioration in renal function.

Drugs that may cause interstitial nephritis include penicillins, cephalosporins, sulphonamides, thiazide diuretics, furosemide, NSAIDs and rifampicin.

Therefore, care should be taken when administering medications to patients with renal problems. Always check with the pharmacist or consult the British National Formulary for drug interactions before administering medications.

See Azhar et al. (2019)

Episodes of Care Child

Beatrice has presented with her mother to the out of hours service at her local GP surgery. She is 3 years old and is visibly lethargic and hot. On assessment she has a raised temperature and she is clammy to touch. Her mother brought her in as she hasn't eaten anything in the last 24 hours and is only taking sips of water. On further discussion her mum states that Beatrice has been crying when she passes urine. A urine analysis is undertaken, and it shows that leucocytes and nitrates are present.

Multiple Choice Questions

1. What does the presence of leucocytes and nitrates in a urinalysis mean?
   (a) presence of glucose
   (b) presence of protein
   (c) indicator of infection
   (d) indicator of acidosis
2. What do you think might be the problem with Beatrice?
   (a) she has a respiratory tract infection
   (b) she has a urine infection
   (c) she is teething
   (d) not sure
3. What other test would help with identifying the correct antibiotics?
   (a) electro-cardiogram
   (b) CT scan
   (c) peak flow
   (d) urine sample for culture
4. Beatrice's urine is a dark colour. What does this tell us about her hydration status?
   (a) she is drinking the right amount
   (b) she is drinking too little
   (c) she is drinking too much
   (d) she is haemorrhaging
5. Why are females more likely to have a urinary tract infection?
   (a) shorter urethra
   (b) longer urethra
   (c) shorter ureters
   (d) longer ureters

Blood Supply of the Kidney

The role of the kidney is to filter at least 20–25% of blood during the resting cardiac output. Approximately 1200 mL of blood flows through the kidney each minute. Each kidney receives its blood supply directly from the aorta via the renal artery (see Figure 11.4), which is divided into anterior and posterior renal arteries. There are several arteries that deliver blood to the kidneys:

- renal artery – arises from the abdominal aorta at the level of first lumbar vertebra;
- segmental artery – branch of the renal artery;
- interlobar artery – branch of the segmental artery;
- arcuate artery – renal columns leading to the corticomedullary junction;
- interlobular arteries – divisions of the arcuate arteries.

Skills in Practice Taking a Urine Sample for Urinalysis or Culture

When undertaking a urinalysis, it is important to understand the relevance of certain findings. There are many reasons to undertake a urinalysis but importantly in can help aid in diagnosis of certain conditions such as urinary tract infection (under 65 years of age), diabetes and kidney disease.

Urine should appear clear and straw like in colour. Frothy urine could indicate the presence of protein or glucose in the urine, and cloudy urine could indicate the presence of infection. Urinalysis can be undertaken with reagent strip or an electronic urinalysis device.

When collecting a sample for microscopy, to avoid contamination of the sample it is advised to take a mid-stream sample. Ask the patient to wash their hands and to clean the urethral meatus (usually with soap and water). Use a wipe to clean front to back (to avoid faecal contamination).

Ask the patient to begin voiding and use a sterile container collect urine without interrupting the flow. Ask the patient to finish voiding and wash hands. The urine sample can then be transferred to a sterile universal container and sent as soon as possible for microscopy, culture and sensitivity to the laboratory. This will aid in identifying the type of bacteria causing an infection and administering appropriate antibiotics.

At all times local policy and procedure must be adhered to.

See Dougherty *et al.* (2015).

The branches of the interlobular artery enter the nephrons as afferent arterioles. Each nephron receives one afferent arteriole, which further subdivides into a tuft of capillaries called the glomerulus. The glomerular capillaries reunite and leave Bowman's capsule as efferent arterioles. Efferent arterioles unite to form peritubular capillaries and then interlobular veins that unite to form the arcuate veins and finally interlobar veins. Blood leaves the kidneys through the renal vein, which then flows into the inferior vena cava. The diameter of the afferent arteriole is larger than the diameter of the efferent arteriole.

Urine Formation

Three processes are involved in the formation of urine:

- filtration
- selective reabsorption
- secretion.

Filtration

Urine formation begins with the process of filtration, which goes on continually in the renal corpuscles. Filtration takes place in the glomerulus which lies in Bowman's capsule. The blood for filtration is supplied by the renal artery. In the kidney the renal artery divides into smaller arterioles. The arteriole entering Bowman's capsule is called the afferent arteriole, which further subdivides into a cluster of capillaries called the glomerulus.

As blood passes through the glomeruli, much of its fluid, containing both useful chemicals and dissolved waste materials, soaks out of the blood through the membranes (by osmosis and diffusion) where it is filtered and then flows into Bowman's capsule. This process is called glomerular filtration. The water, waste products, salt, glucose and other chemicals that have been filtered out of the blood are known collectively as glomerular filtrate.

The fluid from the filtered blood is protein free but contains electrolytes such as sodium chloride, potassium and waste products of cellular metabolism; for example, urea, uric acid and creatinine (McCance and Huether, 2018). The filtered blood then returns into circulation via the efferent arteriole and finally into the renal vein.

Selective Reabsorption

Selective reabsorption processes ensure that any substances in the filtrate that are essential for body function are reabsorbed into the plasma. Substances such as sodium, calcium, potassium and chloride are reabsorbed to maintain fluid and electrolyte balance and the pH of blood. However, if these substances are in excess to body requirements, they are excreted in the urine. Only 1% of the glomerular filtrate actually leaves the body; 99% is reabsorbed into the bloodstream. The reabsorption occurs via three processes:

- osmosis
- diffusion
- active transport.

See Table 11.2 for a summary.

Blood glucose is entirely reabsorbed into the blood from the proximal tubules. In fact, it is actively transported out of the tubules and into the peritubular capillary blood. None of this valuable nutrient is wasted by

293

Table 11.2 Summary of filtration, reabsorption and excretion in the nephron and collecting ducts.

REABSORPTION	EXCRETION
Proximal convoluted tubule	
Water, approximately 65%	Hydrogen ions
Sodium and potassium, 65%	Urea
Glucose, 100%	Creatinine
Amino acids, 100%	Ammonium ions
Chloride, approximately 50%	
Bicarbonate, calcium and magnesium	
Urea	
Loop of Henle	
Water	Urea
Sodium and potassium, approximately 30%	
Chloride, approximately 35%	
Bicarbonate, approximately 20%	
Calcium and magnesium	
Distal convoluted tubule	
Water, approximately 15%	Potassium, depending on serum values
Sodium and chloride, approximately 5%	Hydrogen ions, depending on pH of blood
Calcium	
Some urea	
Collecting duct	
Bicarbonate, depending on serum values	Potassium, depending on serum values
Urea	Hydrogen ions, depending on pH of blood
Water, approximately 9%	
Sodium, approximately 4%	

Source: Adapted from Tortora et al. (2014)

being lost in the urine. Sodium (Na$^+$) and other ions are only partially reabsorbed from the renal tubules into the blood. For the most part, however, sodium ions are actively transported back into blood from the tubular fluid. The amount of sodium reabsorbed varies; it depends largely on how much salt we take in from the foods that we eat.

As a person increases the amount of salt intake into the body, kidneys decrease the amount of sodium reabsorption into the blood. That is, more sodium is retained in the tubules. Therefore, the amount of salt excreted in the urine increases. The process works the other way as well. The less the salt intake, the greater the amount of sodium reabsorbed into the blood, and the amount of salt excreted in the urine decreases.

Excretion

Any substances not removed through filtration are secreted into the renal tubules from the peritubular capillaries (see Figure 11.7) of the nephron (Martini *et al.*, 2017) these include drugs and hydrogen ions. Tubular secretion mainly takes place by active transport. Active transport is a process by which substances are moved

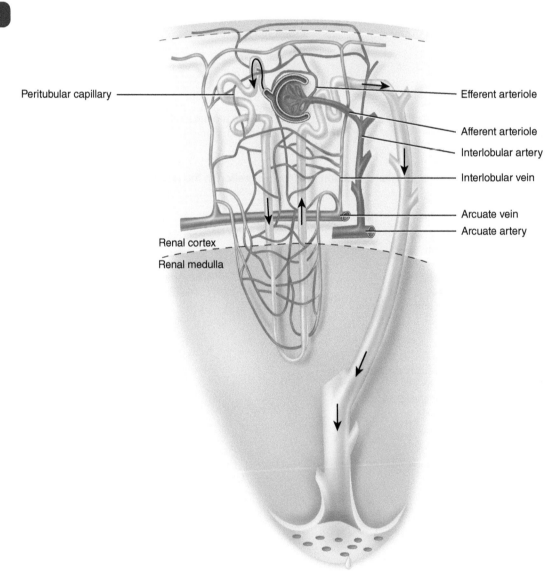

Peritubular capillary

Efferent arteriole

Afferent arteriole

Interlobular artery

Interlobular vein

Arcuate vein

Arcuate artery

Renal cortex

Renal medulla

Figure 11.7 **Nephron with capillaries.** *Source:* Tortora and Derrickson (2009). Reproduced with permission of John Wiley & Sons.

across biological membranes. Tubular secretion occurs from epithelial cells lining the renal tubules and the collecting ducts. Substances secreted into the tubular fluid include:

- potassium ions (K^+)
- hydrogen ions (H^+)
- ammonium ions (NH_4^+)
- creatinine
- urea
- some hormones.

It is the tubular secretion of hydrogen and ammonium ions that helps to maintain the pH of blood. See Table 11.2 for a summary.

Hormonal Control of Tubular Reabsorption and Secretion

Four hormones play a role in the regulation of fluid and electrolytes:

- angiotensin II
- aldosterone
- ADH
- atrial natriuretic peptide.

Angiotensin and Aldosterone
As the blood volume and blood pressure decrease, the juxtaglomerular cells secrete a hormone called renin. Juxtaglomerular cells are found near the glomerulus, and these cells synthesise, store and secrete the hormone renin. Renin acts on a plasma protein called angiotensinogen and converts it into angiotensin I. Angiotensinogen is produced by the hepatocytes of the liver. Angiotensin I is transported by the blood to the lungs. In the lung capillaries there are enzymes called ACE. ACE is predominantly found in the lung capillaries, but this enzyme is also found throughout the body. ACE converts angiotensin I into angiotensin II. Angiotensin II is a short acting, powerful vasoconstrictor, thus increasing blood pressure. Angiotensin II promotes the reabsorption of sodium, chloride and water in the proximal convoluted tubule. It also has an effect on the release of aldosterone.

Aldosterone is a steroid hormone secreted by the adrenal glands. It serves as the principal regulator of the salt and water balance of the body and thus is categorised as a mineralocorticoid. It also has a small effect on the metabolism of fats, carbohydrates and proteins. Aldosterone is synthesised in the body from corticosterone, a steroid derived from cholesterol. Production of aldosterone (in adult humans, about 20–200 µg per day) in the zona glomerulosa of the adrenal cortex is regulated by the rennin–angiotensin system.

Antidiuretic Hormone
The third principal hormone is ADH, which is produced by the hypothalamus gland and is stored by the posterior pituitary gland. This hormone increases the permeability of the cells in the DCT and the collecting ducts. In the presence of ADH, more water is reabsorbed from the renal tubules; therefore, the patient will pass less urine. In the absence of ADH, less water is reabsorbed and the patient will pass more urine. Thus, ADH plays a major role in the regulation of fluid balance in the body.

The most important variable regulating ADH secretion is plasma osmolarity, or the concentration of solutes in blood. Osmolarity is sensed in the hypothalamus by neurones known as an osmoreceptors, and those neurones, in turn, stimulate secretion from the neurones that produce ADH. When plasma osmolarity is below a certain threshold, the osmoreceptors are not activated and the secretion of ADH is suppressed. When osmolarity increases above the threshold, the osmoreceptors recognise this and stimulate the neurones that secrete ADH.

Atrial Natriuretic Peptide
The fourth hormone involved in tubular secretion and reabsorption is atrial natriuretic peptide (ANP) hormone. ANP is a powerful vasodilator and is a protein produced by the myocytes of the atria of the heart in response to increased blood pressure. ANP stimulates the kidneys to excrete sodium and water from the renal tubules, thus decreasing blood volume, which in turn lowers blood pressure. The hormone also inhibits the secretion of aldosterone and ADH.

ANP is involved in the long-term regulation of sodium and water balance, blood volume and arterial pressure. There are two major pathways of natriuretic peptide actions: vasodilator effects and renal effects, which lead to natriuresis and diuresis. ANP directly dilates veins (increases venous compliance) and thereby decreases central venous pressure, which reduces cardiac output by decreasing ventricular preload. ANP also dilates arteries, which decreases systemic vascular resistance and systemic arterial pressure.

Medicines Management Polypharmacy

 Polypharmacy is the term that is used to describe patients who take multiple medications (Payne, 2016). It is identified that people over the age of 65 are more likely to have multiple medications due to multimorbidity. There are some drugs that can be bought over the counter – including paracetamol, ibuprofen and aspirin – which can interact with some medications such as warfarin and prednisolone. Problems can occur in patients when multiple health care professionals are involved, especially if there is no oversight of what is being prescribed.

Common drug interactions in patients with renal disease include cardiovascular agents, antibiotics, anticholinergics and nonsteroidal anti-inflammatory drugs.

Composition of Urine

Urine is a sterile and clear fluid of nitrogenous waste and salts. It is translucent with an amber or light yellow colour. Its colour is due to the pigments from the breakdown of haemoglobin. Concentrated urine tends to be darker in colour than normal urine. However, other factors, such as diet, medications and certain diseases, may affect the colour of the urine. It is slightly acidic, and the pH may range from 4.5 to 8. The pH is affected by an individual's dietary intake and state of health. Diet that is high in animal protein tends to make the urine more acidic, while a vegetarian diet may make the urine more alkaline. The volume of urine produced depends on the circulating volume of blood. ADH regulates the amount of urine passed by the individual. If the person is dehydrated, more ADH is released from the posterior pituitary gland, resulting in water reabsorption and less urine being produced. On the other hand, if the person has consumed a large amount of fluid, which increases the circulating volume, less ADH is released and more water is passed as urine.

Urine is 96% water and approximately 4% solutes derived from cellular metabolism. The solutes include organic and inorganic waste products and unwanted substances such as drugs. Normally there is no protein or blood present in the urine; if these are present, then the person may have medical condition.

Characteristics of Normal Urine

The volume produced is one of the physical characteristics of urine. Other physical characteristics that can apply to urine include colour, turbidity (transparency), smell (odour), pH (acidity/alkalinity) and density.

- **Colour:** Typically yellow–amber, but varies according to recent diet, medication and the concentration of the urine. Drinking more water generally tends to reduce the concentration of urine, and therefore causes it to have a lighter colour. However, if a person does not drink a large amount of fluid, this may increase the concentration and the urine will have a darker colour. See Table 11.3 for foods, medications and illnesses that may affect the colour of the urine.
- **Smell:** The smell, or odour, of urine may provide health information. For example, the urine of diabetics may have a sweet or fruity odour due to the presence of ketones (organic molecules of a particular structure). Generally, fresh urine has a mild smell, but stale urine or infected urine has a stronger odour, similar to that of ammonia. Cloudy urine can indicate infection in the urine whereas foamy urine can indicate the presence of protein and glucose.
- **Acidity:** pH is a measure of the acidity (or alkalinity) of a solution. The pH of a substance (solution) is usually represented as a number in the range 0 (strong acid) to 14 (strong alkali, also known as a 'base'). Pure water is 'neutral', in the sense that it is neither acid nor alkali; it therefore has a pH of 7. The pH of normal urine is generally in the range 4.5–8, a typical average being around 6.0. Much of the variation is due to diet. For example, high protein diets result in more acidic urine, but vegetarian diets generally result in more alkaline urine.
- **Specific gravity:** Specific gravity is also known as 'relative density'. This is the ratio of the weight of a volume of a substance compared with the weight of the same volume of distilled water. Given that urine is mostly water, but also contains some other substances dissolved in the water, its relative density is expected to be close to, but slightly greater than, 1.000.

Table 11.3 Colours of urine.

Food that changes colour of urine

These are some of the foods that may change the colour of urine.

Dark yellow or orange:	carrots
Green:	asparagus
Pink or red:	beetroot, blackberries, rhubarb
Brown:	fava beans, rhubarb

Medicines and vitamins that may change the colour of urine

Yellow or yellow–green:	cascara, sulfasalazine, the B vitamins
Orange:	rifampicin, sulfasalazine, vitamin B, vitamin C
Pink or red:	phenolphthalein, propofol, rifampicin, laxatives containing senna
Green or blue:	amitriptyline, cimetidine, indomethacin, promethazine, propofol, triamterene, several multivitamins
Brown or brownish-black:	levodopa, metronidazole, nitrofurantoin, some antimalarial agents, methyldopa, laxatives containing cascara or senna

Medical conditions that may change the colour of urine

Yellow:	concentrated urine caused by dehydration
Orange:	a problem with the liver or bile duct
Pink or red:	blood in the urine, haemoglobinuria (a condition linked to haemolytic anaemia), myoglobinuria (a condition linked to the destruction of muscle cells)
Deep purple:	porphyria, a rare inherited red blood cell disorder
Green or blue:	urinary tract infection may cause green urine if caused by *Pseudomonas* bacteria; familial hypercalcaemia, a rare genetic condition, can cause blue urine
Brown or dark brown:	blood in the urine, a liver or kidney disorder

Source: Mayo Clinic Staff (2019)

297

Episodes of Care Adult

Mohammed is a 56-year-old man who was been diagnosed with chronic kidney disease 3 years ago after a routine blood test. Over the last year his bloods (urea and creatinine) have been getting worse and as a result his renal team have advised him he will need to commence dialysis in the next 6 months. He was asked to have blood tests every week to check bloods to see what his renal function was. His glomerular filtration rate (an estimate of kidney function) was 18 mL/min/$1.73m^2$ and is considered stage 4 chronic kidney disease (CKD). Stage 5 CKD is anything less than 15 mL/min/$1.73m^2$ and is termed '*end stage*' which means renal replacement therapy will be required in order for the patient to survive.

At the appointment, Mohammed's wife attended and said that Mohammed was suffering with itching of the skin, headaches and was lethargic and disinterested in things. His haemoglobin was only 85 g/L and he was taking multiple medications to improve this. He has also been signed off work with depression and anxiety. She is concerned about how he will cope when he has to start dialysis.

Multiple Choice Questions

1. Why do you think Mohammed might be feeling anxious?
   (a) he is finding it hard to come to terms with the change in his lifestyle
   (b) because his kidneys are not working very well, he is accumulating toxins in the blood and this is affecting how he feels.
   (c) a and b
   (d) another reason
2. One of the problems Mohammed is suffering as a result of CKD is itching. What is causing the itching?
   (a) dry skin
   (b) accumulation of toxins and urea
   (c) allergy
   (d) insect bites

3. Looking at the functions of the kidney. Consider what might be making Mohammed lethargic.
   (a) calcium levels
   (b) vitamin D levels
   (c) erythropoietin levels
   (d) sodium levels
4. Why might Mohammed be suffering from headaches? Look at the functions of the kidney to identify a potential cause.
   (a) raised blood pressure
   (b) fluid accumulation
   (c) increased level of urea
   (d) all of the above
5. In order to improve Mohammed's haemoglobin levels, what medications could be given?
   (a) iron and erythropoietin
   (b) iron and alfacalcidol
   (c) erythropoietin and alfacalcidol
   (d) erythropoietin and calcichew

Ureters

The ureters are tubular organs that run from the renal pelvis to the posterolateral base of the urinary bladder. The ureters are approximately 25–30 cm in length and 5 mm in diameter (Martini *et al.*, 2017). The ureters terminate at the bladder and enter obliquely through the muscle wall of the bladder. They pass over the pelvic brim at the bifurcation of the common iliac arteries (see Figure 11.8).

The ureters have three layers:

- transitional epithelial mucosa (inner layer);
- smooth muscle layer (middle layer);
- fibrous connective tissue (outer layer).

Urine is transported through the ureters via muscular movements of the urinary tract's peristaltic muscular waves. When the renal pelvis becomes laden with urine, the peristaltic wave action encourages urine to leave the body. The amount of urine in the renal pelvis determines the frequency of the peristaltic wave action, which can range from one to every few minutes to one to every few seconds. This action creates a pressure force that moves the urine through the ureters and into the bladder in small spurts.

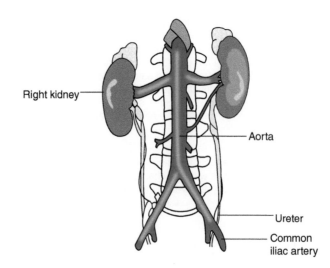

Right kidney

Aorta

Ureter

Common iliac artery

Figure 11.8 **Common iliac vessels and ureter.** *Source:* Nair and Peate (2009). Reproduced with permission of John Wiley & Sons.

Urinary Bladder

The urinary bladder is a hollow muscular organ and is located in the pelvic cavity posterior to the symphysis pubis. In the male the bladder lies anterior to the rectum, and in the female it lies anterior to the vagina and inferior to the uterus (Martini *et al.,* 2017); it is a smooth muscular sac that stores urine. Although the shape of the bladder is spherical, the shape is altered from pressure of surrounding organs. When the bladder is empty, the inner section of the bladder forms folds, but as the bladder fills with urine the walls of the bladder become smoother. As urine accumulates, the bladder expands without a significant rise in the internal pressure of the bladder. The bladder normally distends and holds approximately 350–750 mL of urine. In females the bladder is slightly smaller because the uterus occupies the space above the bladder.

The inner lining of the urinary bladder is a mucous membrane of transitional epithelium that is continuous with that in the ureters. When the bladder is empty, the mucosa has numerous folds called rugae. The rugae and transitional epithelium allow the bladder to expand as it fills. The second layer in the walls is the submucosa, which supports the mucous membrane. It is composed of connective tissue with elastic fibres.

The inner floor of the bladder includes a triangular section called the trigone. The trigone is formed by three openings in the floor of the urinary bladder. Two of the openings are from the ureters and form the base of the trigone. Small flaps of mucosa cover these openings and act as valves that allow urine to enter the bladder but prevent it from backing up from the bladder into the ureters. The third opening, at the apex of the trigone, is the opening into the urethra (see Figure 11.9). A band of the detrusor muscle encircles this opening to form the internal urethral sphincter.

The walls of the bladder consist of muscle fibres:

- transitional epithelial mucosa;
- a thick muscular layer;
- a fibrous outer layer.

The urinary tract can become blocked or obstructed (e.g. from a kidney stone, tumour, expanding uterus during pregnancy or enlarged prostate gland). The build-up of urine can lead to infection and injury of the

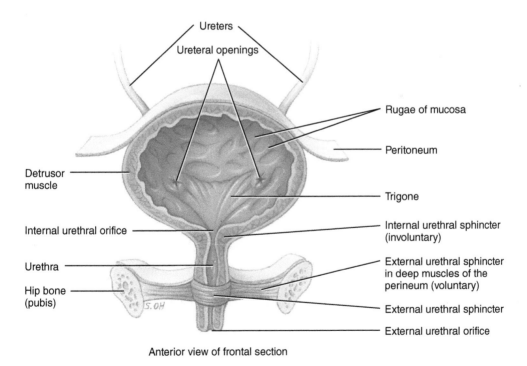

Anterior view of frontal section

Figure 11.9 **Layers of the urinary bladder.** *Source:* Tortora and Derrickson (2009). Reproduced with permission of John Wiley & Sons.

299

kidney. With a kidney stone, the blockage is often painful. Other obstructions may produce no symptoms and be detected only when a blood or urine test is abnormal or when an imaging procedure, such as an X-ray or ultrasound, detects it.

Urinary tract infections, such as cystitis (an infection of the bladder), can lead to more serious infections further up the urinary tract. Symptoms include pyrexia, frequent urination, sudden and urgent need to urinate, and pain or a burning feeling during urination (dysuria). There is often pressure or pain in the lower abdomen or back. Sometimes the urine has a strong or foul odour or is bloody. Pyelonephritis is an infection of kidney tissue; most often, it is the result of cystitis that has been transmitted to the kidney. An obstruction in the urinary tract can make a kidney infection more likely. Infections elsewhere in the body, including, for example, streptococcal infections, the skin infection impetigo or a bacterial infection in the heart, can also be carried through the bloodstream to the kidney and cause a problem there.

Clinical Considerations Prostatic Hyperplasia and Urinary Problems

Enlargement of the prostate gland is a common condition in older men. The prostate is located beneath the bladder with the urethra passing directly through it. As the prostate enlarges it can partially or fully occlude the urethra leading to urinary symptoms.

These symptoms may include frequency, urgency and difficulty in commencing urination. Occasionally the occlusion can lead to an inability to urinate. This will need to be managed urgently to relieve the pressure and prevent damage to the kidney. A catheter may be inserted into the bladder to allow urine to be excreted. Prolonged retention of urine can lead to the development of AKI.

Urethra

The urethra is a muscular tube that drains urine from the bladder and conveys it out of the body. It contains three coats, and they are muscular, erectile and mucous; the muscular is the continuation of the bladder muscle layer. The urethra is encompassed by two separate urethral sphincter muscles. The internal urethral sphincter muscle is formed by involuntary smooth muscles, while the lower voluntary muscles make up the external sphincter muscles. The internal sphincter is created by the detrusor muscle. The urethra is longer in males than in females. Sphincters keep the urethra closed when urine is not being passed. The internal urethral sphincter is under involuntary control and lies at the bladder–urethra junction. The external urethral sphincter is under voluntary control.

Male Urethra

The male urethra passes through four different regions:
- Prostatic region – passes through the prostate gland.
- Membranous portion – passes through the pelvis diaphragm.
- Bulbar urethra – located inside the perineum and scrotum, extends from the external distal urinary sphincter to the peno-scrotal junction, and is surrounded by the corpus spongiosum. It contains the opening of the ducts of the Cowper glands, and differs in length from person to person.
- Penile region – extends the length of the penis.

In the male, the urethra not only excretes fluid waste products but is also part of the reproductive system. Rather than the straight tube found in the female body, the male urethra is S-shaped to follow the line of the penis. It is approximately 20 cm long. The male urethra can be segregated into various portions: the spongy portion, the prostatic portion and the membranous portion. The spongy urethra can be subdivided into fossa navicularis, pendulous urethra and bulbous (bulbar) urethra. The proximal portion, which is also the prostatic portion, is only about 2.5 cm long and passes along the neck of the urinary bladder through the prostate gland. This section is designed to accept the drainage from the tiny ducts within the prostate and is equipped with two ejaculatory tubes (see Figure 11.10).

Female Urethra

The female urethra is bound to the anterior vaginal wall. The external opening of the urethra is anterior to the vagina and posterior to the clitoris. In the female, the urethra is approximately 4 cm long and leads out of

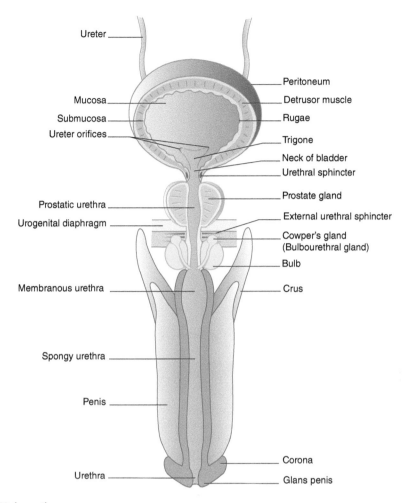

Ureter

Mucosa

Submucosa

Ureter orifices

Prostatic urethra

Urogenital diaphragm

Membranous urethra

Spongy urethra

Penis

Urethra

Peritoneum

Detrusor muscle

Rugae

Trigone

Neck of bladder

Urethral sphincter

Prostate gland

External urethral sphincter

Cowper's gland
(Bulbourethral gland)

Bulb

Crus

Corona

Glans penis

Figure 11.10 **Male urethra.**

the body via the urethral orifice. In the female, the urethral orifice is located in the vestibule in the labia minora. This can be found located in between the clitoris and the vaginal orifice. In the female body the urethra's only function is to transport urine out of the body (see Figure 11.11).

Micturition

When the volume of urine in the bladder reaches about 300 mL, stretch receptors in the bladder walls are stimulated and excite sensory parasympathetic fibres that relay information to the sacral area of the spine. This information is assimilated in the spine and relayed to two different sets of neurones. Parasympathetic motor neurones (in the pons) are excited and act to contract the detrusor muscles in the bladder so that bladder pressure increases and the internal sphincter opens. At the same time, somatic motor neurones supplying the external sphincter via the pudendal nerve are inhibited, allowing the external sphincter to open and urine to flow out, assisted by gravity.

A person usually has great control over bladder function. They can increase or decrease the rate of flow of urine, and stop and start at will (unless there are physiological problems), thus making micturition a simple reflex action.

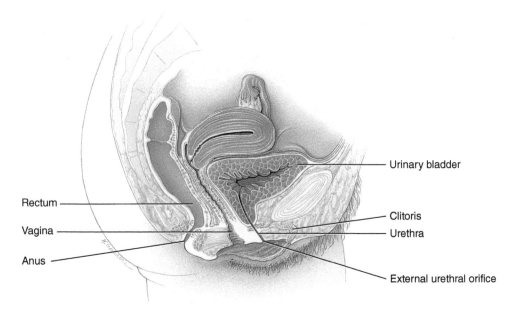

Figure 11.11 **Location of female urethra.** *Source:* Nair and Peate (2013). Reproduced with permission of John Wiley & Sons.

Conclusion

The renal system consists of the kidneys, ureters, urinary bladder and the urethra. These systems collectively play an important role in maintaining homeostasis. They remove the waste products of metabolism, secrete hormones, regulate fluid balance and maintain homeostasis. Some of the functions it carries out include:

- regulating blood volume through urine production and blood pressure by releasing renin;
- regulating the electrolyte balance in the body through hormones such as aldosterone;
- maintaining the acid–base balance by regulating the secretion of hydrogen and bicarbonate ions;
- excreting waste products (e.g. urea and uric acid) and conserving valuable nutrients essential for the body.

Urine is formed by filtration, selective reabsorption and secretion. The selectivity of the glomerular filtrate is determined by the size of the opening of the filter and blood pressure. There are other factors that regulate urine production and electrolyte balance; they include hormone regulation such as ADH, aldosterone and ANP hormones and neuronal regulation through the autonomic nervous system.

The urinary bladder is a storage organ for urine and is located in the pelvic cavity. It contains three layers: the muscular, erectile and mucous layers. Urine is stored in the bladder until the person gets the urge to empty their bladder. The process of micturition is under the control of the sympathetic and parasympathetic system. During micturition, strong muscles in the bladder walls (the detrusor muscles) compress the bladder, pushing its contents into the urethra, thus voiding urine.

Glossary

Anterior: Front.
Bifurcation: Dividing into two branches.
Calyces: Small, funnel-shaped cavities formed from the renal pelvis.
Diuresis: Excess urine production.
Erythropoietin: Hormone produced by the kidneys that regulates red blood cell production.
Excretion: The elimination of waste products of metabolism.

Filtration: A passive transport system.

Glomerulus: A network of capillaries found in Bowman's capsule.

Hilum (hilus): An indention near to the centre of the concave area of the kidney, where its vessels, nerves and ureter enter/leave.

Kidneys: Organs situated in the posterior wall of the abdominal cavity.

Nephron: Functional unit of the kidney.

Posterior: Behind.

Renal artery: Blood vessel that takes blood to the kidney.

Renal cortex: The outermost part of the kidney.

Renal medulla: The middle layer of the kidney.

Renal pelvis: The funnel-shaped section of the kidney.

Renal pyramids: Cone-shaped structures of the medulla.

Renal vein: Blood vessel that returns filtered blood into circulation.

Renin: A renal hormone that alters systemic blood pressure.

Sphincter: A ring-like muscle fibre that can constrict.

Ureter: Membranous tube that drains urine from the kidneys to the bladder.

Urethra: Muscular tube that drains urine from the bladder.

References

Azhar, A., Hussain, K. and Majid, A. (2019) Drug management in patients with reduced kidney function. *Prescriber* (February): 18–22.

Dougherty, L., Lister, S. and West-Oram, A. (2015) *The Royal Marsden Manual of Clinical Nursing Procedures: Student Edition*. Hoboken, NJ: John Wiley & Sons, Incorporated.

Marieb, E.N.H.K. (2016) *Human Anatomy & Physiology*. Boston: Pearson Education.

Martini, F., Nath, J.L. and Bartholomew, E.F. (2017) *Fundamentals of Anatomy & Physiology, Global Edition*. Boston: Pearson Education.

Mayo Clinic Staff. (2019). Urine Color. Retrieved from http://www.mayoclinic.org/diseases-conditions/urine-color/basics/causes/con-20032831 (accessed 26 February 2020).

McCance, K.L. and Huether, S.E. (2018) *Pathophysiology - E-Book: The Biologic Basis for Disease in Adults and Children*. St Louis: Mosby.

Payne, R.A. (2016) The epidemiology of polypharmacy. *Clinical medicine (London, England)* **16**(5): 465–469. doi:10.7861/clinmedicine.16-5-465.

Think Kidneys (2017) Acute Kidney Injury Best Practice Guidance for Undergraduate Nurse Educators. Retrieved from https://www.thinkkidneys.nhs.uk/aki/wp-content/uploads/sites/2/2016/05/Guidance_for_UG-nurse-educators-FINAL.pdf

Thomas, N. (2019) *Renal Nursing: Care and Management of People with Kidney Disease*. London: Wiley.

Tortora, G.J., Derrickson, B. and Tortora, G.J. (2014) *Principles of Anatomy & Physiology*. Hoboken, NJ: Wiley.

Further Reading

NCEPOD (2009) Acute Kidney Injury: Adding insult to Injury. In NCEPOD (Series Ed.) National Confidential Enquiry into Patient Outcome and Death (Ed.) Retrieved from http://www.ncepod.org.uk/2009report1/Downloads/AKI_report.pdf.

NICE (2013) Acute kidney injury: prevention, detection and management (CG169). Retrieved from London: https://www.nice.org.uk/guidance/cg169/resources/acute-kidney-injury-prevention-detection-and-management-35109700165573.

NICE (2014) Chronic kidney disease in adults: assessment and management (CG182). Retrieved from https://www.nice.org.uk/guidance/cg182/resources/chronic-kidney-disease-in-adults-assessment-and-management-pdf-35109809343205.

Royal College of Physicians (2015) Acute kidney injury and intravenous fluid therapy. Retrieved from London: https://www.rcplondon.ac.uk/guidelines-policy/acute-care-toolkit-12-acute-kidney-injury-and-intravenous-fluid-therapy.

Think Kidneys (2017) Acute Kidney Injury Best Practice Guidance for Undergraduate Nurse Educators. Retrieved from https://www.thinkkidneys.nhs.uk/aki/wp-content/uploads/sites/2/2016/05/Guidance_for_UG-nurse-educators-FINAL.pdf.

Thomas, N. (2019) *Renal Nursing: Care and Management of People with Kidney Disease*. London: Wiley.

Activities

Multiple Choice Questions

1. Urine is produced in which part of the urinary system?
   (a) the pelvis of the kidney
   (b) the bladder
   (c) the nephron
   (d) the ureter
2. Filtration of fluid from the blood occurs in which area of the nephron?
   (a) distal convoluted tubule
   (b) Bowman's capsule
   (c) loop of Henle
   (d) proximal convoluted tubule
3. The kidneys produce renin when:
   (a) blood pressure is low
   (b) blood pressure is high
   (c) pH of blood is low
   (d) pH of blood is high
4. What is the name of the hormone that stimulates haemoglobin production?
   (a) thyroxin
   (b) aldosterone
   (c) parathyroid hormone
   (d) erythropoietin
5. The medulla contains the:
   (a) renal pelvis
   (b) the renal artery
   (c) tubules and blood vessels
   (d) glomerulus
6. Which part of the nephron is urine concentrated in:
   (a) Loop of Henle
   (b) glomerulus
   (c) collecting ducts
   (d) renal pelvis
7. The average pH of normal urine is generally:
   (a) acidic
   (b) alkaline
   (c) neutral
8. A sweet fruity smell in the urine can indicate:
   (a) infection
   (b) stale urine
   (c) ketones in the urine
   (d) proteins in the urine
9. The glomerular filtration rate:
   (a) is the amount of filtrate produced in the kidney each hour
   (b) is the amount of filtrate produced in the kidney each minute
   (c) is the amount of filtrate produced in the kidney each day
   (d) is the amount of filtrate found in the bladder each hour
10. How much blood flows through the kidney each minute:
    (a) 4800 mL
    (b) 2400 mL
    (c) 1200 mL
    (d) 600 mL

11. Which gland is situated above each kidney?
    (a) adrenal
    (b) pituitary
    (c) pancreas
    (d) pineal
12. Which hormone is secreted in response to increased osmolarity in the blood?
    (a) calcitriol
    (b) erythropoietin
    (c) renin
    (d) antidiuretic hormone
13. Urea is a by-product of the breakdown of:
    (a) proteins
    (b) muscle
    (c) ketones
    (d) glucose
14. Bicarbonate is reabsorbed in:
    (a) the glomerulus
    (b) the distal convoluted tubule
    (c) the proximal convoluted tubule
    (d) the collecting ducts
15. What is the normal pH of blood?
    (a) 7.35–7.45
    (b) 7.0
    (c) 7.15–7.25
    (d) 7.45–7.55

305

Conditions

The following is a list of conditions that are associated with the renal system. Take some time and write notes about each of the conditions. You may make the notes taken from text books or other resources (e.g. people you work with in a clinical area), or you may make the notes as a result of people you have cared for. If you are making notes about people you have cared for, you must ensure that you adhere to the rules of confidentiality.

Acute Kidney Injury

Chronic Kidney Disease

Pyelonephritis

Vasculitis

Nephrotic syndrome

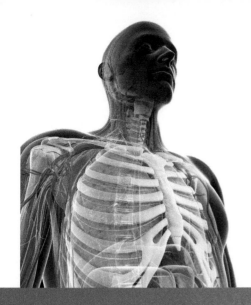

12

The Respiratory System

Anthony Wheeldon

Test Your Prior Knowledge

- List five major structures of the upper and lower respiratory tract.
- What is the main function of the respiratory system?
- Describe the physiological process of breathing – which muscles are utilised?
- How is oxygen transported to body tissue?
- What factors may increase or decrease a person's rate and depth of breathing?

Learning Outcomes

After reading this chapter you will be able to:

- List the main anatomical structures of both the upper and lower respiratory tract.
- Describe the events of pulmonary ventilation.
- Explain how the body is able to control the rate and depth of breathing.
- Discuss the principles of external respiration.
- Describe how oxygen and carbon dioxide are transported around the body.

Visit the student companion website at www.wileyfundamentalseries.com/anatomy where you can test yourself using flashcards, multiple-choice questions and more. Instructor companion site at www.wiley.com/go/instructor/anatomy where instructors will find valuable materials such as PowerPoint slides and image bank designed to enhance your teaching.

Fundamentals of Anatomy and Physiology: For Nursing and Healthcare Students, Third Edition. Edited by Ian Peate and Suzanne Evans.
© 2020 John Wiley & Sons Ltd. Published 2020 by John Wiley & Sons Ltd.
Student companion website: www.wileyfundamentalseries.com/anatomy
Instructor companion website: www.wiley.com/go/instructor/anatomy

Body Map

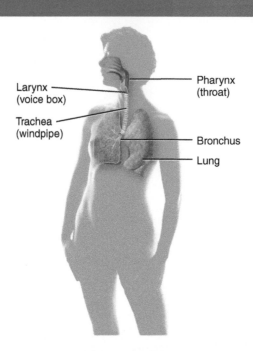

Larynx
(voice box)

Pharynx
(throat)

Trachea
(windpipe)

Bronchus

Lung

Introduction

Human cells can only survive if they receive a continuous supply of oxygen. As cells use oxygen, a waste gas, carbon dioxide, is produced. If allowed to build up, carbon dioxide can disrupt cellular activity and disturb homeostasis. The principal function of the respiratory system, therefore, is to ensure that the body extracts enough oxygen from the atmosphere and disposes of the excess carbon dioxide. The collection of oxygen and removal of carbon dioxide is referred to as respiration. Respiration involves the following four distinct processes: pulmonary ventilation, external respiration, transport of gases and internal respiration. Although all four are examined in this chapter, only pulmonary ventilation and external respiration are the sole responsibility of the respiratory system. As oxygen and carbon dioxide are transported around the body in blood, effective respiration is also reliant upon a fully functioning cardiovascular system.

Organisation of the Respiratory System

The respiratory system is divided into the upper and lower respiratory tract (see Figure 12.1). All structures found below the larynx form part of the lower respiratory tract. The respiratory system can also be said to be divided into conduction and respiratory regions. The upper respiratory tract and the uppermost section of lower respiratory tract form the conduction region, in which air is conducted through a series of tubes and vessels. The respiratory region is the functional part of the lungs, in which oxygen diffuses into blood. The structures within the respiratory region are microscopic, very fragile and easily damaged by infection. For this reason, both the upper and lower respiratory tracts are equipped to fight off any invading airborne bacterial or viral pathogens.

The Upper Respiratory Tract

Air enters the body via the nasal and oral cavities. The nasal cavity is divided into two equal sections by the nasal septum, a structure formed out of the ethmoid bones and the vomer of the skull. The space where air enters the nasal cavity just inside the nostrils is referred to as the vestibule. Beyond each vestibule the nasal

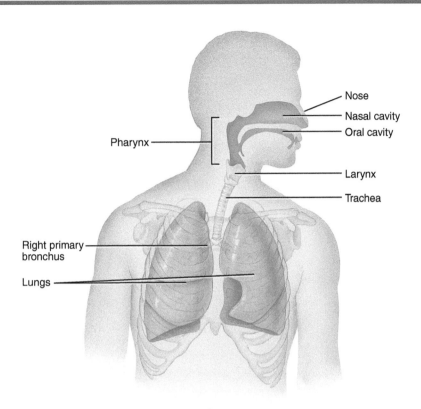

Anterior view showing organs of respiration

Figure 12.1 **Major structures of the upper and lower respiratory tract.** *Source:* Tortora and Derrickson (2017). Reproduced with permission of John Wiley & Sons.

cavities are subdivided into three air passageways, the meatuses, which are formed by three shelf-like projections called the superior, middle and inferior nasal conchae (see Figure 12.2). The region around the superior conchae and upper septum contains olfactory receptors, which are responsible for our sense of smell. The pharynx connects the nasal and oral cavity with the larynx. The pharynx is divided into three regions called the nasopharynx, the oropharynx and the laryngopharynx. The nasopharynx sits behind the nasal cavity and contains two openings that lead to the auditory (Eustachian) tubes. The oropharynx and laryngopharynx sit underneath the nasopharynx and behind the oral cavity. The oropharynx and oral cavity are divided by the fauces (see Figure 12.2). Both the oropharynx and the laryngopharynx are passageways for food and drink as well as air. To protect them from abrasion by food particles they are lined with non-keratinised stratified squamous epithelium (see Chapter 4).

As well as providing the sense of smell, the upper respiratory tract also ensures that the air entering the lower respiratory tract is warm, damp and clean. The vestibule is lined with coarse hairs that filter incoming air, ensuring that large dust particles do not enter the airways. The conchae are lined with a mucous membrane made from pseudostratified ciliated columnar epithelium, which contains a network of capillaries and a plentiful supply of mucus-secreting goblet cells. The blood flowing through the capillaries warms the passing air, while the mucus moistens it and traps any passing dust particles. The mucus-covered dust particles are then propelled by the cilia towards the pharynx, where they can be swallowed or expectorated.

To add further protection, the upper respiratory tract is lined with irritant receptors, which when stimulated by invading particles (dust or pollen, for example) force a sneeze, ensuring the offending material is ejected through the nose or mouth. The pharynx also contains five tonsils. The two tonsils visible when the mouth is open are the palatine tonsils; behind the tongue lie the lingual tonsils, and the pharyngeal tonsil or adenoid sits on the upper back wall of the pharynx. Tonsils are lymph nodules and part of the body's defence system. The epithelial lining of their surface has deep folds, called crypts. Inhaled bacteria or particles become entangled within the crypts and are then engulfed and destroyed.

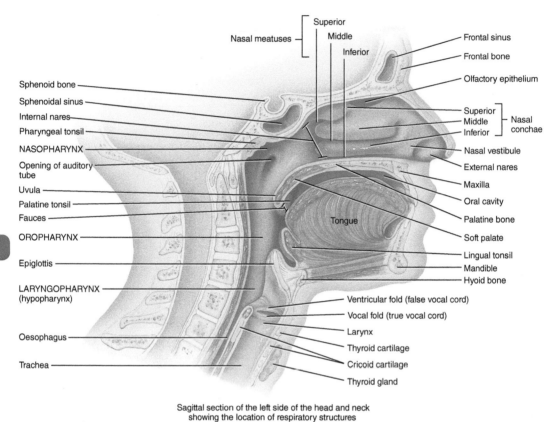

Superior
Middle
Inferior

Nasal meatuses

Frontal sinus

Frontal bone

Olfactory epithelium

Sphenoid bone

Sphenoidal sinus

Internal nares

Pharyngeal tonsil

NASOPHARYNX

Opening of auditory
tube

Uvula

Palatine tonsil

Fauces

OROPHARYNX

Epiglottis

LARYNGOPHARYNX
(hypopharynx)

Oesophagus

Trachea

Superior
Middle   Nasal
Inferior   conchae

Nasal vestibule

External nares

Maxilla

Oral cavity

Palatine bone

Tongue

Soft palate

Lingual tonsil

Mandible

Hyoid bone

Ventricular fold (false vocal cord)

Vocal fold (true vocal cord)

Larynx

Thyroid cartilage

Cricoid cartilage

Thyroid gland

Sagittal section of the left side of the head and neck
showing the location of respiratory structures

Figure 12.2 **Structures of the upper respiratory tract.** *Source:* Tortora and Derrickson (2017). Reproduced with permission of John Wiley & Sons.

The Lower Respiratory Tract

The lower respiratory tract includes the larynx, the trachea, the right and left primary bronchi and all the constituents of both lungs (see Figure 12.3). The lungs are two cone-shaped organs that almost fill the thorax. They are protected by a framework of bones, the thoracic cage, which consists of the ribs, sternum (breastbone) and vertebrae (spine). The tip of each lung, the apex, extends just above the clavicle (collarbone), and their wider bases sit just above a concave muscle called the diaphragm. The larynx (voice box) connects the trachea and the laryngopharynx. The remainder of the lower respiratory tract divides into branches of airways. For this reason, the structure of the lower respiratory tract is often referred to as the bronchial tree.

Larynx

The larynx consists of nine pieces of cartilage tissue: three single pieces and three pairs (see Figure 12.4). The single pieces of cartilage are the thyroid cartilage, the epiglottis and the cricoid cartilage. The thyroid cartilage is more commonly known as the Adam's apple and, together with the cricoid cartilage, protects the vocal cords. The cricothyroid ligament, which connects the thyroid and cricoid cartilage, is the landmark of an emergency airway or tracheostomy (McGrath, 2014). The epiglottis is a leaf-shaped piece of elastic cartilage attached to the top of the larynx. Its function is to protect the airway from food and water. On swallowing,

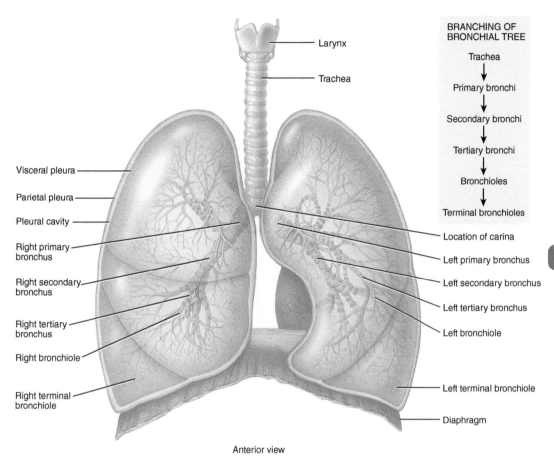

BRANCHING OF BRONCHIAL TREE

Trachea
↓
Primary bronchi
↓
Secondary bronchi
↓
Tertiary bronchi
↓
Bronchioles
↓
Terminal bronchioles

Larynx

Trachea

Visceral pleura

Parietal pleura

Pleural cavity

Right primary bronchus

Right secondary bronchus

Right tertiary bronchus

Right bronchiole

Right terminal bronchiole

Location of carina

Left primary bronchus

Left secondary bronchus

Left tertiary bronchus

Left bronchiole

Left terminal bronchiole

Diaphragm

Anterior view

Figure 12.3 Gross anatomy of the lower respiratory tract. *Source:* Tortora and Derrickson (2017). Reproduced with permission of John Wiley & Sons.

the epiglottis blocks entry to the larynx and food and liquids are diverted towards the oesophagus, which sits nearby. Inhalation of solid or liquid substances can block the lower respiratory tract and cut off the body's supply of oxygen – this medical emergency is referred to as aspiration and necessitates the swift removal of the offending substance.

The three pairs of cartilage are the arytenoid, cuneiform and corniculate cartilages (see Figure 12.4). The arytenoid cartilages are the most significant as they influence the movement of the mucous membranes (true vocal folds) that generate the voice. Speaking, therefore, is reliant upon a fully functioning respiratory system. Many obstructive lung disorders, such as asthma, reduce a person's ability to speak a full sentence without drawing a new breath (Wheatley, 2018).

Trachea

The trachea (or windpipe) is a tubular vessel that carries air from the larynx down towards the lungs. The trachea is also lined with pseudostratified ciliated columnar epithelium so that any inhaled debris is trapped and propelled upwards towards the oesophagus and pharynx to be swallowed or expectorated. The trachea and the bronchi also contain irritant receptors, which stimulate a cough, forcing larger invading particles upwards. The outermost layer of the trachea contains connective tissue that is reinforced by a series of 16–20 C-shaped cartilage rings. The rings prevent the trachea from collapsing during an active breathing cycle.

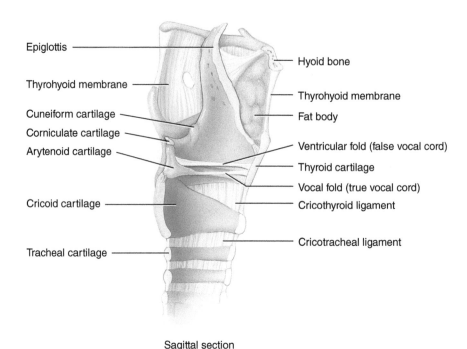

Epiglottis

Thyrohyoid membrane

Cuneiform cartilage

Corniculate cartilage

Arytenoid cartilage

Cricoid cartilage

Tracheal cartilage

Hyoid bone

Thyrohyoid membrane

Fat body

Ventricular fold (false vocal cord)

Thyroid cartilage

Vocal fold (true vocal cord)

Cricothyroid ligament

Cricotracheal ligament

Sagittal section

Figure 12.4 **Anatomy of the larynx.** *Source:* Tortora and Derrickson (2017). Reproduced with permission of John Wiley & Sons.

Skills in Practice Removal of Bronchial Secretions (Suction)

The insertion of a tracheostomy will irritate the airways and stimulate the production of bronchial secretions, which the patient will find difficult to expectorate. Suction is a method of removing bronchial secretions and keeping the airways clear.

When clearing bronchial secretions via a tracheostomy the nurse inserts a sterile catheter, which is attached to suction, into the stoma. The suction then removes the bronchial secretions. It is paramount that the procedure is executed quickly and aseptically and with care to minimise the chances of trauma and hypoxia.

Before suctioning can commence the nurse must select an appropriate catheter size and ensure the suction pressure is set at a safe level (ideally 11–16 kPa). Once the procedure has been explained to the patient, the nurse, using aseptic technique, gently inserts the suction catheter into the tracheostomy and pushes it down the airway until the patient coughs or resistance is felt. The nurse should then withdraw the catheter by 1–2 cm before applying the suction. The suction catheter is then withdrawn, while continually suctioning until it is removed. Whilst the catheter is in place, the suction pressure will remove excess secretions and dispose of them safely. The process should not take more than 15 seconds and twisting and pushing back and forth should be avoided. Oxygen saturations must be monitored throughout the procedure and if the patient is receiving oxygen it must be replaced immediately afterwards. Local policy and procedures must be adhered to at all time.

Bronchial Tree

The lungs are divided into distinct regions called lobes. There are three lobes in the right lung and two in the left. The heart, along with its major blood vessels, sits in a space between the two lungs called the cardiac notch. Each lung is surrounded by two thin protective membranes called the parietal and visceral pleura (see Figure 12.3). The parietal pleura lines the wall of the thorax, whereas the visceral pleura lines the lungs themselves. The space between the two pleurae, the pleural space or cavity, is minute and contains a thin film of lubricating fluid. This reduces friction between the two pleurae, allowing the two layers to slide over one another during breathing. The fluid also helps the visceral and parietal pleura to adhere to each other, in the same way two pieces of glass stick together when wet. However, should any substance enter the pleural space the parietal and visceral pleura may separate, causing the lung to collapse. Substances that can enter the pleural cavity include blood or fluid and in most cases air. A collection of air in the pleural cavity is called a pneumothorax or collapsed lung. Blood in the pleural cavity is a referred to as a haemothorax and fluid collecting between the pleura is called a pleural effusion.

Skills in Practice Nursing Care and Management of a Chest Drain

A chest drain is a plastic tube inserted into the pleural cavity to remove air or fluid that may have collected there as a result of disease or trauma. The plastic tube is connected to a container, which collects the air or fluid. When chest drains are used to collect air, the container will contain water, which provides a seal or valve that allows gas to exit the lungs but not to re-enter. When used to extract air, chest drains can be attached to suction pressure to aid lung reinflation.

The main care responsibilities when nursing a person with a chest drain are monitoring both the individual and the drain. Attention should be paid to the position of both the patient and the chest drain. The patient should wherever possible remain in an upright position so as to encourage drainage and chest expansion. The position of the drain itself is equally important as it must be kept below the patient's chest level to prevent fluid re-entering the pleural space. The nurse must also check that the drain is not coiled or looped as this will impede drainage.

The nurse must monitor the chest drain closely and observe for signs of 'swinging' and 'bubbling'. The level of the water seal in the container should fluctuate between 5 and 10 cm, in sync with the patient's breathing. This movement is referred to as swinging and absence of swinging could indicate that there is a kink or blockage in the tubing. 'Bubbling' is the presence of bubbles in the water seal. 'Bubbling' normally occurs when the patient coughs or exhales. Continuous 'bubbling', however, could indicate a problem with the drain or insertion site.

Chest drain insertion can be very painful and nurses must talk with their patients about their pain and administer prescribed analgesics to keep pain levels to a minimum. Furthermore, nurses must regularly assess for signs of infection, such as redness, swelling and heat around the insertion site.

313

Within the lungs the primary bronchi divide into the secondary bronchi, each serving a lobe (three secondary bronchi on the right and two on the left). The secondary bronchi split into tertiary bronchi (see Figures 12.3 and 12.5), of which there are 10 in each lung. Tertiary bronchi continue to divide into a network of bronchioles, which eventually lead to a terminal bronchiole. The section of the lung supplied by a terminal bronchiole is referred to as a lobule, and each lobule has its own arterial blood supply and lymph vessels. The bronchial tree continues to subdivide, with the terminal bronchiole leading to a series of respiratory bronchioles, which in turn generate several alveolar ducts. The airways terminate with numerous sphere-like structures called alveoli, which are clustered together to form alveolar sacs (see Figure 12.6). Human lungs contain an average of 480 million alveoli (Ochs *et al.*, 2004). The transfer of oxygen from air to blood only occurs from the respiratory bronchiole onwards. The airways found between the trachea and the respiratory bronchioles form the conduction region of the lungs. The airways found beyond the respiratory bronchioles constitute the functional respiratory region of the lungs. This region accounts for two-thirds of the lungs' surface area (Tortora and Derrickson, 2017).

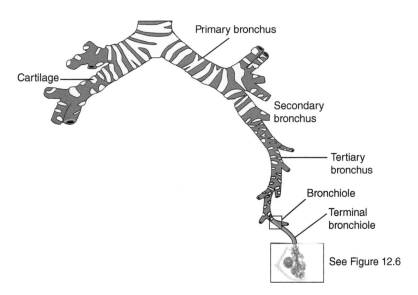

Figure 12.5 **The bronchial tree.** *Source:* Peate (2017). Reproduced with permission of John Wiley & Sons.

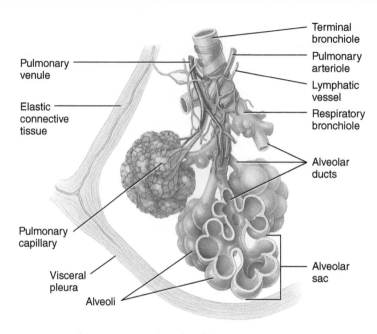

Diagram of a portion of a lobule of the lung

Figure 12.6 **Microscopic anatomy of a lobule.** *Source:* Tortora and Derrickson (2017). Reproduced with permission of John Wiley & Sons.

Episodes of Care Child

Asthma is a chronic inflammatory disorder of the lungs. It causes the bronchi and bronchioles to become inflamed and constricted. As a result, airflow becomes obstructed, often resulting in a characteristic wheeze and a cough.

Amy is 4 years old and has had a troublesome cough for 4 weeks. At first her mother and father thought she had a common cold, but as the symptoms of the cold abated, the cough remained. Amy's father takes her to the GP and explains that the cough is worse at night and stops Amy from sleeping. He also states that Amy's cough is exacerbated by running and playing with her friends.

Asthma is triggered by exposure to substances or situations that wouldn't normally cause airway irritation. Substances such as pollen and dust are common triggers, but asthma can be caused by situations such as inhaling cold air, exercise, stress and upper airway infections such as the common cold. Asthma can develop at any stage of life but is common in childhood, with 1 in every 11 children in the UK living with the condition (British Lung Foundation, 2019). However, asthma is very difficult to diagnose in children, especially in the under 5s, as the symptoms could be caused by other common childhood conditions, such as rhinitis, sinusitis or reflux. When caring for a child under the age of 5, GPs and practice nurses are advised to use their clinical judgement and treat the child as having asthma if they have asthma like symptoms. They should also be closely monitored and if they still have asthma-like symptoms when they turn 5, GPs should consider diagnostic tests such as fractional exhaled nitric oxide test, spirometry or peak flow.

The practice nurse listens to Amy's chest and asks her to blow into a peak flow meter. The practice nurse concludes that Amy has asthma-like symptoms and prescribes a short acting beta2 agonist inhaler and asks that Amy comes back to the surgery in two weeks. A practice nurse spends time with Amy and her father explaining how to take her inhaler properly, using a device called a spacer to ensure as much of the medication as possible enters Amy's airways. The nurse also asks Amy's father to monitor the effectiveness of the inhaler (see Medicines Management – salbutamol).

When Amy returns in 2 weeks her father states that the inhaler makes the cough better, but it still remains, especially at night. In response the practice nurse prescribes an inhaled corticosteroid inhaler to be taken twice a day and for her to be reviewed in 8 weeks' time (see Medicines Management – corticosteroid therapy).

Multiple Choice Questions

1. Which of the following are characteristic asthma-like symptoms?
   (a) cough
   (b) wheeze
   (c) breathlessness on exercise
   (d) all of the above
2. How many children in the UK live with asthma?
   (a) 1 in 2
   (b) 1 in 101
   (c) 1 in 11
   (d) 1 in 1000
3. Which of the following conditions could cause asthma-like symptoms?
   (a) chicken pox
   (b) reflux
   (c) head lice
   (d) threadworm
4. What test can be used to confirm a diagnosis of asthma in children?
   (a) dkin-prick test
   (b) Heaf test
   (c) fractional exhaled nitric oxide test
   (d) oxygen saturation reading
5. What device can enhance the inhalation of beta2 agonist therapies?
   (a) syringe
   (b) mask
   (c) peak flow meter
   (d) spacer

Medicines Management Salbutamol

 Salbutamol is a Beta-2 (β_2) agonist bronchodilator therapy used to reverse airway constriction caused by obstructive airways diseases, such as asthma. Asthma is a chronic inflammatory airway disease in which individuals are said to have hypersensitive or hyper-responsive airways. People living with asthma experience periods of reversible inflammation and constriction in the bronchi and bronchioles, which causes breathlessness and a characteristic wheeze. When encountering a trigger (e.g. allergy, infection or stress), mast cells on the walls of the bronchi and bronchioles release several cytokines (chemical messengers) that cause increased mucus production and increased capillary permeability. Very soon the airways become full of mucus and fluid leaking from blood vessels and airflow becomes obstructed. β_2 agonists such as salbutamol stimulate β_2 receptor cells on the walls of the bronchi and bronchioles, causing bronchodilation.

Salbutamol can be inhaled, injected or taken orally. The most common route is via an inhaler and given its effectiveness in reducing airway constriction it is often referred to by health professionals as a 'reliever'. In emergency situations, salbutamol can be nebulised. A nebuliser forces a jet stream of air or oxygen through a liquid preparation of salbutamol, producing a mist that the patient inhales via a special mask or pipe. While salbutamol is an effective pharmacological treatment, the nurse must be aware of the following side effects, especially when nebulised:

- tachycardia and other arrhythmias
- hand shaking and tremors
- headache
- nervous tension.

Other β_2 agonist therapies include terbutaline, fenoterol and salmeterol.
See British Thoracic Society and Scottish Intercollegiate Guidelines Network (2016).

Medicines Management Corticosteroid Therapy

Corticosteroids are potent anti-inflammatory agents that are often used to reduce bronchial hyperactivity in people living with chronic inflammatory airway diseases, such as asthma and chronic obstructive pulmonary disease. Corticosteroids reduce airway inflammation and therefore are very effective in the treatment of airway obstruction. Corticosteroids are a first-line treatment for moderate, severe and life-threatening asthma. Common corticosteroids include:

- prednisolone
- hydrocortisone.

Patients taking the above corticosteroids will need careful monitoring as they may cause the following side effects:

- osteoporosis
- diabetes
- mood swings
- weight gain
- increased body hair.

Inhaled corticosteroids are used very effectively for the prophylaxis of asthma and are often referred to as 'preventers' by health care professionals. Preparations such as beclamethasone, budesonide and fluticasone are often prescribed for patients living with asthma to be used daily to minimise the potential for exacerbation.

See British Thoracic Society and Scottish Intercollegiate Guidelines Network (2016).

Blood Supply

The conduction and respiratory regions of the lungs receive blood from different arteries. Deoxygenated blood is delivered to the lobules via capillaries that originate from the right and left pulmonary arteries. Once reoxygenated, blood is sent back to the left-hand side of the heart via one of four pulmonary veins, ready to be ejected into systemic circulation (see Figure 12.7). The conduction region of the lungs receives oxygenated blood from capillaries that stem from the bronchial arteries, which originate from the aorta. Some of the bronchial arteries are connected to the pulmonary arteries, but most blood returns to the heart via the pulmonary or bronchial veins.

Respiration

The process by which oxygen and carbon dioxide are exchanged between the atmosphere and body cells is called respiration. Respiration follows the following four distinct phases:

- **pulmonary ventilation** – how air gets in and out of the lungs;
- **external respiration** – how oxygen diffuses from the lungs to the bloodstream and how carbon dioxide diffuses from blood and to the lungs;
- **transport of gases** – how oxygen and carbon dioxide are transported between the lungs and body tissues;
- **internal respiration** – how oxygen is delivered to and carbon dioxide collected from body cells.

The understanding of all four processes is reliant upon the appreciation of a series of gas laws, which are summarised in Table 12.1.

Pulmonary Ventilation

The Mechanics of Breathing

Pulmonary ventilation describes the process more commonly known as breathing. For air to pass in and out of our lungs, a change in pressure needs to occur. Before inspiration the intrapulmonary pressure, the pressure within the lungs, is the same as atmospheric pressure. During inspiration the thorax expands, and the intrapulmonary pressure falls below atmospheric pressure. Because intrapulmonary pressure is now less than

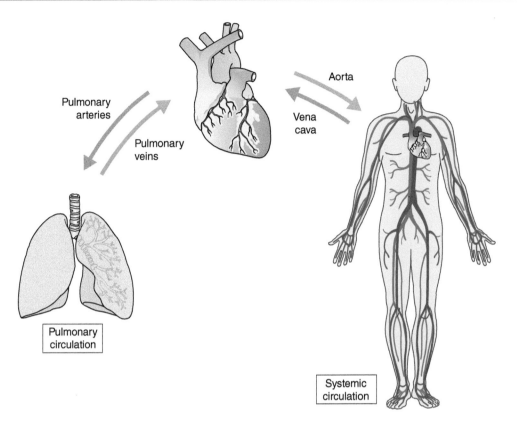

Figure 12.7 **The flow of blood between the lungs, the heart and the body.**

Table 12.1 **Summary of important gas laws.**

GAS LAW	SUMMARY	CLINICAL APPLICATION
Boyle's law	At a fixed temperature the pressure exerted by gas is inversely proportional to its volume	As the thorax expands, intrapulmonary pressure falls below atmospheric pressure
Dalton's law	In a mixture of gases each gas will exert its own individual pressure, as if no other gases are present	Differences in partial pressure govern the movement of oxygen and carbon dioxide between the atmosphere, the lungs and blood
Henry's law	The quantity of gas that will dissolve in a liquid is proportional to its pressure and its solubility	Oxygen and carbon dioxide are soluble in water and are transported in blood. Nitrogen is highly insoluble and, despite accounting for 79% of the atmosphere, very little is dissolved in blood
Fick's law	The rate a gas will diffuse across a permeable membrane will depend upon pressure difference, surface area, diffusion distance and molecular weight and solubility	Helps explain how altitude, exercise and respiratory disease can influence the amount of oxygen that is diffused into blood

Source: Adapted from Davies and Moores (2010).

atmospheric pressure, the air will naturally enter our lungs until the pressure difference no longer exists. This phenomenon is explained by Boyle's law and Dalton's law. Gases exert pressure, and Boyle's law states that at a fixed temperature the amount of pressure exerted by a given mass of gas is inversely proportional to the size of its container. Larger volumes provide greater space for the circulation of gas molecules, and therefore less pressure is exerted. In smaller volumes the gas molecules are more likely to collide with the walls of the container and exert a greater pressure as a result (see Figure 12.8). Dalton's law explains that in a mixture of gases each gas exerts its own individual pressure proportional to its size. For example, atmospheric air contains a mixture of gases. Each individual gas will exert its own pressure dependent upon its quantity. Nitrogen, for example, will exert the greatest pressure as it is the most abundant gas. Collectively, all the gases in the atmosphere exert a pressure, atmospheric pressure, which is 101.3 kPa (kilopascals) at sea level (see Table 12.2). On inhalation the thorax expands, intrapulmonary pressure falls below 101.3 kPa and, because air flows from areas of high pressure to low pressure, air enters the lungs (Hickin *et al.*, 2015).

A range of respiratory muscles are used to achieve thoracic expansion during inspiration (see Figure 12.9). The major muscles of inspiration are the diaphragm and external intercostal muscles. The diaphragm is a dome-shaped skeletal muscle found beneath the lungs at the base of the thorax. There are 11 external inter-costal muscles, which sit in the intercostal spaces – the spaces between the ribs. During inspiration the dia-phragm contracts downwards, pulling the lungs with it. Simultaneously, the external intercostal muscles pull the rib cage outwards and upwards. The thorax is now bigger than before, and intrapulmonary pressure is reduced below atmospheric pressure as a result. The most important muscle of inspiration is the diaphragm; 75% of the air that enters the lungs is as a result of diaphragmatic contraction. Expiration is a more passive process. The external intercostal muscles and the diaphragm relax, allowing the natural elastic recoil of the lung tissue to spring back into shape, forcing air back into the atmosphere (see Figure 12.10).

Other respiratory muscles can also be utilised. The abdominal wall muscles and internal intercostal mus-cles, for instance, are utilised to force air out beyond a normal breath, for example, when playing a musical instrument or blowing out candles on a birthday cake. The sternocleidomastoids, the scalenes and the pecto-ralis can also be used to produce a deep forceful inspiration. These muscles are referred to as accessory mus-cles, so called because they are rarely used in normal, quiet breathing (Rolfe, 2019).

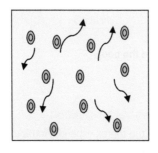

In larger volumes gases exert less pressure

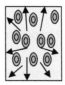

In smaller volumes gases exert more pressure

Figure 12.8 **Boyle's law: the volume of a gas varies inversely with its pressure.**

Table 12.2 **The proportion of gases that constitute the atmosphere (partial pressures are expressed as P_{gas}).**

GAS	VOLUME (%)	PRESSURE (KPA)
Nitrogen $\left(P_{N_2}\right)$	78.084	79.055
Oxygen $\left(P_{O_2}\right)$	20.946	21.218
Carbon dioxide $\left(P_{CO_2}\right)$	0.035	0.0355
Argon (P_{Ar})	0.934	0.946
Other gases[a]	0.001	0.001
Total atmospheric pressure (P_B)	100	101.3

Sources: Adapted from Brimblecombe (1995), Lumb (2016) and Lutgens and Tarbuck (2018)
[a] Neon, helium, methane, krypton, nitrous oxide, hydrogen, ozone, xenon.

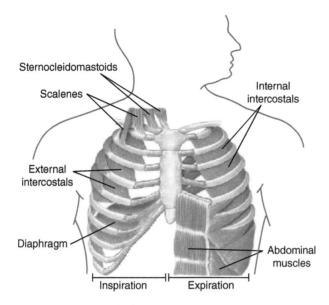

Figure 12.9 **The muscles involved in pulmonary ventilation.** *Source:* Peate (2017). Reproduced with permission of John Wiley & Sons.

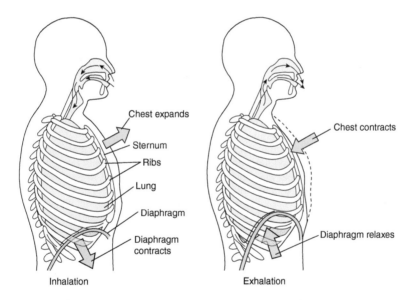

Figure 12.10 **Movements of inspiration and expiration.** *Source:* Peate (2017). Reproduced with permission of John Wiley & Sons.

Work of Breathing

During inspiration, respiratory muscles must overcome various factors that hinder thoracic expansion. The natural elastic recoil of lung tissue, the resistance to airflow through narrow airways and the surface tension forces at the liquid–air interface in the lobule all oppose thoracic expansion. The energy required by the respiratory muscles to overcome these hindering forces is referred to as work of breathing. The amount of energy expended is kept to a minimum by the ease with which lungs can be stretched. This ease of stretch is called lung compliance. Because of lung compliance, an inhalation of around 500 mL of air is achievable without any noticeable effort. Blowing a similar amount of air into a balloon would take a much greater effort. Lung compliance is aided by the production of a detergent-like substance called surfactant. Whenever a liquid and gas come into close contact with one another, surface tension is generated. Surfactant reduces the surface tension that occurs where the alveoli meet pulmonary capillary blood flow in the lobule, thereby reducing the amount of energy required to inflate the alveoli. Surfactant is manufactured by type II alveolar cells, found in the alveoli.

Work of breathing is also required to overcome airway resistance. As air flows through the bronchial tree, resistance to airflow occurs as the gas molecules begin to collide with one another in the increasingly narrow airways. Despite these opposing forces, work of breathing accounts for less than 5% of total body energy expenditure. However, many lung diseases can affect lung compliance and airway resistance and, therefore, increase work of breathing. In asthma, for example, airway inflammation reduces the diameter of the airways and increases airway resistance. If the diameter of an airway is halved, resistance increases 16-fold. Lung diseases that damage lung tissue can also affect lung compliance. Any increase in airway resistance and lung compliance will inevitably increase work of breathing. In acute respiratory disease, work of breathing could account for up to 30% of total body energy expenditure (Levitzky *et al.*, 1990).

Episodes of Care Learning Disabilities

Pneumonia is an infection of the alveoli and small airways. Inflammation and oedema cause the alveoli to fill with debris and exudate until a solid mass called consolidation is formed. The consolidation can be patchy and spread throughout both lungs or concentrated in one mass affecting one or more lobes. Symptoms of pneumonia include fever, painful breathing, cough, expectoration of sputum, dehydration and lethargy. Community acquired pneumonia is most commonly treated in the community, but it can develop into a severe infection, which will require admission to hospital.

Howard is a 30-year-old man who has Down syndrome. Howard has been brought into the GP surgery by Mike, a care support worker who works at Garden House Care Home, where Howard resides. Mike is concerned about Howard as his mood has changed significantly over the past week. Instead of being his happy and cheerful self, Howard is much quieter than normal, isn't eating or drinking and becomes angry and agitated. When asked, Howard stated that it hurt when he took a deep breath and that he felt very tired. On listening to Howard's chest, the GP can hear rales, a cracking and bubbling sound indicative of mild pneumonia, on the right side. She prescribes a 5-day course of amoxicillin and paracetamol for pain. She also advises Howard to get plenty of rest and to drink plenty of fluid. She asked Howard to come back to the surgery in 1 week's time unless he began to feel worse or saw no improvement after 3 days, in which case he should come back to the surgery sooner.

Respiratory disease is the most common cause of death in people with a learning disability. This is due to differences in the structure and function of the airways associated with poor muscle tone. Pneumonia is also common in people with Down syndrome, this is thought to be due to their under-development immune system. Pneumonia is treatable with antibiotics, analgesia, bed rest and fluids, but if left untreated people can develop a severe infection, which could lead to a hospital admission. Early detection is key. However, patients with a learning disability often find communicating or understanding their health difficult, which makes accessing health services challenging. Nurses need to be acutely aware of this as often the health needs of people with learning disabilities, like Howard, are overlooked and their respiratory symptoms deteriorate and ultimately make their treatment more complex.

After three days of treatment Mike was pleased to see Howard was much more like his old self, and although Howard stated he still felt a little poorly, he was less agitated and irritable, a little more active and had started to eat a little more. After 1 week, the GP was happy to see that Howard was cheerful and talkative. When she listened to his chest, she could not hear any added breath sounds.

Multiple Choice Questions

1. What is the solid mass that forms in pneumonia infections called?
   (a) clotting
   (b) constipation
   (c) plugging
   (d) consolidation
2. Which of the following are symptoms of pneumonia?
   (a) fever
   (b) painful breathing
   (c) dehydration
   (d) all of the above

3. Which of the following is an antibiotic, commonly used to treat mild pneumonia?
    (a) paracetamol
    (b) amoxicillin
    (c) levothyroxine
    (d) furosemide
4. Which of the following statements is true?
    (a) people with learning disabilities are less likely to contract a respiratory disease
    (b) respiratory diseases such as asthma and COPD are uncommon in people with a learning disability
    (c) respiratory disease is the most common cause of death in people with learning disabilities
    (d) all of the above
5. Which of the following statements is false?
    (a) the health needs of people with a learning disability are often overlooked
    (b) people with Down's syndrome are at an increased risk of contracting pneumonia
    (c) pneumonia, if left untreated, can be severe and necessitate an admission to hospital.
    (d) none of the above

Volumes and Capacities

Lung volumes and capacities measure or estimate the amount of air passing in and out of the lungs. Everyone has a total lung capacity (TLC), which is the total amount of air their lungs are capable of housing. Everyone's TLC will be dependent upon their age, sex and height. TLC can be subdivided into a range of potential or actual volumes of air. For example, the amount of air that passes in and out of the lungs during one breath is called the tidal volume V_T. After a normal, quiet breath the lungs will still have room for a deeper inspiration that could fill the lungs. This potential capacity for inspiration is referred to as inspiratory reserve volume (IRV). Likewise, after a normal, quiet breath, there remains the potential for a larger exhalation. This potential capacity of exhalation is referred to as expiratory reserve volume (ERV). If tidal volume increases, due to exercise for example, IRV and ERV would be reduced. Tidal volume, IRV and ERV can all be measured. However, because a small volume of air always remains in the lungs – even after maximal exhalation – TLC can only be estimated. This small volume of remaining air is called residual volume (RV). Because RV cannot be exhaled, the total amount of air that could possibly pass in and out of an individual's lungs is a combination of tidal volume, IRV and ERV, which collectively is referred to as vital capacity (see Figure 12.11).

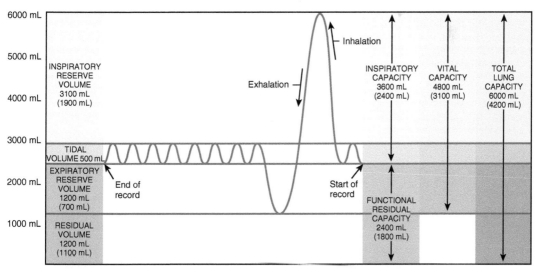

Figure 12.11 Diagrammatic description of the major lung volumes and capacities. *Source:* Tortora and Derrickson (2017). Reproduced with permission of John Wiley & Sons.

Table 12.3 Important lung volumes.

VOLUME	CALCULATION
Minute volume V_E	Tidal volume (T_V) × Respiration rate e.g. 500 (T_V) × 12 = 6000 mL (V_E)
Alveolar minute ventilation V_A	[Tidal volume (T_V) – Anatomical dead space (V_D)] × Respiration rate e.g. [500 (T_V) – 150 (V_D)] × 12 = 4000 mL (V_A)

Source: Martini and Nath (2018). Reproduced with permission of Pearson Education Limited.

Other important measures of lung volume include minute volume V_E, alveolar minute ventilation V_A and anatomical dead space V_D (see Table 12.3). Minute volume V_E is the amount of air breathed in each minute and is calculated by multiplying tidal volume V_T by respiration rate. In health, minute volume is around 6–8 mL per minute. However, only the air that travels beyond the terminal bronchioles will take part in gaseous exchange. For this reason, the air present in the rest of the lungs is referred to as anatomical dead space V_D. Therefore, in order to ascertain exactly how much air is available for gaseous exchange, anatomical dead space must be accounted for. Alveolar minute ventilation V_A is calculated by subtracting anatomical dead space from minute volume, which in health would be approximately 4–6 mL per minute (Hickin *et al.,* 2015).

Episodes of Care Mental Health

COPD has been defined as airflow obstruction that is progressive, not fully reversible and does not change markedly over several months. It has one major cause – smoking. COPD is a term now used to describe the traditional diagnosis of chronic bronchitis or emphysema. People with chronic asthma are also at risk of developing fixed airway obstruction as airways become re-modelled over time. Their symptoms may be indistinguishable from COPD and many COPD patients may also have asthma.

Leonard is a 77-year-old man living with chronic obstructive pulmonary disease. Recently, Leonard had been experiencing increased levels of breathlessness, fatigue and general feelings of being unwell. Leonard's daughter made him an appointment with the respiratory nurse as she was increasingly concerned about his well-being, his low mood and his general lack of interest in his garden, which was normally his pride and joy. On examination the nurse noted Leonard was experiencing breathlessness on mild exertion but that there were no signs of infection or moderate exacerbation. The nurse and Leonard chatted about the steps he takes to manage his condition and it was clear that he often felt sad and had lost interest in 'most things'. Leonard stated that he felt he had become a burden on his daughter and that he preferred to stay at home rather than visit her and his grandchildren. Based on what she had been told, the respiratory nurse informed Leonard that she felt he was depressed.

Depression is very common in people living with long term respiratory diseases, like COPD. However, diagnosing depression in people living with COPD can be challenging as many of the symptoms, such as disturbed sleep and lack of appetite, can overlap. One of the main nursing considerations for the management of depression in people living with COPD is the promotion of coping strategies and fostering self-management techniques.

The respiratory nurse recommended that Leonard attend pulmonary rehabilitation sessions as they had been positively evaluated and been shown to effectively reduce depression and anxiety in patients like Leonard. There was a local group that met once a week at the local hospital and she was happy to refer him to the nurse that ran it. Pulmonary rehabilitation services are run by specialist nurses, physiotherapists and specialist pulmonary rehabilitation practitioners. Leonard agreed to give it a try and when he was home read the leaflet which the nurse had given him. The leaflet explained that the aims of the service were to reduce symptoms of breathlessness, help him manage his condition and keep him out of hospital as much as possible, increase his fitness and reduce the frequency of exacerbations and reduce levels of depression and anxiety.

Leonard attended his first pulmonary rehabilitation session the following week. He was introduced to the service by a physiotherapist who explained that he would attend 8 classes of 2 hours duration, in which he would learn exercises, which he could do at home and techniques to help him cope with his breathlessness.

Multiple Choice Questions

1. COPD is an umbrella term for which two diseases?
   (a) chronic bronchitis and emphysema
   (b) emphysema and lung cancer
   (c) fibrosing alveolitis and chronic bronchitis
   (d) asthma and pneumonia
2. What is the main cause of COPD?
   (a) depression
   (b) infection
   (c) smoking
   (d) all of the above
3. Which of the following are symptoms of depression?
   (a) low mood
   (b) lack of interest in hobbies and pastimes
   (c) social isolation
   (d) all of the above
4. The nursing priorities for people living with COPD are:
   (a) administration of prescribed antibiotics
   (b) monitoring of respiratory rate and oxygen saturations
   (c) promotion of coping skills and self-management techniques
   (d) ensuring safe administration of oxygen
5. The aim of pulmonary rehabilitation is:
   (a) reduction of breathlessness
   (b) reduce hospital admissions
   (c) treat depression and anxiety
   (d) all of the above

323

Clinical Considerations Spirometry and Peak Flow

Spirometry measures the force and volume of a maximum expiration after a full inspiration. The air the patient forces out is referred to as forced vital capacity (FVC). The volume the patient expires after 1 second is called forced expiratory volume in the first second (FEV_1). By comparing FEV_1 with FVC, the FEV_1:FVC ratio, the severity of airway obstruction can be ascertained. An FEV_1:FVC ratio of less than 80% is indicative of obstructive airways disease (Scanlon and Heuer, 2017).

Peak expiratory flow rate (PEFR), or 'peak flow', measures the extent of airway resistance. PEFR is the force of expiration in litres per minute. It measures the patient's maximum expiratory flow rate via their mouth. An inability to meet a predicted value based on age, sex and height could indicate increased airway resistance, as occurs during an asthma attack. PEFR provides a quick and simple assessment of the airways; however, regular peak flow measurements are more revealing than single arbitrary readings, and nurses should be mindful that PEFR is effort dependent (Talley and O'Connor, 2017).

Control of Breathing

The rate and depth of breathing are controlled by the respiratory centres, which are found in the brainstem, within the areas called the medulla oblongata and pons (see Figure 12.12). The rate of breathing is set by the inspiratory centre of the medulla oblongata. The expiratory centre is thought to play a role in forced expiration. Also within the medulla oblongata are specialised chemoreceptors that continually analyse carbon dioxide levels within cerebrospinal fluid. As levels of carbon dioxide rise, messages are sent via the phrenic and intercostal nerves to the diaphragm and intercostal muscles instructing them to contract more frequently and harder, increasing respiratory rate and depth. Another set of chemoreceptors found in the aorta and carotid arteries analyse levels of oxygen as well as carbon dioxide. If oxygen falls or carbon dioxide rises, messages are sent to the respiratory centres via the glossopharyngeal and vagus nerves, stimulating further contraction to produce faster, deeper breathing. An increase in CO_2 levels has a more powerful effect on respiratory rate than a reduction in oxygen level.

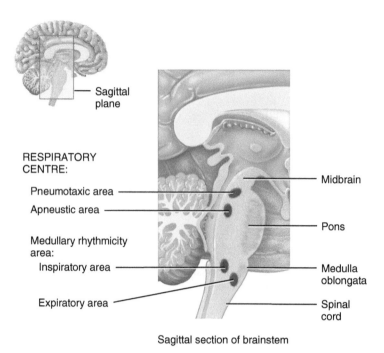

RESPIRATORY
CENTRE:

Pneumotaxic area

Apneustic area

Medullary rhythmicity
area:
    Inspiratory area

Expiratory area

Sagittal
plane

Midbrain

Pons

Medulla
oblongata

Spinal
cord

Sagittal section of brainstem

Figure 12.12 **The respiratory centres of the brainstem.** Source: Tortora and Derrickson (2017). Reproduced with permission of John Wiley & Sons.

Breathing is refined by the actions of the pneumotaxic and apneustic centres of the pons (see Figure 12.12). The pneumotaxic centre sends inhibitory signals to the medulla to slow breathing down, while the apneustic centre stimulates the inspiratory centres, lengthening inspiration. Both these actions fine-tune breathing and prevent the lungs from becoming overinflated. Throughout the day, whether at work, rest or play, respiration rate will change in order to meet the body's oxygen needs.

Clinical Considerations Respiratory Rate

In health, an adult's respiratory rate is normally between 12 and 16 respirations per minute. Although breathing is essentially a subconscious activity, the rate and depth of breathing can be controlled voluntarily or even stopped altogether, when swimming underwater for example. However, this voluntary control is limited, as the respiratory centres have a strong urge to keep breathing. Breathing can also be influenced by state of mind. The inspiratory area of the respiratory centres can be stimulated by both the limbic system and hypothalamus, two areas of the brain responsible for processing emotion. Fear, anxiety or even the anticipation of stressful activities can cause an involuntary increase in the rate and depth of breathing. Other factors that can influence breathing include pyrexia and pain. In summary, while the rate and depth of breathing can be consciously altered, subconscious respiratory centre control will over-ride voluntary control in order to maintain homeostasis. Any changes in respiratory rate are, therefore, clinically significant (Hogan, 2006).

External Respiration

Gaseous Exchange

External respiration only occurs beyond the respiratory bronchioles. External respiration is the diffusion of oxygen from the alveoli into pulmonary circulation (blood flow through the lungs) and the diffusion of carbon dioxide in the opposite direction. Diffusion occurs because gas molecules always move from areas of high concentration to low concentration. Each lobule of the lung has its own arterial blood supply; this blood supply originates from the pulmonary artery, which stems from the right ventricle of the heart. The blood present in the pulmonary artery has been collected from systemic circulation and is therefore low in oxygen and relatively

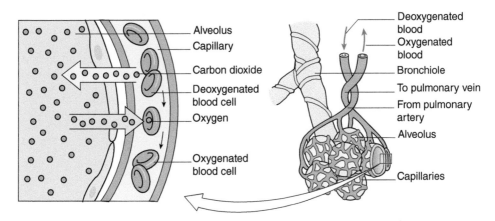

Figure 12.13 External respiration: exchange of oxygen and carbon dioxide within the lungs.

high in carbon dioxide. The amount (and therefore pressure) of oxygen in the alveoli is far greater than in the passing arterial blood supply. Oxygen, therefore, moves passively out of the alveoli and into pulmonary circulation and on towards the left-hand side of the heart. Because there is less carbon dioxide in the alveoli than in pulmonary circulation, carbon dioxide transfers into the alveoli ready to be exhaled (see Figure 12.13).

Factors Influencing Diffusion

It takes approximately 0.25 s for an oxygen molecule to diffuse from the alveoli into pulmonary circulation. However, there are various influencing factors that determine the rate by which oxygen and carbon dioxide diffuse between alveoli and pulmonary circulation. This is best explained using Fick's law of diffusion, which uses an equation to determine the rate of diffusion (see Box 12.1). According to Fick's law, the rate of diffusion is determined by gas solubility/molecular weight, surface area, concentration difference and membrane thickness. The more soluble a gas is in water the easier it is for diffusion to occur. Oxygen and carbon dioxide are both soluble in water and therefore easily diffused; indeed, carbon dioxide is 20 times more soluble than oxygen. The most abundant gas in the atmosphere is nitrogen; however, nitrogen is highly insoluble in water and therefore very little diffuses into the bloodstream. The larger the surface area available for diffusion the greater the rate of diffusion will be. Large inhalations will recruit more alveoli, and a greater rate of diffusion occurs as a result. The greater the gas concentration difference between the alveoli and pulmonary circulation, the faster that gas will diffuse. Because blood travelling towards the alveoli is deoxygenated, there always remains a large difference in concentration of oxygen between the alveoli and pulmonary circulation. However, the rate of diffusion can be enhanced if this concentration difference is increased, by administering prescribed oxygen therapy for example. The final factor for consideration is membrane thickness. The further the distance gases must travel, the slower the diffusion will be. Conditions such as pulmonary oedema, in which fluid collects in the alveoli, result in an increased membrane thickness. The distance between alveoli and pulmonary circulation slows the rate of diffusion.

Box 12.1 Fick's Law of Diffusion

$$J = \frac{S}{wt_{mol}} \times A \times \frac{\Delta C}{t}$$

where

J is the rate of diffusion
S is the solubility
wt_{mol} is the molecular weight
A is the surface area
ΔC is the concentration difference
t is the membrane thickness.

Source: Hickin *et al.* (2015).

Clinical Considerations Sputum

Often, the nurse has the responsibility to examine and observe the sputum (sometimes this is called phlegm, secretions or expectorate) that a person may produce. At times the nurse is required to obtain a specimen of the person's sputum for microbiological analysis. The nurse must be able to carry out these important tasks safely and effectively. The skills required to do this include the ability to determine what is sputum and what are oral secretions (spit), the application of infection control activities and the ability to document findings accurately and report any concerns.

The production of sputum is an important part of a person's immune system. You may be required to ask the person you are caring for about their sputum production. The following questions can help generate important information:

- Is there anything that causes (provokes) you to produce sputum?
- When do you produce it?
- How often do you produce it?
- Can you describe it – what does it look like?
- Does your sputum have any smell?
- How much do you produce?
- The sputum you are producing now, has this changed recently? If so, tell me about that.

It can be difficult for the person to provide you with answers concerning their sputum production. You can help them by asking them to measure it in relation to teaspoons, tablespoons or an egg cup. Understanding the sputum produced and describing and reporting its characteristics – for example, the consistency, the amount produced, the odour and its colour – can provide you with much information about the person you are caring for. Also note if the person producing the sputum did this with ease or difficulty, and if, after the specimen was produced, they became breathless or cyanotic.

If the person you are caring for needs to use a sputum pot, you must make sure that it is placed within their reach and that you offer them tissues and a receptacle to dispose of the used tissues. Disposing of sputum safely can help prevent and control infection; sputum is potentially an infectious body fluid. Care interventions include ensuring that the sputum pot is changed daily and that the lid is firmly closed when it is not in use. Used tissues and sputum pots must be carefully disposed of regardless of the care setting. Disposable, one-use-only sputum pots must be provided. Incineration is needed if sputum is infectious. Local policy and procedures must be adhered to.

Medicines Management Oxygen

Oxygen is a drug, which must be prescribed. Oxygen is used to treat hypoxaemia, not breathlessness. There is no evidence that oxygen relieves breathlessness in patients with normal or near normal oxygen saturation readings.

The aim of oxygen therapy is to maintain a normal or near-normal oxygen saturation level and that this should be achieved on the lowest possible concentration of oxygen. The target oxygen saturation levels for acutely ill adults are 94–98% and 88–92% for those at risk of hypercapnic (excess carbon dioxide) failure – that is, patients living with chronic obstructive pulmonary disease.

Oxygen should only be administered by competent clinicians, and each patient receiving oxygen should have their oxygen saturations monitored regularly. For this reason, it is essential that oxygen saturation reading equipment should be within easy reach of patients receiving oxygen therapy.

It is important that nurses use the correct delivery method in order to ensure the patient receives the correct prescription. Many oxygen prescriptions come in the form of a percentage. Venturi masks ensure that the patient receives the correct percentage of oxygen by mixing room air with pure oxygen. Venturi masks are available in the following concentrations – please ensure you include the correct flow rate to ensure the patient receives the correct dose:

24% – 2 L of oxygen per minute
28% – 4 L of oxygen per minute
35% – 8 L of oxygen per minute
40% – 10 L of oxygen per minute
60% – 15 L of oxygen per minute.

Simple oxygen masks do not deliver oxygen with such accuracy. They can deliver between 40% and 60% oxygen with a flow rate of 5–10 L of oxygen per minute. Flow rates of less than 5 L of oxygen per minute may lead to the build-up of carbon dioxide within the mask. Re-breather oxygen masks can deliver up to 90% oxygen and are very effective in emergency situations.

Nasal cannula ensure a steady delivery of oxygen into the nasal cavity. Flow rates between 1 and 4 L of oxygen per minute will provide the patient with 24–40% oxygen. However, the actual volume of oxygen delivered will vary from patient to patient, as mouth breathing may dilute delivery. Flow rates greater than 4 L of oxygen per minute will provide greater concentrations of oxygen, but this may cause nasal dryness and discomfort.

Oxygen in the atmosphere is moist and humidified. Medical oxygen, on the other hand, is dry. Patients on long-term oxygen therapy may encounter nasal or oral dryness, which can cause discomfort. In such situations the team caring for the patient may consider using humidified (passed through water) oxygen.

Documentation and administration must comply with local policy and procedure.

See British Thoracic Society Emergency Oxygen Guideline Development Group (2017).

Ventilation and Perfusion

External respiration is most effective where there is an adequate supply of both oxygen and blood. In order to ensure a good enough supply of oxygen, the alveoli must be adequately ventilated. In health, an alveolar minute ventilation V_A of around 4 L is required. In order to ensure that an adequate supply of blood is reoxygenated, a plentiful supply of blood must be delivered to the lungs from the right ventricle of the heart; in other words, a pulmonary blood flow of around 5 L per minute. This ideal delivery of adequate amounts of both air and blood is referred to as the ventilation V_A:perfusion Q ratio. A normal V_A:Q ratio would be 4:5 or 0.8. Any disruption to either ventilation or pulmonary blood flow would lead to a V_A:Q mismatch and less oxygen diffusing into blood. For example, if someone hypoventilates and V_A falls below 4 L, then less blood would be reoxygenated. This would be described as a low V_A:Q ratio (i.e. 3:5 or 0.3). Another potential problem would be an inadequate pulmonary blood flow, due to an embolism, for example. In such an instance, less blood is available to be reoxygenated and the V_A:Q ratio would become high (i.e. 4:3 or 1.34). However, the V_A:Q ratio differs throughout the lungs and depends upon a person's position (Margereson, 2001).

Transport of Gases

Both oxygen and carbon dioxide are transported from the lungs to body tissues in blood. Both gases travel in blood plasma and haemoglobin, which is found within erythrocytes (red blood cells). Key gas transport terminology is summarised in Table 12.4.

Table 12.4 Definitions of important gas transport terminology.

GAS TRANSPORT TERM	DEFINITION
Oxygen saturation (SaO_2)	The percentage of arterial haemoglobin carrying oxygen molecules SpO_2 = SaO_2 measured by a pulse-oximeter
Partial pressure of arterial oxygen (PaO_2)	The amount of oxygen dissolved in arterial blood plasma measured in kilopascals
Partial pressure of carbon dioxide ($PaCO_2$)	The amount of carbon dioxide dissolved in arterial blood plasma measured in kilopascals
Oxygen capacity	The potential space for oxygen transported by haemoglobin (Hb) per 100 mL of blood Hb × 1.39 = oxygen capacity per 100 mL of blood
Arterial oxygen content (CaO_2)	The actual amount of oxygen in arterial blood carried by haemoglobin per 100 mL of arterial blood Arterial oxygen saturation (SaO_2) × oxygen capacity = oxygen content per 100 mL of arterial blood
Oxygen delivery (DO_2)	The actual amount of oxygen being delivered to body tissues based on cardiac output. Arterial oxygen content (CaO_2) × cardiac output = oxygen delivery (DO_2)
Oxygen consumption (VO_2)/ oxygen extraction ratio	The amount of oxygen utilised by body tissues each minute

Transport of Oxygen

Most of the oxygen, around 98.5%, is transported attached to haemoglobin in the erythrocyte (red blood cell). Each erythrocyte contains around 280 million haemoglobin molecules and each haemoglobin molecule has the potential to carry four oxygen molecules. The percentage of haemoglobin carrying oxygen is measured as oxygen saturation (SaO_2). The remaining 1.5% of oxygen is dissolved in blood plasma, and is often measured in kilopascals (PaO_2), which in health is around 11–13.5 kPa (82–101 mmHg). The delivery of oxygen, therefore, is also reliant upon the presence of an adequate supply of erythrocytes and haemoglobin. In health, the average male would possess between 15 and 18 g of haemoglobin for every 100 mL of blood. Each gram of haemoglobin can carry approximately 1.34 mL of oxygen. Therefore, a male with a haemoglobin of 16 g per dL would have the capacity to carry 21.44 mL of oxygen for every 100 mL of blood ($16 \times 1.34 = 21.44$). This volume of oxygen is referred to as oxygen capacity. However, it is rare for an individual's haemoglobin to be fully saturated with oxygen. The actual amount of oxygen being transported by haemoglobin is called oxygen content (CaO_2). Oxygen content is determined by oxygen saturation levels. In health, an individual's oxygen saturation level (SaO_2) would normally be between 97% and 99%. Therefore, a male with a haemoglobin of 16 g per dL and an SaO_2 of 98% would have an oxygen content of 21.01 mL (0.98×21.44). CaO_2 only provides the amount of available oxygen per 100 mL of blood. Multiplying CaO_2 by cardiac output will provide the amount of oxygen being delivered to all body tissues each minute. This volume of oxygen is called oxygen delivery (DO_2). In other words, if cardiac output is 5000 mL per minute, the aforementioned individual would have an oxygen delivery (DO_2) of 1050 mL per minute (21.01 mL per 100 mL of blood $\times$ 5000).

The relationship between oxygen attached to arterial haemoglobin (SaO_2) and oxygen dissolved in plasma (PaO_2) is described by the oxyhaemoglobin dissociation curve (see Figure 12.14). As PaO_2 falls, SaO_2 decreases in an S-shaped curve. If PaO_2 falls as low as 8 kPa (60 mmHg), SaO_2 will remain around 90%. Therefore, natural fluctuations in oxygenation, such as occur when singing, laughing and talking, will not result in dramatic reductions in oxygen saturations. The release of oxygen from haemoglobin can be increased by 2,3-diphosphoglycerate, which is released during hypoxia and high temperatures.

Clinical Considerations Measuring Oxygen Levels

Pulse oximeters measure, via a sensor, the oxygen content of arterial blood flowing through parts of the body that are furthest from your heart, i.e. fingers, feet and earlobes. The oxygen content is expressed as a percentage of haemoglobin carrying oxygen and is called 'oxygen saturation' (SpO_2). In health, SpO_2 should be between 95 and 99%; however, tremors, anaemia, polycythaemia, cold extremities, nail varnish and acrylic nails can all jeopardise an accurate reading. Pulse oximeters also rely on adequate pulsatile blood flow to the area where the sensor is placed. For this reason, SpO_2 should only be used in conjunction with other nursing observations (Clark *et al.*, 2006).

For a more accurate measure, practitioners use an arterial blood gas reading. In such instances a sample of the patient's arterial blood is placed into a blood gas analyser. A printed or visual result is produced within seconds. Arterial blood gas readings provide information on pH, carbon dioxide and bicarbonate as well as oxygen. An oxygen saturation produced via blood gas analysis is referred to as SaO_2. In addition to an oxygen saturation, blood gas analysis measures the pressure exerted by the oxygen dissolved in plasma. In health, arterial oxygen should be around 11–13.5 kPa (82–101 mmHg) and is expressed as PaO_2 (partial pressure of arterial oxygen).

Hypoxia and Hypoxaemia

Hypoxia is defined as a lack of oxygen within body tissues. Hypoxaemia is defined as a lack of oxygen within arterial blood. Naturally, hypoxaemia will lead to hypoxia as the tissues are receiving less oxygen. However, as respiration also relies on a fully functioning cardiovascular system, hypoxia can also occur even when arterial blood is fully oxygenated – see Table 12.5.

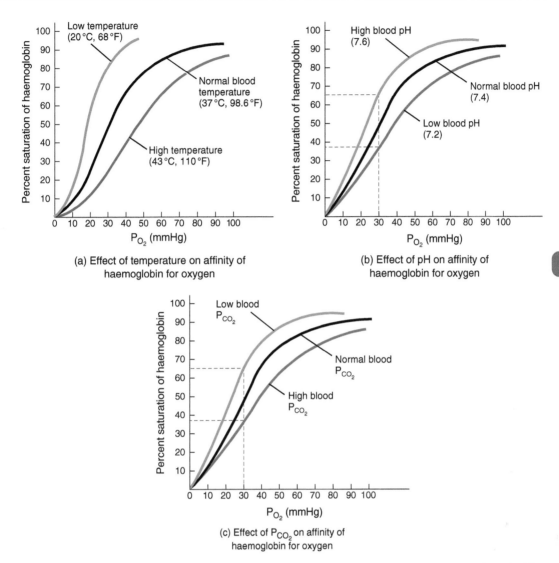

Figure 12.14 The oxyhaemoglobin dissociation curve: (a) at normal body temperature, arterial carbon dioxide levels and normal arterial blood pH; (b) with high or low arterial blood pH; (c) with high or low arterial carbon dioxide levels. *Source:* Tortora and Derrickson (2017). Reproduced with permission of John Wiley & Sons.

Table 12.5 The major types of hypoxia and their causes.

TYPE OF HYPOXIA	CAUSE
Stagnant or circulatory hypoxia	Heart failure, lack of cardiac output, leads to hypoxia
Haemic hypoxia	Lack of blood or haemoglobin (e.g. haemorrhage)
Histotoxic hypoxia	Poisoning (e.g. carbon monoxide inhalation)
Demand hypoxia	May occur when the demand for oxygen is high (e.g. during fever)
Hypoxic hypoxia	Hypoxia as a result of hypoxaemia

Transport of Carbon Dioxide

Just like oxygen, a small amount of carbon dioxide, around 10%, is transported in plasma. Carbon dioxide is also transported attached to haemoglobin, although only around 30% is transported that way. Nevertheless, haemoglobin has a greater affinity for carbon dioxide than for oxygen. Within the tissues this facilitates the release of oxygen as carbon dioxide is being created. However, as carbon dioxide levels increase (hypercapnia), the amount of oxygen binding to haemoglobin will be reduced. Any build-up of carbon dioxide will affect the oxyhaemoglobin dissociation curve by pulling the natural curve to the right, resulting in a greater risk of hypoxaemia. Conversely, a fall in carbon dioxide (hypocapnia) has the opposite effect (see Figure 12.14).

Acid–Base Balance

The majority of carbon dioxide is transported as bicarbonate ions (HCO_3^-). As carbon dioxide enters the erythrocyte it combines with water to form carbonic acid (H_2CO_3). H_2CO_3 then quickly dissociates into hydrogen ions (H^+) and bicarbonate ions (HCO_3). The formation of H_2CO_3 is very slow in plasma; in the red blood cell this reaction is speeded up by the presence of the enzyme carbonic anhydrase. The newly produced H^+ combines with haemoglobin, whereas HCO_3^- leaves the erythrocyte and enters blood plasma. For this reason, increased and decreased levels of H^+ can also influence the oxyhaemoglobin dissociation curve (see Figure 12.14). Within the lungs, as carbon dioxide leaves the pulmonary circulation and enters the alveoli this process is reversed. The transport of carbon dioxide as HCO_3^- is summarised by the following equation:

$$\underset{\text{carbon dioxide}}{CO_2} + \underset{\text{water}}{H_2O} \leftrightarrow \underset{\text{carbonic acid}}{H_2CO_3} \leftrightarrow \underset{\text{hydrogen ions}}{H^+} + \underset{\text{bicarbonate ions}}{HCO_3^-}$$

Note that the arrow symbols indicate that the equation moves both ways. For example, at a tissue level the equation moves from left to right, whereas within the lungs it moves in the opposite direction.

Arterial blood pH is mainly influenced by the levels of H^+. If blood pH falls out of its optimum range of 7.35–7.45 an acid–base imbalance may occur. The respiratory system can help to maintain acid–base balance by controlling the expulsion and retention of carbon dioxide. When pH falls (acidosis), respiratory rate increases, and more carbon dioxide is expelled. This results in greater amounts of hydrogen ions H^+ and HCO_3^- combining to form hydrogen ions (H^+) and bicarbonate ions (HCO_3^-) combining to form carbonic acid (H_2CO_3). In other words, the above equation moves from right to left. H^+ levels are reduced, and as a result pH increases. H_2CO_3 is a weak acid and has only a minimal effect on blood pH. If blood pH rises, respiratory rate and depth may fall, resulting in the retention of carbon dioxide. The above equation will now move from left to right and more H^+ will be created.

Internal Respiration

Internal respiration describes the exchange of oxygen and carbon dioxide between blood and tissue cells, a phenomenon governed by the same principles as external respiration. Cells utilise oxygen when manufacturing the cells' prime energy source, adenosine triphosphate (ATP). In addition to ATP the cells produce water and carbon dioxide. Because cells are continually using oxygen, its concentration within tissues is always lower than within blood. Likewise, the continual use of oxygen ensures that the level of carbon dioxide within tissue is always higher than within blood. As blood flows through the capillaries, oxygen and carbon dioxide follow their pressure gradients and continually diffuse between blood and tissue (see Figure 12.15). The concentration of oxygen in blood flowing away from the tissues back towards the heart is described as deoxygenated. In reality, if measured, the oxygen saturation of venous blood would probably be around 75%. This means that only around 25% of oxygen content (CaO_2) leaves the bloodstream, leaving a plentiful supply. The actual amount of oxygen used by the tissues every minute is referred to as oxygen consumption (VO_2) or oxygen extraction ratio (see Table 12.4).

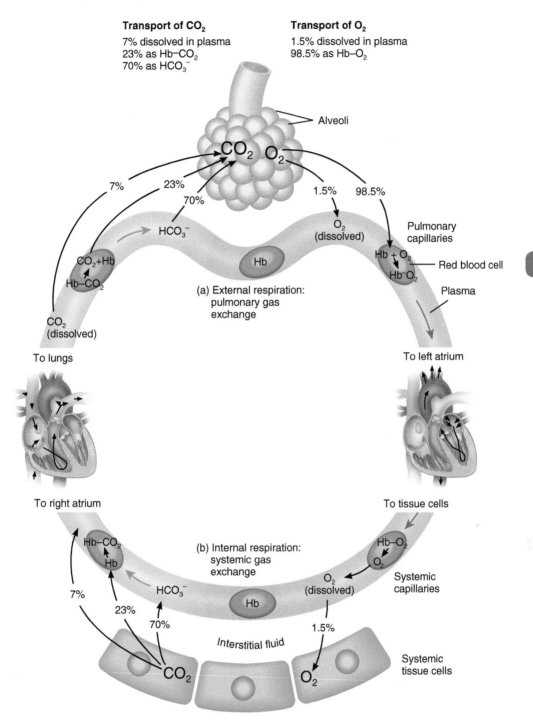

Transport of CO$_2$
7% dissolved in plasma
23% as Hb–CO$_2$
70% as HCO$_3^-$

Transport of O$_2$
1.5% dissolved in plasma
98.5% as Hb–O$_2$

Alveoli

CO$_2$ O$_2$

7%   23%
70%

1.5%   98.5%

HCO$_3^-$

O$_2$
(dissolved)

Pulmonary
capillaries

CO$_2$+Hb

Hb

Hb + O$_2$

Red blood cell

Hb–CO$_2$

Hb–O$_2$

(a) External respiration:
pulmonary gas
exchange

Plasma

CO$_2$
(dissolved)

To lungs

To left atrium

To right atrium

To tissue cells

Hb–CO$_2$

(b) Internal respiration:
systemic gas
exchange

Hb–O$_2$

Hb

O$_2$

7%   Hb

HCO$_3^-$

O$_2$
(dissolved)

Systemic
capillaries

23%

Hb

70%

1.5%

Interstitial fluid

CO$_2$

O$_2$

Systemic
tissue cells

Figure 12.15 (a, b) External and internal respiration: oxygen and carbon dioxide follow their pressure gradients (Hb: haemoglobin). *Source:* Tortora and Derrickson (2017). Reproduced with permission of John Wiley & Sons.

331

Conclusion

This chapter has examined the anatomy and physiology of the respiratory system. The respiratory system is divided into the upper and lower respiratory tracts. The lower respiratory tract consists of lung tissue and major airways. The structures within the lower respiratory tract are fragile and susceptible to infection, the main function of the upper respiratory tract therefore is the protection of the lower respiratory tract. The main function of the lower respiratory tract is the reoxygenation of arterial blood and the expulsion of excess carbon dioxide – a process called respiration. Respiration involves four distinct physiological processes: pulmonary ventilation (breathing), external respiration (gaseous exchange), transport of gases and internal respiration. Only the first two processes are the sole responsibility of the respiratory system, and effective respiration is also reliant upon a fully functioning cardiovascular system.

Glossary

Accessory muscles: Muscles not normally involved in respiration that can be utilised to increase inspiration.

Acid–base balance: The mechanisms by which the body maintains arterial blood pH between 7.35 and 7.45.

Alveolar minute ventilation: The amount of air reaching the respiratory portion of the lungs each minute.

Anatomical dead space: The portion of the airway not involved in the exchange of oxygen and carbon dioxide (also referred to as the conducting zone).

Aorta: First major blood vessel of arterial circulation. Emerges from the left ventricle of the heart.

Apex: The tip or highest point of a structure.

Apneustic centre: Area of the pons (brainstem), which influences inspiration.

Arytenoid cartilage: Cartilage tissue involved in the production of the voice.

Aspiration: The inhalation of solid or liquid substances.

Asthma: A chronic inflammatory disorder of the lungs. It causes the bronchi and bronchioles to become inflamed and constricted. As a result, airflow becomes obstructed, often resulting in a characteristic wheeze.

Bronchial artery: Artery that delivers oxygenated blood from the aorta to the bronchi and bronchioles.

Bronchial tree: The lower respiratory tract.

Bronchial veins: Veins that carry deoxygenated blood from the bronchi and bronchioles to the superior vena cava.

Bronchiole: Section of the lower respiratory tract found beyond the tertiary bronchus.

Cardiac notch: The space between the right and left lung occupied by the heart and its major blood vessels.

Carotid artery: Major artery supplying the brain, stems from the aorta.

Cartilage: Type of connective tissue that contains collagen and elastic fibres. Cartilage can stand up to both tension and compression.

Cerebrospinal fluid: Fluid found within the brain and spinal cord.

Chemoreceptors: Sensory cells sensitive to specific chemicals.

Chronic obstructive pulmonary disease: An umbrella term that encompasses chronic bronchitis, emphysema and chronic asthma – respiratory diseases which obstruct airflow.

Cilia: Hair-like extensions to the plasma membrane.

Clavicle: Anatomical term for the collarbone.

Conducting zone: Section of the airways which plays no part in the exchange of oxygen and carbon dioxide (also referred to as anatomical dead space).

Corniculate cartilage: Cartilage tissue involved in the production of the voice.

Cricoid cartilage: Ring of cartilage that forms the lower part of the larynx (voice box).

Cricothyroid ligament: Tissue that connects the thyroid cartilage and the cricoid cartilage, the main structures found in the larynx (voice box).

Cuneiform cartilage: Cartilage tissue involved in the production of the voice.

Diaphragm: Concave respiratory muscle that separates the lungs and the abdomen.

Diffusion: The passive movement of molecules or ions from a region of high concentration to low concentration until a state of equilibrium is achieved.

Embolism: Blockage of a blood vessel by a foreign substance or blood clot.

Epiglottis: Leaf-shaped piece of cartilage that sits atop the larynx.

Ethmoid bone: Sponge-like bone found in the skull. Forms part of the nasal septum.

Expectorate: To cough up and spit out mucus or sputum.

Expiratory reserve volume: The potential capacity for exhalation beyond a normal breath out.

External respiration: The process by which oxygen and carbon dioxide are exchanged between the lungs and blood.

Fauces: The opening into the pharynx from the oral cavity.

Glossopharyngeal nerve: Cranial nerve IV – nerve that communicates with tongue and pharynx. Also transmits information on oxygen and carbon dioxide levels.

Goblet cells: Mucus-secreting cells found in epithelial tissue.

Hypothalamus: Region of the diencephalon area of the brain. Responsible for the maintenance of homeostasis.

Hypoxaemia: A reduced amount of oxygen within arterial blood.

Hypoxia: A reduced amount of oxygen within the tissues.

Hypoventilation: Decreased ventilation – lack of air entering the alveoli.

Inspiratory reserve volume (IRV): The potential capacity for inspiration beyond a normal breath in.

Intercostal nerves: Nerves that link the respiratory centre in the brainstem with the intercostal muscles.

Intercostal spaces: The anatomical spaces found between the ribs.

Internal respiration: The process by which oxygen is exchanged for carbon dioxide within the tissues.

Intrapulmonary pressure: The pressure exerted by all the gases present within the lungs.

Laryngopharynx: The lower section of the pharynx (throat).

Larynx: The physiological term for the voice box.

Limbic system: Part of the functional brain, which processes emotion.

Lingual tonsils: Tonsils found underneath the tongue.

Lobes: Distinct regions of the lungs. There are three lobes in the right lung and two in the left lung.

Lobule: Minute portion of lung tissue served by its own capillary.

Lower respiratory tract: All respiratory passages found below the larynx.

Lung compliance: The ease with which the lungs can be inflated.

Lymph nodules: Egg-shaped masses of lymph tissues that provide an immune response.

Lymph vessel: A vessel that carries lymphatic fluid. Part of the lymphatic system which forms part of the immune system.

Meatuses: Three passageways found within the nasal cavity.

Medulla oblongata: Area of the brainstem.

Minute volume (V_E): The amount of air breathed in one minute.

Nasal cavity: Anatomical space within the nose.

Nasal conchae: Bones found within the nasal cavity.

Nasal septum: Structure that divides the nose into two nostrils.

Nasopharynx: The upper section of the pharynx (throat).

Non-keratinised stratified squamous epithelium: Cuboid or columnar-shaped cells that line and protect wet surfaces such as the mouth, oesophagus, epiglottis, tongue and vagina.

Oesophagus: Tubular vessel that carries food and liquid from the pharynx to the stomach.

Olfactory: Pertaining to the sense of smell.

Oropharynx: The middle section of the pharynx (throat).

Oxyhaemoglobin dissociation curve: An S-shaped curve that describes the relationship between the volume of oxygen attached to haemoglobin and the amount of oxygen dissolved in plasma.

Palatine tonsils: Tonsils found towards the rear of the oral cavity. Usually visible when the mouth is open.

Parietal pleura: Protective membrane which attaches the walls of the thorax to the lungs.

Pharyngeal tonsil: Tonsil that sits on the back wall of the pharynx. Also known as the adenoid.

Pharynx: Passageway for food and air, which links the nasal and oral cavity with the larynx. More commonly called the throat.

Phrenic nerve: Nerve that links the diaphragm to the respiratory centre in the brainstem.

Pleural space: The minute space between the visceral and parietal pleura.

Pneumotaxic centre: Portion of the medulla oblongata (brainstem) that influences inspiration.

Pons: Area of the brainstem.

Pseudostratified ciliated columnar epithelium: Covering or lining of internal body surface that contains cilia and mucus-secreting goblet cells.

Pulmonary artery: Artery that carries deoxygenated blood from the right-hand side of the heart towards the lungs.

Pulmonary oedema: A condition characterised by the leakage of fluid into the alveoli.

Pulmonary veins: Veins that carry oxygenated blood from the lungs back to the left-hand side of the heart.

Pulmonary ventilation: The process by which air enters and exits the lungs (breathing).

Pyrexia: Elevated temperature associated with fever.

Residual volume (RV): A small amount of air that permanently remains in the lungs.

Respiratory zone: The portion of lung tissue involved in the exchange of oxygen and carbon dioxide.

Sternum: Flat bone which forms part of the thoracic cage. Protects the heart and lungs. Commonly referred to as the breastbone.

Surfactant: A detergent-like substance manufactured by cells of the alveoli, which reduces surface tension and increases lung compliance.

Systemic circulation: The flow of blood from the left ventricle and right atrium delivering oxygen to and collecting carbon dioxide from body tissues.

Thoracic cage: Framework of bones, which consists of the ribs, sternum (breastbone) and vertebrae (spine).

Thorax: The body trunk above the diaphragm and below the neck.

Thyroid cartilage: The outer wall of the larynx (voice box).

Tidal volume (V_T): The volume of air that passes in and out of the lungs during one breath.

Tonsils: Lymph nodules found within the upper respiratory tract. They form part of the body's defence.

Total lung capacity (TLC): The maximum amount of air that a person's lungs can accommodate.

Tracheostomy: A procedure in which an incision is made in the trachea to facilitate breathing.

Transport of gases: The process by which oxygen and carbon dioxide are delivered between the lungs and the tissues.

Upper respiratory tract: All structures of the respiratory system situated between the oral and nasal passageways and the larynx.

Vagus nerve: Cranial nerve X – major nerve in parasympathetic function. Also transmits information on oxygen and carbon dioxide levels.

Ventilation V_A: perfusion Q ratio: The ratio of blood and air delivery to the lungs every minute. Ideally 4 L of air to 5 L of blood.

Vestibule: The space inside the nasal cavity, just inside the nostrils.

Visceral pleura: Protective membrane that lines the lungs.

Vital capacity: The maximum potential for inspiration and expiration, measured in litres.

Vomer: Triangular-shaped bone that forms the base of the nasal cavity.

References

Brimblecombe, P. (1995) *Air Composition and Chemistry*, 2nd edn. Cambridge: Cambridge University Press.

British Lung Foundation (2019) What is asthma in children? Online. https://www.blf.org.uk/support-for-you/asthma-in-children/what-is-it (accessed 16th June 2019).

British Thoracic Society and Scottish Intercollegiate Guidelines Network (2016) *SIGN 141: British Guideline on the Management of Asthma: A National Clinical Guideline*. London: BTS.

British Thoracic Society Emergency Oxygen Guideline Development Group (2017) Guideline for oxygen use in adults in healthcare and emergency settings. *Thorax* **72**(supplement 1).

Clark, A.P., Giuliano, K. and Chen, H. (2006) Pulse oximetry revisited: 'but his O₂ sat was normal!' *Clinical Nurse Specialist* **20**(6): 268–272.

Davies, A. and Moores, C. (2010) *The Respiratory System: Basic Science and Clinical Conditions*. 2nd edn. Edinburgh: Churchill Livingstone.

Hickin, S., Renshaw, J. and Williams, R. (2015) *Crash Course: Respiratory System*, 4th edn. Edinburgh: Mosby.

Hogan, J. (2006) Why don't nurses monitor the respiratory rates of patients? *British Journal of Nursing* **15**(9): 489–492.

Levitzky, M.G., Cairo J.M. and Hall, S.M. (1990) *Introduction to Respiratory Care*. London: W.B. Saunders.

Lumb, A.B. (2016) *Nunn's Applied Respiratory Physiology*, 8th edn. Edinburgh: Elsevier.

Lutgens, F.K. and Tarbuck, E.J. (2018) *The Atmosphere: An Introduction to Meteorology*, 14th edn. New York: Pearson.

Margereson, C. (2001) Anatomy and physiology. In Esmond, G. (ed.), *Respiratory Nursing*. Edinburgh: Baillière Tindall.

Martini, F.H. and Nath, J.L. (2018) *Fundamentals of Anatomy and Physiology*, 11th edn. Harlow: Pearson.

McGrath, B. (2014) *Comprehensive Tracheostomy Care: The National Tracheostomy Safety Project Manual*. Chichester: John Wiley & Sons, Ltd.

Ochs, M., Nyengaard, A.J., Knudsen, L. Voigt, M., Wahlers, T., Richter, J. and Gundersen, H.J. (2004) The number of alveoli in the human lung. *American Journal of Respiratory and Critical Care Medicine* **169**: 120–124.

Peate, I. (2017) *Fundamentals of Applied Pathophysiology: An Essential Guide for Nursing Students*, 3rd edn. Oxford: John Wiley & Sons, Ltd.

Rolfe, S. (2019) The importance of respiratory rate monitoring. *British Journal of Nursing* **28**(8): 504–508.

Scanlon, C.L. and Heuer, A.J. (2017) *Wilkin's Clinical Assessment in Respiratory Care*, 8th edn. St Louis: Elsevier.

Talley, N.J. and O'Connor, S. (2017) *Clinical Examination: A Systematic Guide to Physical Diagnosis*, 8th edn. Chatswood: Elsevier.

Tortora, G.J. and Derrickson, B.H. (2017) *Principles of Anatomy and Physiology*, 15th edn. Hoboken, NJ: John Wiley & Sons, Inc.

Wheatley, I. (2018) Respiratory rate 3: How to take an accurate measurement. *Nursing Times* **114**(7): 21–22.

Further Reading

British Lung Foundation
https://www.blf.org.uk/Home

The British Lung Foundation website provides a wealth of information for patients with respiratory disease. By accessing this site, you can gain insight into the support available for people living with lung disease, which may help you in practice and in your academic studies.

British Thoracic Society
https://www.brit-thoracic.org.uk

The British Thoracic Society website provides a range of information and clinical guidance that is based on best available evidence. Their guidance is essential for all health professionals that wish to provide gold-standard care for their respiratory patients. British Thoracic Society guidance will also ensure that your academic work is up to date.

Respiratory Education UK
https://www.educationforhealth.org/REUK/

The Respiratory Education UK website has access to a range of courses and information, which you may wish to utilise for your studies. There are also quizzes and exercises, which can test your understanding.

Activities

Multiple Choice Questions

1. Which of the following structures is not found in the upper respiratory tract?
   - (a) palatine tonsils
   - (b) turbinates
   - (c) carina
   - (d) fauces

2. Which of the following is more commonly known as the voice box?
   - (a) larynx
   - (b) epiglottis
   - (c) carina
   - (d) acinus

3. Which of the following structures is found in the respiratory zone?
   - (a) alveolar ducts
   - (b) terminal bronchioles
   - (c) tertiary bronchus
   - (d) trachea

4. How many lobes are there in the left lung?
   - (a) 1
   - (b) 2
   - (c) 3
   - (d) 4

5. Which of the following statements on pulmonary ventilation is true?
   - (a) the diaphragm is responsible for 75% of thoracic expansion
   - (b) expiration is dependent upon external intercostal muscle activity
   - (c) intrapulmonary pressure is always greater than atmospheric pressure
   - (d) the diaphragm and external intercostal muscles are two major accessory muscles

6. Which of the following statements on work of breathing is true?
   (a) increased airway diameter increases airway resistance
   (b) surfactant increases alveolar surface tension
   (c) lung disease can increase work of breathing
   (d) in health, work of breathing accounts for 50% of total body energy expenditure

7. Where are the respiratory centres?
   (a) the medulla oblongata and pons
   (b) the hypothalamus
   (c) the limbic system
   (d) cerebral cortex

8. Which of the following could increase the rate of breathing?
   (a) increased carbon dioxide levels
   (b) decreased oxygen levels
   (c) pyrexia
   (d) all of the above

9. Which of the following statements on external respiration is true?
   (a) the concentration of oxygen is greater in pulmonary circulation than in the alveoli
   (b) the concentration of carbon dioxide is greater in the alveoli than in pulmonary circulation
   (c) carbon dioxide diffuses from the alveoli into pulmonary circulation
   (d) oxygen diffuses from the alveoli into pulmonary circulation

10. Reduced levels of oxygen in blood is called:
    (a) hypoxaemia
    (b) hypercapnia
    (c) hypocapnia
    (d) hypoxia

11. Increased carbon dioxide levels in blood is referred to as:
    (a) hypoxaemia
    (b) hypercapnia
    (c) hypoxia
    (d) apnoea

12. Which of the following can be transported attached to haemoglobin?
    (a) oxygen
    (b) carbon dioxide
    (c) hydrogen ions
    (d) all of the above

13. The majority of carbon dioxide is transported by which method?
    (a) attached to haemoglobin
    (b) dissolved in plasma
    (c) as carbonic acid
    (d) as carbon monoxide

14. Which of the following will influence the release of oxygen from haemoglobin?
    (a) carbon dioxide
    (b) heat
    (c) hydrogen ions
    (d) all of the above

15. The amount of oxygen utilised by cells is referred to as:
    (a) oxygen content (CaO_2)
    (b) oxygen delivery (DO_2)
    (c) oxygen consumption (VO_2)
    (d) oxygen capacity

Conditions

The following is a list of conditions that are associated with the respiratory system. Take some time and write notes about each of the conditions. You may make the notes taken from textbooks or other resources (e.g. people you work with in a clinical area), or you may make the notes as a result of people you have cared for. If you are making notes about people you have cared for, you must ensure that you adhere to the rules of confidentiality.

Asthma

Chronic obstructive
pulmonary disease

Pneumoconiosis

Lung cancer

Cystic fibrosis

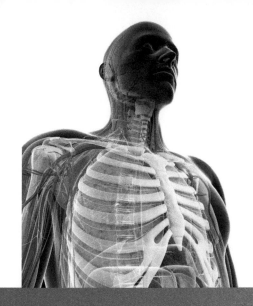

The Reproductive Systems

Karen Mate

Test Your Prior Knowledge

- **Where does fertilisation occur?**
- **What is the inner layer of the uterus called?**
- **What is the role of the hormone testosterone?**
- **A woman is most fertile at what stage of the menstrual cycle?**
- **What is the function of the prostate gland and the testes?**

Learning Outcomes

After reading this chapter you will be able to:

- **Describe the male and female reproductive organs.**
- **Understand the role and functions of the male reproductive system.**
- **Understand the role and functions of the female reproductive system.**
- **Provide an overview of the role and functions of the various hormones associated with the male and female reproductive systems.**
- **Outline the phases of the uterine cycle.**

Visit the student companion website at www.wileyfundamentalseries.com/anatomy where you can test yourself using flashcards, multiple-choice questions and more. Instructor companion site at www.wiley.com/go/instructor/anatomy where instructors will find valuable materials such as PowerPoint slides and image bank designed to enhance your teaching.

Fundamentals of Anatomy and Physiology: For Nursing and Healthcare Students, Third Edition. Edited by Ian Peate and Suzanne Evans.
© 2020 John Wiley & Sons Ltd. Published 2020 by John Wiley & Sons Ltd.
Student companion website: www.wileyfundamentalseries.com/anatomy
Instructor companion website: www.wiley.com/go/instructor/anatomy

Body Map

Mammary
gland

Uterine
(fallopian)
tube

Ovary

Uterus

Vagina

Penis

Testis

Ductus
(vas)
deferens

Seminal
vesicle

Prostate

Introduction

Reproduction is one of the most important and essential attributes of living organisms; all living organisms reproduce to create new individuals of their own kind, thereby giving rise to the next generation. Although not necessary for survival of the individual, reproduction is essential for survival of the species. Human reproduction is sexual; the male gamete (sperm) and female gamete (ovum) combine at fertilisation resulting in a new and unique combination of parental genes. The structure and function of the reproductive systems is a major point of difference between men and women.

The gametes are produced by gonads; testes produce sperm in the male, and the ovaries produce ova in the female. The gonads also produce hormones required for the development, upkeep and performance of the reproductive organs and other sexual characteristics. Fertilisation occurs inside the body of the female to form a zygote, which goes on to develop into an embryo and then a fetus. The female reproductive organs take on the responsibility for nurturing the developing fetus until birth. After birth, the mother continues to provide nutritional support for the child through lactation and breastfeeding.

This chapter provides an overview of the structure and functions of the male and female reproductive systems, which includes the gonads and a number of accessory organs and structures. The male reproductive system includes the testes, accessory ducts, accessory glands and the penis. The female reproductive system includes the uterus, uterine tubes, ovaries, vagina, vulva and mammary glands.

The Male Reproductive System

The male reproductive system, being located partially outside of the body cavity, is more visually obvious than the female reproductive system; there are, however, internal and external structures. Testes are the male gonads that working in unison with other body systems (e.g. the neuroendocrine system), produce the hormones that are essential for development of the male reproductive tract, sexual behaviour, performance and actions. The male reproductive tract shares some structures with the urinary system including the urethra and penis. The male reproductive system is shown in Figure 13.1.

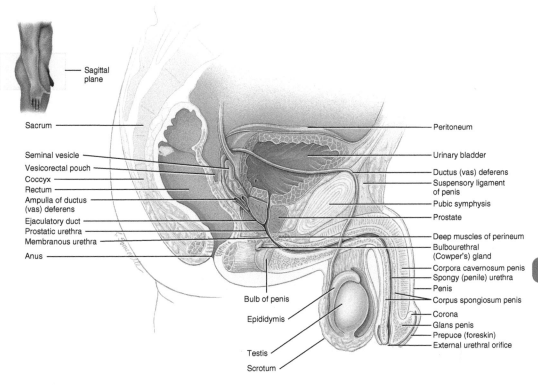

Figure 13.1 **The male reproductive system.** *Source:* Tortora and Derrickson (2009). Reproduced with permission of John Wiley & Sons.

The functions associated with the male reproductive system include:

- production, maintenance and transport of sperm (the male reproductive cells);
- production of the fluid components of semen;
- ejection of sperm from the penis;
- production and secretion of the male sex hormones.

The major structures of the male reproductive system include the testes and other external genitalia (penis and scrotum); a number of ducts responsible for the transportation of the sperm from the testes to the penis (epididymis and vas deferens) and outside the body (ejaculatory duct and urethra); and two seminal vesicles, bulbourethral glands and the prostate gland.

The Scrotum

The scrotal sac can be likened to a loose bag of skin suspended from the root of the penis. From the outside the scrotum usually appears as a single sac of skin that is separated into two portions by a ridge in the middle known as the raphe. From the inside, the scrotum is divided into two sacs separated by a scrotal septum with a testicle in each (see Figure 13.2).

The location of the scrotum outside of the pelvic cavity, and its association with muscle fibres assists with maintaining the temperature of the testes at approximately 2–3 °C below core body temperature, which is the most favourable temperature for sperm production. The cremaster and dartos muscles respond to changes in temperature to regulate the temperature of the testes. In response to cold temperatures, the cremaster muscle contracts, moving the testes upwards towards the body where more body heat can be absorbed. Contraction of the dartos muscle tightens the scrotum around the testes to reduce heat loss. Conversely, when cooling is required, the cremaster muscle loosens and the testes are subsequently moved away from the heat of the body and cool down. The dartos muscle also loosens allowing for increased heat exchange and cooling.

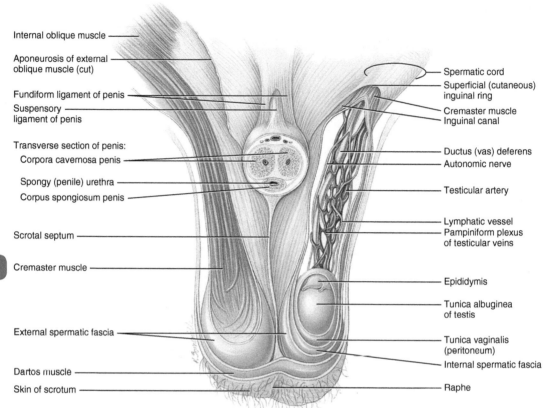

Internal oblique muscle

Aponeurosis of external oblique muscle (cut)

Fundiform ligament of penis

Suspensory ligament of penis

Transverse section of penis:
  Corpora cavernosa penis

  Spongy (penile) urethra
  Corpus spongiosum penis

Scrotal septum

Cremaster muscle

External spermatic fascia

Dartos muscle

Skin of scrotum

Spermatic cord
Superficial (cutaneous) inguinal ring
Cremaster muscle
Inguinal canal

Ductus (vas) deferens
Autonomic nerve

Testicular artery

Lymphatic vessel
Pampiniform plexus of testicular veins

Epididymis

Tunica albuginea of testis

Tunica vaginalis (peritoneum)
Internal spermatic fascia

Raphe

Anterior view of scrotum and testes and transverse section of penis

Figure 13.2 **The scrotum and testes.** *Source:* Tortora and Derrickson (2009). Reproduced with permission of John Wiley & Sons.

Episodes of Care Child

Anil, a 17-year-old, has been playing squash, and during the game his opponent's racquet hit him in the groin with some force. This winded Anil, who fell to the ground but recovered in order to continue playing the game. After the game ended he went for a shower, and the pain in the scrotal region was excruciating. He then noticed his left testicle was swollen and very tender to touch. He vomited and his lower abdomen 'felt like it was going to bust'. He was taken to the accident and emergency department where he was examined by a nurse practitioner who tried to manually rotate what he thought was torsion of the left testicle. However, the pain was so intense that a colour Doppler examination was performed. Anil was given intramuscular pain relief and an antiemetic. The findings confirmed the nurse's diagnosis of left testicular torsion. Anil then underwent detorsion and orchidopexy.

It is important that once diagnosis has been confirmed that surgery takes place as soon as possible to reduce ischaemia and to preserve function and fertility. Complications of an untreated or delayed torsion include infarction of the testicle along with subsequent atrophy, infection and cosmetic deformity. There is evidence that the contralateral (not torted) testis can also be negatively affected after unilateral testicular torsion and detorsion (Shimizu *et al.*, 2016).

Multiple Choice Questions

1. Testicular torsion occurs most commonly in
    (a) neonates
    (b) adolescents
    (c) middle-aged men
    (d) elderly men

342

2. The primary role of the cremasteric reflex is
   (a) prevention of testicular torsion
   (b) to assist with ejaculation
   (c) to prevent chaffing during walking and running
   (d) thermoregulation and temperature control
3. Which of the following urological disorders requires emergency care?
   (a) urinary tract infection
   (b) orchitis
   (c) testicular torsion
   (d) all of the above
4. A 17-year-old male presents with sudden onset of pain and swelling of the right testis. He reports having regular unprotected sex with multiple partners. Physical examination finds an absent cremasteric reflex. What is the next step in management of this patient?
   (a) urinalysis and culture
   (b) antibiotic treatment for sexually transmitted diseases
   (c) ice pack and scrotal support
   (d) colour Doppler examination
5. Which of the following statements about testicular torsion is TRUE?
   (a) manual detorsion is commonly used as a definitive treatment
   (b) it is often caused by epididymitis
   (c) it is a surgical emergency
   (d) it can be treated with high doses of antibiotics

The Testes

During the development of male fetuses *in utero*, the testes first appear in the abdominal cavity, then before birth they traverse the inguinal canal and enter the scrotal sac. The testes are suspended in the scrotal sac, hanging one on either side of the penis, usually with one hanging lower than the other. Production of viable sperm requires a temperature approximately 2 °C lower than the normal body temperature, and for this reason the testes in the scrotal sac are external to the body.

The key functions of the testes are to:

- produce sperm (spermatozoa);
- produce the male sex hormones (e.g. testosterone).

The testes are small oval-shaped organs measuring approximately 5 cm long and 2.5 cm wide with a layer of serous fibrous connective tissue surrounding them. There are three layers that cover the testes:

1. tunica vaginalis
2. tunica albuginea
3. tunica vasculosa.

The testes are divided into approximately 250–300 compartments or lobules. Inside each compartment is a collection of tightly coiled hollow tubes known as the seminiferous tubules, which are the site of sperm production (see Figure 13.3). There are spaces located between the tubules, and in these spaces is a cluster of cells called the interstitial or Leydig cells that synthesise and secrete the hormone testosterone, as well as other androgens.

The seminiferous tubules have an outer layer of smooth muscle and an inner layer composed of Sertoli cells and developing sperm cells. Sperm cells, in their various stages of development, slowly make their way through the spaces between adjacent Sertoli cells until they are released into the lumen of the seminiferous tubule. Sertoli cells nurture and control the developing sperm, and are therefore sometimes referred to as the nurse cells or mother cells. Some of the key functions of Sertoli cells include stimulation of sperm proliferation and differentiation, provision of nutrients for developing sperm, phagocytosis of defective sperm, and secretion of fluid and proteins into the lumen of the seminiferous tubule.

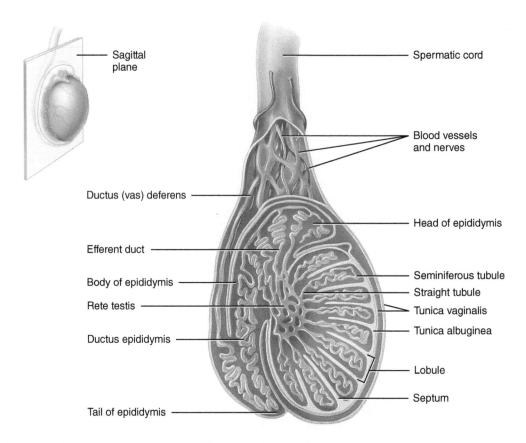

Sagittal plane

Spermatic cord

Blood vessels and nerves

Ductus (vas) deferens

Head of epididymis

Efferent duct

Body of epididymis

Seminiferous tubule

Straight tubule

Rete testis

Tunica vaginalis

Tunica albuginea

Ductus epididymis

Lobule

Septum

Tail of epididymis

Figure 13.3 **A testicle demonstrating seminiferous tubules.** *Source:* Tortora and Derrickson (2009). Reproduced with permission of John Wiley & Sons.

Spermatogenesis

Sperm production occurs in the seminiferous tubules of the testes and is called spermatogenesis (see Figure 13.4). Spermatogenesis usually commences around puberty and continues for the rest of a man's life, with most men producing between 50–200 million sperm every day.

Spermatogenesis is a complex activity that takes approximately 74 days in humans. Spermatogenesis begins with the mitotic division of spermatogonia, undifferentiated stem cells that are located close to the basement membrane. Spermatogonia contain the diploid ($2n = 46$) number of chromosomes and divide continually by mitosis to produce primary spermatocytes that are also diploid ($2n = 46$). Some spermatogonia remain close to the basement membrane of the seminiferous tubule, acting as a pool of undifferentiated stem cells for future sperm production.

Primary spermatocytes (with 46 chromosomes) then undergo the first division of meiosis to form haploid secondary spermatocytes with 23 chromosomes each. Each secondary spermatocyte then undergoes a second meiotic division to form spermatids. As a result of these meiotic divisions, each primary spermatocyte (containing 46 chromosomes) has gone on to produce four spermatids, each containing 23 chromosomes. The final stage of spermatogenesis is the differentiation of round spermatids into elongated sperm cells that are released into the lumen of the seminiferous tubule.

The sperm cells have 23 chromosomes each, which is half the number of a normal human cell. When the sperm unites with an ovum (also containing 23 chromosomes) at fertilisation, the result of conception (conceptus) will have the required 46 chromosomes.

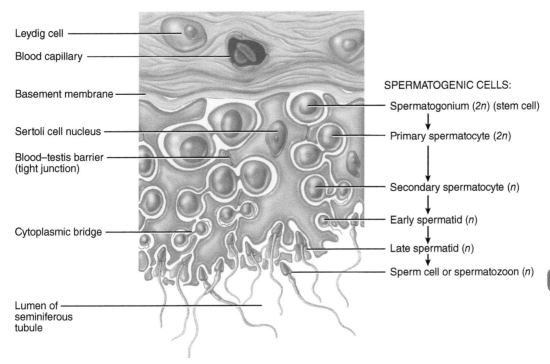

Leydig cell

Blood capillary

Basement membrane

Sertoli cell nucleus

Blood–testis barrier (tight junction)

Cytoplasmic bridge

Lumen of seminiferous tubule

SPERMATOGENIC CELLS:

Spermatogonium (2n) (stem cell)

Primary spermatocyte (2n)

Secondary spermatocyte (n)

Early spermatid (n)

Late spermatid (n)

Sperm cell or spermatozoon (n)

345

Figure 13.4 **Stages of spermatogenesis.** *Source:* Tortora and Derrickson (2009). Reproduced with permission of John Wiley & Sons.

Clinical Considerations Cryptorchidism

Undescended testes (cryptorchidism) is a common childhood condition where the child is born without both testes in the scrotal sac. In the majority of cases no action will be required, as the testes will migrate down into the scrotum during the first 3–6 months. There are, however, a small number of cases where the testes remain undescended unless treated. Current recommendations are that a diagnosis of congenital cryptorchidism should be confirmed at 3–6 months of age and orchidopexy done at 6–12 months of age (Holland et al., 2016).

In utero the testes develop inside the child's abdomen prior to slowly moving down into the scrotal sac from about 2 months before birth. The exact reason why some boys are born with undescended testes is not fully understood, but risk factors that have been identified include a relationship with low birth weight, being born prematurely (before the 37th week of pregnancy) and having a family history of undescended testicles.

In most cases, the testicle(s) will move down into the scrotum naturally; if this is not the case, treatment is usually recommended (e.g. orchidopexy). Boys with undescended testicles may have problems associated with fertility, and there is also an increased risk of the boy developing testicular cancer.

Sperm

There are approximately 200 million sperm produced every day (Tortora and Derrickson, 2012). Each sperm cell is equipped with structural specialisations that allow it to reach the site of fertilisation and penetrate the ovum; the elongated tail assists with movement, the midpiece contains the mitochondria necessary to provide energy; the head contains the genetic material and is covered by an acrosomal cap that contains enzymes to assist the sperm with penetration of the egg cellular and non-cellular coverings that surround the ovum (see Figure 13.5).

After sperm are released into the lumen of the seminiferous tubules, they move towards the rete testes, a network of interconnected tubes that empty into a single tube called the epididymis.

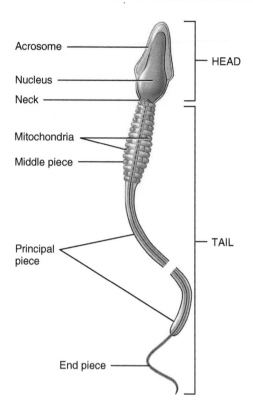

Figure 13.5 **Components of a sperm.** *Source:* Tortora and Derrickson (2009). Reproduced with permission of John Wiley & Sons.

Epididymis

The epididymis is a long and highly coiled duct that is loosely attached to the testis; it is lined with pseudostratified columnar epithelium and surrounded by a layer of smooth muscle. If it were fully uncoiled, each human epididymis would stretch to approximately 5 metres in length. As sperm travel, they travel through highly coiled duct that constitutes the epididymis they develop the ability to move spontaneously and actively (motility).

Transport of sperm through the epididymis usually takes 1–2 weeks in humans and is required in order for sperm to develop motility and the ability to fertilise an ovum. Sperm can also be stored in the epididymis and then released via peristaltic activity as the smooth muscle contracts during sexual arousal, moving the sperm along the epididymis into the vas deferens. Sperm stored in the epididymis can remain there for several weeks; those sperm that are not ejaculated are eventually reabsorbed.

The epididymis leads to the larger and more muscular duct called the vas deferens.

The Vas Deferens, Spermatic Cord and Ejaculatory Duct

The vas deferens (plural vasa deferentia), also referred to as the ductus deferens, is less convoluted than the epididymis and has a larger diameter, and the length of the vas deferens is approximately 45 cm (Tortora and Derrickson, 2012). This tube contains ciliated epithelium and is surrounded by a thick muscle layer. The vas deferens carries sperm from the scrotum, through a slit-like passage in the abdominal wall called the inguinal canal, to the abdominal cavity. Between the scrotal sac and the inguinal canal is the spermatic cord, a supporting structure consisting of the vas deferens as it ascends through the scrotum, blood vessels and nerves (Colbert *et al.*, 2012).

There are two vasa deferentia, one arising from each testicle, that join at the base of the urinary bladder. Each vas deferens merges with one seminal vesicle to form the ejaculatory ducts. The ejaculatory ducts connect to the urethra, where the sperm will be ejaculated during orgasm as a result of sexual intercourse or masturbation. After the sperm are ejaculated it is unusual for it to survive longer than 48 hours within the female reproductive tract.

The Seminal Vesicles and Prostate Gland

The seminal vesicles and prostate gland also secrete most of the fluids that are found in the ejaculate. The fluid secreted is a milky alkaline fluid providing a friendly environment for sperm to survive, preparing them for survival in the acidity of the vagina.

There are a pair of seminal vesicles, each about 5 cm in length, that lie at the base of the urinary bladder. Secretions from the seminal vesicles are released into the ejaculatory duct and account for approximately two-thirds of the volume of semen. The secretions include fructose (a sugar) as an energy source for sperm and a clotting protein that helps semen to coagulate after ejaculation.

The prostate is a single doughnut-shaped gland approximately the size of a walnut, measuring about 4 cm. It goes around the urethra under the urinary bladder and is made of 20–30 glands enclosed in smooth muscle (Marieb, 2012).

The prostate consists of three distinct zones:

- the central zone
- the peripheral zone
- the transition zone.

Secretions of the prostate gland compose approximately one-third of the volume of the semen; the fluid helps sperm motility and to maintain viability. Prostatic fluid is slightly acidic (pH 6.5). Prostatic secretions enter the urethra via a number of ducts during ejaculation.

The Penis

The penis is the male copulatory organ. The penis encloses the urethra and is a highly vascular organ. This organ is the passageway for excretion of urine as well as the ejaculation of semen. The penis has a shaft and a tip known as the glans, and in the uncircumcised male this is covered by the prepuce (also called the foreskin). The attached portion of the penis is known as the root, and the freer moving part is called the shaft or the body.

The penis is cylindrical in shape, composed of three cylindrical masses of tissues surrounded by fibrous tissue called the tunica albuginea. There are two masses of corpora cavernosa, and the corpus spongiosum which contains the spongy urethra (see Figure 13.6).

The penis is usually flaccid and hangs down, but during sexual excitation it becomes erect (an erection), swollen, engorged with blood, firmer and straighter. The erection reflex depends upon stimulation of the

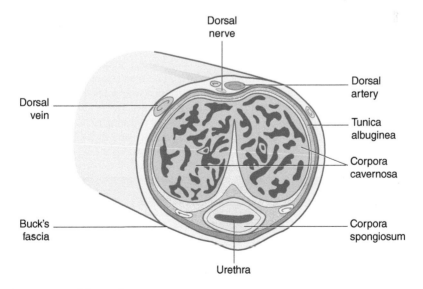

Figure 13.6 **The anatomy of the penis.** *Source:* Peate (2009). Reproduced with permission of John Wiley & Sons.

parasympathetic nervous system can be incited by sight, touch, pressure, sounds, smells or visions of a sexual encounter. Following parasympathetic stimulation, the penis becomes erect as a result of blood filling erectile tissue in the corpora cavernosa and corpus spongiosum, permitting the penis to penetrate the vagina and deposit sperm (ejaculation) as close to the site of fertilisation as possible.

When ejaculation has occurred, the arterioles vasoconstrict and the penis becomes flaccid.

Medicines Management Erectile Dysfunction

 Erectile dysfunction occurs when a man cannot get or maintain an erection that allows sexual activity with penetration. There are a number of treatments for this condition. One works by preventing the action of a chemical in the body called phosphodiesterase type 5. Viagra (sildenafil) is one example; it improves the blood flow to the penis following sexual stimulation. Before taking sildenafil, the prescriber needs to know if the person has:

- any disease, injury or deformity of the penis;
- any heart or blood vessel disease;
- a gastric condition that causes bleeding;
- an eye condition causing loss of vision;
- hypotension or angina;
- liver or kidney problems;
- had a stroke or a heart attack;
- sickle-cell disease;
- ever had an allergic reaction to sildenafil or to any other medicine.

Sildenafil should be taken as prescribed:

One (25–100 mg) tablet should be taken 1 h before the man plans to have sex. The medication can be taken before or after food, but may take longer to work if taken with food. Sildenafil should not be taken more frequently than once a day.

See Hackett *et al.* (2018); Australian Medicines Handbook (2019).

Hormonal Control of Male Reproduction

Testicular functions, including sperm production are under hormonal control.

The male sex hormones are known as androgens. The majority of androgens are produced in the testes, although the cortical region of the adrenal gland is also responsible for producing a small amount. Testosterone is the main androgen produced by the testes. This hormone is essential for the growth and maintenance of the male sexual organs as well as the secondary sex characteristics (e.g. pitch of voice, musculature and body hair) and for effective spermatogenesis. It also encourages metabolism, growth of muscles and bone, as well as libido (sexual desire).

Apart from a small amount of testosterone secreted by the testes *in utero, testosterone levels remain low throughout childhood,* until the male reaches puberty. With the onset of puberty the hypothalamus intensifies its secretion of gonadotrophin-releasing hormone (GnRH). The release of GnRH stimulates the anterior pituitary gland to release luteinising hormone (LH), which in turn stimulates the Leydig cells in the testis to produce testosterone. As the levels of testosterone increase, it has a negative feedback effect on the hypothalamus resulting in reduced secretion of GnRH, and on the pituitary resulting in reduced secretion of LH. This negative feedback mechanism involving the hypothalamus, pituitary and testes controls the levels of secretion of testosterone in the blood and the production of sperm (spermatogenesis) (see Figure 13.7).

The Female Reproductive System

The female reproductive system is designed to produce ova, receive the penis during intercourse and the sperm that has been ejaculated, store, contain and nourish a foetus, and feed the newborn after birth with breast milk. Usually, each month, a woman's body (during puberty to menopause) prepares itself to become pregnant. If pregnancy does not happen then a menstrual period occurs and the cycle recommences.

The organs of the female reproductive system include the ovaries, oviducts (fallopian tubes), uterus, vagina, and the external genitalia known collectively as the vulva.

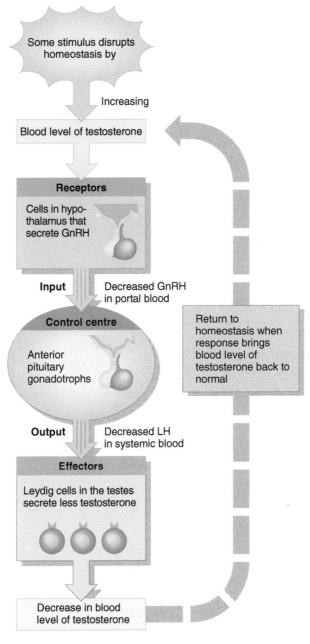

Figure 13.7 **Negative feedback system associated with the control of testosterone in the blood.** *Source:* Tortora and Derrickson (2009). Reproduced with permission of John Wiley & Sons.

The breasts are also a part of the female reproductive organs. Unlike in men, the urethra and urinary meatus are not part of the reproductive organs in women; nevertheless, they are very close in proximity and, as such, health problems that may affect one can often affect the other. Figure 13.8 demonstrates the location of the female reproductive organs.

The Ovaries

The ovaries are the female gonads; they are paired almond-shaped glands located on either side of the uterus. A collection of ligaments holds them in position; the ovarian ligament attaches the ovaries to the uterus, and

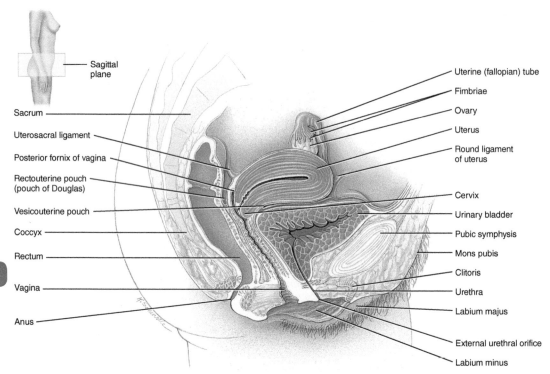

Figure 13.8 **The female reproductive system.** *Source: Tortora and Derrickson (2009). Reproduced with permission of John Wiley & Sons.*

the suspensory ligament attaches them to the pelvic wall. The ovaries provide a space of storage for the female germ cells; they also produce the female hormones oestrogen and progesterone. A woman's total number of ova is present at her birth; when a girl reaches puberty she usually ovulates each month.

The ovary contains a number of small structures called ovarian follicles. Each follicle contains an immature ovum, called an oocyte. Monthly, follicles are stimulated by two hormones, follicle-stimulating hormone (FSH) and luteinizing hormone (LH), which stimulate the follicles to mature, leading to the release of a mature ovum at ovulation.

Follicles are not evenly distributed throughout the ovary; they are restricted to the ovarian cortex or outer region of the ovary, surrounded by dense irregular connective tissue. The ovarian medulla, or inner portion of the ovary, contains blood vessels, nerves and lymphatic tissues surrounded by loose connective tissue. There is an unclear border between the ovarian cortex and medulla.

Oogenesis and Follicular Development

The term oogenesis refers to the formation of the female gametes in the ovary. Oogonia are diploid ($2n$) stem cells (Stanfield, 2017) that form during foetal development; they go on to increase in size to form primary oocytes that begin the first stage of meiosis before birth (Figure 13.9). Females are therefore born with their entire lifetime supply of gametes, unlike males that continue to produce spermatozoa throughout their adult life. Primary oocytes remain arrested in the first stage of meiosis until puberty, when the correct hormonal conditions are established for further development of the follicle and the ovum that it contains. At this stage the primary oocyte is surrounded by a single layer of follicle cells, and the structure is known as a primordial follicle (see Figure 13.10).

Every month, from puberty until menopause, FSH and LH are released by the anterior pituitary gland and stimulate follicle growth and maturation. A few primordial follicles start growing each month in response to FSH and LH, developing into a secondary follicle with increased numbers of follicle cells that secrete fluid that builds up in a cavity within the follicle (figure 13.10). The fluid filled cavity within the developing follicle is called an antrum. Follicles at this stage of development are called Graafian follicles. It is at this stage, just before ovulation, that the diploid primary oocyte completes the first meiotic division to produce a haploid secondary oocyte and a polar body. The polar body contains very little cytoplasm, and essentially acts as a dumping site for the nuclear material not required by the developing ovum. The secondary oocyte becomes arrested during the second meiotic division, which is only completed if the ovum becomes fertilised.

The Graafian follicle also manufactures oestrogen; this stimulates the growth of endometrium. Usually only one Graafian follicle will reach the maturity required to release an oocyte each month. This is called ovulation.

Episodes of Care Learning Disabilities

Women with learning disabilities face the same reproductive and sexual health issues as other women, and have the right to make their own informed decisions about contraception and other aspects of their sexual health care. Some of the barriers that women with a learning disability face when acessing reproductive health care include lack of information about their options and difficulty communicating with clinicians, raising the topic of sexual health and privacy issues (Greenwood et al., 2014).

It is important to broach the topic of sexual health primary when treating women with a learning disability, and to respect their autonomy and privacy by requesting family members to leave the room if it is appropriate and desired by the patient. Women with an ID are at a higher risk for sexual abuse, so it is appropriate to include a discussion of consensual sexual activity versus sexual abuse. With regard to contraception, it is important to determine whether it is requested for prevention of pregnancy or other reasons such as management of the menstrual cycle in order to identify the most approriate method for each woman. This discussion will also be useful in making a decision about whether to screen for cervical cancer and sexually transmitted infections. More information and recommendations for providing sexual and reproductive health services to women with an learning disabilites in primary care can be found in Greenwood and Wilkinson (2013).

The most important principle when providing reproductive health care for women with a learning disability is to respond to patients with repect with careful attention to the individual's needs and priorities. The American College of Obstetricians and Gynecologists (2009) hosts an interactive site for clinicians serving women with disabilities to assist with their provision of reproductive health services.

Multiple Choice Questions

1. When offering care and support with regards to the sexual health needs of people with learning disabilities, the nurse should:
   (a) ensure the parent(s) are present during the consultation
   (b) use clear, plain, language, large text and photographs
   (c) never use terms that are considered to be 'street talk'
   (d) never use explicit illustrations
2. In providing sexual health advice to an adult person with a learning disability:
   (a) you must always seek the written permission of the parent(s)
   (b) you should never offer the person emergency contraception unless the parent(s) have agreed with this and in writing
   (c) you should always have another health care provider with you as you offer any advice
   (d) it is important to try to match the educator to the person's gender, culture, ethnicity or sexuality
3. People with learning disabilities:
   (a) have the same sexual needs as the rest of the population
   (b) find the expression of sexuality complex
   (c) have individual needs
   (d) all of the above
4. People with learning disabilities tend to have:
   (a) an inability to make decisions about their sexual relationships
   (b) poor sexual knowledge and their sexual experiences tend to occur in unsafe environments due to restrictions in, and the prohibition of, relationships
   (c) a reduced libido
   (d) more STIs than the population as a whole
5. Traditionally, the sexual rights of people with learning disabilities have:
   (a) been unacknowledged and neglected
   (b) been acknowledged and provided for
   (c) always been given the consideration that they deserve
   (d) been found to meet the needs of this population

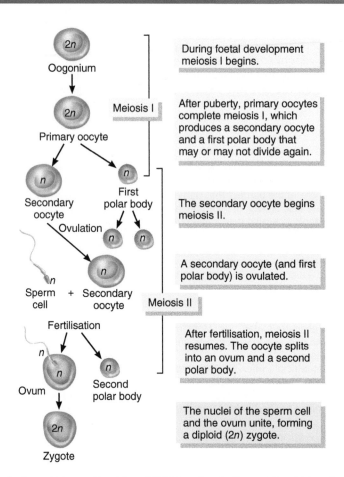

During foetal development meiosis I begins.

After puberty, primary oocytes complete meiosis I, which produces a secondary oocyte and a first polar body that may or may not divide again.

The secondary oocyte begins meiosis II.

A secondary oocyte (and first polar body) is ovulated.

After fertilisation, meiosis II resumes. The oocyte splits into an ovum and a second polar body.

The nuclei of the sperm cell and the ovum unite, forming a diploid (2n) zygote.

Figure 13.9 **Oogenesis.** *Source:* Tortora and Derrickson (2009). Reproduced with permission of John Wiley & Sons.

Corpus Luteum

The remnants of a large ruptured follicle become a new structure called the corpus luteum.

The corpus luteum produces two hormones, oestrogen and progesterone, with the aim of supporting the endometrium until conception takes place or the cycle starts again. The corpus luteum gradually disintegrates and a scar is left on the outside of the ovary that is called the corpus albicans.

The Role of the Female Sex Hormones

Oestrogens, progesterone and androgens are produced by the ovaries in a repetitive pattern. Although oestrogens are secreted all the way through the menstrual cycle, they are at their highest level just prior to the ovulation stage of the cycle.

Oestrogens are essential for the development and maintenance of secondary sex characteristics; and, working in combination with a number of other hormones, they stimulate the female reproductive system to prepare for growth of a foetus (LeMone and Burke, 2011). Oestrogens have a key role to play in the usual structure of the skin and blood vessels. They also help to reduce the rate of bone resorption (bone breakdown), enhance increased high-density lipoproteins, decrease cholesterol levels and increase blood clotting.

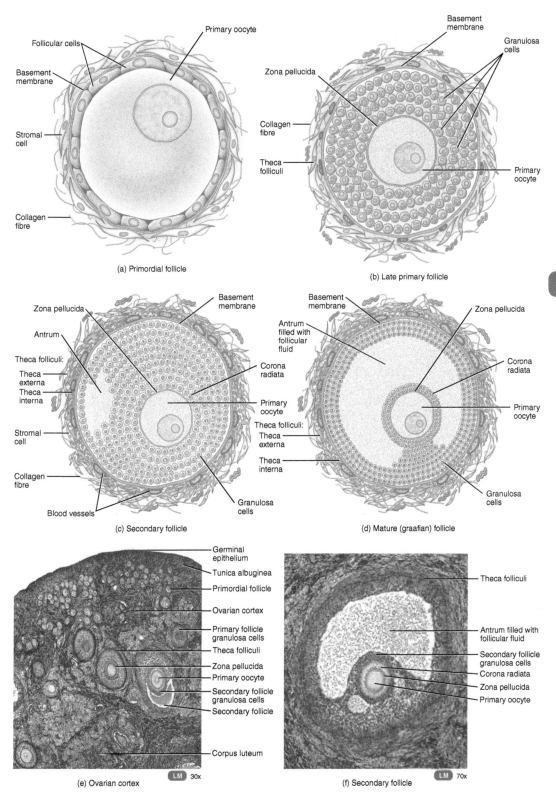

(a) Primordial follicle

(b) Late primary follicle

(c) Secondary follicle

(d) Mature (graafian) follicle

(e) Ovarian cortex

(f) Secondary follicle

Figure 13.10 (a–f) The developmental sequences associated with maturation of an ovum. *Source:* Tortora and Derrickson (2009). Reproduced with permission of John Wiley & Sons.

Medicines Management Contraception

The combined oral contraceptive pill (the pill) contains two hormones: an oestrogen and a progestogen. If taken correctly, it is a very effective form of contraception.

The pill alters the body's hormone balance so that ovulation does not occur. It causes the mucus made by the cervix to thicken and form a mucous plug. This makes it difficult for sperm to get through to the uterus to fertilise an egg. The pill also makes the lining of the uterus thinner. This makes it less likely that a fertilised egg will be able to attach to the uterus. Before taking the combined oral contraceptive pill the prescriber needs to know if the person has:

- unexplained vaginal bleeding
- current or recent breast cancer
- migraine, with or without aura
- diabetes mellitus
- smoking
- BMI>30
- systemic lupus erythematosus
- antiphospholipid syndrome
- hereditary angiodema
- recently given birth.

The pill should be taken at the same time every day.

See Australian Medicines Handbook (2019).

The Internal Organs

The internal organs of the female reproductive system are the vagina and cervix, uterus, oviducts (also known as fallopian tubes or uterine tubes) and ovaries. The ovaries (discussed earlier) are the primary reproductive organs in women, as well as producing female sex hormones. The vagina, uterus and fallopian tubes act as an accessory channel for the ovaries and the growing foetus.

The Uterus

This hollow organ is also known as the womb. It is a very muscular organ lying in the pelvic cavity posterior and superior to the urinary bladder; it lies anterior to the rectum (Figure 13.11 outlines the uterus and associated structures).

The uterus is approximately 7.5 cm long. There are three principal parts associated with the uterus:

- the **fundus**, a thick muscular region situated above the fallopian tubes;
- the **body**, the main portion of the uterus, joined to the cervix by an isthmus;
- the **cervix**, the narrowest part of the uterus opening out into the vagina.

As well as having three aspects or parts, the uterus also has three layers. The perimetrium is the outer serous layer, merging with the peritoneum. The middle layer is the myometrium and comprises most of the uterine wall. There are a number of muscle fibres in this layer running in a number of various directions; this arrangement allows contractions to occur during menstruation or childbirth and an increase in size as the foetus grows. The endometrium, the innermost layer, lines the uterus, and this layer is shed during menstruation. The three layers are summarised in Table 13.1.

The Fallopian Tubes

The paired Fallopian tubes (also known as oviducts, salpinges, or uterine tubes) are delicate, thin cylindrical structures approximately 8–14 cm long (Marieb, 2012). They are affixed to the uterus at one end and are supported by the broad ligaments. The lateral ends of the Fallopian tubes are open and made of projections called fimbriae that drape over the ovary. The fimbriae pick up the ovum after it is discharged from the ovary.

The Fallopian tubes have a layer of smooth muscle and are lined with ciliated, mucus-producing epithelial cells. The actions of the cilia and contractions of the smooth muscle transport the ovum along the tubes onwards to the uterus. It is in the end of the fallopian tube closest to the ovary where the fertilisation of the ovum by the sperm usually occurs.

The term adnexa is used collectively when discussing the Fallopian tubes, ovaries and supporting tissues.

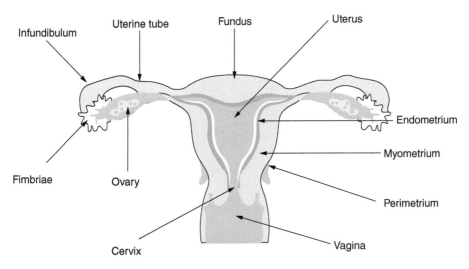

Figure 13.11 **The uterus and associated structures.** *Source:* Nair and Peate (2009). Reproduced with permission of John Wiley & Sons.

Table 13.1 **The layers of the uterus.**

LAYER	COMMENTS
Perimetrium	A serous membrane enveloping the uterus; this is the outer layer. It provides support to the uterus located within the pelvis. This may also be known as the parietal peritoneum.
Myometrium	This layer is the middle layer and is composed of smooth muscle. During pregnancy and childbirth, the uterus is required to stretch and the muscular layer allows this to happen. The muscle will contract during labour, and postnatally this muscular layer contracts forcefully to force out the placenta. The contractions also help to control potential blood loss after birth.
Endometrium	The endometrium is the mucous membrane lining the inside of the uterus. The endometrium changes throughout the menstrual cycle. It becomes thick and rich with blood vessels to prepare for pregnancy. If the woman does not become pregnant then, part of the endometrium is shed, resulting in menstrual bleeding.

Source: Adapted from McGuinness (2010) and Waugh and Grant (2018).

Clinical Considerations Insertion of Intrauterine Contraceptive Device

An intrauterine device (IUD) is a small T-shaped plastic and copper device that is inserted into the uterus by a specially trained nurse or a doctor. The IUD works by preventing the sperm and egg from surviving in the uterus or fallopian tubes; it can also prevent a fertilised egg from implanting in the uterus.

There are different types of IUD; some contain more copper than others. Those IUDs with more copper are more than 99% effective. Copper changes the make-up of the fluids in the uterus and fallopian tubes. IUDs with less copper will be less effective. There are types and sizes of IUD to suit different women; they can be inserted at the GP surgery, local contraception clinic or sexual health clinic. An IUD can be inserted at any time, though it may be easier when the woman is menstruating, as the cervix is slightly open at that time.

A metal or plastic speculum is gently inserted into the vagina in order to see the cervix. The cervix is wiped with a special cleanser. Next, a small 'sound' (probe-like instrument) is inserted to measure the length of the uterus. The IUD is then inserted using a very small straw. The IUD has a string attached to one end. The nurse or doctor will trim the IUD string that is coming through the cervix into the vagina. The string allows the woman to check that the IUD is in place (see Figure 13.12).

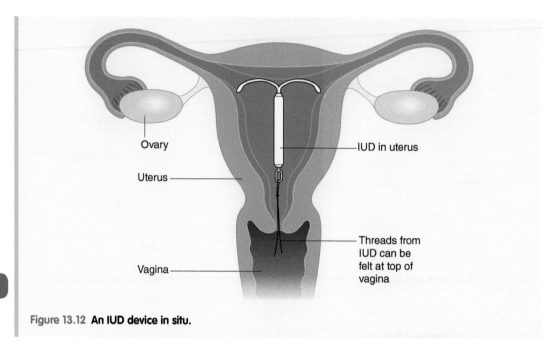

Figure 13.12 **An IUD device in situ.**

The Vagina

The vagina is a tubular, fibromuscular structure approximately 8–10 cm in length (Jenkins and Tortora, 2012) with several functions; it is the receptacle for the penis during sexual intercourse, an organ of sexual response, the canal that allows the menstrual flow to leave the body, and the passage for the birth of the child. The vagina is situated posterior to the urinary bladder and urethra; it is anterior to the rectum. The upper element contains the uterine cervix in an area that is known as the fornix. The vaginal walls are made of membranous folds of tissue called the rugae. These membranes are made up of mucus-secreting stratified squamous epithelial cells.

Usually, the walls of the vagina are moist and have a pH ranging from 3.8 to 4.2. This pH inhibits the growth of bacteria (it is bacteriostatic) and is maintained by the action of the hormone oestrogen and healthy vaginal microorganisms (the normal vaginal flora). Oestrogen stimulates the growth of vaginal mucosal cells, making them thicken and develop and increase glycogen content. The glycogen is fermented to lactic acid by lactobacilli (organisms that produce lactic acid) that usually live in the vagina, causing slight acidifying of the vaginal fluid (LeMone and Burke, 2011).

Medicines Management Atrophic Vaginitis

Many women notice changes in their vagina and genital area after the menopause. These changes may include dryness (atrophic vaginitis) and discomfort during sex. These can often be improved with treatment. Treatment options include hormone replacement therapy (HRT), oestrogen cream or pessaries and lubricating gels.

HRT means taking oestrogen in the form of a tablet, gel or patches. This is often the best treatment for relieving symptoms. As with all medications, there are advantages and disadvantages of using HRT. Precaution with use of HRT is advised for women with:

- breast cancer or other oestrogen dependent tumour
- unexplained vaginal bleeding
- history of endometriosis or uterine fibroids
- migraine
- diabetes mellitus
- epilepsy

- smoking
- systemic lupus erythematosus
- hereditary angioedema.

Sometimes a cream, pessary or vaginal tablet or ring containing oestrogen is prescribed. A pessary is inserted into the vagina using a small applicator. The ring is a soft, flexible ring with a centre containing oestrogen, releasing a steady, low dose of oestrogen, it lasts for 3 months. Oestrogen creams and pessaries can damage latex condoms and diaphragms.

If vaginal dryness is the only problem, or hormone creams are not recommended, lubricating gels may help, e.g. Replens®, Sylk® and Hyalofemme®.

See Australian Medicines Handbook (2019).

The Cervix

The cervix projects into the vagina and forms a pathway between the uterus and the vagina. The uterine opening of the cervix is known as the internal os, and the vaginal opening called the external os. The space between these openings, the endocervical canal, acts as a conduit for the discharge of menstrual fluid, the opening for sperm and delivery of the infant during birth. The cervix is a rigid structure, protected by mucus that alters in consistency and quantity during the uterine cycle and during pregnancy.

Skills in Practice Vaginal Swab

A vaginal swab test involves taking a sample of vaginal secretions to test for the presence of a genital tract infection. The secretions are collected with a device that looks like a cotton bud; it is then placed in a special container and sent to the microbiology laboratory for further analysis. This procedure can be used to test for chlamydia and gonorrhea, as well as fungal and bacterial infections such as candida albicans and bacterial vaginosis.

A full medical and sexual history should be obtained, and the procedure must be explained. Offer a chaperone to all women and obtain informed consent before the procedure is commenced.

Ensure that the patient's bladder is empty and position her in a dorsal position with knees flexed and hips abducted. Depending upon local protocols, a speculum may be used. The sterile swab is carefully inserted into the inside opening of the vagina, and gently rotated against the sides of the vagina for 10–30 seconds. The sterile swab is inserted approximately 5 cm into the vagina for a high vaginal swab, and approximately 1–2 cm for a low vaginal swab. The patient may prefer to collect her own low vaginal swab, with instructions from the medical or nursing staff. The swab is then withdrawn without touching the skin and placed into a collection tube containing transport medium. The samples should reach the pathology lab within 24 hours for optimal culture results.

The External Genitalia

Collectively, the external genitalia are known as the vulva. They include the mons pubis, the labia, the clitoris, the vaginal and urethral openings, and glands (LeMone and Burke, 2011).

The mons pubis is a pad of elevated adipose tissue covered with skin that lies anteriorly to the symphysis pubis to provide cushioning. After puberty, the mons is covered with coarse pubic hair.

The labia are divided into two structures. The labia majora are the outermost folds of skin that begin at the base of the mons pubis and terminate at the anus. They are covered with pubic hair and contain an abundance of adipose tissue. The labia minora, situated between the clitoris and the base of the vagina, are enclosed by the labia majora. They are made of skin, adipose tissue and some erectile tissues with a number of sebaceous glands. They are usually light pink and are devoid of pubic hair.

The clitoris is composed of two small erectile bodies, the corposa cavernosa and several nerves and blood vessels. The glans clitoris is covered by a layer of skin called the clitorial prepuce (or clitoral hood) that is formed where the labia minora unite. The glans clitoris is the exposed portion of the clitoris and is likened to the glans penis in the male. This aspect of the external genitalia is capable of enlargement and has a role to play in sexual excitement in the woman.

Episodes of Care Adult

Patient X has arrived at the sexual health clinic complaining of discharge 'down below'. The nurse takes a history from the lady and is informed that five days ago she had her clitoral hood pierced and yesterday she was feeling very warm, generally unwell, nauseous and she has noticed a discharge from the vulval area and her underwear is stained. The nurse examines the patient and observes a yellow discharge, redness and swelling in the vulval area.

It is likely that this patient has a bacterial infection as a result of the piercing; she may also be having an allergic reaction to the metal that has been used.

Other complications associated with genital piercings can include haemorrhage, nerve damage and thick scarring at the piercing site. There is also the risk of contracting HIV, hepatitis B and C, sexually transmitted infections or other infections. These risks can be minimised with the use of a new, sterile needle as well using a reputable piercer. Using proper jewellery made out of metals such as surgical stainless steel or titanium can reduce the risk of infection and allergic reaction.

Persons with piercings should take care when using condoms – do not use the teeth to open the packet, and avoid damaging the condom with nails, jewellery or piercings.

See British Association for Sexual Health and HIV (2012) and Lee *et al.* (2018).

Multiple Choice Questions

1. The term vulva refers to the:
   (a) area covering the pubic bone
   (b) external genitals of the female
   (c) outer labial folds
   (d) inner labial folds
2. The labia minora join at the anterior of the vulva to form the
   (a) vaginal opening
   (b) labia majora
   (c) clitoral hood
   (d) external urethral orifice
3. HIV can be spread from contaminated needles when:
   (a) piercing ears
   (b) injecting steroids
   (c) piercing genitals
   (d) all of the above
4. Genital piercing may compromise the contraceptive efficacy of:
   (a) combined oral contraceptive
   (b) condoms
   (c) IUD
   (d) both b and c
5. The most common causative agents of infection associated with genital piercing include:
   (a) staphylococcus aureus
   (b) molluscum contagiosum
   (c) HIV
   (d) *N. gonorrhoeae* and *C. trachomatis*

The Breasts

The breasts are dome-shaped protrusions that differ in size between individuals; they are also sometimes called the mammary glands. The breasts are located between the third and seventh ribs on the anterior aspect chest wall. The breasts are supported by the pectoral muscles and are provided with a rich supply of nerves, blood vessels and lymph (see Figure 13.13). A pigmented area known as the areola is situated a little below the centre of each breast and contains glands that secrete sebum – a thick substance composed of fat and cell debris (sebaceous glands) – and a nipple. The nipple is usually protruding, becoming erect in response to cold and stimulation.

The breasts are made of adipose (fat) tissue, fibrous connective tissue and milk-producing glandular tissue. There are bands of fibrous tissue that support the breast and extend from the outer breast tissue to the nipple, dividing the breast into 15 to 25 lobes. The lobes are comprised of alveolar glands joined by ducts that open out on to the nipple. A hormone called prolactin controls the production of milk.

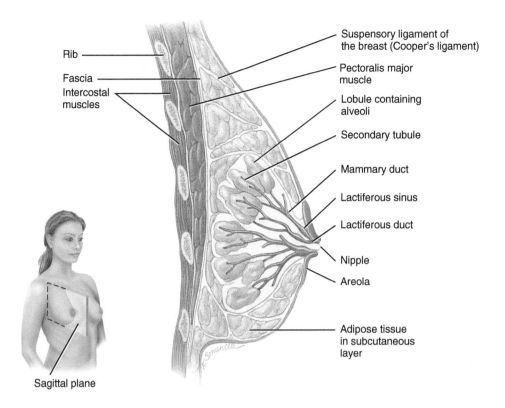

Rib

Fascia

Intercostal
muscles

Suspensory ligament of
the breast (Cooper's ligament)

Pectoralis major
muscle

Lobule containing
alveoli

Secondary tubule

Mammary duct

Lactiferous sinus

Lactiferous duct

Nipple

Areola

Adipose tissue
in subcutaneous
layer

Sagittal plane

Sagittal section

Figure 13.13 **The breast.** *Source:* Tortora and Derrickson (2009). Reproduced with permission of John Wiley & Sons.

Skills in Practice Breast Examination

A clinical breast examination is an essential step to evaluate any woman with a breast symptom or lump and is therefore an important skill for medical and nursing practitioners. Women who present with breast pain, skin changes, nipple discharge, lumps or changes in size, shape or texture should undergo a thorough breast examination.

A thorough breast examination requires the woman to be undressed down to the waist, firstly in a seated position for visual inspection followed by laying in a supine position for palpation. The visual inspection is conducted with the woman in several positions (e.g. hands on hips and raised overhead) so that the size, shape, symmetry, texture and colour of the whole breast and nipple can be assessed. The palpation phase requires a meticulous and systematic approach to cover the entire extent of breast tissue, which usually covers most of the anterior chest wall. A variety of techniques exist to ensure complete palpation of the breast tissue including the 'spoke' or 'wagon wheel' method and the concentric circles method. The nipple areolar area should also be palpated for abnormalities, and for expressible nipple discharge.

After examination of the breast, the axilla and supraclavicular area should be palpated for lymph node enlargement.

See Powell (2009) and Henderson and Ferguson (2019).

The Uterine Cycle

The endometrium of the uterus responds to changes in oestrogen and progesterone during the ovarian cycle as it prepares for the implantation of a fertilised embryo. The endometrium is receptive to implantation of the embryo for only a brief period every month, coinciding with the time when the embryo would normally reach the uterus from the uterine tube (usually 7 days after ovulation).

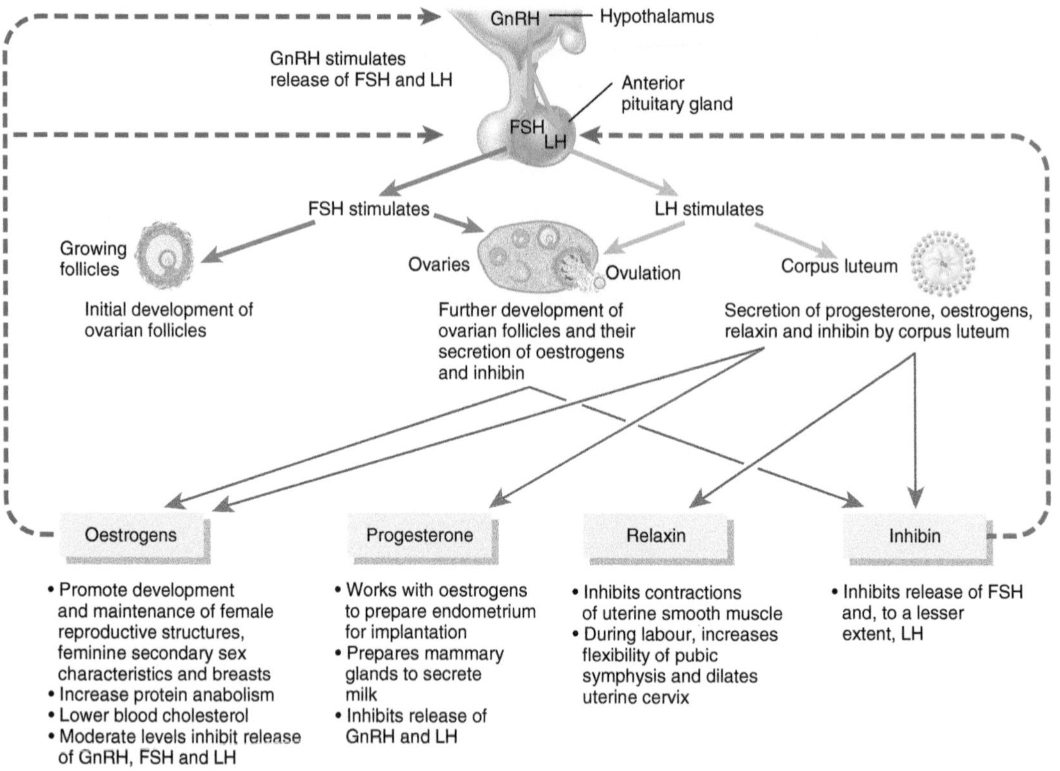

Figure 13.14 **The ovarian and uterine cycles.** *Source:* Tortora and Derrickson (2009). Reproduced with permission of John Wiley & Sons.

The menstrual cycle begins with the menstrual phase which lasts from days 1 to 5. During this time the inner functionalis layer of the uterine endometrium is released as menstrual fluid. As the growing follicle in the ovary begins to produce the hormone oestrogen (days 6 to 14), the proliferative phase of the uterine endometrium commences. During this time the functionalis layer thickens while at the same time spiral arteries multiply and tubular glands form (LeMone and Burke, 2011). Cervical mucus is produced in increasing amounts and becomes thin and stretchy, enabling sperm to penetrate it easily and travel up into the uterus.

The final phase of the uterine cycle, lasting from days 14 to 28, is the secretory phase. As the corpus luteum produces progesterone, the rising levels act on the endometrium, resulting in an increased vascularity, changing the inner layer to secretory mucosa, stimulating the secretion of glycogen into the uterine cavity. It also causes the cervical mucus to become thick again, blocking the passage of sperm. If an embryo has not implanted into the uterus by this stage, hormone levels will fall. Spasm of the spiral arteries causes hypoxia (lack of oxygen) of the endometrial cells, which begin to degenerate and then slough off. As with the ovarian cycle, the process begins again with the sloughing of the functionalis layer. Figure 13.14 demonstrates the ovarian and uterine cycles.

Episodes of Care Adult

An ectopic pregnancy occurs when an early embryo implants in a location other than the uterus, most commonly the uterine tubes. The symptoms of an ectopic pregnancy can include vaginal bleeding, lower left or right side abdominal pain and feeling faint or lightheaded.

Alice Smethwick has undergone laparoscopic surgery for ectopic pregnancy – a right salpingectomy. Alice is at home 2 days post-procedure and experiencing abdominal discomfort; she is also complaining of neck and shoulder pain. She makes an appointment to see the practice nurse.

The practice nurse explains to Alice that the gas (carbon dioxide) that was pumped into her abdominal cavity to allow the surgeon to identify the fallopian tubes has caused the abdominal discomfort. The neck and shoulder pain experienced by some people is also related to the laparoscopy and the carbon dioxide gas. The gas irritates the diaphragm and the phrenic nerve. It is explained to Alice that this pain will go away as the gas is absorbed. She is also told that lying down can also help decrease the pain.

See National Institute of Health and Care Excellence (2019).

Multiple Choice Questions

1. What is an ectopic pregnancy?
   (a) a pregnancy occurring in the uterine tubes
   (b) a pregnancy occurring in the abdominal cavity
   (c) a pregnancy occurring in the cervix
   (d) all of the above
2. The symptoms of an ectopic pregnancy commonly include
   (a) diarrhoea
   (b) dysuria
   (c) back pain
   (d) fainting
3. The risk factors for ectopic pregnancy include:
   (a) previous genital surgery
   (b) irritable bowel syndrome
   (c) polycystic ovary syndrome
   (d) body mass index of 35 or more
4. Following an ectopic pregnancy, a woman:
   (a) should not use a Mirena IUD
   (b) should not use the combined oral contraceptive pill
   (c) has a 3 fold increased risk of caesarian section compared to women who have not had a previous ectopic pregnancy
   (d) can try for another pregnancy when psychologically ready, with no time limit
5. Which of the following statements about laparoscopic surgery for ectopic pregnancy is true?
   (a) shoulder pain is common after surgery as diaphragmatic irritation causes referred pain
   (b) oxygen is usually used to inflate the abdominal cavity as it is safer than medicinal air
   (c) hydrotherapy in a hot tub will ease pain and reduce recovery time
   (d) most women will experience post-operative vaginal bleeding

Conclusion

The male and female reproductive systems are complex. All living things reproduce; fundamentally, organisms make more organisms akin to themselves. Without these reproductive systems human life would end; these systems are essential for life. In the human reproductive process, two types of sex cells, or gametes, are required. The male gamete, or sperm, and the female gamete, the egg or ovum, meet in the female's reproductive system to begin the creation of a new individual. Anatomical and physiological processes are required to ensure this marvel works effectively.

Sexual reproduction, the process of producing offspring for the survival of the species and passing on hereditary traits from one generation to the next, is the key function of the male and female reproductive systems. The male and female reproductive systems contribute to the events leading to fertilisation. The female organs take on responsibility for the developing human, birth and nourishment. The systems also provide pleasure, sexual pleasure and sexual excitement; for a number of people this is an important aspect of their being.

Glossary

Adrenal cortex: The outer portion of an adrenal gland.
Androgens: Masculinising male sex hormones produced by the testes in the male and the adrenal cortex in both sexes.
Anterior: Near to the front.

Anti-emetic: Anti-sickness medication.

Broad ligament: A double fold of parietal peritoneum attaching the uterus to the side of the pelvic cavity.

Canal: A channel or passageway, a narrow tube.

Connective tissue: The most prominent type of tissue in the body; this tissue provides support.

Corpus albicans: A whitish fibrous patch in the ovary formed after the corpus luteum regresses.

Corpus luteum: A yellowish body found in the ovary when a follicle has discharged its secondary oocyte.

Endometrium: The mucous membrane lining the uterus.

Foetus: The developing organism *in utero*.

Fimbriae: Finger-like structures found at the end of the fallopian tubes.

Follicle: A secretory sac or cavity containing a group of cells that contains a developing oocyte in the ovary.

Follicle-stimulating hormone: Secreted by the anterior pituitary gland; initiates the development of an ovum.

Gamete: A male or female sex cell.

Glans penis: The enlarged region at the end of the penis.

Gonad: A gland that produces hormones and gametes – in men the testes, in females the ovaries.

Gonadotrophic hormone: Anterior pituitary hormone affecting the gonads.

Haploid: Having half the number of chromosomes.

Hormone: A secretion of endocrine cells that alters the physiological activity of target cells.

Human chorionic gonadotrophin: A hormone produced by the developing placenta.

Inguinal canal: Passage in the lower abdominal wall in the male.

Inhibin: A hormone secreted by the gonads inhibiting the release of FSH by the anterior pituitary.

In utero: Within the uterus.

Isthmus: A narrow strip of tissue or a narrow passage connecting to bigger parts.

Lateral: Farthest from the midline of the body.

Leydig cell: A type of cell that secretes testosterone.

Ligament: Dense regular connective tissue.

Luteinising hormone: A hormone secreted by the anterior pituitary stimulates ovulation and prepares glands in the breast to produce milk. Stimulates testosterone secretion in the testes.

Meatus: A passage or opening.

Meiosis: A kind of cell division occurring during the production of gametes.

Menopause: The termination of the menstrual cycles.

Myometrium: The smooth muscle layer of the uterus.

Oestrogens: Feminising sex hormones produced by the ovaries.

Orchidopexy: Surgery to move an undescended testicle into the scrotum and permanently fix it there

Oocyte: An immature egg cell.

Oogenesis: Formation and development of the female gametes.

Ovarian cycle: The ovarian cycle is a series of events in the ovaries that occur during and after the maturation of the oocyte.

Ovarian follicle: A general name for immature oocytes.

Ovary: The female gonad.

Ovulation: The rupture of a mature Graafian follicle with discharge of a secondary oocyte after penetration by sperm.

Ovum: The female egg cell.

Penis: The organ of urination and copulation.

pH: A measure of acidity and alkalinity.

Phagocytosis: The process by which phagocytes ingest and destroy microbes, cell debris and other foreign matter.

Placenta: An organ attached to the lining of the uterus during pregnancy.

Progesterone: A female sex hormone produced by the ovaries.

Prolactin: A hormone secreted by the anterior pituitary that initiates and maintains milk production.

Rete: The network of ducts in the testes.

Scrotum: The skin-covered pouch containing the testes.

Semen: Fluid discharged by ejaculation.

Spermatogenesis: The maturation of spermatids into sperm.

Testes: The male gonads.

Testosterone: Male sex hormone.

Urethra: The tube from the urinary bladder to the exterior of the body that conveys urine in females and urine and semen in males.

Uterus: Hollow muscular organ in the female, also called the womb.

Vagina: A muscular tubular organ in the female leading from the uterus to the vestibule.

Vas deferens: The main secretory duct of the testicle, through which semen is carried from the epididymis to the prostatic urethra, where it ends as the ejaculatory duct.

Vulva: The female external genitalia.

References

American College of Obstetricians and Gynecologists (2009) Interactive site for clinicians serving women with disabilities https://www.acog.org/About-ACOG/ACOG-Departments/Women-with-Disabilities/Interactive-site-for-clinicians-serving-women-with-disabilities (accessed 13 May 2019).

Australian Medicines Handbook (2019) Australian Medicines Handbook Pty Ltd; Adelaide.

British Association for Sexual Health and HIV (2012) A BASHH Guide to Condoms. https://www.bashh.org/public/condoms/ (accessed 7 May 2019).

Colbert, B.J., Ankney, J. and Lee, K.T. (2012) *Anatomy and Physiology for Health Professionals. An Interactive Journey*, 2nd edn. Upper Saddle River, NJ: Pearson.

Greenwood, N.W. and Wilkinson, J. (2013) Sexual and reproductive health care for women with intellectual disabilities: a primary care perspective. *International Journal of Family Medicine* 2013: 642472. doi:10.1155/2013/642472

Greenwood, N.W., Ferrari, B., Bhakta, S., Ostrach, B. and Wilkinson, J. (2014) Experiences, beliefs and needs of women with intellectual disabilities in accessing their reproductive rights. *Contraception* 90: 348–349.

Hackett, G., Kirby, M., Wylie, K., Heald, A., Ossei-Gerning, N., Edwards, D. and Muneer A. (2018) British Society for Sexual Medicine Guidelines on the Management of Erectile Dysfunction in Men – 2017. *Journal of Sexual Medicine* 15: 430–457.

Henderson, J.A. and Ferguson, T. (2019) *Breast Examination Technique.* Treasure Island FL: StatPeals Publishing https://europepmc.org/books/NBK459179;jsessionid=9E47EC89EA23040DBC95267EA887C9C4 (accessed February 2020).

Holland, A.J., Nassar, N. and Schneuer, F.J. (2016) Undescended testes: an update. *Current Opinion in Pediatrics* 28(3): 388–394.

Jenkins, G.W. and Tortora, G.J. (2012) *Anatomy and Physiology. From Science to Life*, 3rd edn. Hoboken, NJ: John Wiley & Sons, Inc.

Lee, B., Vangipuram, R., Petersen, E., Tyring, S.K. (2018) Complications associated with intimate body piercings. *Dermatology Online Journal* 24(7): 2.

LeMone, P. and Burke, K. (2011) *Medical–Surgical Nursing. Critical Thinking in Client Care*, 5th edn. Upper Saddle River, NJ: Pearson.

Marieb, E.N. (2012) *Human Anatomy and Physiology*, 9th edn. San Francisco, CA: Pearson.

McGuinness, H. (2010) *Anatomy and Physiology. Therapy Basics*, 4th edn. London: Hodder.

Nair, M. and Peate, I. (2009) *Fundamentals of Applied Pathophysiology: An Essential Guide for Nursing Students.* Oxford: John Wiley & Sons, Ltd.

National Institute of Health and Care Excellence (2019) *Ectopic Pregnancy and Miscarriage: Diagnosis and Initial Management.* NICE guideline [NG126]. https://www.nice.org.uk/guidance/ng126 (accessed 7 May 2019).

Peate, I. (2009) *Men's Health.* Oxford: John Wiley & Sons, Ltd.

Powell RW (1990) Breast Examination. In: Walker HK, Hall WD, Hurst JW, editors. *Clinical Methods: The History, Physical, and Laboratory Examinations.* 3rd edition. Boston: Butterworths; Chapter 176. https://www.ncbi.nlm.nih.gov/books/NBK285/ (accessed 13 May 2019).

Shimizu, S., Tsounapi, P., Dimitriadis, F., Higashi, Y., Shimizu, T. and Saito, M. (2016) Testicular torsion–detorsion and potential therapeutic treatments: A possible role for ischemic postconditioning. *International Journal Urology* 23: 454–463.

Stanfield, C.L. (2017) *Principles of Human Physiology*, 6th edn. Boston, MA: Pearson.

Tortora, G.J. and Derrickson, B.H. (2009) *Principles of Anatomy and Physiology*, 12th edn. Hoboken, NJ: John Wiley & Sons, Inc.

Tortora, G.J. and Derrickson, B. (2012) *Essentials of Anatomy and Physiology*, 9th edn. New York: John Wiley & Sons, Inc.

Waugh, A. and Grant, A. (2018) *Ross and Wilson Anatomy and Physiology in Health and Illness*, 13th edn. Edinburgh: Churchill Livingstone.

Further Reading

Endometriosis
http://www.endometriosis-uk.org
https://www.endometriosisaustralia.org/
Charities dedicated to providing information on endometriosis and support for those affected by endometriosis.

Family Planning Associations
http://www.fpa.org.uk
https://www.fpnsw.org.au
Family Planning Associations provide straightforward information, advice and support on sexual health, sex and relationships.

Prostate Cancer

http://prostatecanceruk.org

https://www.ausprostatecancer.com.au/

Prostate Cancer UK and Prostate Cancer Australia aim to help men survive prostate cancer and enjoy a better quality of life. They offer support to men and provide information, fund research, raise awareness and improve care.

Women's Health

https://jeanhailes.org.au/

An Australian not-for-profit organisation dedicated to improving the knowledge of women's health throughout the various stages of their lives.

Activities

Multiple Choice Questions

1. The cell that is created by fertilisation is:
   - (a) the oocyte
   - (b) the zygote
   - (c) the sperm
   - (d) the semen

2. The sperm are stored and mature in:
   - (a) the epididymis
   - (b) the ova
   - (c) the testes
   - (d) the seminal vesicles
3. The primary male sex hormone is:
   - (a) testosterone
   - (b) oestrogen
   - (c) progesterone
   - (d) all of the above
4. The gland that releases a small amount of fluid prior to ejaculation is:
   - (a) the ejaculatory duct
   - (b) the prostate gland
   - (c) Cowper's gland
   - (d) the bulbourethral gland
5. The seminiferous tubules produce:
   - (a) semen
   - (b) inhibin
   - (c) follicle-stimulating hormone
   - (d) none of the above
6. The membranous walls of the vagina that form folds are called:
   - (a) vestibule
   - (b) fornix
   - (c) mons
   - (d) rugae
7. The surge in luteinising hormone that occurs during the middle of the ovarian cycle triggers:
   - (a) follicle maturation
   - (b) menopause
   - (c) menstruation
   - (d) ovulation
8. In which part of the breast is the milk actually produced?
   - (a) milk ducts
   - (b) areola
   - (c) alveoli
   - (d) Montgomery glands

9. What is the principal hormone secreted by the corpus luteum?
    (a) gonadotrophin releasing hormone (GnRH)
    (b) progesterone
    (c) testosterone
    (d) follicle Stimulating Hormone (FSH)
10. At what phase of the uterine cycle is endometrium is ready to receive the developing embryo?
    (a) follicular
    (b) proliferative
    (c) secretory
    (d) menstrual
11. The interstitial (or Leydig) cells produce _____.
    (a) testosterone
    (b) androgen binding protein
    (c) spermatocytes
    (d) spermatogonia
12. When are primary oocytes formed?
    (a) as the woman reaches puberty
    (b) this varies
    (c) as the woman reaches the menopause
    (d) before the birth of the woman
13. If pregnancy does not occur, what happens to the corpus luteum?
    (a) it degenerates
    (b) it causes ectopic pregnancy
    (c) it remains and develops into a new secondary oocyte
    (d) it causes infection
14. Endometriosis can be defined as:
    (a) cancer
    (b) a sexually transmitted infection
    (c) a type of allergy
    (d) tissue from the endometrium found outside of the uterus
15. How does the contraceptive pill containing estrogen and progesterone prevent pregnancy?
    (a) it causes the endometrium to hypertrophy
    (b) it suppresses follicle-stimulating hormone and luteinising hormone, preventing ovulation
    (c) it liquefies the semen
    (d) it causes a decrease in the amount of testosterone the woman produces

Find Out More

1. What does the surgical procedure circumcision entail?
2. Discuss the various methods of contraception.
3. What advice should be given to a man who is considering using Viagra for the first time?
4. What is the role and function of the nurse in respect to protecting vulnerable people?
5. How can the nurse ensure that the information provided to various communities is appropriate and informative?
6. Outline the barriers that may be encountered when conducting an assessment of a person's sexual health.
7. How may the nurse reduce the impact of the barriers identified above?
8. Describe the changes that can occur in the normal ageing process in relation to the female reproductive system.
9. List the issues a man may have to face post-prostatectomy.
10. Discuss the services and support systems available to young mums in the area where you live.

Conditions

The following is a list of conditions that are associated with the reproductive systems. Take some time and write notes about each of the conditions. You may make the notes taken from textbooks or other resources (e.g. people you work with in a clinical area), or you may make the notes as a result of people you have cared for. If you are making notes about people you have cared for, you must ensure that you adhere to the rules of confidentiality.

Prostatitis

Cervicitis

Uterine cancer

Endometriosis

Premature ejaculation

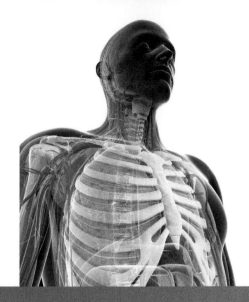

The Nervous System

Louise McErlean and Janet G. Migliozzi

Test Your Prior Knowledge

- Which other system does the nervous system work closely with?
- List the structures of the central nervous system.
- How many pairs of cranial nerves are there?
- Name the two divisions of the autonomic nervous system.
- Differentiate between sensory information and motor information.

Learning Outcomes

After reading this chapter you will be able to:

- Describe the structures of the nervous system the functions of each of these structures.
- Describe the conduction of nerve impulses.
- Identify the function of different areas of the brain.
- Understand the structure and function of the spinal cord.
- Differentiate between the sympathetic and parasympathetic nervous systems.

Visit the student companion website at www.wileyfundamentalseries.com/anatomy where you can test yourself using flashcards, multiple-choice questions and more. Instructor companion site at www.wiley.com/go/instructor/anatomy where instructors will find valuable materials such as PowerPoint slides and image bank designed to enhance your teaching.

Fundamentals of Anatomy and Physiology: For Nursing and Healthcare Students, Third Edition. Edited by Ian Peate and Suzanne Evans.
© 2020 John Wiley & Sons Ltd. Published 2020 by John Wiley & Sons Ltd.
Student companion website: www.wileyfundamentalseries.com/anatomy
Instructor companion website: www.wiley.com/go/instructor/anatomy

Body Map

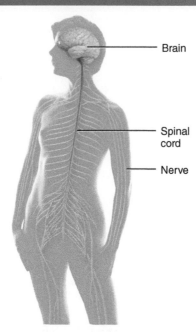

Brain

Spinal cord

Nerve

Introduction

The nervous system is a major communicating and control system within the body. It works with the endocrine system to control many body functions. The nervous system provides a rapid and short-acting response, and the endocrine system provides a slower but often more sustained response. The two systems work together to maintain homeostasis.

The nervous system interacts with all of the systems of the body. This system is large and complex. In order to facilitate understanding of the nervous system it has to be divided into smaller functional and anatomical parts. This chapter outlines the divisions of the nervous system; it discusses the structure and function of the nervous system and how it influences other structures of the body. Having such an important role in maintaining homeostasis, the nervous system possesses additional protection, and that too will be investigated.

Organisation of the Nervous System

The nervous system can be divided into two parts: the central nervous system and the peripheral nervous system. The central nervous system consists of the brain and spinal cord and is the control and integration centre for many body functions.

The peripheral nervous system carries sensory information to the central nervous system and motor information out of the central nervous system. The direction of information flow to and from the nervous system is important and is shown in Figure 14.1.

Sensory Division of the Peripheral Nervous System

Sensory information (stimuli) is gathered from both inside and outside of the body. This sensory input is delivered to the central nervous system via the peripheral nerves. Sensory nerve fibres are also called afferent fibres. Sensory information always travels from the peripheral nervous system towards the central nervous

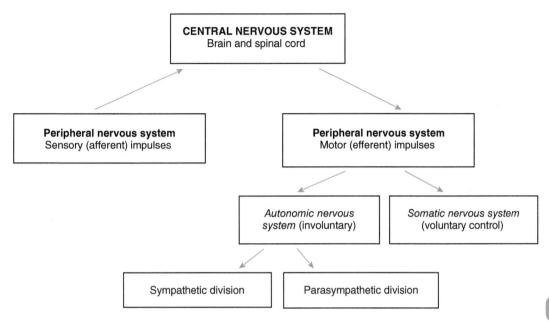

Figure 14.1 **Organisation of the nervous system.**

system. There are many different kinds of sensory information, including pain, pressure, temperature, chemical levels and more. Consider the maintenance of body temperature. As warm-blooded animals, it is important that body temperature is maintained between 36.5 and 37.5 °C. Temperature receptors in the skin called thermoreceptors detect changes in temperature, and as temperature changes have the potential to cause damage to cells and tissues, this information must be relayed to the central nervous system and, if required, acted upon.

Central Nervous System

The central nervous system consists of the brain and spinal cord. The central nervous system processes and integrates sensory information. The received information has to be interpreted, it can be stored to be dealt with later or it can be acted upon immediately with one or more motor responses. For example, the sensation of temperature change would be received and interpreted by the hypothalamus (a structure of the central nervous system) and an appropriate action would be initiated.

Motor Division of the Peripheral Nervous System

The motor division of the peripheral nervous system always carries impulses away from the central nervous system, usually to effector organs. Motor nerve fibres are also called efferent fibres. There are two types of motor information. Motor information to the somatic nervous system or to the autonomic nervous system.

Somatic Nervous System

The somatic nervous system is under voluntary control, and the effector (tissue or organ responding to instruction from the central nervous system) is skeletal (voluntary) muscle.

The central nervous system's response to sensory information may be to activate the somatic nervous system, eliciting a voluntary response involving skeletal muscle movement. So, from the example of temperature, if an increase in temperature is detected, then it might require the removal of a coat or the opening of a window – this is the motor response that involves the somatic nervous system. It is a voluntary activity that the person chooses to do.

Autonomic Nervous System

The central nervous system's response to sensory information may be to activate the autonomic nervous system. This would lead to an involuntary action. The autonomic nervous system is responsible for involuntary motor responses. The effector may be smooth or cardiac muscle (both involuntary muscles) or a gland.

In the example of increased temperature, the involuntary response is to lose heat through the skin – so warm blood is directed to the skin when peripheral blood vessels vasodilate. Vasodilatation is an example of an involuntary autonomic nervous system response. The individual cannot control this response.

The autonomic nervous system is further divided into the sympathetic (fight or flight) and the parasympathetic (rest and digest) divisions. The autonomic nervous system will be discussed later in the chapter. A fine balance between both of these divisions is required for the maintenance of homeostasis.

Neurones

The functional unit of the nervous system is the neurone or nerve cell. It has many features in common with other cells, including a nucleus and mitochondria, but because of its vital role is well protected and has some specialist modifications. Two specialist characteristics of neurones are:

- irritability, in response to a stimulus – the ability to initiate a nerve impulse;
- conductivity – the ability to conduct an impulse.

Neurones consist of an axon, dendrites and a cell body. Their function is to transmit nerve impulses. Nerve impulses only travel in one direction: from the receptive area – the dendrites – to the cell body, and down the length of the axon (see Figure 14.2).

Axons bundled together are called nerves. Neurones rely on a constant supply of oxygen and glucose. Once the neurones of the brain and spinal cord have matured after birth they will not be replaced or regenerated if they become damaged. Peripheral neurones can regenerate if the cell body is not damaged and the alignment of the neurone is not disrupted.

Dendrites

Dendrites are short branching processes that receive information and conduct it toward the cell body. Their branching processes provide a large surface area for this function. In sensory neurones the dendrites may form the part of the sensory receptors, and in motor neurones they can form part of the synapse between one neurone and the next.

Cell body

Most of the neurone cell bodies are located inside the central nervous system and form the grey matter. When clusters of cell bodies are grouped together in the central nervous system they are called nuclei. Cell bodies located in the peripheral nervous system are called ganglia.

Axons

Each neurone has only one axon that conducts information away from the cell body. The axon can branch to form an axon collateral (see Figure 14.2). The axon will also branch at its terminal into many axon terminals. The axon delivers the impulse to another neurone or a gland or a muscle.

The axon length can vary quite significantly from very short to 100 cm long (Marieb and Hoehn, 2015).

Myelin Sheath

Peripheral nerve axons and long or large axons are covered in a myelin sheath. Myelin is a fatty material whose purpose is to protect the neurone and to electrically insulate it, speeding up impulse transmission. Within the peripheral nervous system Schwann cells wrapped in layers around the neurone form the myelin

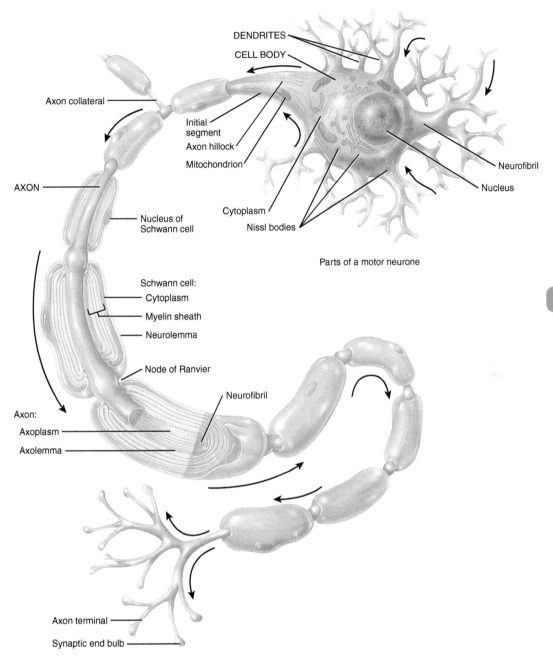

DENDRITES

CELL BODY

Axon collateral

Initial segment

Axon hillock

Mitochondrion

AXON

Neurofibril

Nucleus

Cytoplasm

Nucleus of Schwann cell

Nissl bodies

Parts of a motor neurone

Schwann cell:
Cytoplasm
Myelin sheath
Neurolemma

Node of Ranvier

Neurofibril

Axon:
Axoplasm
Axolemma

Axon terminal

Synaptic end bulb

Figure 14.2 **Motor neurone.** *Source:* Tortora and Derrickson (2009). Reproduced with permission of John Wiley & Sons.

sheath. The outermost part of the Schwann cell is its plasma membrane, and this is called the neurilemma. There is a regular gap (about 1 mm) between adjacent Schwann cells. The gaps are called the nodes of Ranvier. Collateral axons can occur at the node (see Figure 14.2). Some nerve fibres are unmyelinated, and this makes nerve impulse transmission significantly slower.

371

> **Clinical Considerations** Multiple Sclerosis
>
> Multiple sclerosis is a condition where areas of demyelination of the white matter (myelinated fibres form white matter) can occur. Areas of demyelination are called plaques. Multiple sclerosis affects the 20–40 years age range and is most frequently seen in temperate climates. The cause is unknown but it is suspected that there may be a genetic link; viral infection has also been implicated. Neuronal damage caused by the demyelination leads to:
> - skeletal muscle weakness, often progressing to paralysis
> - visual disturbances
> - uncoordinated movements
> - burning or tingling sensations.
>
> Multiple sclerosis can be a chronic disease characterised by periods of remission or the disease can progress rapidly, leading to death.

Sensory (Afferent) Nerves

The dendrites of sensory neurones are often sensory receptors, and when they are stimulated the impulse generated travels towards the spinal cord and brain. There are different types of sensory receptors:

- special senses (as discussed in Chapter 15);
- somatic sensory receptors, located in the skin, such as touch, temperature and pain;
- autonomic nervous system receptors, located throughout the body, such as baroreceptors monitoring blood pressure, chemoreceptors monitoring blood pH and visceral pain receptors;
- proprioceptors, monitoring muscle movement, stretch and pain.

Motor (Efferent) Nerves

Information from the central nervous system is delivered to the peripheral nervous system via the motor nerves. Information transmitted through a voluntary somatic nerve may result in skeletal muscle contraction or the information may be autonomic in nature, not under voluntary control, and may lead to smooth muscle contraction or the release of the products of a gland.

The Action Potential

The nervous system is a vast communicating network sending information from the internal and external environment to the central nervous system and from the central nervous system to the muscles and glands. The way that the functional unit, the neurone, achieves this is by the generation and conduction of impulses or action potentials.

Generation of the action potential occurs due to the movement of ions into and out of the neurone and the electrical charge associated with this movement.

Two principal ions are involved:

- sodium – normally found outside of the cell (principal extracellular cation);
- potassium – normally found inside the cell (principal intracellular cation).

Simple Propagation of Nerve Impulses

When there is no impulse being transmitted the cell is in its resting state – the nerve cell membrane is said to be polarised. When stimulated by an impulse, the cell membrane changes its permeability and the extracellular sodium ions move into the cell – this is called depolarisation. The movement of these ions changes the electrical charge on either side of the cell membrane from more positive extracellularly to more negative extracellularly as the impulse travels the length of the axon. This activity creates the action potential. This process happens in a wave along the length of the neurone from the active part of the neurone to the resting part of the neurone, always in one direction. At the same time, potassium ions move out of the neurone into the extracellular space, returning the electrical charge associated with the polarised neurone back to more positive outside the cell and more negative inside. This is the repolarising phase. The sodium–potassium pump is activated to return sodium to the extracellular space in exchange for potassium (see Figure 14.3).

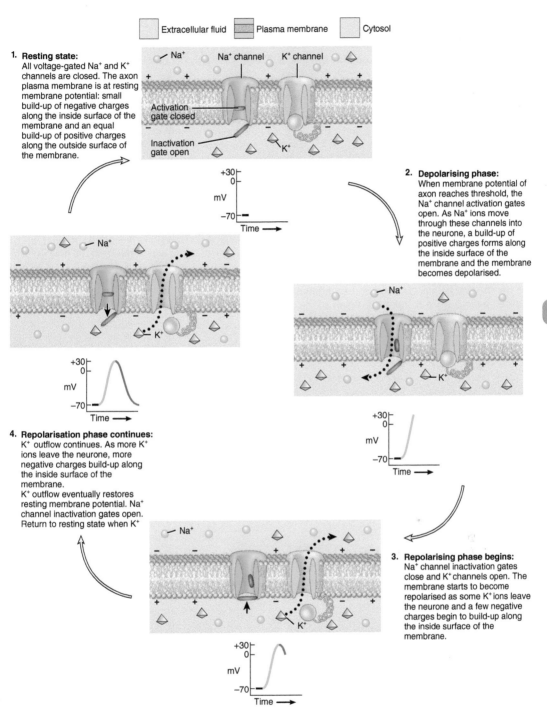

Figure 14.3 **Action potential.** *Source:* Tortora and Derrickson (2009). Reproduced with permission of John Wiley & Sons.

Saltatory Conduction

Saltatory conduction occurs in myelinated neurones as the electrical charge associated with the nerve impulse jumps between one node of Ranvier and the next. This occurs much faster than simple propagation. Conduction is also faster when the neurone has a larger diameter.

The Refractory Period

When the action potential is stimulated, the neurone cannot accept another impulse or generate another action potential no matter how strong the impulse is. This is known as the refractory period.

Episode of Care Child

Epilepsy is a neurological condition that can affect children and young people. It is associated with a disruption of the electrical activity within the neurons in the brain. Epilepsy affects 1 in 200 children.

Symptoms of epilepsy include staring, loss of consciousness, difficulty breathing, jerky movements of the limbs, loss of bladder and/or bowel control. Children with symptoms of epilepsy are referred to a paediatrician. Tests to diagnose epilepsy include electroencephalogram (EEG). Some tests (for example CT or MRI) are important to rule out other conditions such as brain tumour. Treatments include ketogenic diet, antiepileptic medication or surgery.

Mansoor Khan is 6 years old when his parents suspect he is having an epileptic seizure. There is no family history of epilepsy. His parents ring an ambulance, but the seizure is over before the ambulance arrived. Mansoor is admitted to hospital and investigations cannot find any abnormalities to account for the seizure activity. Mansoor's parents are advised to take Mansoor home and to return to the hospital if there is any further seizure activity.

On further investigation, Mansoor's teachers had noted that he was daydreaming during the afternoon on the day that he has the seizure. They attributed this to tiredness, however Mansoor's parents have also noticed periods when he appears vague, so they return to the GP for some further investigations.

Multiple Choice Questions

1. Which of the following are symptoms of epilepsy?
   (a) memory loss
   (b) uncontrollable shaking and jerking movements
   (c) dilated pupils
   (d) hemiparesis
2. Which of the following can lead to epilepsy?
   (a) the misuse of alcohol
   (b) a head injury
   (c) following a stroke
   (d) all of the above
3. Which medication can be used to treat epilepsy?
   (a) sodium valporate
   (b) ranitidine
   (c) amilodipine
   (d) baclofen
4. Which is true of a focal seizure?
   (a) it affects both hemispheres of the brain
   (b) it affects one hemisphere of the brain
   (c) it lasts longer than a generalised seizure
   (d) there is always a loss of consciousness
5. What ketogenic diet is sometimes used as a treatment for epilepsy?
   (a) high protein, low carbohydrate
   (b) low fat, high carbohydrate
   (c) low protein, high carbohydrate
   (d) high fat, low carbohydrate

Neurotransmitters

Neurones do not come into contact with one another. Where one neurone ends and another begins, there is a space called the synapse. In order for communication to occur between neurones or between the neurone and a muscle or gland, a chemical messenger called a neurotransmitter is secreted by the neurone into the extracellular space at the synapse. Those effector cells or neurones in close proximity to the neurotransmitter will either be stimulated or inhibited by the neurotransmitter, depending upon which neurotransmitter is secreted. The action of the neurotransmitter is short-lived, and any neurotransmitter not used is absorbed by the neurone to be recycled and used again or deactivated by enzymes.

Some examples of neurotransmitters are:

- acetylcholine, released within the central nervous system and also at the neuromuscular junction;
- norepinephrine, released within the central nervous system and also at autonomic nervous system synapses;
- dopamine, released within the central nervous system and also at autonomic nervous system synapses.

Clinical Considerations EEG

An EEG records brain activity. It is particularly useful for diagnosing conditions such as epilepsy, dementia and encephalopathy.

Electrodes are placed on the head and attached to an EEG machine. The electrical activity generated by nerve impulses is then measured. During the EEG, the patient may be asked to breathe deeply or blink several times. There are different types of EEG used to ascertain triggers that may lead to seizure activity, and these include sleep EEG, sleep-deprived EEG, ambulatory EEG and strobe lighting EEG.

The test can usually be carried out in an out-patient department (apart from sleep EEG), and the outcome could lead to a treatment plan being implemented or altered.

Episode of Care Mental Health

Alzheimer's disease is a form of dementia. It is a progressive neurodegenerative disease which affects the brain cells. Neurofibrillary tangles are formed within the neurons and amyloid plaques are formed around the neurons. There is also a reduction in the neurotransmitter acetylcholine. Contributing factors to the condition include:

- Increasing age – the disease usually affects those over 65 years old.
- Untreated depression.
- Family history of the condition.
- Lifestyle factors.
- Cardiovascular disease.

Initial symptoms of Alzheimer's include memory loss; forgetting recent conversations; getting lost in familiar places; losing items which are found in unusual places; repeating the same conversations; difficulty judging spaces; difficulty concentrating and disorientation. These symptoms progress as the disease progresses. Acetylcholinestrase inhibitors help increase acetylcholine and therefore can help to manage symptoms. Other treatments could include antidepressants, cognitive behavioural therapy and cognitive rehabilitation.

Grace is 75 years old. Her family have brought her to see her GP. Both Grace and her family have noticed a decrease in memory with Grace reporting that she frequently forgets where she has put things or family anniversaries. Grace is concerned as her mother developed dementia at a young age and she recognises some of the symptoms she feels she has developed. Grace has previously sought treatment for depression after her husband died 10 years ago. She did not take the prescribed anti-depressants and her family suspect that her alcohol consumption increased at this time.

The GP orders some routine bloods to rule out other conditions and assesses Grace using the General Practitioner Assessment of Cognition test. The GP refers Grace to a psychiatrist for ongoing treatment.

Multiple Choice Questions

1. Which neurotransmitter is associated with Alzheimer's disease?
   (a) dopamine
   (b) adrenaline
   (c) acetylcholine
   (d) insulin
2. Which of the following is a type of dementia?
   (a) Parkinson's disease
   (b) Alzheimer's disease
   (c) motor neurone disease
   (d) all of the above

3. Which of the following are symptoms of Alzheimer's disease?
   (a) low blood pressure
   (b) memory loss
   (c) weight gain
   (d) increased intracranial pressure
4. Which of the following are risk factors for Alzheimer's disease?
   (a) age
   (b) gender
   (c) lifestyle
   (d) all of the above
5. Which of these is present in Alzheimer's disease?
   (a) lack of oxygen to the brain
   (b) Lewy bodies
   (c) loss of microglia
   (d) neurofibrillary tangles

Neuroglia

Neuroglia (see Figure 14.4) are cells that support neurones. They are more numerous than neurones. Within the central nervous system the neuroglial cells account for more than half of the weight of the brain (Marieb and Hoehn, 2015). Neuroglia can multiply in order to support the neurones. Because of this, nervous system tumours often originate from neuroglia.

Within the peripheral nervous system, two types of neuroglia have been identified:

1. Schwann cells, responsible for forming the myelin sheath;
2. Satellite cells, whose function is not known.

Within the central nervous system; four type of neuroglial cell have been identified:

1. Astrocytes are star-shaped cells which occur in large quantities between neurones and blood vessels, supporting and anchoring them to each other. They help form the blood–brain barrier, which gives the neurones an extra layer of protection from any toxic substances within the blood.
2. Microglia lie close to neurones and can move closer if they need to fulfil their function as nervous system macrophages. They phagocytose pathogens or cell debris.
3. Oligodendrocytes are found close to myelinated neurones. They help to form and maintain the myelin sheath.
4. Ependymal cells are often ciliated and are found lining cavities, such as the spinal cord or the ventricles of the brain. Their role is to circulate cerebrospinal fluid (CSF) (Waugh and Grant, 2018).

The Meninges

Nervous tissue is easily damaged by pressure and therefore needs to be protected. The hair, skin and bone offer an outer layer of protection. Adjacent to the nervous tissue are the meninges (see Figure 14.5). The meninges cover the delicate nervous tissue, providing further protection. They also protect the blood vessels that serve nervous tissue and they contain CSF.

The meninges consist of three connective tissue layers:

- Dura mater – this layer lies closest to the bone of the skull and is a double layer of tough, fibrous, connective tissue. The outer layer is called the periosteal layer (the spinal cord lacks this layer), and the meningeal layer lies closest to the brain.
- Arachnoid mater – between the dura mater and the arachnoid mater there is a space called the subdural space. The arachnoid mater is a delicate serous membrane (Seeley et al., 2016). The subarachnoid space is below the arachnoid mater and above the pia mater. The subarachnoid space contains CSF and is also home to some of the larger blood vessels serving the brain.
- Pia mater – this is a delicate connective tissue layer that clings tightly to the brain. It contains many tiny blood vessels that serve the brain.

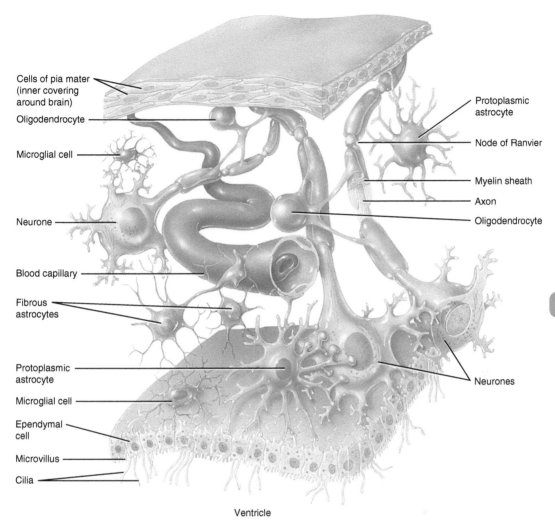

Cells of pia mater (inner covering around brain)

Oligodendrocyte

Microglial cell

Neurone

Blood capillary

Fibrous astrocytes

Protoplasmic astrocyte

Microglial cell

Ependymal cell

Microvillus

Cilia

Protoplasmic astrocyte

Node of Ranvier

Myelin sheath

Axon

Oligodendrocyte

Neurones

Ventricle

Figure 14.4 **Neuroglia.** *Source:* Tortora and Derrickson (2009). Reproduced with permission of John Wiley & Sons.

Clinical Considerations Meningitis

Meningitis is inflammation of the meninges caused by either bacteria or viruses. It can be diagnosed through symptoms that include photophobia, headache, nausea and vomiting and also by a procedure called a lumbar puncture. In lumbar puncture a small amount of CSF is removed and examined in the laboratory for the presence of microbes. A lack of prompt treatment can have fatal consequences.

Cerebrospinal Fluid

CSF is produced by the choroid plexus in the ventricles of the brain (see Figure 14.6). There is approximately 150 mL of CSF circulating around the brain, in the ventricles and around the spinal cord. The CSF is replaced every 8 h (Marieb and Hoehn, 2015). It is a thin fluid similar to plasma and has several important functions:

- it acts as a cushion, supporting the weight of the brain and protecting it from damage;
- it helps to maintain a uniform pressure around the brain and spinal cord;
- there is a limited exchange of nutrients and waste products between neurones and CSF.

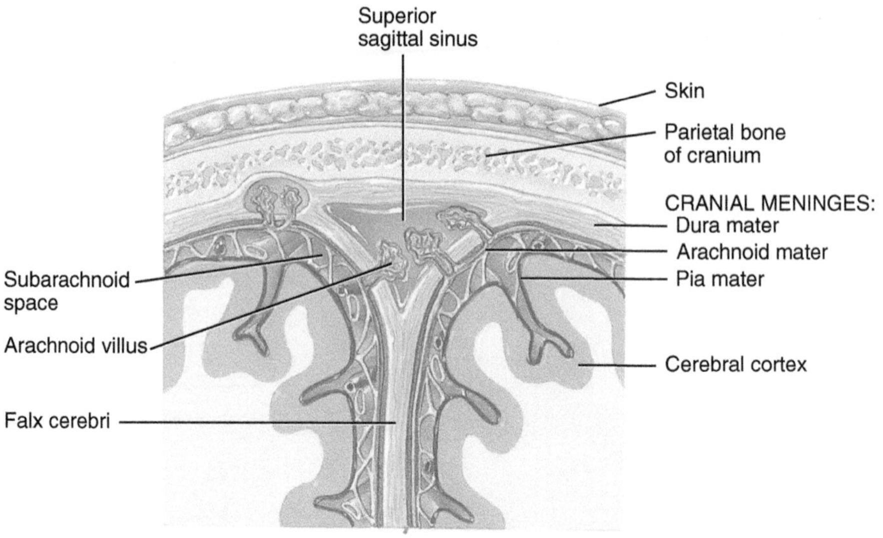

Superior
sagittal sinus

Skin

Parietal bone
of cranium

CRANIAL MENINGES:
Dura mater
Arachnoid mater
Pia mater

Subarachnoid
space

Arachnoid villus

Cerebral cortex

Falx cerebri

Figure 14.5 The meninges. *Source:* Tortora and Derrickson (2009). Reproduced with permission of John Wiley & Sons.

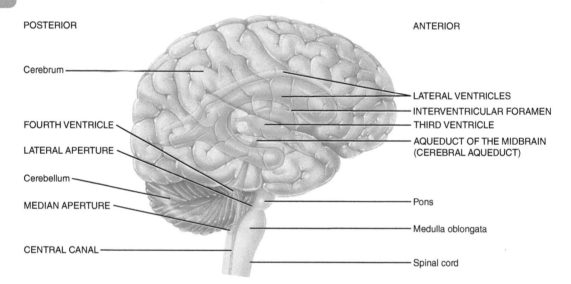

POSTERIOR

ANTERIOR

Cerebrum

LATERAL VENTRICLES
INTERVENTRICULAR FORAMEN
THIRD VENTRICLE
AQUEDUCT OF THE MIDBRAIN
(CEREBRAL AQUEDUCT)

FOURTH VENTRICLE

LATERAL APERTURE

Cerebellum

MEDIAN APERTURE

Pons

Medulla oblongata

CENTRAL CANAL

Spinal cord

Figure 14.6 The ventricles (right lateral view of the brain). *Source:* Tortora and Derrickson (2009). Reproduced with permission of John Wiley & Sons.

There are four ventricles in the brain: the paired lateral ventricles, one in each cerebral hemisphere; the third ventricle, situated below this; and the fourth ventricle, located inferior to the third. The third and fourth ventricles communicate via the central canal and CSF circulates through the central canal and into the spinal cord.

Any additional pressure applied to the brain caused by swelling (cerebral oedema), tumour or haemorrhage (through trauma) can lead to a reduced volume of CSF being produced.

Clinical Considerations Lumbar Puncture

Lumbar puncture is often used to diagnose conditions such as meningitis and multiple sclerosis. A sample of CSF is removed and sent for laboratory analysis. The sample is taken by inserting a needle between the third and fourth lumbar vertebrae and the CSF is removed from the subarachnoid space. This procedure is usually carried out under local anaesthetic.

The CSF circulates around the brain and spinal cord. The pressure exerted by the CSF is known as intracranial pressure (ICP). Normal ICP is 8–20 cm H_2O. If the ICP is raised this could be for a variety of reasons, including cerebral oedema in the brain as might be seen in head injury, head trauma or meningitis. It could also be raised because of the additional white cells, protein or myelin within the CSF, as in multiple sclerosis.

The CSF should be colourless. Cloudy CSF may indicate the presence of infection. CSF is usually watery in viscosity. If it is more viscous then this could indicate the presence of infection or tumour. Laboratory analysis will give a more accurate interpretation than a visual inspection.

Laboratory analysis will show the amount of glucose protein and immunoglobulins, for example, present in CSF. The white cells can be analysed, and the presence of bacteria and viruses is also investigated.

There are side effects associated with lumbar puncture, and these include back pain from the site of the puncture and headache. The headache is relieved by lying down.

The Brain

The brain lies in the cranial cavity and weighs between 1450 and 1600 g (Marieb and Hoehn, 2015). It receives 15% of the cardiac output and has a system of autoregulation ensuring the blood supply is constant despite positional changes. The arrangement of the arteries serving the brain is unique, and they are connected to each other by a structure called the circle of Willis (see Figure 14.7). This arrangement ensures that blood pressure remains equal in both halves of the brain. Should one of the arteries serving the brain become narrowed by arterial disease or thrombus then there will be an alternative route available, maintaining the essential supply of oxygen and glucose required by the brain.

The brain can be divided into four anatomical regions. Each region contains one or more structures (see Figure 14.8):

- cerebrum
- cerebral hemispheres
- diencephalon
- thalamus
- hypothalamus
- epithalamus
- brainstem
- midbrain
- pons

379

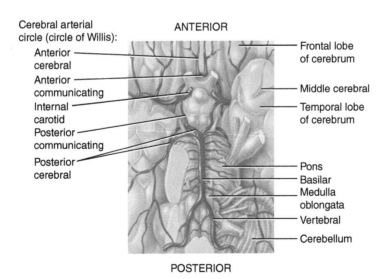

Figure 14.7 **Circle of Willis.** *Source:* Tortora and Derrickson (2009). Reproduced with permission of John Wiley & Sons.

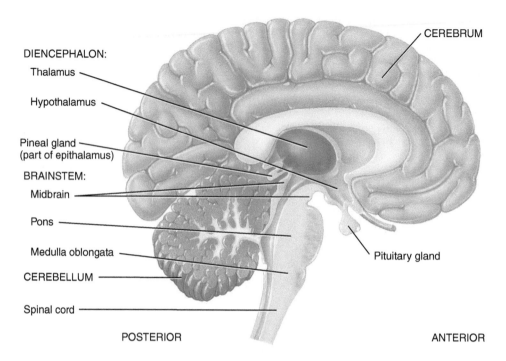

DIENCEPHALON:
Thalamus
Hypothalamus
Pineal gland
(part of epithalamus)
BRAINSTEM:
Midbrain
Pons
Medulla oblongata
CEREBELLUM
Spinal cord

CEREBRUM

Pituitary gland

POSTERIOR   ANTERIOR

Figure 14.8 **The structures of the brain.** *Source:* Tortora and Derrickson (2009). Reproduced with permission of John Wiley & Sons.

- medulla oblongata
- reticular formation
- cerebellum.

Cerebrum

This is the largest brain structure. It is divided into the left and right hemispheres by the longitudinal cerebral fissure. Each hemisphere can be divided into lobes – occipital, frontal, parietal and temporal. The outer layer of the cerebrum is called the cerebral cortex and is made of grey matter (nerve cell bodies). The layers below this are white matter (nerve fibres). The cerebral cortex is responsible for our conscious mind and consists of interneurones (the neurones that lie between sensory and motor neurones). The cerebral cortex can be divided into functional areas, which were mapped by Brodmann in 1906 (see Figure 14.9). The circled numbers on the diagram represent important areas on Brodmann's map. While functional and structural areas of the brain have been identified, it is important to remember that the areas do not function independently from one another, and damage to one structure may have consequences for another.

The first of the functional areas is the motor area and it is subdivided as follows:

- the primary motor area – responsible for contraction of skeletal muscles;
- the premotor area – involved in fine skeletal muscle movement creating the manual dexterity associated with repetitive or learned motor movement (e.g. tying a shoelace, learning to paint, giving an injection);
- Broca's area – responsible for the motor movement required to produce speech;
- the frontal eye field area – controls voluntary movement of the eyes.

The second functional area is the sensory area, responsible for awareness of sensation. It can be divided as follows:

- the primary somatosensory area – receives sensory information from the skin and also from proprioceptors in skeletal muscles;
- the somatosensory association area – integrates the sensory information being relayed to the primary somatosensory area and provides information about size, texture, previous experience;
- the visual areas – the primary visual area receives information from the eye and the visual association area helps to connect this information with past visual experiences;

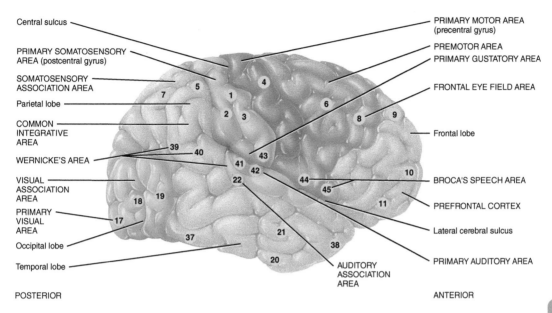

Figure 14.9 **Right cerebral hemisphere.** *Source:* Tortora and Derrickson (2009). Reproduced with permission of John Wiley & Sons.

- the auditory areas – associated with the interpretation of sounds;
- the olfactory area – interprets smell information received from the nose via the olfactory nerves;
- the gustatory area – interprets taste information.

There are many other association areas within the cerebrum that act as communication areas between different functional regions in the cerebrum, such as Wernicke's area, which is responsible for understanding written and spoken language and is closely associated with Broca's speech area.

Diencephalon

This part of the brain is surrounded by the cerebrum and contains three paired structures:

- Thalamus – acts as a relay station for sensory impulses going to the cerebral cortex for integration and motor impulses entering and leaving the cerebral hemispheres. It also has a role in memory.
- Hypothalamus – is closely associated with the pituitary gland and produces two hormones: antidiuretic hormone (ADH) and oxytocin. The hypothalamus has many functions and these include:
  - control of body temperature
  - control of the autonomic nervous system
  - control of fluid balance and thirst
  - control of appetite
  - associated with the limbic system dealing with emotional reactions
  - control of sexual behaviours.
- Epithalamus – this structure is linked to the pineal gland, which secretes the hormone melatonin responsible for sleep–wake cycles.

Brainstem

The structures that form the brainstem are involved in many activities that are essential for life. The brainstem is associated with the cranial nerves.

- Midbrain – conduction pathway that connects the cerebrum with the lower brain structures and spinal cord.
- Pons – also a conduction pathway communicating with the cerebellum. The pons works with the medulla oblongata to control depth and rate of respiration.
- Medulla oblongata – relay station for sensory nerves going to the cerebrum. The medulla contains autonomic centres such as the cardiac centre, the respiratory centre, the vasomotor centre and the coughing, sneezing and vomiting centre. The medulla is also the site of decussation of the pyramidal tracts – this means that the right side of the body is controlled by the left cerebral hemisphere and vice versa.

Clinical Considerations Concussion

Concussion is a minor head injury and is defined as a brief period of unconsciousness. It is also termed mild traumatic brain injury (VanMeter and Hubert, 2014). Signs and symptoms include nausea, headaches, dizziness, impaired concentration, amnesia (memory loss), extreme tiredness, and intolerance to light and noise. The symptoms usually only last for 24 h.

Cerebellum

The cerebellum coordinates voluntary muscle movement, balance and posture. It ensures that muscle movements are smooth, coordinated and precise.

The Limbic System and the Reticular Formation

The limbic system and reticular formation are functional systems as they consist of networks of neurones that can be located close to many anatomical structures.

The limbic system is located close to the cerebrum and the diencephalon. It is known as the emotional brain and is responsible for the interpretation of facial expression, helping identify fear and danger.

The reticular formation is a functional system located in the core of the brainstem and consists of a collection of neurones that have several functions:

- contains the reticular activating system that is responsible for alertness;
- filters or blocks repetitive stimuli, such as background noise;
- regulates skeletal muscle activity;
- coordinates visceral activity controlled by the autonomic nervous system.

The brain is a well-protected control and integration centre that receives information from the peripheral sensory nervous system and sends motor information to the peripheral nervous system through a comprehensive network of pathways via the spinal cord.

Medicines Management Midazolam

Midazolam is a medication classified as a benzodiazepine. Benzodiazepines act on central nervous system receptors and produce a sedative effect. Midazolam is thought to produce amnesia and is therefore useful in procedures that require the patient to be awake and cooperative despite the unpleasant nature of the procedure, such as endoscopy (Galbraith et al., 2007). The intention is that the patient will not remember the procedure.

Midazolam is a short-acting benzodiazepine and has a half-life of 2–3 h (Galbraith et al., 2007). It is available for administration via a variety of routes, including intravenous and intramuscular.

Midazolam has a number of side effects, and these include:

- respiratory failure
- respiratory depression
- hypotension
- anaphylaxis
- convulsions
- dry mouth
- constipation
- nausea
- euphoria
- hiccups
- headache.

As benzodiazepines can be addictive in some instances their use has been abused. An antagonist called flumazenil is available to reverse the effects of the medication.

Benzodiazepines should be prescribed with caution.

Medicines Management Phenytoin

John is 34 years old and experiences seizures following his recovery from a head injury. He has been prescribed phenytoin sodium 100 mg orally three times a day for this. This medicine works during the action potential. It promotes the removal of sodium during the refractory period, thus reducing the hyperexcitability of neurones that can lead to seizure (McFadden, 2019). John has been advised to avoid alcohol and to maintain good oral hygiene practices, as this medicine has a known side effect of gingival hyperplasia (gum overgrowth).

The Peripheral Nervous System

The peripheral nervous system includes all the tissues that lie outside of the central nervous system:

- cranial nerves
- spinal nerves
- spinal cord
- autonomic nervous system.

The peripheral nervous system is subdivided into the efferent or motor system and the afferent or sensory system. The somatic sensory system serves the skeletal muscles, joints, tendons and the skin and includes the senses of vision, hearing, smell and taste (Logenbaker, 2016). The internal organs of the body are supplied by the visceral sensory system. Both the somatic and visceral sensory systems take information from peripheral sensory receptors towards the central nervous system.

Commands from the central nervous system to the skeletal muscles are carried by the somatic motor system. The autonomic motor system predominantly regulates the activity of smooth and cardiac muscles and glands (Logenbaker, 2016).

Cranial Nerves

There are 12 pairs of cranial nerves that emerge from the brain and supply various structures, most of which are associated with the head and neck. Figure 14.10 provides an overview of the location and function of the cranial nerves.

The 12 pairs of cranial nerves differ in their functions: some are sensory nerves (i.e. contain sensory fibres), some are motor nerves (i.e. contain only motor fibres) and some are mixed nerves (i.e. contain both sensory and motor nerves).

Table 14.1 provides a summary of the cranial nerves, their different components and function.

The Spinal Cord

The average adult spinal cord (see Figure 14.11) is between 42 and 45 cm long and extends from the medulla oblongata (lower part of the brain) to the upper part of the second lumbar vertebra. The spinal cord is enclosed within the vertebral canal, which forms a protective ring of bone around the cord. Other protective coverings include the spinal meninges, which are three layers of connective tissue coverings that extend around the spinal cord. The spinal meninges consist of:

- the pia mater – the innermost layer;
- the arachnoid mater – the middle layer;
- the dura mater – the outermost layer, which consists of a dense, irregular connective tissue.

The spinal cord consists of a central canal and grey and white matter. The central canal and the spinal meninges contain CSF. The grey matter consists mostly of cell bodies and their dendrites, and the whiter areas consist of the axons of neurones, which carry signals up and down the cord via ascending and descending tracts. These tracts cross as they enter and exit the brain, and this explains why the right side of the brain controls the left side of the body and the left side of the brain controls the right side of the body.

The spinal cord is divided into the right and left halves by the deep anterior median fissure and the shallow posterior median sulcus (Tortora and Derrickson, 2014).

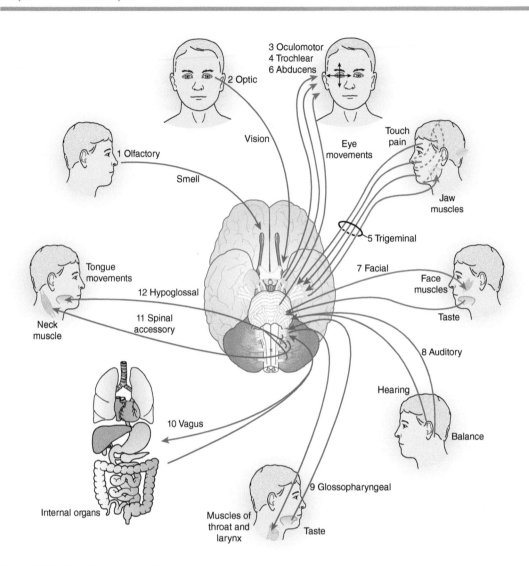

Figure 14.10 Functions of cranial nerves.

Functions of the Spinal Cord

The spinal cord provides a means of communication between the brain and the peripheral nerves that leave the spinal cord (Logenbaker, 2016) and has two major functions in maintaining homeostasis (Tortora and Derrickson, 2014):

- The tracts of the white matter of the spinal cord carry sensory impulses to the brain and motor impulses from the brain to the skeletal muscles and other effector muscles.
- The grey matter of the spinal cord is a site for integration of reflexes, which is a rapid, involuntary action in relation to a particular stimulus.

Spinal Nerves

There are 31 pairs of spinal nerves attached to the spinal cord within the human body, which are named and numbered according to the region and level of the vertebral column from which they emerge (Figure 14.12).

Each nerve innervates a group of muscles (myotome) and an area of skin (dermatome), and most also innervate some of the thoracic and abdominal organs (Figure 14.13).

Table 14.1 **The cranial nerves.**

NUMBER	NAME	COMPONENTS	LOCATION/FUNCTION
I	Olfactory	Sensory	Olfactory receptors for sense of smell
II	Optic	Sensory	Retina (sight)
III	Oculomotor	Motor	Eye muscles (including eyelids and lens, pupil)
IV	Trochlear	Motor	Eye muscles
V	Trigeminal	Sensory and motor	Teeth, eyes, skin, tongue for sensation of touch, pain and temperature
VI	Abducens	Motor	Jaw muscles (chewing)
			Eye muscles
VII	Facial	Sensory and motor	Taste buds
			Facial muscles, tear and salivary glands
VIII	Vestibulocochlear	Sensory	Inner ear (hearing and balance)
IX	Glossopharyngeal	Sensory and motor	Pharyngeal muscles (swallowing)
X	Vagus	Sensory and motor	Internal organs
XI	Spinal accessory	Motor	Neck and back muscles
XII	Hypoglossal	Motor	Tongue muscles

385

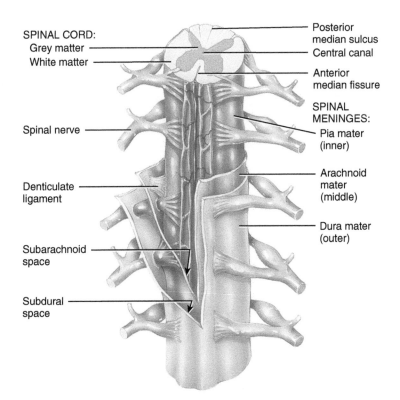

Figure 14.11 **The spinal cord.** *Source:* Tortora and Derrickson (2009). Reproduced with permission of John Wiley & Sons.

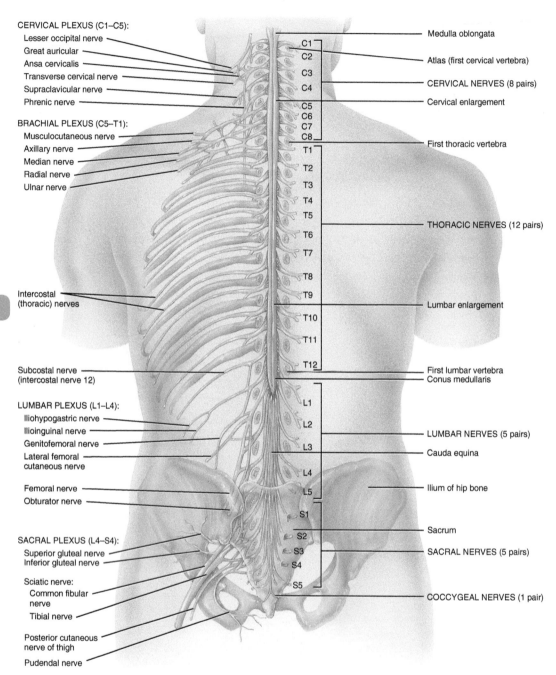

CERVICAL PLEXUS (C1–C5):
Lesser occipital nerve
Great auricular
Ansa cervicalis
Transverse cervical nerve
Supraclavicular nerve
Phrenic nerve

BRACHIAL PLEXUS (C5–T1):
Musculocutaneous nerve
Axillary nerve
Median nerve
Radial nerve
Ulnar nerve

Intercostal
(thoracic) nerves

Subcostal nerve
(intercostal nerve 12)

LUMBAR PLEXUS (L1–L4):
Iliohypogastric nerve
Ilioinguinal nerve
Genitofemoral nerve
Lateral femoral
cutaneous nerve

Femoral nerve
Obturator nerve

SACRAL PLEXUS (L4–S4):
Superior gluteal nerve
Inferior gluteal nerve

Sciatic nerve:
Common fibular
nerve
Tibial nerve

Posterior cutaneous
nerve of thigh
Pudendal nerve

C1
C2
C3
C4
C5
C6
C7
C8
T1
T2
T3
T4
T5
T6
T7
T8
T9
T10
T11
T12
L1
L2
L3
L4
L5
S1
S2
S3
S4
S5

Medulla oblongata
Atlas (first cervical vertebra)
CERVICAL NERVES (8 pairs)
Cervical enlargement

First thoracic vertebra

THORACIC NERVES (12 pairs)

Lumbar enlargement

First lumbar vertebra
Conus medullaris

LUMBAR NERVES (5 pairs)
Cauda equina

Ilium of hip bone

Sacrum
SACRAL NERVES (5 pairs)

COCCYGEAL NERVES (1 pair)

Posterior view of entire spinal cord and portions of spinal nerves

Figure 14.12 **The spinal cord and spinal nerves.** *Source:* Tortora and Derrickson (2009). Reproduced with permission of John Wiley & Sons.

The spinal nerves provide the paths of communication between the spinal cord and specific regions of the body as they connect the central nervous system to sensory receptors, muscles and glands in all the parts of the body. A typical spinal nerve (Figure 14.14) has two connections to the spinal cord – a posterior root and an anterior root, which unite to form a spinal nerve at the intervertebral foramen. A spinal nerve is an example of a mixed nerve as it contains both sensory (posterior root) and motor (anterior root) nerves.

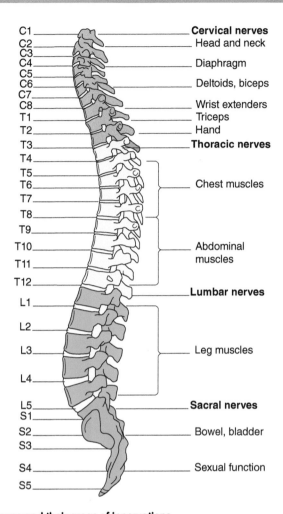

C1 — **Cervical nerves**
C2 — Head and neck
C3
C4 — Diaphragm
C5
C6 — Deltoids, biceps
C7
C8 — Wrist extenders
T1 — Triceps
T2 — Hand
T3 — **Thoracic nerves**
T4
T5
T6 — Chest muscles
T7
T8
T9
T10 — Abdominal muscles
T11
T12
L1 — **Lumbar nerves**
L2
L3 — Leg muscles
L4
L5 — **Sacral nerves**
S1
S2 — Bowel, bladder
S3
S4 — Sexual function
S5

Figure 14.13 **The spinal nerves and their areas of innervations.**

Episodes of Care Learning Disabilities

A spinal cord injury (SCI) is a devastating and life altering injury that, due to each body system being innervated by the spinal cord, affects nearly all body systems. The commonest cause of SCIs in the UK is road traffic collision (RTC), followed by falls, sport-related injuries and violence. The number of people being injured or diagnosed with a spinal cord injury each year in the UK is now estimated to be around 2500 – this equates to approximately 35 individuals per week or a paralysis every four hours (Aspire, 2019).

Josh is a 15 year old with a learning disability who enjoys horse riding and plays horse-ball for his local club. During a recent match, Josh was thrown from his horse, landed awkwardly and sustained a SCI to his thoracic region which has resulted in paralysis from the waist down. Josh has experienced intense grief because of his condition and has become very depressed. Due to his learning disability, Josh, at times cannot communicate clearly and becomes very anxious, frustrated and agitated often refusing to participate in his care.

The psychosocial needs of the patient with an SCI should never been overlooked and requires skilled interventions by health professionals to improve health and well-being. In the case of an individual with a learning disability the assessment of mental health is fraught with difficulties, and without accurate assessment and diagnosis, the selection of appropriate treatment can be very difficult, or almost impossible (Gates et al., 2014). Josh was seen and assessed by a psychiatrist and specialist learning disabilities nurse. A diagnosis of exogenous depression was made and Josh was commenced on antidepressant medication in the form of a selective serotonin reuptake inhibitor (SSRI), in this case Citalopram 20 mg once a day. The specialist learning disabilities nurse also supported Josh and his family with psychological interventions to help manage Josh's current psychological difficulties.

Multiple Choice Questions

1. Which of the following describes exogenous depression:
   (a) has no easily identifiable or known cause
   (b) is severe in nature
   (c) can be explained by external 'triggers'
   (d) is caused by internal biological factors

2. Selective serotonin reuptake inhibitors (SSRIs):
   (a) increase uptake of dopamine
   (b) can increase anxiety
   (c) are quick acting
   (d) require the avoidance of certain foodstuffs

3. Spinal cord injury (SCI): Select all that apply:
   (a) is always irreversible
   (b) is most likely, in the UK, to be caused by a fall.
   (c) can lead to premature death
   (d) accounts for 2500 UK hospital admissions each year

4. Which of the following factors increases the risk of spinal cord injury? Select all that apply:
   (a) male gender
   (b) car driver
   (c) playing rugby
   (d) over 65 years old

5. A spinal cord injury sustained at T12 is likely to result in:
   (a) the patient requiring artificial support in order to breathe
   (b) paralysis to the arms
   (c) some movement in the legs
   (d) loss of sensation below the waist

388

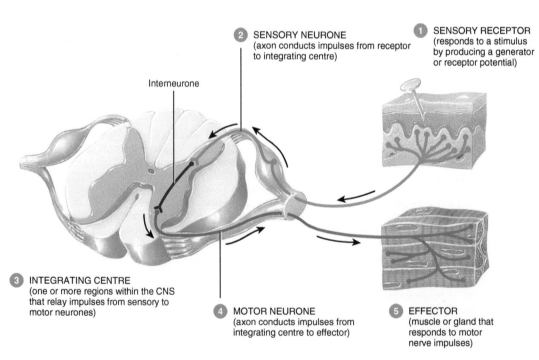

Figure 14.14 **A typical spinal nerve (CNS: central nervous system).** *Source:* Tortora and Derrickson (2009). Reproduced with permission of John Wiley & Sons.

Clinical Considerations Acute Spinal Cord Compression

Acute spinal cord compression is a neurological emergency that requires rapid diagnosis and treatment if permanent loss of function is to be avoided. Common causes of spinal cord compression include:

- trauma (car accidents, sports injury and falls);
- tumours, both benign and malignant;
- a prolapsed intervertebral disc (L4–L5 and L5–S1 are the most common levels of disc prolapse);
- an epidural or subdural haemorrhage;
- inflammatory disease (e.g. rheumatoid arthritis);
- infection.

Signs and symptoms include sensory loss, paraesthesia, disturbance of gait, loss of power or paralysis.

Medicines Management Paracetamol

Paracetamol (acetaminophen) is a common over-the-counter medication used to treat mild to moderate pain and is also effective as a fever reducer. The exact mechanism of action of is not known; however, it is thought that the analgesic mechanism of paracetamol involves the metabolites of paracetamol, which act on receptors in the spinal cord and are thought to suppress the signal transduction from the superficial layers of the dorsal horn to alleviate pain (Farquhar-Smith et al., 2018).

In relation to its fever-reducing properties, it has been proposed that the main mechanism of action is the inhibition of the enzyme cyclooxygenase (COX), and recent findings suggest that it is highly selective for COX-2. The COX family of enzymes is responsible for the metabolism of compounds that encourage inflammatory responses. Paracetamol is thought to reduce the oxidised form of the COX enzyme, preventing it from forming pro-inflammatory chemicals. This leads to a reduced amount of prostaglandins S, thus lowering the hypothalamic set-point in the thermoregulatory centre.

Paracetamol is used to treat many conditions, such as headache, muscle aches, arthritis, backache, toothache, colds and fevers.

Overdosage of paracetamol is particularly dangerous as it may cause liver damage, which may not be apparent for 4–6 days after ingestion. Treatment includes infusing acetylcysteine, which protects the liver. However, it is most effective if given within 8 h of ingestion, after which effectiveness declines.

Clinical Considerations Panic Attack

A panic attack is a rush of intense psychological and physical symptoms. These symptoms of panic can be frightening and happen suddenly, often for no clear reason.

Panic attacks usually last between 5 and 20 min, and the individual may experience unpleasant psychological and physical symptoms; however, these are usually short-lived and will not cause harm (NHS Choices, 2019). Psychological symptoms can include an overwhelming sense of fear and a sense of unreality, as if the individual is detached from the world around them. Physical symptoms of panic can include sweating, trembling, shortness of breath, a choking sensation, chest pain, a feeling of nausea and palpitations.

The physical symptoms of a panic attack are caused by the body's sympathetic response to something that the individual perceives as a threat and causes the release of hormones, such as adrenaline, resulting in an increased heart rate and muscle tension.

Sufferers of panic attacks can be helped to manage their condition through learning breathing and relaxation techniques and avoiding substances such as caffeine, nicotine and alcohol (NHS Choices, 2019).

The Autonomic Nervous System

The autonomic nervous system plays a major role in the maintenance of homeostasis by regulating the body's automatic, involuntary functions. In common with the rest of the nervous system, it consists of neurones, neuroglia and other connective tissue. However, its structure is unique, in that it is divided into two: namely, the sympathetic division and the parasympathetic division. These two divisions have several common features (Logenbaker, 2016):

- they innervate all internal organs;
- they utilise two motor neurones and one ganglion to transmit an action potential;
- they function automatically and usually in an involuntary manner.

Sympathetic Division (Fight or Flight)

The sympathetic division (see Figure 14.15) includes nerve fibres that arise from the 12 thoracic and first two lumbar segments of the spine; hence, it is also referred to as the thoracicolumbar division. The sympathetic division takes control of many internal organs when a stressful situation occurs. This can take the form of

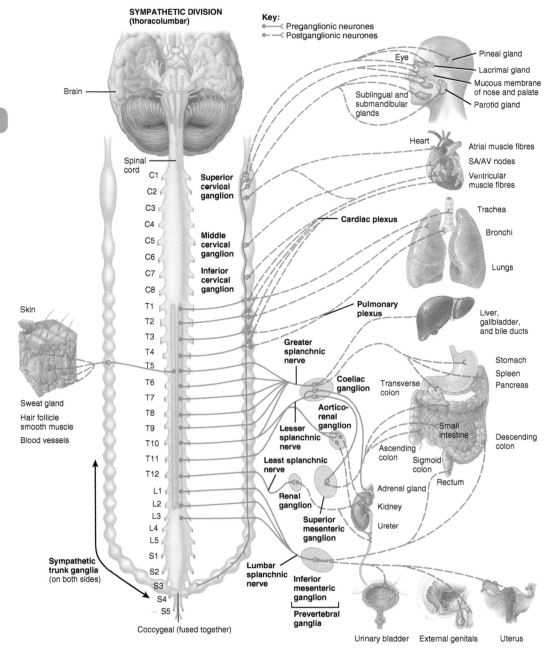

Figure 14.15 **Sympathetic nervous system.** *Source:* Tortora and Derrickson (2009). Reproduced with permission of John Wiley & Sons.

physical stress if undertaking strenuous exercise or emotional stress at times of anger or anxiety. In emergency situations, the sympathetic nervous system releases norepinephrine, which assists in the 'fight or flight' response (Migliozzi, 2017).

Parasympathetic Division (Rest and Digest)

The parasympathetic division includes fibres that arise from the lower end of the spinal cord and several cranial nerves; hence, it is often referred to as the craniosacral division. The parasympathetic division is most active when the body is at rest; it utilises acetylcholine to control all the internal responses associated with a state of relaxation (Figure 14.16) and, therefore, has many opposite effects on the body to the sympathetic nervous system (Migliozzi, 2017).

Table 14.2 provides a summary of the physiological effects of the sympathetic and parasympathetic divisions of the nervous system.

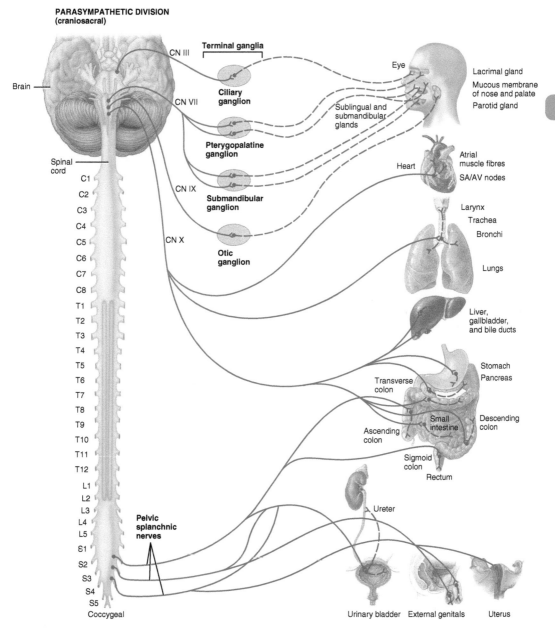

391

Figure 14.16 Parasympathetic nervous system. *Source:* Tortora and Derrickson (2009). Reproduced with permission of John Wiley & Sons.

Table 14.2 **Effects of the parasympathetic and sympathetic divisions of the autonomic nervous system.**

ORGAN/SYSTEM	SYMPATHETIC EFFECTS	PARASYMPATHETIC EFFECTS
Cell metabolism	Increases metabolic rate, stimulates fat breakdown and increases blood sugar levels	No effect
Blood vessels	Constricts blood vessels in viscera and skin	
	Dilates blood vessels in the heart and skeletal muscle	No effect
Eye	Dilates pupils	Constricts pupils
Heart	Increases rate and force of contraction	Decreases rate
Lungs	Dilates bronchioles	Constricts bronchioles
Kidneys	Decreases urine output	No effect
Liver	Causes the release of glucose	No effect
Digestive system	Decreases peristalsis and constricts digestive system sphincters	Increases peristalsis and dilates digestive system sphincters
Adrenal medulla	Stimulates cells to secrete epinephrine and norepinephrine	No effect
Lacrimal glands	Inhibits the production of tears	Increases the production of tears
Salivary glands	Inhibits the production of saliva	Increases the production of saliva
Sweat glands	Stimulates to produce perspiration	No effect

Medicines Management Carbamazepine

Carbamazepine is an anticonvulsant primarily used in the treatment of epileptic seizures. Carbamazepine works by blocking the sodium channels of nerve cells in the brain and so reduces the increased excitability and firing activity of neurones that occur during an epileptic seizure.

Antiepileptic hypersensitivity syndrome has been associated with some antiepileptic drugs and usually starts between 1 and 8 weeks after commencing treatment, and signs and symptoms include fever, rash, lymphadenopathy liver and haematological dysfunction. If signs of hypersensitivity syndrome occur, the drug should be withdrawn immediately (Joint Formulary Committee, 2018).

Patients with epilepsy may drive a car but not larger vehicles, e.g. passenger-carrying vehicles or lorries (Driver and Vehicle Licensing Agency – *DVLA 2019*). However, patients are advised not to drive during medication changes or withdrawal of antiepileptic drugs, and for 6 months afterwards. Similarly, patients who have had a first or single epileptic seizure must not drive for 6 months after the seizure (Joint Formulary Committee, 2018).

Conclusion

In conclusion, the nervous system is a highly organised network of cells and structures that include the brain and cranial nerves and the spinal cord and spinal nerves, which play a major role in maintaining homeostasis. The nervous system responds to external and internal stimuli through three basic functions: the sensory, integrative and motor functions, which generate responses and create changes in bodily functions as required. Conditions affecting the nervous system can have a devastating effect on the quality of life and the functions essential for survival.

Glossary

Action potential: Conduction along a nerve or muscle cell membrane caused by a large, transient depolarisation.

Antidiuretic hormone (ADH): Hormone that acts on the kidneys to reabsorb more water, thus reducing urine output.

Afferent fibres: Carry nerve impulses towards the central nervous system.

Arachnoid mater: Middle layer of the meninges.

Astrocyte: Neuroglial cell that helps the blood–brain barrier.

Autonomic nervous system: Involuntary motor division of the motor nervous system.

Axon: Process of a neurone that carries impulses away from the cell body.

Brainstem: Collective name given to the pons, medulla and midbrain.

Cation: An ion with a positive charge.

Central nervous system: Brain and spinal cord.

Cerebellum: Anatomical region of the brain responsible for coordinated and smooth skeletal muscle movements.

Cerebral hemispheres: Division of the cerebrum.

Cerebrospinal fluid: Fluid that surrounds the central nervous system.

Cerebrum: Large anatomical region of the brain which is divided into the cerebral hemispheres.

Circle of Willis: Part of arterial blood supply to the brain.

Cranial nerves: Twelve pairs of nerves that leave the brain and supply sensory and motor neurones to the head, neck, part of the trunk and the viscera of the thorax and abdomen.

Dendrite: Part of a neurone that transmits impulses towards the cell body.

Diencephalon: Anatomical region of the brain consisting of the thalamus, hypothalamus and epithalamus.

Dura mater: Tough outer layer of the meninges.

Effector: Muscle, gland or organ stimulated by the nervous system.

Efferent fibres: Carry nerve impulses away from the central nervous system.

Ependymal cells: Neuroglial cells that line the cavities of the central nervous system.

Epinephrine: Hormone produced by the adrenal medulla that is also a neurotransmitter.

Epithalamus: Part of the brain that forms the diencephalon.

Ganglia: A group of neuronal cell bodies lying outside the central nervous system.

Hypothalamus: Part of the diencephalon with many functions.

Lobe: A clear anatomical division or boundary within a structure.

Medulla oblongata: Part of the brainstem.

Meninges: Three layers of tissue that cover and protect the central nervous system (dura, arachnoid and pia maters).

Midbrain: Part of the brainstem that links the brainstem to the diencephalon.

Microglia: Neuroglia that has the ability to phagocytose material.

Motor area: The area located in the cerebral cortex that controls voluntary motor function.

Motor nerves: Neurones that conduct impulses to effectors which may be either muscle or glands.

Myelin sheath: Fatty insulating layer that surrounds nerve fibres responsible for speeding up impulse conduction.

Neuroglia: Cells of the nervous system that protect and support the functional unit – the neurone.

Neuromuscular junction: Region where skeletal muscle comes into contact with a neurone.

Neurone: Functional unit of the nervous system responsible for generating and conducting nerve impulses.

Nuclei: Cluster of cell bodies within the central nervous system.

Oligodendrocytes: Glial cell that helps produce the myelin sheath.

Peripheral nervous system: All nerves located outside of the brain and spinal cord (the central nervous system).

Pia mater: Innermost layer of the meninges.

Pineal gland: Part of the diencephalon that has an endocrine function.

Pituitary gland: An endocrine gland located next to the hypothalamus that produces many hormones.

Receptor: Sensory nerve ending or cell that responds to stimuli.

Refractory period: The period immediately after a neurone has fired when it cannot receive another impulse.

Reticular formation: Area located throughout the brainstem that is responsible for arousal, regulation of sensory input to the cerebrum and control of motor output.

Saltatory conduction: Transmission of an impulse down a mylelinated nerve fibre where the impulse moves from node of Ranvier to node.

Sensory area: An area of the cerebrum responsible for sensation.

Sensory nerves: Neurones that carry sensory information from cranial and spinal nerves into the brain and spinal cord.

Somatic nervous system: Voluntary motor division of the peripheral nervous system.

Spinal nerves: Thirty-one pairs of nerves that originate on the spinal cord.

Synapse: Junction between two neurones or neurones and effector site.

Thalamus: Part of the diencephalon.

Ventricle: Cavity in the brain.

White matter: Myelinated nerve fibres.

References

Aspire (2019) *Supporting people with spinal injury* https://www.aspire.org.uk/ (accessed May 2019).

Driver and Vehicle Licensing Agency (DVLA) – GOV.UK https://www.gov.uk/government/organisations/driver-and-vehicle-licensing-agency (accessed June 2019).

Farquhar-Smith, P., Beaulieu, P. and Jaggar, S. (2018) *Landmark Papers in Pain: Seminal Papers in Pain with Expert Commentaries.* Oxford: Open University Press.

Galbraith, Bullock, S., Manias, E., Hunt, B. and Richards, A. (2007) *Fundamentals of Pharmacology.* Harlow: Pearson.

Gates, B., Fearns, D. and Welch, J. (2014) *Learning Disability Nursing at a Glance.* Oxford: Wiley-Blackwell.

Joint Formulary Committee (2018) *BNF 75.* London: Pharmaceutical Press.

Logenbaker, S.N. (2016) *Mader's Understanding Human Anatomy and Physiology,* 9th edn. London: McGraw-Hill.

Marieb, E.N. and Hoehn, K. (2015) *Human Anatomy and Physiology,* Global edn. San Francisco, CA: Pearson Benjamin Cummings.

McFadden, R., (2019) *Introducing Pharmacology: For Nursing and Healthcare,* 3rd edn. England: Routledge.

Migliozzi, J.G. (2017) The nervous system and associated disorders. In Nair, M. and Peate, I. (eds) *Fundamentals of Applied Pathophysiology: An Essential Guide For Nursing And Healthcare Students,* 3rd edn. Oxford: John Wiley & Sons, Ltd.

NHS Choices (2019) Panic Disorder. https://www.nhs.uk/conditions/panic-disorder/ (accessed February 2019).

Seeley, R.R., Stephens T.D. and Vanputte, C. (2016) *Anatomy and Physiology,* 11th edn. New York: McGraw-Hill.

Tortora, G.J. and Derrickson, B.H. (2014) *Principles of Anatomy and Physiology,* 15th edn. Hoboken, NJ: John Wiley & Sons, Inc.

VanMeter, K.C. and Hubert, R.J. (2014). *Gould's Pathophysiology for Health Professions,* 5th edn. St Louis: Elsevier Saunders.

Waugh, A. and Grant, A. (2018) *Ross and Wilson Anatomy and Physiology in Health and Illness,* 13th edn. Edinburgh: Elsevier Churchill Livingstone.

Further Reading

Epilepsies: Diagnosis and Management
http://www.nice.org.uk/guidance/cg137
Link to clinical guidance on the epilepsies. The epilepsies, the diagnosis and management of the epilepsies in adult and children in primary and secondary care.

Head Injury: Assessment and Early Management
http://www.nice.org.uk/guidance/cg176
Link to clinical guidance on head injury: triage, assessment, investigation and early management of head injury in children, young people and adults.

Parkinson's UK
A UK charity supporting those affected by Parkinson's disease and supporting Parkinson's disease research http://www.parkinsons.org.uk/

The Stroke Association
A UK charity that helps those affected by stroke and their families.
http://www.stroke.org.uk/

Activities

Multiple Choice Questions

1. Which part of the brain is responsible for thinking, reasoning and intelligence?
   (a) cerebellum
   (b) hypothalamus
   (c) cerebrum
   (d) epithalamus

2. Which structures are involved in the control of respiration?
   (a) pons and medulla
   (b) thalamus and epithalamus
   (c) somatic and sensory nervous system
   (d) cerebellum and cerebrum

3. Which neuroglial cell acts as a macrophage?
   (a) oligodendrocyte
   (b) astrocyte
   (c) microglia
   (d) Schwann cell

4. Which layer of the meninges is closest to the skull bone?
   (a) dura mater
   (b) arachnoid mater
   (c) pia mater
   (d) subarachnoid space

5. Which neurotransmitter is associated with the neuromuscular junction?
   (a) dopamine
   (b) norepinephrine
   (c) acetylcholine
   (d) CSF

6. Which part of the brain is closely associated with the pituitary gland?
   (a) thalamus
   (b) epithalamus
   (c) hypothalamus
   (d) pons

7. Which is true of the autonomic nervous system?
   (a) it has two divisions – the somatic and voluntary divisions
   (b) it is housed in the cerebrum
   (c) it helps regulate heart rate and blood pressure
   (d) it does not influence any other system of the body

8. Nerves that carry impulses towards the central nervous system are:
   (a) afferent nerves
   (b) efferent nerves
   (c) motor nerves
   (d) mixed nerves

9. Sympathetic stimulation of the nervous system would lead to all but which of the following responses:
   (a) bronchioles dilate
   (b) urine output increases
   (c) heart rate increases
   (d) epinephrine (adrenaline) is released

10. Nerves that carry impulses away from the central nervous system are:
    (a) afferent nerves
    (b) efferent nerves
    (c) motor nerves
    (d) mixed nerves

11. Cerebrospinal fluid:
    (a) contains white blood cells
    (b) is secreted by the choroid plexus
    (c) contains fat
    (d) is an opaque body fluid
12. The trigeminal nerve:
    (a) provides taste sensations
    (b) is the seventh cranial nerve
    (c) controls the muscles of facial expression
    (d) supplies the muscles of mastication
13. The spinal cord:
    (a) passes through the foramen magnum
    (b) gives origin to cranial nerves
    (c) has a central canal
    (d) has grey matter on the outside
14. The parasympathetic nervous system:
    (a) includes the vagus nerve
    (b) provides actions for immediate responses
    (c) causes vasoconstriction
    (d) can increase blood pressure
15. The spinal nerves:
    (a) have two connections to the spinal cord
    (b) consist of 34 pairs of nerves
    (c) can regenerate if damaged
    (d) branch into five plexuses

Find Out More

1. Name the two major divisions of the nervous system.
2. Differentiate between the parasympathetic nervous system and the sympathetic nervous system.
3. Identify the functions of the neuroglia.
4. Describe the action potential.
5. Identify the functions of the different regions of the brain.
6. Describe to a patient's relative what the acronym FAST in relation to stoke means.
7. Explain the difference between stroke and transient attacks.
8. Define the term saltatory conduction.
9. What is the difference between the term afferent and efferent?
10. What is the function of brainstem?

Conditions

The following is a list of conditions that are associated with the nervous system. Take some time and write notes about each of the conditions. You may make the notes taken from textbooks or other resources (e.g. people you work with in a clinical area), or you may make the notes as a result of people you have cared for. If you are making notes about people you have cared for, you must ensure that you adhere to the rules of confidentiality.

Multiple sclerosis

Botulism

Fibromyalgia

Parkinson's disease

Epilepsy

Raised intracranial pressure

Alzheimer's disease

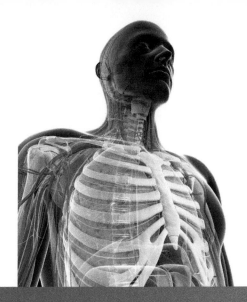

15

The Senses

Carl Clare

Test Your Prior Knowledge

- Which cranial nerve is responsible for conveying information about perceived smells to the brain?
- Name the main components of the ear involved in the sense of balance.
- What part of the tongue is involved in the sense of taste?
- Name the two substances that fill the eye chambers and help to maintain the shape of the eye.
- What is the name for short-sightedness?

Learning Outcomes

After reading this chapter you will be able to:

- Describe the process by which we perceive smell.
- Explain the mechanisms responsible for the perception of different tastes.
- Describe the way in which human beings maintain a sense of balance.
- Explore the mechanisms that lead to sound information being converted into action potentials to be relayed to the brain.
- Describe the difference between rods and cones in the eye.
- Explain how a visual image is focused on the retina.

Visit the student companion website at www.wileyfundamentalseries.com/anatomy where you can test yourself using flashcards, multiple-choice questions and more. Instructor companion site at www.wiley.com/go/instructor/anatomy where instructors will find valuable materials such as PowerPoint slides and image bank designed to enhance your teaching.

Fundamentals of Anatomy and Physiology: For Nursing and Healthcare Students, Third Edition. Edited by Ian Peate and Suzanne Evans.
© 2020 John Wiley & Sons Ltd. Published 2020 by John Wiley & Sons Ltd.
Student companion website: www.wileyfundamentalseries.com/anatomy
Instructor companion website: www.wiley.com/go/instructor/anatomy

Introduction

The senses are usually thought of as the five senses of smell, taste, hearing, vision and touch. However, in physiology the sense of touch is excluded from the senses as it is considered a somatic sense. Thus the 'senses' is a term used to refer to the senses of:

- smell
- taste
- hearing
- sight.

Also included in this list of senses is the sense of

- equilibrium.

This chapter will explore these five senses in three sections:

- the 'chemical' senses of smell and taste;
- the senses associated with the ear: those of equilibrium and hearing;
- the sense of sight.

In all these sections there will be a review of the anatomy of the particular organs involved in these senses, followed by a discussion of the physiology of how these senses are monitored and create action potentials to be transmitted to the brain. Finally, the pathways these action potentials take to the brain will be reviewed, along with a brief discussion of the processing of this information in the brain itself.

The Chemical Senses

With regard to the senses, the chemical senses are the senses of smell and taste, which rely on chemoreceptors. There are two main types of chemoreceptor:

- distance chemoreceptors – for instance, the olfactory (smell) receptors;
- direct chemoreceptors – for instance, the sense of taste, which relies on the taste buds.

The Sense of Smell (Olfaction)

In evolutionary terms the sense of smell is one of the oldest senses. The sense of smell is useful to us for the identification of food that is safe to eat and that which has gone rotten; it helps us to identify dangers such as hazardous chemicals and gives us pleasure through the smell of flowers and perfume. Olfaction (the sense of smell) is dependent on receptors that respond to airborne particles. In the nasal cavity either side of the nasal septum there are paired olfactory organs made up of two layers (Figure 15.1):

- Olfactory epithelium – this layer contains the olfactory receptor cells, supporting cells and regenerative basal cells (stem cells) that mature into receptor cells to replace those that die.
- Lamina propria – a layer of areolar tissue containing numerous blood vessels and nerves. This layer also contains the olfactory glands, which secrete a lipid-rich substance that absorbs water to form a thick mucus that covers the olfactory epithelium.

The olfactory region of each of the two nasal passages is about 2.5 cm^2 (Jenkins and Tortora, 2013) and between them they contain approximately 50 million receptor cells.

When air is inhaled through the nose the air in the nasal cavity is subject to turbulent flow and this ensures that airborne smell particles (odorant molecules) are brought to the olfactory organs. Approximately 2% of the inhaled air in an average inspiration passes the olfactory organs; the act of sniffing increases this percentage by a large amount. The olfactory receptors can only be stimulated by compounds that are soluble in water or lipid and can therefore diffuse through the mucus that overlies the olfactory epithelium.

Olfactory Receptors

The olfactory receptors are highly modified neurones contained within the olfactory epithelium. The tip of each receptor projects beyond the surface of the epithelium (Figure 15.1). This projection forms the base for up to 20 cilia (hair-like structures) that extend into the surrounding mucus. These cilia lie laterally in the

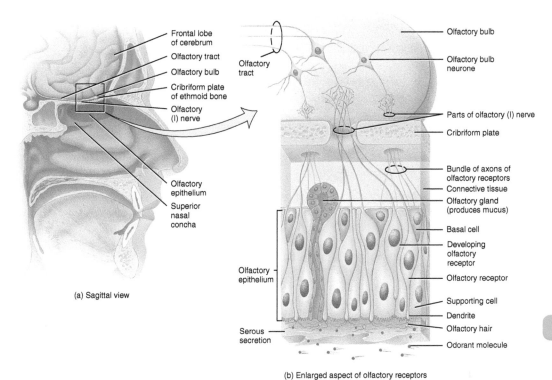

(a) Sagittal view

(b) Enlarged aspect of olfactory receptors

Figure 15.1 **(a, b) Gross and microscopic anatomy of olfaction.** *Source:* Tortora and Derrickson (2009). Reproduced with permission of John Wiley & Sons.

mucus (they lie relatively flat rather than upright), thus exposing a larger surface area to any compound that is dissolved into the mucus.

Dissolved chemicals interact with odorant-binding proteins on the surface of the cilia; a local depolarisation occurs by the opening of sodium channels in the cell membrane. If enough local depolarisations occur, then an action potential is generated within the receptor cell.

Medicines Management Flixonase

Flixonase (fluticasone propionate) is a topical glucocorticoid medicine that is commonly used for the treatment of allergic rhinitis (inflammation of the inside of the nose) and nasal polyps.

Flixonase is available as a nasal spray or nasal drops. The methods for instilling nasal drops and nasal sprays vary slightly and are detailed below. The nurse should adhere to local policy and procedure at all times.

Nasal spray technique:

- Blow the nose to clear it.
- Shake the bottle.
- Close off one nostril and put the nozzle in the open nostril.
- Tilt the head forward slightly and keep the bottle upright.
- Squeeze a fine mist into the nose while breathing in slowly. The person should not sniff hard.
- Breathe out through the mouth.
- Take a second spray in the same nostril then repeat this procedure for the other nostril if prescribed.

Nasal drops technique:

- Blow the nose to clear it.
- Shake the container.
- Tilt the head backwards.

(Continued)

401

- Place the drops in the nostril.
- Keep the head tilted and sniff gently to let the drops penetrate.
- Repeat for the other nostril if prescribed.

The side effects of flixonase include nose bleed (a very common side effect) and dryness or irritation of the nose or throat. Minimising the side effects of flixonase medications can be done by:

- Prescribing a nasal spray instead of drops. If nasal drops are indicated or preferred, ensure that they are used correctly.
- Prescribing the weakest potency possible, for the shortest period of time.

See National Institute for Health and Care Excellence (2015).

The Olfactory Pathway

The olfactory system is very sensitive and as little as four molecules can lead to the activation of a receptor. However, activation of a receptor cell does not mean there will be awareness of the smell. There is a significant amount of convergence along the olfactory nervous pathway and inhibition at intervening synapses can prevent the signal from reaching the olfactory cortex in the brain. However, the olfactory threshold remains very low; for instance, humans can detect very low concentrations of the chemicals added to the odourless natural gas used in the home, making it 'smell' and thus ensuring leaks are detected by the homeowner.

On each side of the nose, axons leaving the olfactory epithelium receptor cells collect into 20 or more bundles that penetrate the cribriform plate of the ethmoid bone (Figure 15.2); these bundles comprise the right and left olfactory nerves until they reach the olfactory bulbs in the brain. At the olfactory bulbs the axons converge to connect with postsynaptic (mitral) cells in large synaptic structures called glomeruli. Efferent fibres of cells elsewhere in the brain also innervate the olfactory bulb, thus allowing for the potential inhibition of the signalling pathways, for instance in central adaptation (Box 15.1).

Box 15.1 Central Adaptation

Have you ever noticed that when meeting someone during the day you will smell their perfume or aftershave, but having spent some time with them you will no longer be aware of that smell? Humans tend to 'habituate' to persistent smells to the point that they are no longer perceived. This is not due to the local receptors adapting to the persistent stimuli; it is a function of central adaptation. That is, higher centres in the brain are responsible for our reduced perception of a persistent smell. The transmission of the sensory information for that particular smell is inhibited at the level of the olfactory bulb by nerve impulses from the centres in the brain.

Axons exiting from the olfactory bulbs travel along the olfactory nerves (cranial nerve I, which is a paired nerve) to reach the olfactory cortex, the hypothalamus and portions of the limbic system via the olfactory tracts. Olfactory stimulation is the only sensory information that reaches the cerebral cortex directly; all other senses are processed by the thalamus first. The fact that the limbic system and hypothalamus receive olfactory input helps to explain the profound emotional response that can be triggered by certain smells.

Olfactory Discrimination

The olfactory system can make distinctions among some 2000–4000 chemical stimuli; however, there are no reasons that can be found to explain this in the structure of the receptor cells themselves. Though the epithelium is divided into areas of receptors with particular sensitivity for certain smells, it appears that the central nervous system interprets each smell by analysing the overall pattern of receptor activity (Tortora and Derrickson, 2012). It has been proposed that smell is perceived in primary odours (Haehner et al., 2013); the exact number remains a source of contention and estimates vary from 7 to 30. Some of the smells that we perceive are not detected by the olfactory receptors at all; some of what we sense is actually pain. The nasal cavity contains pain receptors that respond to certain irritants such as ammonia, chillies and menthol. As we get older, smell discrimination and sensitivity reduce as we lose receptors compared with the total number we had when younger and the receptors that remain become less sensitive.

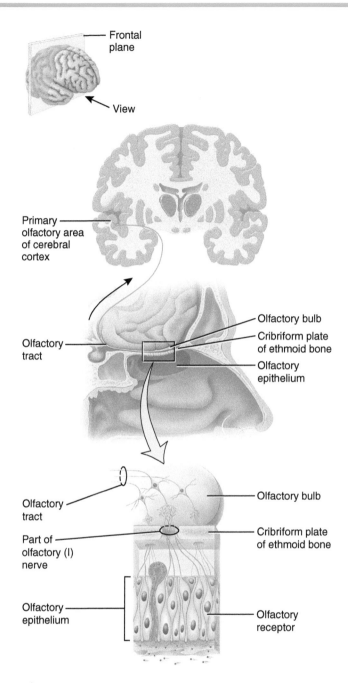

Figure 15.2 **Olfactory pathway.** *Source:* Tortora and Derrickson (2009). Reproduced with permission of John Wiley & Sons.

Clinical Considerations Loss of the Sense of Smell (Anosmia)

The loss of the sense of smell (known as anosmia) is normally an acquired disorder due to either trauma to the nose or brain injury, but some people are born without a sense of smell (congenital anosmia).

While appearing to be a minor problem, the loss of the sense of smell is often associated with feelings of depression and a reduced quality of life (Neuland et al., 2011).

While temporary anosmia is common with conditions such as rhinitis, the common cold and hay fever, permanent anosmia is often related to trauma, surgery and degenerative conditions such as Alzheimer's and Parkinson's.

> Anosmia is noted to be an early indicator of Parkinson's with 95% of patients presenting with anosmia years before motor-related symptoms appear (Haehner et al., 2011).
>
> Patients with anosmia are advised to take certain safety measures:
>
> - install smoke alarms;
> - clearly mark expiry dates on food and leftovers;
> - read the warning labels on chemical agents and cleaners to avoid potentially harmful gases;
> - switch from gas to electric.
>
> See NHS Choices (2015).

The Sense of Taste

Like the sense of smell, the sense of taste helps to protect us from poisons but also drives our appetite. There are five basic tastes:

- sweet
- sour
- bitter
- salt
- umami.

The first four tastes are already common knowledge, but the fifth was relatively unknown in the western hemisphere until recently. Umami is the taste associated with the proteins found in meat and fish (Osawa, 2012) and has been known as a concept of taste to the Japanese for many years.

The sense of taste is associated with the taste buds, which are the sensory receptor for taste and found primarily in the oral cavity. There are approximately 10,000 taste buds in the oral cavity; most are found on the tongue, but a few are on the soft palate, the inner surface of the cheeks and the pharynx and epiglottis.

Most of the taste buds are found in peg-like projections of the tongue's mucosa. These projections are known as papillae (singular is papilla) and gives the tongue its slightly rough feel. The papillae are found in four major forms (Figure 15.3):

- Fungiform – mushroom-shaped papillae found scattered over the tongue surface but most abundant at the tip and sides. They usually contain 1–18 taste buds, which are located on the top of these papillae.
- Circumvallate (otherwise known as vallate) – the largest of the papillae and found in the least number. Seven to 12 of them are found in an inverted 'V' shape at the back of the tongue. They contain approximately 250 taste buds, which are located in the side walls of these papillae.
- Foliate – 'leaf-like' papillae found on the sides of the rear of the tongue, which contain around 100 taste buds.
- Filiform – thread-like structures that contain no taste buds. They provide friction to aid the movement of food by the tongue.

Taste Buds

Each taste bud is globular in structure and consists of 40–60 epithelial cells of three major types (Figure 15.4):

- Supporting cells form the greatest part of the taste bud. They help to insulate the receptor cells from each other and the epithelium of the tongue.
- Gustatory (or taste) cells – the chemoreceptor responsible for sensing taste.
- Basal cells – stem cells that mature into new receptor cells to replace those that die.

Both the supporting cells and the gustatory cells have long microvilli (protrusions of the cell membrane that increase its surface area) called gustatory hairs. These gustatory hairs project from the tip of the cell and protrude through a 'taste pore' in the epithelium to allow them to be bathed in saliva. The gustatory hairs are the sensitive portion of the gustatory cell.

Coiling around the gustatory cells are the sensory dendrites, which are the initial part of the gustatory pathway. Each afferent nerve fibre receives nerve signals from several receptor cells.

The Taste Receptor

The activation of the taste receptor requires the chemical compound (known as a tastant; Jenkins and Tortora, 2013) that is to be tasted to dissolve in the saliva, then diffuse into the taste pore and come into contact with

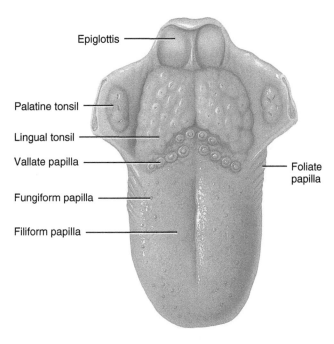

Figure 15.3 **Tongue and the location of the papillae.** *Source:* Tortora and Derrickson (2009). Reproduced with permission of John Wiley & Sons.

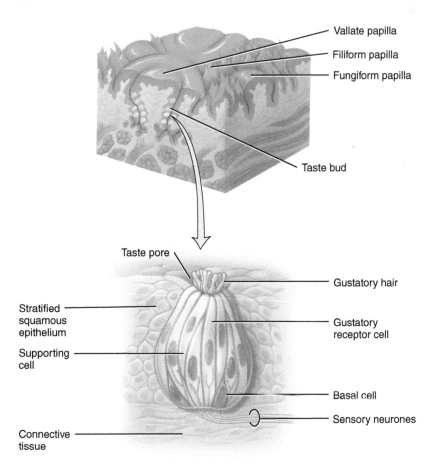

Figure 15.4 **Cross-section of part of the tongue and microscopic view of a taste bud.** *Source:* Tortora and Derrickson (2009). Reproduced with permission of John Wiley & Sons.

the gustatory hairs. Depending on the type of taste, this has one of four potential effects (the exact mechanism that is involved in the sensing of umami is unknown):

- salt – salty taste initiates an influx of sodium into the cell;
- sour – sour taste leads to a hydrogen ion blockade of sodium and potassium channels in the cell membrane;
- bitter – bitter taste leads to an influx of calcium ions into the cell;
- sweet – sweet taste leads to an inactivation of potassium channels.

All these effects lead to the depolarisation of the cell and the release of neurotransmitters. Salt taste and sour taste have direct effects on the cell membrane. Bitter taste, sweet taste and umami exert their action on the cell by the use of messenger systems activated by G-protein-coupled receptors.

It appears that we have various sensitivities to different tastes. We are most sensitive to bitter tastes, then sour and then sweet and salty. To an extent this makes evolutionary sense as poisons tend to taste bitter, whereas acids and food that has 'gone off' often taste sour. Thus, we are most sensitive to those tastes that may indicate something that could harm us.

It should be noted that the taste buds are not the only methods by which we experience the taste of a food. It is clear that the sense of smell is also of vital importance to how we experience taste – just think of how food tastes when your nose is blocked due to a cold; 80% of the sense of taste is actually smell. As with the sense of smell, there are also pain receptors involved with the sense of taste and certain tastes will elicit a pain stimulus as opposed to a gustatory one.

The Gustatory Pathway

The release of neurotransmitters by the gustatory cells creates an action potential in related afferent nerve fibres. The sensory information from the tongue is transmitted along two cranial nerve pairs:

- chorda tympani –a branch of the facial nerve (cranial nerve VII) relays impulses from the anterior two-thirds of the tongue;
- lingual branch of the glossopharyngeal nerve (cranial nerve IX) – carries the sensory information of the posterior third of the tongue.

Sensory information from the taste buds in the epiglottis and pharynx is transmitted by the vagus nerve (cranial nerve X). All the afferent fibres terminate in the solitary nucleus of the medulla. The sensory messages are then transmitted, ultimately, to the thalamus and the gustatory cortex in the parietal lobes. Afferent fibres also project into the hypothalamus and limbic system. Ultimately, many of the branches of afferent nerves that divert to various parts of the brain, apart from the cortex, are involved in the triggering of reflexes involved with digestion (for instance, salivation).

The gustatory pathway is unique among the senses because if the taste buds lose their afferent nerve fibres (for instance, are cut) the taste bud then degenerates. As we get older, we lose the sense of taste as there is a reduction in the number of taste buds; gustatory cells die and are not replaced at the same rate as they die and those cells that remain become less sensitive.

Episode of Care Mental Health

Jennifer is a 36-year-old currently being treated for severe depression with fluoxetine (Prozac). She has come to her outpatient appointment and is complaining of a constantly dry mouth which is affecting her sense of taste and her appetite as well as severe halitosis (bad breath) and recurrent gum infections. Jennifer has been looking on the internet and knows that a dry mouth is a known side effect of fluoxetine, as the constantly dry mouth is making her very unhappy, she is becoming non-concordant with her medication and is saying she is going to stop taking it altogether.

Saliva is an essential body fluid and contains substances that:

- protect, lubricate and cleanse the oral mucosa;
- aid chewing, swallowing and talking;
- protect the teeth against decay;
- protect the mouth, teeth and throat from infection by bacteria, yeasts and viruses;
- support and facilitate our sense of taste.

Dry mouth (xerostomia) is a known side effect of many medications (Mohammed, 2014) used in the treatment of depression and psychosis including the selective serotonin reuptake inhibitors, tricyclic antidepressants and many antipsychotic medications (especially clozapine). The effects of dry mouth are unpleasant and can exacerbate feelings of depression. The effects include:

- altered taste sensation;
- difficulty eating (especially dry food);
- gum disease and dental decay;
- halitosis (bad breath);
- thirst;
- thick stringy saliva;
- sores in the mouth.

The symptoms can be so upsetting that patients may stop taking their medication to avoid the side effects.

The medical treatment of dry mouth remains limited but there are several things patients can do to help:

- Drink water, especially at mealtimes. Acidic drinks should be avoided as they have an effect on dental enamel and increase the chances of dental caries.
- Avoid caffeine as it can exacerbate the feeling of dry mouth.
- Chewing sugar free chewing gum or sucking sugar free sweets to promote saliva production.
- Stopping smoking.
- Using proprietary saliva sprays and oral rinses.
- Using lip balm to protect lips.
- Clean teeth regularly and ensure they have regular dental checks.
- Using a humidifier in the bedroom to try and reduce the dry mouth feeling at night.

The medical treatment of dry mouth is possible using medications such as pilocarpine and cevimeline, but these medications also have side effects that may be just as unpleasant.

Multiple Choice Questions

1. Which drugs can cause xerostomia?
   (a) selective serotonin reuptake inhibitors
   (b) antipsychotics
   (c) tricyclic antidepressants
   (d) all of the above
2. The effects of xerostomia lead to difficulty eating. To aid with eating the patient should:
   (a) sip water when drinking
   (b) eat sugar free foods
   (c) eat foods with a strong taste
   (d) only eat liquid foods
3. Patients with xerostomia should avoid drinking:
   (a) sugar free drinks
   (b) caffeine
   (c) alcohol
   (d) hot drinks
4. The dental effects of xerostomia include dental decay, therefore patients should be advised to:
   (a) brush their teeth every hour
   (b) use mouthwash every hour
   (c) have regular dental check-ups.
   (d) have fluoride treatment monthly
5. Why are the medications used for xerostomia not commonly prescribed?
   (a) doctors don't know about them
   (b) they are expensive
   (c) they are not licensed for that use
   (d) they have side effects that can be just as unpleasant

Clinical Considerations Taste Disorders

Taste disorders are relatively common in the general population and can be split into three types:

- Ageusia – the complete loss of taste. Although ageusia is rare.
- Hypogeusia – this is much more common and is the reduced ability to taste the five main tastes of salt, sweet, bitter, sour and umami.
- Dysgeusia – this is usually characterised as a foul, salty, rancid or metallic taste that persists in the mouth.

The causes of altered taste sensations are varied and include:

- upper respiratory and middle ear infections;
- radiation therapy for cancers of the head and neck;
- exposure to certain chemicals, such as insecticides and some medications, including some common antibiotics and antihistamines;
- head injury;
- some types of surgery to the ear, nose and throat (such as middle-ear surgery) or extraction of the wisdom teeth;
- poor oral hygiene and dental problems.

Alteration in taste can affect the appetite and especially in the elderly can lead to a reduced food intake. The advice for improving appetite for patients with a taste disorder is:

- prepare foods with a variety of colours and textures;
- use aromatic herbs and hot spices to add more flavour – however, avoid adding more sugar or salt to foods;
- if the diet permits, add small amounts of cheese, bacon bits, butter, olive oil or toasted nuts on vegetables;
- avoid combination dishes, such as casseroles, that can hide individual flavours and dilute taste.

The Senses of Equilibrium and Hearing

The ear is divided into three sections: external, middle and inner (see Figure 15.5).

Each of these three sections is integral in the process of hearing and the inner ear is also essential in the maintenance of the sense of balance.

The Structure of the Ear
The Outer Ear

The outer ear consists of:

- auricle (pinna)
- external auditory canal
- tympanic membrane.

The auricle is the shell-shaped projection surrounding the external auditory canal. It is made of elastic cartilage covered with skin. The auricle can be further broken down into the rim, known as the helix and the earlobe, which lacks supporting cartilage and so is soft. The function of the auricle is to direct sound waves into the external auditory canal.

The external auditory canal (meatus) is a short, S-shaped, narrow passage about 2.5 cm long and 0.6 cm wide, which extends from the auricle to the tympanic membrane (Figure 15.5). At the end closest to the auricle the external auditory ear canal is made of elastic cartilage; the rest of the canal is a channel through the temporal bone and thus needs no supporting cartilage. The entire canal is lined with skin with associated hairs, sebaceous (oil) glands and modified sweat glands called ceruminous glands. The ceruminous glands secrete a yellow-brown waxy cerumen (ear wax). The purpose of the oils and the wax is to lubricate the ear canal, kill bacteria and, in conjunction with the hairs, keep the canal free of debris.

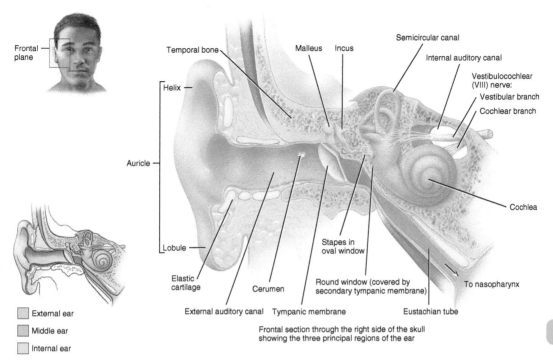

Figure 15.5 **Structure of the ear.** *Source:* Tortora and Derrickson (2009). Reproduced with permission of John Wiley & Sons.

Episode of Care Learning Disabilities

Stephen is a 21-year-old gentleman who lives with his parents. He attends college 3 days a week where he is studying horticulture and a day centre 2 days a week. His parents have received reports that Stephen has become less and less attentive in college and has become more withdrawn from his friends in both college and the day centre. Staff at the college have noticed that they have to give Stephen instructions several times and that his speaking voice has become louder. Concerned, Stephen's parent's take him to see the GP. Examining Stephen, the GP notices that he has difficulty assessing Stephen's ears as the ear canal is very narrow, but the GP can definitely see a lot of ear wax. Unwilling to try and clean Stephen's ears due to the narrowed ear canal the GP refers Stephen to the local ENT clinic. In the clinic it is confirmed that Stephen does have a narrow ear canal (a common finding in children with Down syndrome but usually this resolves by the age of 3 (Shott, 2006)). Following cleaning of the impacted ear wax using microsuction Stephen's hearing does improve but it is recommended that he is kept under review by the clinic as many of the otolaryngological features of Down syndrome predispose the patient to chronic otitis media (middle ear infections).

From birth the person with Down syndrome will often have external ear canal stenosis but this usually resolves by the age of 3 years. However, even after this age the patient with Down syndrome will be predisposed to chronic problems with the ear. Upper respiratory tract infections are common and thus predispose the patient to developing otitis media, potentially leading to 'glue ear' (otitis media with effusion) which is less likely to self-limit in those with Down syndrome. The reasons for this predisposition to respiratory and ear infections are not entirely clear but probably include anatomical differences in the structure of the mid face, a reduction in T and B lymphocytes (Shott, 2006) thus reducing the effectiveness of the immune system, differences in the shape and size of the eustachian tube and hypotonia of the muscles controlling the eustachian tube leading to eustachian tube collapse.

Microsuction is one of the safest methods of earwax removal with few potential side effects. Patients may report feeling dizzy afterwards, but this quickly passes (within minutes). Patients prone to the build up of ear wax should be advised of a few simple precautions to prevent the impaction of the wax in the ear canal (which makes the wax less likely to drain naturally).

• Never put anything into the ear canal, especially cotton buds, keys, or tissues to either clean them or to dry them.

- If there is an ear infection present, try to avoid water entering the ear canal. Use a small amount of cotton wool soaked in white soft paraffin placed just inside the opening of the ear to prevent water entering the ear canal when having a bath or shower. Do not push the cotton wool into the ear canal.
- If there is a possibility that there is a hole in the ear drum do no use any over the counter preparations for ear wax removal, consult with the practice nurse or GP.

Multiple Choice Questions

1. Otitis media is:
    (a) infection of the ear drum
    (b) infection of the inner ear
    (c) infection of the middle ear
    (d) infection of the outer ear
2. A common potential side effect of micro-suction treatment for ear wax is:
    (a) dizziness
    (b) fainting
    (c) perforation of the ear drum
    (d) loss of hearing
3. A narrow ear canal in those with Down syndrome usually resolves by:
    (a) adulthood
    (b) age 3 years
    (c) age 10 years
    (d) age 16 years
4. What should a patient put in their ear to try and clear ear wax:
    (a) cotton bud
    (b) special scraper
    (c) tissues
    (d) none of the above
5. In patients with Down syndrome, why are ear infections more common than in the general population?
    (a) they produce more ear wax
    (b) the eustachian tube is often a different shape and size
    (c) the ear drum is often broken
    (d) the outer ear is higher up

Medicines Management Antibiotic Ear Drops

Infections of the outer ear are relatively common and can be treated with antibiotic ear drops; however, with the increase in antibiotic resistance, current NICE guidelines suggest that antibiotics should be the last resort in treating ear infections (NICE, 2018). The first line treatment for any ear infection should be pain relief, placing a warm or cold flannel on the ear and removing any discharge by wiping the outside of the ear (never placing anything in the ear canal).

Outer ear infections usually present with the following symptoms:

- pain inside the ear
- a high temperature of 38 °C or above
- being sick
- a lack of energy
- difficulty hearing
- discharge running out of the ear
- a feeling of pressure or fullness inside the ear
- itching and irritation in and around the ear.

If the infection does not clear after 3 days, the patient develops a very high temperature, a sore throat, or inflammation around the ear then the patient should seek advice from a doctor or pharmacist.

If the infection is associated with significant inflammation the GP may prescribe antibiotic eardrops with steroids to reduce the inflammation. In severe cases oral antibiotics may be required. As with all antibiotics it is important that they are used correctly and the entire course of treatment is taken.

Skills in Practice Instillation of Ear Drops

David is a 76-year-old gentleman who has been suffering with the build up of ear wax in his ear canals leading to hearing loss. Prior to microsuction removal of the wax he has been asked to instill olive oil into his ears to help soften the wax. He is to do this once a day for 7 days. You have been asked to teach David's partner how to put the olive oil into David's ears.

1. Gather the equipment, he will need a bottle of olive oil, an eye dropper with bulb (available from the local chemist – preferably with a small bottle to put the olive oil in), some cotton wool.
2. He should wash his hands with soap and water.
3. If the olive oil is in the eye dropper bottle, hold it in your hands for a few minutes to warm it up – this prevents the shock of a cold fluid entering the ear canal.
4. David must lie on one side with the ear up and have 2–3 drops of olive oil dripped into the ear using the eye dropper (do not put the dropper into the ear). He then stays on his side for 5 minutes to allow the oil to seep down the canal. In the meantime, he can massage the ear just in front of the tragus (the small flap at the front of the ear) and pull the top of the ear upwards and backwards, this helps the olive oil work its way down the ear canal.
5. After 5 minutes wipe any excess olive oil from the outside of the ear and be prepared to wipe away olive oil draining from the ear, but do not put anything in the ear canal.
6. Repeat on the other side.

Sound waves entering the external auditory canal travel along until they reach the tympanic membrane (ear drum), a thin translucent connective tissue membrane covered by skin on its external surface and internally by mucosa and shaped like a flattened cone protruding into the middle ear. Sound waves that reach the tympanic membrane make it vibrate and this vibration is transmitted to the bones of the middle ear.

Hearing Aids

Hearing aids work by converting speech and other sounds to acoustic signals; they then amplify these. There are some hearing aids that depress lower frequency sounds and others that amplify higher frequency sounds. With advances in technology, increasingly smaller, more efficient hearing aids are now being produced. There are several different types, informally named by their placement in or around the ear: behind-the-ear, in-the-ear, or in-the-canal hearing aids. Although hearing aids can amplify sounds, they cannot make words clearer or speech any easier to understand, except by making the sounds louder.

Hearing aids can pick up the sound that is entering the ear, process it to match the hearing loss and then release the signal back into the ear instantaneously. A digital hearing aid is much more advanced than an analogue aid. It contains a silicon chip made up of millions of electrical components, continuously processing incoming sound, converting it into clearer and more audible sounds and then releasing these at the appropriate sound level into the ear. The digital hearing aid helps the user distinguish between sounds that need to be amplified and unwanted noise that needs to be reduced.

Digital hearing aids can be modified in order to work with an individual's personal degree of hearing loss and lifestyle needs. They have a number of preset programmes, which can be used in various situations; for example, quiet conversations, when at concerts, or at parties where there is much background noise. The user can watch the TV while taking part in conversations, identify where sounds are coming from, eliminate whistling and feedback while on the telephone and can link up via wireless technology to the TV, mobile telephone, computer or stereo system.

Middle Ear

Otherwise known as the tympanic cavity, this is a small, air-filled cavity lined with mucosa and contained within the temporal bone. It is enclosed at both ends, by the ear drum at the lateral end and medially by a bony wall with two openings:

- oval (vestibular) window
- round (cochlear) window.

The middle ear is connected to the nasopharynx by the eustachian (auditory) tube, a 4 cm long tube that consists of two portions:

- the section near the connection to the middle ear, which is relatively narrow and is supported by elastic cartilage;
- the section near the nasopharynx, which is relatively broad and funnel-shaped.

When open, the eustachian tube allows the passage of air and thus ensures the equalisation of the pressures on both sides of the tympanic membrane so both are subject to the same atmospheric pressure. The eustachian tube is normally closed at the end nearest the nasopharynx, but opens during yawning and swallowing (Jenkins and Tortora, 2013). If equalisation of pressures does not happen, then the difference in pressures between the two sides can lead to reduced hearing as the tympanic membrane cannot move freely.

Within the middle ear there are three bones known as the ossicles or ossicular chain. These three bones connect the tympanic membrane with the receptor complexes of the inner ear:

- the malleus (hammer) attaches at three points to the inner surface of the tympanic membrane;
- the incus (anvil) attaches the malleus to the stapes;
- the stapes (stirrup) – the edges of the base of the stapes are bound to the edge of the oval window.

The joints between these three bones are the smallest synovial joints in the body and each has its own tiny capsule and supporting extracapsular ligaments.

Vibration in the tympanic membrane is the first stage in the perception of sound; this vibration converts the sound waves into mechanical movement (the vibration). The ossicles act as levers and conduct the vibrations to the inner ear. They are connected in such a way that the in–out movement of tympanic vibration is converted into a rocking motion of the stapes. The ossicles collect the force applied to the tympanic membrane, amplify it and transmit it to the oval window. This amplification explains why humans can hear even very quiet noises, but can also be a problem in very noisy environments. In order to protect the tympanic membrane and the ossicular chain from violent movement resulting from extreme noises, they are supported by two small muscles:

- The tensor tympani muscle is a short ribbon of muscle connected to the 'handle' of the malleus. When it contracts, the malleus is pulled medially (towards the inner ear), stiffening the tympanic membrane.
- The stapedius muscle is attached to the stapes and pulls it, reducing the movement against the oval window.

Inner Ear

The senses of equilibrium (part of the sense of balance) and hearing are provided by the receptors in the inner ear.

The inner ear is also known as the labyrinth owing to the complicated series of canals it contains. The inner ear is composed of two main, fluid-filled parts:

- bony labyrinth – a series of cavities within the temporal bone that contain the main organs of balance (the semicircular canals and the vestibule) and the main organ of hearing (the cochlea);
- membranous labyrinth – a series of fluid-filled sacs and tubes that are contained within the bony labyrinth.

Between the bony and membranous labyrinth flows perilymph, a liquid that is rather like cerebrospinal fluid; the fluid within the membranous labyrinth is known as endolymph.

As noted above, the bony labyrinth can be divided into three parts (Figure 15.6):

- The vestibule consists of a pair of membranous sacs: the saccule and the utricle. Receptors in these two sacs provide the sensations of gravity and linear acceleration.
- The semicircular canals enclose slender semicircular ducts. Receptors in these ducts are stimulated by the rotation of the head. The combination of the vestibule and the semicircular canals is known as the vestibular complex.
- The cochlea is a spiral-shaped, bony chamber that contains the cochlear duct of the membranous labyrinth. Receptors within this duct give us the sense of hearing.

Equilibrium

The sense of equilibrium is part of the sense of balance and is controlled by receptors in the semicircular ducts, the utricle and the saccule of the inner ear. The sensory receptors in the semicircular ducts are active

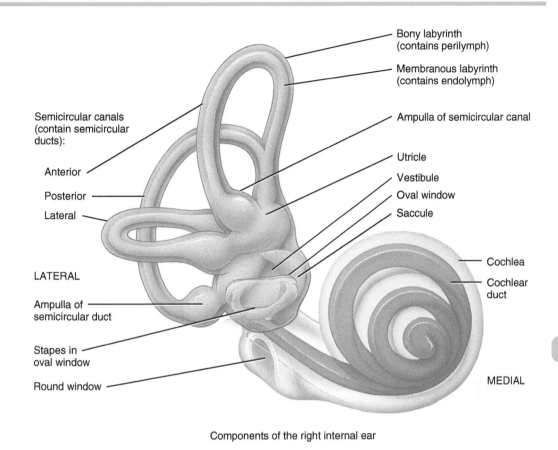

Bony labyrinth
(contains perilymph)

Membranous labyrinth
(contains endolymph)

Semicircular canals
(contain semicircular
ducts):

Ampulla of semicircular canal

Utricle

Anterior

Vestibule

Posterior

Oval window

Lateral

Saccule

LATERAL

Cochlea

Cochlear
duct

Ampulla of
semicircular duct

Stapes in
oval window

Round window

MEDIAL

Components of the right internal ear

Figure 15.6 **Inner ear.** *Source:* Tortora and Derrickson (2009). Reproduced with permission of John Wiley & Sons.

during movement but inactive when the body is motionless. The sensory receptors in the ducts respond to rotational movements of the head. There are three of these ducts: lateral, posterior and anterior.

The ducts are continuous with the utricle. Each semicircular duct contains an ampulla, an expanded region that contains the majority of the receptors. The area in the wall of the ampulla that contains the receptors is known as the crista and each crista is bound to a cupula – a gelatinous structure that extends the full width of the ampulla. The hair cells (receptors) are surrounded by supporting cells and are monitored by the dendrites of sensory neurones.

The free surfaces of the hair cells are covered with stereocilia, which resemble very long microvilli. Along with the fine stereocilia, the hair cell will also have one kinocilium – a single, large and thick cilium. When an external force pushes against the cilia the distortion of the plasma membrane of the hair cell alters the rate that the cell releases chemical transmitters. So, for instance, if a person moves their head to look to the left the cilia of the lateral semicircular canal are subject to pressure and thus the cell membranes are distorted, leading to an altered release of neurotransmitters and the perception of rotational movement (Figure 15.7). Any movement of the head can be perceived by varying combinations of stimulation of the three ducts and their receptors.

In contrast to the semicircular canals, the utricle and the saccule provide equilibrium information whether the body is moving or stationary. The two chambers are connected by a narrow passageway that is also connected to the endolymphatic duct. The hair cells of the utricle and saccule are clustered in oval structures called maculae. As with the hair cells of the ampullae, the cilia of the hair cells in the utricle and saccule are embedded in a gelatine-like substance. However, the surface of this substance contains densely packed calcium carbonate crystals called statoconia. This combination of gelatine-like substance and calcium carbonate crystals is known as an otolith (Figure 15.8).

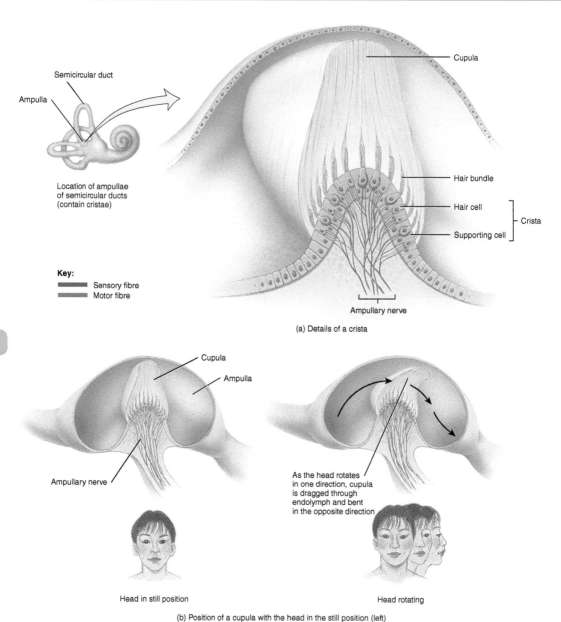

Key:
Sensory fibre
Motor fibre

414

(a) Details of a crista

(b) Position of a cupula with the head in the still position (left)
and when the head rotates (right)

Figure 15.7 **(a, b) Ampulla at rest and in response to movement.** *Source:* Tortora and Derrickson (2009). Reproduced with permission of John Wiley & Sons.

When the head is in a neutral position, the statoconia sit on top of the macula. The pressure they generate is therefore downwards and the hair cell microvilli are pushed down. When the head is tilted, the pull of gravity on the statoconia shifts and the microvilli are moved to one side or the other. This distorts the cell membrane and triggers altered neurotransmitter release (Figure 15.9).

A similar type of activity happens when the body is subject to linear acceleration; for example, as a car speeds up, the otolith lags behind due to inertia. The brain would normally differentiate between the action of gravity and the action of acceleration by integrating the information from the receptors with visual information.

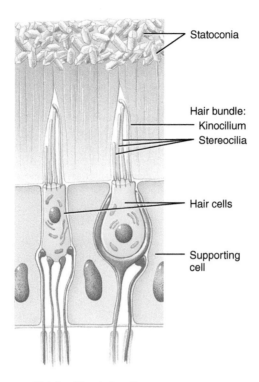

Details of two hair cells

Figure 15.8 **Hair cells and otolith.** *Source:* Tortora and Derrickson (2009). Reproduced with permission of John Wiley & Sons.

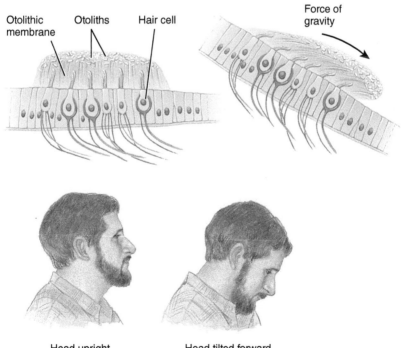

Position of macula with head upright (left) and tilted forward (right)

Figure 15.9 **Action of gravity on the otolith.** *Source:* Tortora and Derrickson (2009). Reproduced with permission of John Wiley & Sons.

Pathways for the Equilibrium Sensations

The hair cells in the semicircular canals, the vestibule and the saccule are monitored by sensory neurones located in the vestibular ganglia. Sensory fibres from these ganglia form the vestibular branch of the vestibulocochlear nerve (cranial nerve VIII). These fibres feed into neurones within the vestibular nuclei at the boundary of the pons and the medulla oblongata in the brain.

The vestibular nuclei have four functions:

- Integrating sensory information about equilibrium received from both sides of the head.
- Relaying information to the cerebellum.
- Relaying information to the cortex.
- Sending commands to motor nuclei in the brainstem and the spinal cord. The motor commands are reflex-type commands for eye, head and neck movements, such as the movement of the eyes that occurs in response to sensations of motion.

Hearing

The sense of hearing is provided by receptors in the cochlear duct; they are hair cells similar to those of the semicircular canals and vestibule. However, their positioning within the cochlear duct and the organisation of the surrounding structures protect them from stimuli generated by anything other than sound waves.

The ossicular chains transmit and amplify pressure waves from the air into pressure waves in the perilymph of the cochlea. These waves stimulate the hair cells along the cochlear spiral:

- the **frequency** of the perceived sound is detected by the part of the cochlear duct that is stimulated;
- the **intensity** (volume) of the sound is detected by the number of hair cells that are stimulated at the particular point in the cochlea.

Within the bony labyrinth of the cochlea there are three ducts (Figure 15.10):

- the vestibular duct (scala vestibuli) connects to the oval window;
- the tympanic duct (scala tympani) connects to the round window;
- the cochlear duct (scala media) is separated from the tympanic duct by the basilar membrane.

Both the vestibular and the tympanic duct are connected at the tip of the cochlear spiral and therefore make up one continuous perilymphatic chamber (Figure 15.11).

Between the vestibular and the tympanic ducts is the cochlear duct; the hair cells of this duct are located in a structure called the organ of Corti (Figure 15.12). The organ of Corti sits on the basilar membrane and its hair cells are arranged in a series of longitudinal rows.

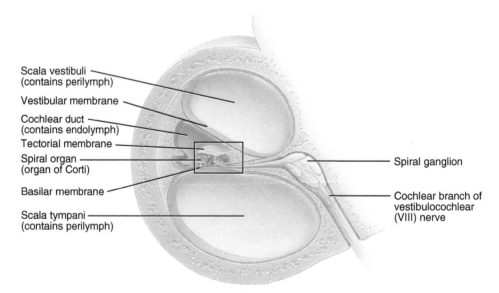

Scala vestibuli (contains perilymph)

Vestibular membrane

Cochlear duct (contains endolymph)

Tectorial membrane

Spiral organ (organ of Corti)

Basilar membrane

Scala tympani (contains perilymph)

Spiral ganglion

Cochlear branch of vestibulocochlear (VIII) nerve

Section through one turn of the cochlea

Figure 15.10 Cross-section of the cochlea (highlighted section is shown in detail in Figure 15.12). *Source:* Tortora and Derrickson (2009). Reproduced with permission of John Wiley & Sons.

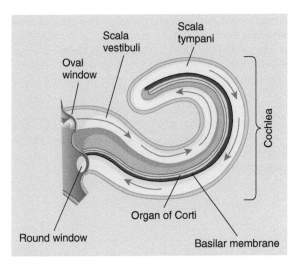

Figure 15.11 **Cochlea showing the continuous nature of the vestibular and tympanic ducts.**

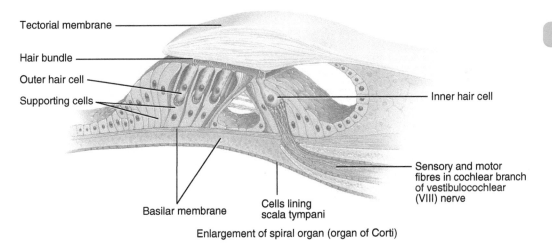

Enlargement of spiral organ (organ of Corti)

Figure 15.12 **Organ of Corti.** *Source:* Tortora and Derrickson (2009). Reproduced with permission of John Wiley & Sons.

The hair cells of the organ of Corti do not have kinocilia and their stereocilia are in contact with the overlying tectorial membrane; this membrane is attached to the inner wall of the cochlear duct. When a portion of the basilar membrane bounces up and down in response to pressure waves in the perilymph the stereocilia of the hair cells are pressed against the tectorial membrane and become distorted.

The Hearing Process

1. Sound waves travel down the external auditory canal and arrive at the tympanic membrane.
2. Movement is created in the tympanic membrane, which leads to the movement of the ossicles and the amplification of the movement.
3. Movement of the stapes at the oval window creates pressure waves in the perilymph of the vestibular duct.
4. The pressure waves distort the basilar membrane. The location of the maximum distortion depends on the frequency of the sound, as the basilar membrane varies in width and flexibility along its length. Higher pitch sounds create maximum distortion near to the oval window and lower pitch sounds further away from the window. The amount of distortion gives sensory information as to the volume of the sound.
5. Vibration in the basilar membrane leads to vibration of the hair cell cilia against the tectorial membrane, leading to the release of neurotransmitters by the hair cells. As hair cells are arranged in rows, a soft sound may only distort a few hair cells in a single row, but more cells in more rows will be stimulated as the volume increases.

6. Information about the region of stimulation and the intensity of that stimulation is relayed to the brain via the cochlear branch of the vestibulocochlear nerve (cranial nerve VIII). The cell bodies of the neurones that monitor the hair cells of the cochlea are located in the spiral ganglia at the centre of the bony cochlea. The nerve impulses are then transmitted via the cochlear branch of cranial nerve VIII to the cochlear nuclei of the medulla oblongata and then to other centres in the brain.

Medicines Management Ototoxicity

 Ototoxicity is the property of being toxic to the ear. There are over 200 drugs that can lead to ototoxicity, tinnitus and associated hearing loss.

Many of the drugs are used in common practice, such as:

- furosemide
- gentamicin
- metropolol
- ramipril
- sodium valproate.

Patients should be informed that if they do experience any suspected tinnitus or hearing loss with a drug it is important they do not stop taking the drug until they have talked to their doctor.

Avoiding Ototoxicity

Many ototoxic drugs are excreted in the urine and thus it is best to avoid ototoxic drugs in patients with renal impairment and they should be used with caution in the elderly. Furthermore, the patient should be well hydrated to ensure good renal function.

Drugs such as gentamicin and vancomycin are normally given at set times and the nurse should avoid giving these drugs too early as it may cause an excessive blood level. Also, blood levels of these drugs are required at regular intervals and it is important to adhere to medical instructions regarding the administration before and after drug administration.

Furosemide toxicity is related to the speed of administration and therefore, it is essential that the instructions for the speed of delivery of intravenous furosemide are followed.

Clinical Considerations Noise Exposure and Ear Damage

 As noise levels increase, the chance of damage to the ear increases. The following table gives examples of the types of noise levels at certain decibel (dB) levels and the exposure time at which damage may occur.

DB LEVEL	MAXIMUM EXPOSURE PER DAY	EXAMPLES
10		Breathing
20		Rustling leaves
60		Conversation
75		Typical car interior on motorway
85	16 h	City traffic (inside car)
90	9 h	Power drill, food blender
97	3 h	French horn at 10 feet
100	2 h	Farm tractor, outboard motor, jet take-off at 1000 feet
110	0.5 h	Chainsaw, pneumatic drill, car horn at 3 feet
120	0 h	Typical rock concert, loud thunderclap
125	Hearing damage occurring	Pneumatic riveter at 4 feet
132–140	Permanent hearing damage	Gunshot, very loud rock concert 50 feet in front of speakers
150–160	Eardrum rupture	Jet take off at 75 feet, gunshot at 1 foot
190	Immediate death of tissue	Jet engine at 1 foot
194		Loudest sound in air, air particle distortion (sonic boom)

The Sense of Sight

Vision is perhaps the sense that we value the most; we learn more about the world around us through sight than we do with any of the other senses. Without sight many of our daily tasks and pleasures would be impossible and many others would become more difficult. The sense of sight is based on the eyes and around the eyes there are accessory structures that help to keep the eyes safe and working well (Figure 15.13):

- Eyelids (palpebrae) – a continuation of the skin. Continual blinking keeps the surface of the eye lubricated and removes dirt. The gap between them is known as the palpebral fissure.
- Eyelashes – robust hairs that help to keep foreign matter out of the eyes. They are associated with the tarsal glands which produce a lipid-rich secretion that helps to prevent the eyelids from sticking together.
- Lacrimal caruncle – a small collection of soft tissue that contains accessory glands.
- Commissure – the point where the eyelids meet; there are two: the lateral and the medial.
- Conjunctiva – the epithelial cell layer that lines the inside of the eyelids and the outer surface of the eye.

Lacrimal Apparatus

A constant flow of tears washes over the eyes to keep the conjunctiva moist and clean. Tears have several functions:

- reduce friction
- remove debris
- prevent bacterial infection
- provide nutrients and oxygen to parts of the conjunctiva.

The lacrimal apparatus produces, distributes and removes tears. It consists of:

- a lacrimal gland
- lacrimal canaliculi
- a lacrimal sac
- a nasolacrimal duct.

The lacrimal gland (tear gland) creates most of the content of tears (about 1 mL per day). Once the lacrimal secretions reach the eye they mix with the products of the accessory glands and the tarsal glands. This

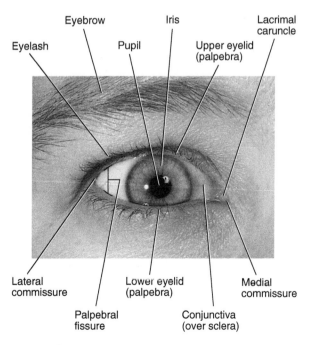

Figure 15.13 **Accessory structures of the eye.** *Source:* Tortora and Derrickson (2009). Reproduced with permission of John Wiley & Sons.

results in a mixture that lubricates the eye and reduces evaporation. The nutrient and oxygen demands of the corneal cells are supplied by diffusion from the lacrimal secretions. The secretions also contain antibacterial enzymes and antibodies to attack pathogens before they enter the body.

Blinking sweeps the tears across the ocular surface and they accumulate at the medial commissure from where they are drained by the lacrimal canaliculi into the lacrimal sac and from there into the nasal cavity through the nasolacrimal duct.

The Eye
The wall of the Eye
The wall of the eye has three layers (Figure 15.14):

- fibrous tunic
- vascular tunic
- neural tunic.

Fibrous Tunic
The fibrous tunic is the outermost layer of the eye and consists of the sclera and the cornea; it has three main functions:

- provides support and some protection;
- is the attachment site for the extrinsic muscles;
- contains structures that assist in the focusing process.

420

Most of the ocular surface is covered by the sclera (the 'white' of the eye), which is made up of dense fibrous connective tissue containing collagen and elastic fibres. The surface of the sclera contains small blood

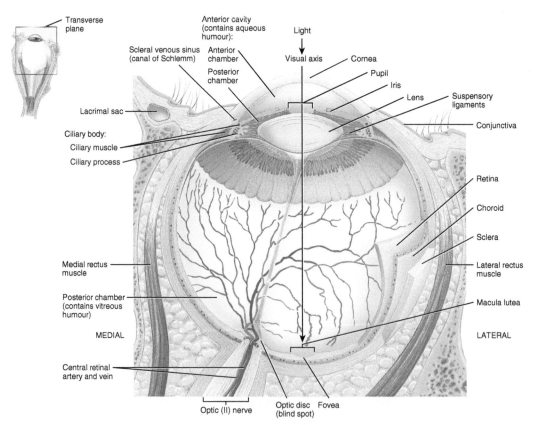

Superior view of transverse section of right eyeball

Figure 15.14 **Anatomy of the eye.** *Source:* Tortora and Derrickson (2009). Reproduced with permission of John Wiley & Sons.

vessels and nerves. The transparent cornea is continuous with the sclera and is made up of a dense matrix of fibres laid down in such a way that they do not interfere with the passage of light.

Vascular Tunic (Uvea)

The vascular tunic is the middle of the three layers of the eye and contains numerous blood vessels, lymph vessels and the smooth muscles involved in eye functioning. The functions of this layer include:

- providing a structure for the blood and lymph vessels that supply the tissues of the eye;
- regulating the amount of light that enters the eye;
- secreting and reabsorbing the aqueous humour;
- controlling the shape of the lens.

  The vascular tunic is made up of:

- the iris
- the ciliary body
- the choroid.

Iris

The iris is the central, coloured portion of the eye (Figure 15.13) and regulates the amount of light entering the eye by adjusting the size of the central opening (the pupil). It is formed of two layers of pigmented cells and fibres and two layers of smooth muscle (the pupillary muscles):

- pupillary constrictor muscles
- pupillary dilator muscles.

421

Both sets of muscles are controlled by the autonomic nervous system; activation of the parasympathetic nervous system leads to constriction of the pupil in response to bright light. Activation of the sympathetic nervous system leads to the dilation of the pupil in response to dim light levels. At its edge the iris attaches to the anterior part of the ciliary body.

Ciliary body

The greatest part of the ciliary body is made up of the ciliary muscle, a smooth muscular ring that projects into the interior of the eye. The epithelial covering of this muscle has many folds called ciliary processes. The suspensory ligaments of the lens attach to the tips of these processes.

Choroid

The choroid is a vascular layer that separates the fibrous and neural tunics. It is covered by the sclera and attached to the outermost layer of the retina. The choroid contains an extensive capillary network that delivers oxygen and nutrients to the retina.

Neural Tunic (Retina)

This is the innermost layer of the eye, consisting of a thin outer layer called the pigmented part and a thicker inner layer called the neural part.

- The pigmented part of the retina absorbs the light that passes through the neural part; this prevents light bouncing back through the neural part and causing 'visual echoes'.
- The neural part of the retina contains light receptors, support cells and is responsible for the preliminary processing and integration of visual information.

Organisation of the Retina

Figure 15.15 shows the two types of receptor cells contained within the outermost layer of the retina (closest to the pigmented part). These receptor cells are the cells that detect light (photoreceptors).

- Rods – these photoreceptors do not discriminate between colours. They are very sensitive and enable us to see in very low light levels. Rods are mostly concentrated in a band around the periphery of the retina and this density reduces towards the centre of the eye.
- Cones – these photoreceptors provide colour vision and give sharper, clearer images than the rods do, but they require more intense light. Cones are mostly situated in the macula lutea and particularly at its centre in an area called the fovea (Figure 15.14).

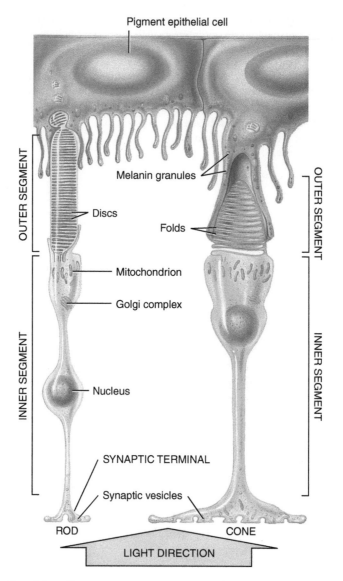

Figure 15.15 **Cross-section of the retina.** *Source:* Tortora and Derrickson (2009). Reproduced with permission of John Wiley & Sons.

The elongated outer sections of the rods and cones contain hundreds to thousands of flattened membranous discs. In the rods the discs are separate and form the shape of a cylinder. In cones the discs are in fact folds of the plasma membrane and the outer segment tapers to a blunt point.

Episode of Care Adult

Daphne is a 70-year-old lady who is reporting difficulty with her vision. She states that her sense of colour is getting worse, she is finding it difficult to read and when she looks at straight lines they look 'crooked'. When asked to view things out of the side of her eye, she states that these problems go away and they seem to only to affect the centre of her vision. On examination it is clear that Daphne is developing age related macular degeneration (AMD), at present it appears this is dry AMD and beyond the recommendations given below there is no treatment currently available for dry AMD.

Age related macular degeneration is a disease that develops in middle to older age. It usually first affects people in their 50s and 60s. AMD is the most common cause of sight loss, affecting approximately 600,000 people in the UK. The symptoms of AMD are:

- Blurred or 'fuzzy' vision.
- Straight lines, such as sentences on a page, appearing wavy or distorted.

- Blurry areas on a printed page.
- Difficulty reading or seeing details in low light levels.
- Extra sensitivity to glare.

   AMD is divided into two types:

- Dry AMD (or early AMD) is the slow degeneration of the cells in the retina, as the cells die they are not replaced leading to a loss in visual acuity. It is a disease that is slow in progression (often months to years). There is no treatment for dry AMD.
- Wet AMD is a disease where new blood vessels grow in the retina and leak blood which leads to scarring. Wet AMD is much quicker in onset but is treatable, so early diagnosis and referral is essential. Currently treatment involves either injections into the eye or laser treatment for those patients who do not respond to the injections. Despite the eye injections sounding unpleasant they are hardly noticed by the patient as the eye is anaesthetised and the injection is into the corner of the eye so the patient does not see the needle.

   The causes of AMD are unknown but seem to be linked to smoking, being overweight, high blood pressure and a family history of AMD.

   Patients with any form of AMD can help to inhibit its progress by:

- Protecting the eyes from the sun by using good quality sunglasses.
- Stopping smoking.
- Having regular eye examinations (this especially helps if dry AMD develops into wet AMD).
- There is some evidence that eating a healthy diet rich in antioxidants, omega 3 and lutein (found in eggs and some fruits and vegetables) may help prevent AMD and inhibit its progression.

   It is important to note that AMD does not mean the patient will become totally blind as the peripheral vision is not affected.

Multiple Choice Questions

1. At what age is AMD likely to appear?
   (a) 30–40 years
   (b) 40–50 years
   (c) 50–60 years
   (d) 70–80 years
2. Approximately how many people in the UK are affected by AMD?
   (a) 300,000
   (b) 400,000
   (c) 500,000
   (d) 600,000
3. AMD leads to the loss of:
   (a) central vision
   (b) peripheral vision
   (c) close vision
   (d) distance vision
4. Which forms of AMD can be treated?
   (a) dry
   (b) wet
   (c) peripheral
   (d) none
5. What foods can help protect against AMD?
   (a) vegetables
   (b) fruits
   (c) fish
   (d) all of the above

   There are three types of cones (red, blue and green) and colour discrimination is based on the integration of information received from the three types of cones. For instance, yellow is shown by highly stimulated green cones, less strongly stimulated red cones and a relative lack of stimulation of the blue cones.

   A narrow connecting stalk links the outer segment to the inner segment, which is the part of the cell that contains all the usual cellular organelles. The inner segment is also the area where synapses with other cells are made and neurotransmitters are released.

The rods and cones synapse with neurones called bipolar cells, which in turn synapse within a layer of neurones called ganglion cells. At both these synapse areas there are associated cells that can stimulate or inhibit the communication between the two cells and therefore alter the sensitivity of the retina (for instance, in response to very bright, or dim, light levels).

Axons from approximately 1 million ganglion cells converge on the optic disc, at which point they turn and penetrate the wall of the eye and proceed to the diencephalon of the brain as the optic nerve. The central retinal artery and vein pass through the centre of the optic nerve. The optic disc contains no photoreceptors and thus this area is known as the blind spot; however, we do not notice the blind spot in our vision as involuntary eye movements keep the visual image moving and the brain can thus supply the missing information.

The Chambers of the Eye

The eye is divided into two main cavities: a large posterior cavity and a smaller anterior cavity. The anterior cavity is further divided into the anterior chamber and the posterior chamber (Figure 15.14).

- The anterior cavity is filled with a substance called aqueous humour that circulates between the anterior and posterior chambers by passing through the pupil and performing a vital role as a transport medium for nutrients and waste products. The fluid pressure created by the aqueous humour in the anterior cavity helps to maintain the shape of the eye. Aqueous humour is produced by the epithelial cells of the ciliary body and within a few hours is drained through the canal of Schlemm to the sclera to be recycled.
- The posterior cavity is the larger of the two cavities of the eye and is filled with a gelatinous mass known as vitreous humour. The vitreous humour helps to stabilise the shape of the eye as the activity of the extraocular muscles would otherwise distort the shape of the eye. Unlike aqueous humour, the vitreous humour is created during the development of the eye and is never replaced. A thin film of aqueous humour infiltrates the posterior chamber, bathing the retina, supplying nutrients and removing waste. The pressure it creates also helps to keep the neural part of the retina against the pigmented part; though the two are close together, they are not fixed to each other and thus this external pressure is required.

Skills in Practice Using Eye Drops

Sarah is a 72-year-old lady who has been to see her optician for new glasses. During routine testing the optician has detected the onset of glaucoma and referred Sarah to her GP. The treatment for early open angle glaucoma is eye drops and the GP has prescribed prostaglandin eye drops to help the flow of aqueous humour from the eye and thus reduce the pressure. At present, glaucoma cannot be cured and the treatment is dependent on early recognition to avoid permanent damage. To use eye drops the patient should be advised to:

- wash their hands;
- ensure the eye drops are in date;
- put their head back;
- use their finger to pull down the lower eyelid;
- hold the bottle and allow a single drop to fall into the pocket made by pulling down the eyelid;
- close the eye and keep it closed for a few minutes.

Tonometry

Measuring intra-ocular pressure (IOP) is an important ophthalmic test and the correct term is tonometry. Tonometry is the objective measurement of IOP and is usually based on the assessment of resistance of the cornea to indent (this is usually a blast of air). Normal IOP is between about 10 and 21 mmHg. There are several types of tonometer available; an applanation tonometer is a tool that measures the amount of force needed to temporarily flatten part of the cornea. The tonometer measures the degree of resistance provided by the cornea to gentle indentation, converting this into a figure. A drop of fluorescein/anaesthetic provides a blue light filter. The procedure does not hurt; the patient has to keep their eyes wide open. While this test is completely painless, many patients find this test very difficult.

There are contraindications to this procedure, such as trauma or corneal ulcer. Measuring IOP is quick and simple and because of this it is routinely performed on all adults who require eye tests.

Focusing Images onto the Retina

In order for a visual image to be useful, it must be focused onto the retina; this is the purpose of the lens of the eye. First, the light entering the eye is subject to refraction and the lens provides the additional, adjustable refraction required to focus the image onto the retina.

Refraction

Light is refracted (bent) when it passes from one medium to another medium with a different density (Figure 15.16).

The majority of the refraction in the eye happens when light enters the cornea from the air; additional refraction occurs when light passes from the aqueous humour into the lens. The lens provides the extra refraction to focus the light onto the retina and can adjust this refraction according to the focal length.

Focal length is the distance between the focal point (e.g. on the retina) and the centre of the lens (Figure 15.17). It is dependent on:

- The distance from the object to the lens. The further away an object is, the shorter the focal length.
- The shape of the lens. The rounder the lens the more refraction occurs. A very round lens has a shorter focal length than a flatter lens.

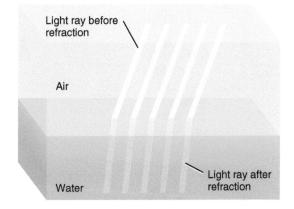

Refraction of light rays

Figure 15.16 **Refraction of light passing from air (less dense) to water (dense).** *Source:* Tortora and Derrickson (2009). Reproduced with permission of John Wiley & Sons.

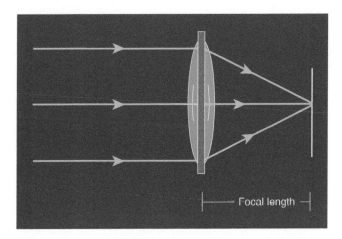

Figure 15.17 **Focal length.**

The lens lies behind the cornea and is held in place by ligaments that are attached to the ciliary body. It is made up of concentric layers of cells that are precisely organised and are covered by a fibrous capsule. Many of the capsule fibres are elastic and if it were not subject to external forces by the ligaments the lens would be spherical. Within the lens are lens fibres, specialised cells that have lost their nucleus and other organelles. They are filled with a protein called crystallin, which is responsible for the transparency and the focusing power of the lens.

The process of changing the shape of the lens to focus an image onto the retina is known as accommodation. The shape of the lens is altered by tension being applied to or relaxed on the suspensory ligaments by smooth muscles within the ciliary body (Figure 15.18).

Myopia, Hyperopia and Presbyopia

In a person who has myopia (short-sightedness) the lens is unable to focus the image onto the retina and the focus of the image falls short (Figure 15.19). With myopia, people can see objects close to them but those that are far away are blurred. Myopia is easily corrected for by the use of corrective lenses, either in the form of glasses or contact lenses.

In the person with hyperopia (long-sightedness) the image is focused onto a point behind the retina (Figure 15.20); therefore, these people can see things at a distance but not near to them.

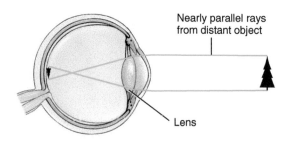

(a) Viewing distant object

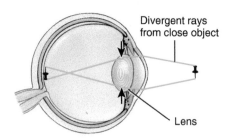

(b) Accommodation close object

Figure 15.18 **Accommodation to (a) far and (b) near objects.** *Source:* Tortora and Derrickson (2009). Reproduced with permission of John Wiley & Sons.

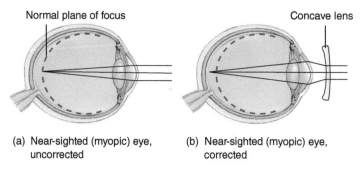

(a) Near-sighted (myopic) eye, uncorrected

(b) Near-sighted (myopic) eye, corrected

Figure 15.19 **(a) Myopic eye uncorrected and (b) corrected by a concave lens.** *Source:* Tortora and Derrickson (2009). Reproduced with permission of John Wiley & Sons.

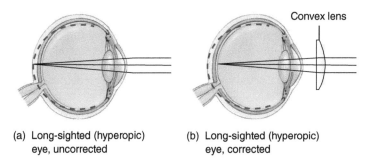

(a) Long-sighted (hyperopic) eye, uncorrected

(b) Long-sighted (hyperopic) eye, corrected

Figure 15.20 (a) Hyperopic eye uncorrected and (b) corrected by a convex lens. *Source: Tortora and Derrickson (2009). Reproduced with permission of John Wiley & Sons.*

Presbyopia is the loss of the ability to focus on close objects as the person ages; the most common theory for this is the loss of elasticity in the lens. The loss of the ability to focus on near objects occurs in everyone, but at different rates and with different effects on vision. The onset of presbyopia is most commonly noticed at 40–50 years of age. Presbyopia is treatable with corrective glasses (usually known as reading glasses, though they are corrective for all tasks that require near vision).

Clinical Considerations 20/20 Vision

The term 20/20 vision refers to a measure of visual acuity. The meaning is that the person being tested can see the same detail from 20 feet away as a person with normal eyesight would see from 20 feet. In other words, 20/20 vision is normal vision. If a person has 20/40 vision they are only able to see detail at 20 feet that a person with normal vision can see at 40 feet. A person with a visual acuity of 20/70 can only see detail at 20 feet that a person with normal sight could see at 70 feet and so on. The visual acuity is not a direct correlation with the prescription for eyeglasses, but the prescribed glasses are intended to achieve 20/20 vision. Visual acuity is tested using a standard size Snellen chart at 20 feet and lit to a standard brightness (Figure 15.21).

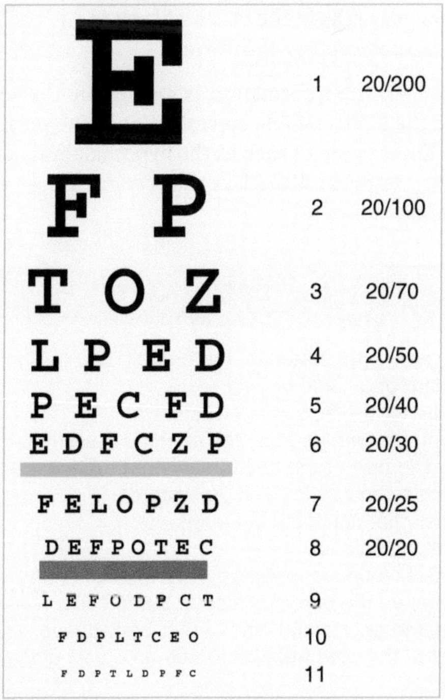

E	1	20/200
F P	2	20/100
T O Z	3	20/70
L P E D	4	20/50
P E C F D	5	20/40
E D F C Z P	6	20/30
F E L O P Z D	7	20/25
D E F P O T E C	8	20/20
L E F O D P C T	9	
F D P L T C E O	10	
F D P T L D P F C	11	

Figure 15.21 Snellen chart.

The Processing of Visual Information

The ganglion cells that monitor the rods in the retina (M cells) supply information about the general form of an object, motion and shadows in dim light. As many as 1000 rods may pass information to one M cell. This convergence leads to a loss of specific information and the activation of an M cell indicates that light has struck a general area rather than a specific point. This loss of specific location-based information is partially compensated for by the fact that the M cells' activity varies depending on the pattern of stimulation in their specific field (area of retina). So, for instance, an M cell would react differently to a stimulus at the edge of its receptive field than from one at its centre.

Cone cells show very little convergence; for instance, in the fovea the ratio of cones to ganglion is 1:1 (Martini and Nath, 2009). The ganglion cells that monitor cones (P cells) are more numerous than M cells and because there is little convergence these cells provide location-specific information. As a result of this, cones supply more precise information about a visual image than do rods.

Central Processing of Visual Information

Once axons from the ganglion cells have exited the eye through the optic disc they proceed to the diencephalon as the optic nerves (cranial nerve II). The two optic nerves (one for each eye) reach the diencephalon at the optic chiasm. From there, half the nerves go to the lateral geniculate nucleus on the same side of the brain and the other half cross over and proceed to the lateral geniculate nucleus on the opposite side. From each lateral geniculate nucleus, visual information also travels to the occipital cortex of the cerebral hemisphere on the same side. Involuntary eye control (such as pupillary reflexes) is processed in the diencephalon and the brainstem.

Conclusion

In this chapter there has been a review of the senses:

- olfaction (smell), which is based in the olfactory receptors of the nose;
- gustation (taste), which is partially based in the gustatory receptors on the tongue, but also has a large input from the olfactory receptors;
- equilibrium, which is a part of the sense of balance and is based in the hair cells of the semicircular canals and the vestibule;
- hearing, which is based in the hair cells in the organ of corti in the cochlea of the inner ear;
- sight, which is based in the photoreceptors of the eye.

With the exception of smell, all the information generated by the senses is processed in the thalamus before being transmitted on to the higher brain centres. Some of the senses (smell and taste) also have direct input into other centres of the limbic system, such as the hypothalamus, and this is an indication of both how ancient they are in evolutionary terms and the fact that certain smells and tastes can evoke subconscious responses, such as salivation and emotions.

Glossary

Afferent: Heading towards a centre (for instance, the brain).
Ampulla: A sac-like enlargement of a canal or duct.
Anterior: Located at, or related to, the front of a structure.
Antibody: Proteins in the blood that are used by the immune system to identify and destroy pathogens.
Autonomic nervous system: The part of the nervous system that controls involuntary functions, made up of the parasympathetic and sympathetic nervous systems.
Axon: Extension of a nerve cell that conducts impulses.
Balance: The ability to control equilibrium.
Cartilage: A supporting connective tissue made up of various cells and fibres.
Cilia: Small, hair-like processes on the outer surface of some cells.
Connective tissue: Tissue that supports and binds other body tissue.
Convergence: The movement of the eyes inwards to see an object close to the face.

Efferent: Heading away from a centre.

Endolymph: The fluid in the membranous labyrinth of the inner ear.

Enzyme: A protein that increases the rate of a chemical reaction.

Equilibrium: Stability at rest or when moving.

Ethmoid bone: A bone in the skull that separates the nasal cavity from the brain.

Extrinsic: Not inherent to the process or object, external.

Focal length: The distance between the focal point (e.g. on the retina) and the centre of the lens of the eye.

Fovea (fovea centralis): A small depression in the retina containing cones and where vision is the most acute.

Ganglion: A mass, or group, of nerve cells.

Glomeruli (glomerulus – singular): In the olfactory pathway, a structure containing a mass of synapses.

Gustatory: Relating to the sense of taste.

Hyperopia: Long-sightedness.

Iris: The central, coloured portion of the eye.

Lacrimal: Relating to tears.

Lateral: Away from the midline of the body (to the left or right).

Ligament: Fibrous tissue that binds joints together and connects bones and cartilage.

Limbic system: A group of structures/centres in the brain associated with various emotions and feelings, such as anger, fear, sadness and pleasure.

Lipid: A group of organic compounds, including the fats, oils, waxes, sterols and triglycerides.

Medial: Towards the midline of the body.

Medulla oblongata: A part of the brainstem that contains the cardiac and respiratory centres.

Microvilli (microvillus – singular): Protrusions of the cell membrane that increase its surface area.

Myopia: Short-sightedness.

Nasopharynx: The part of the airway that begins in the nose and ends at the soft palate.

Neurone: Nerve cell.

Olfaction: The sense of smell.

Olfactory: Pertaining to the sense of smell.

Olfactory bulb: A structure of the brain involved in olfaction, the perception of odours.

Papilla (papillae – plural): Small, nipple-shaped projection.

Parasympathetic nervous system: Part of the autonomic nervous system.

Pathogen: An infectious agent that causes disease (for instance, bacteria or virus).

Perilymph: The clear fluid found between the bony labyrinth and the membranous labyrinth in the inner ear.

Photoreceptor: Light-sensing neurone.

Pons: Part of the brainstem, the pons contains centres that deal with sleep, swallowing, hearing, equilibrium, taste, eye movement and many other functions.

Posterior: Located at, or related to, the rear of a structure.

Presbyopia: The loss of the ability to focus on close objects as the person ages.

Pupil: The opening in the centre of the iris of the eye that allows light to enter.

Pupillary constrictor muscles: Smooth muscles contained within the iris of the eye; when stimulated they lead to the constriction of the pupil.

Pupillary dilator muscles: Smooth muscles contained within the iris of the eye; when stimulated they lead to the dilation of the pupil.

Reflex: Involuntary function or movement in response to a stimulus.

Refraction: The change of direction of light as it passes from one medium to another with a different density.

Snellen chart: Standardised chart for testing visual acuity.

Sympathetic nervous system: Part of the autonomic nervous system.

Synapse: A gap between two neurones or a neurone and an organ across which neurotransmitters diffuse to transmit a nerve impulse.

Synovial joint: A freely moving joint in which bony surfaces are covered with cartilage and connected by ligaments lined with a synovial membrane. The membrane secretes a lubricating fluid and keeps it around the joint.

Thalamus: A pair of structures in the brain that relay messages from most of the senses.

Transparent: Clear, can see through it.

Umami: The 'fifth taste', related to proteins found in meat and fish.

Visual acuity: Detailed central vision.

References

Haehner, A., Hummel, T. and Reichmann, H. (2011) Olfactory loss in Parkinson's disease. *Parkinson's Disease* **2011**: 50939. doi:10.4061/2011/450939.

Haehner, A., Tosch, C., Wolz, M., Klingelhoefer, L., Fauser, M., Storch, A., Reichman, H. and Hummel, T. (2013) Olfactory training in patients with Parkinson's disease. *PLoS ONE* **8**(4), e61680.

Jenkins, G.W. and Tortora, G.J. (2013) *Anatomy and Physiology: From Science to Life*, 3rd edn. Hoboken, NJ: John Wiley & Sons. Inc.

Martini, F.H. and Nath, J.L. (2009) *Fundamentals of Anatomy and Physiology*, 8th edn. San Francisco, CA: Pearson Benjamin Cummings.

Mohammed, A.A. (2014). Update knowledge of dry mouth-A guideline for dentists. *African Health Sciences* **14**(3): 736–742.

National Institute for Health and Clinical Excellence (NICE) (2015) NG91 Otitis media (acute): antimicrobial prescribing. https://www.nice.org.uk/guidance/NG91 (accessed 7 August 2019).

Neuland, C., Bitter, T., Marschner, H., Gudziol, H. and Guntinas-Lichius, O. (2011) Health-related and specific olfaction-related quality of life in patients with chronic functional anosmia or severe hyposmia. *The Laryngoscope* **121**(4): 867–872.

NHS (2015) Lost or changed sense of smell https://www.nhs.uk/conditions/lost-or-changed-sense-smell/ (accessed 7 August 2019).

Osawa, Y. (2012) Glutamate perception, soup stock and the concept of umami: the ethnography, food ecology and history of dashi in Japan. *Ecology of Food and Nutrition* **51**(4): 329–345.

Shott, S.R. (2006) Down syndrome: Common otolaryngologic manifestations. *American Journal of Medical Genetics Part C on Holoprosencephaly* **142C**:131–140.

Tortora, G.J. and Derrickson, B.H. (2009) *Principles of Anatomy and Physiology*, 12th edn. Hoboken, NJ: John Wiley & Sons, Inc.

Tortora, G.J. and Derrickson, B.H. (2012) *Principles of Anatomy and Physiology*, 13th edn. Hoboken, NJ: John Wiley & Sons, Inc.

Further Reading

ENT UK

https://entuk.org/

The website of the British Association of Otorhinolaryngologists and the British Academic Conference in Otolaryngology. This group states its aims as including promoting care, professional education and information for the public. The site has useful information on a variety of conditions of the ear and the nose.

eyeSmart

http://www.geteyesmart.org/eyesmart/index.cfm

This is a website created and maintained by the American Association of Ophthalmology (eye doctors). It contains useful sections on eye conditions, symptoms and lifestyle advice related to eye health.

National Institute on Deafness and Other Communication Disorders

http://www.nidcd.nih.gov/health/Pages/Default.aspx

A useful website maintained by the United States National Institutes of Health detailing various disorders of the ear and mouth, including taste disorders, balance disorders and disorders of the ear.

Royal National Institute of Blind People (RNIB)

http://www.rnib.org.uk/

The RNIB is a UK-based charity offering information, support and advice to people experiencing sight loss. The website is a useful source of information, including sections on eye conditions, tests and coping with sight loss.

Activities

Multiple Choice Questions

1. Approximately how many taste buds does the average person have?
   - (a) 5,000
   - (b) 8,000
   - (c) 10,000
   - (d) 12,000

2. Which cranial nerves transmit the sensory input from the tongue?
   (a) VII and IX
   (b) IX and X
   (c) VII and X
   (d) VIII and IX
3. What percentage of the sense of taste is actually due to the sense of smell?
   (a) 60%
   (b) 70%
   (c) 80%
   (d) 90%
4. What percentage of inhaled air passes the olfactory organs?
   (a) 2%
   (b) 4%
   (c) 5%
   (d) 10%
5. What is the purpose of the eustachian tube?
   (a) to equalise the pressure between the outer ear and the nasopharynx
   (b) to equalise the pressure between the inner ear and the nasopharynx
   (c) to equalise the pressure between the middle ear and the nasopharynx
   (d) to equalise the pressure between the inner ear and middle ear
6. The utricle and saccule of the ear are stimulated by:
   (a) gravity
   (b) linear acceleration
   (c) rotation of the head
   (d) vertical acceleration
7. The organ of Corti is found in:
   (a) the vestibulocochlear duct
   (b) the tympanic duct
   (c) the vestibular duct
   (d) the cochlear duct
8. Information about the volume and pitch of a sound are transmitted to the brain via a branch of which cranial nerve?
   (a) VI
   (b) VIII
   (c) IX
   (d) X
9. The eyelids are made of:
   (a) elastic cartilage
   (b) connective tissue
   (c) muscle tissue
   (d) epithelial tissue
10. The coloured part of the eye is known as:
    (a) the uvea
    (b) the cornea
    (c) the iris
    (d) the choroid body
11. Photoreceptors are found in:
    (a) the fibrous tunic
    (b) the neural part of the neural tunic
    (c) the vascular tunic
    (d) the pigmented part of the neural tunic
12. What is the role of the pigmented part of the retina?
    (a) create vitreous humour
    (b) interpreting colour
    (c) absorbing light
    (d) processing visual information.

13. Rods are mostly found where in the retina?
   (a) centre
   (b) periphery
   (c) optic disc
   (d) fovea
14. The most common age of onset for presbyopia is:
   (a) 30–40
   (b) 40–50
   (c) 50–60
   (d) 70–80
15. The majority of the refraction of light in the eye happens:
   (a) when the light enters the lens of the eye
   (b) when the light enters the pupil
   (c) when the light enters the posterior cavity
   (d) when the light enters the cornea of the eye

Conditions

The following is a list of conditions that are associated with the senses. Take some time and write notes about each of the conditions. You may make the notes taken from text books or other resources (e.g. people you work with in a clinical area), or you may make the notes as a result of people you have cared for. If you are making notes about people you have cared for, you must ensure that you adhere to the rules of confidentiality.

Anosmia

Ageusia

Meniere's disease

Glaucoma

Retinopathy

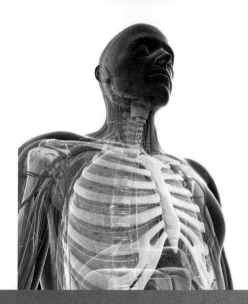

16

The Endocrine System

Carl Clare

Test Your Prior Knowledge

- How are hormones transported in the body?
- What is meant by the 'half-life' of a hormone?
- Name one hormone released by the pituitary gland.
- Where in the body is the thyroid gland found?
- What stimulates the release of insulin?

Learning Outcomes

After reading this chapter you will be able to:

- Name the endocrine glands in the body and the hormones they secrete.
- Discuss the different forms of stimulus for the release of hormones.
- Explain the control of hormone release by the hypothalamus.
- Discuss the hormonal responses to stress.
- Explain the role of insulin and glucagon in the control of blood glucose levels.

Visit the student companion website at www.wileyfundamentalseries.com/anatomy where you can test yourself using flashcards, multiple-choice questions and more. Instructor companion site at www.wiley.com/go/instructor/anatomy where instructors will find valuable materials such as PowerPoint slides and image bank designed to enhance your teaching.

Fundamentals of Anatomy and Physiology: For Nursing and Healthcare Students, Third Edition. Edited by Ian Peate and Suzanne Evans.
© 2020 John Wiley & Sons Ltd. Published 2020 by John Wiley & Sons Ltd.
Student companion website: www.wileyfundamentalseries.com/anatomy
Instructor companion website: www.wiley.com/go/instructor/anatomy

Body Map

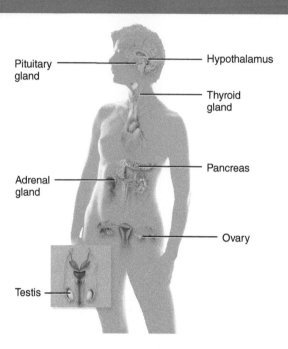

Pituitary gland

Hypothalamus

Thyroid gland

Pancreas

Adrenal gland

Ovary

Testis

Introduction

Homeostasis (from the Greek *homoios*, 'similar'; and *histemi*, 'standing still') refers to the process of maintaining a stable internal environment. In other words, homeostasis refers to the maintenance of normal physiological balance and functioning within the body. There are two major systems in the body for maintaining homeostasis: the nervous system and the endocrine system. Table 16.1 shows the differences between these two systems.

The nervous system reacts rapidly to stimuli and effects its changes over a period of seconds or minutes; thus, it is involved in the immediate and short-term maintenance of homeostasis. Owing to its rapid onset of action, the nervous system is responsible for the control of rapid bodily processes such as breathing and movement. The endocrine system is often responsible for the regulation of longer term processes. The major functions it coordinates are

- homeostasis – maintains the internal body environment;
- storage and utilisation of energy substrates (carbohydrates, proteins and fats);
- regulation of growth and reproduction;
- control of the body's responses to external stimuli (particularly stress).

It should be noted, however, that though these two systems are separate they often act together and complement each other in the maintenance of homeostasis.

The endocrine system is made up of a collection of small organs that are scattered throughout the body, each of which releases hormones into the blood supply ('endo' = within, 'crine' = to secrete). These hormone-releasing organs can be split into three main categories (Jenkins and Tortora, 2013).

Table 16.1 **Nervous system versus endocrine system.**

	NERVOUS SYSTEM	ENDOCRINE SYSTEM
Speed of action	Seconds	Minutes to hours (even days)
Duration of action	Seconds to minutes	Minutes to days
Method of transmitting messages	Electrical	Chemical
Transport method	Neurones	Hormones

- Endocrine glands – organs whose only function is the production and release of hormones. These include:
  - pituitary gland
  - thyroid gland
  - parathyroid gland
  - adrenal gland.
- Organs that are not pure glands (as they have other functions as well as the production of hormones) but contain relatively large areas of hormone-producing tissue. These include:
  - hypothalamus
  - pancreas.
- Other tissues and organs that also produce hormones – areas of hormone-producing cells are found in the wall of the small intestine and the stomach.

There are no cell types, organs or processes that are not influenced by the endocrine system in some way and while there are many hormones that we know of there are probably many more that are yet to be discovered.

The Endocrine Organs

Figure 16.1 shows the endocrine organs and their position within the body. Each of these organs will typically have a rich blood supply delivered by numerous blood vessels. The hormone-producing cells within the organ are arranged into branching networks around this supply. This arrangement of blood vessels and hormone-producing cells ensures that hormones enter the bloodstream rapidly and are then transported throughout the body to the target cells (see Figure 16.2).

435

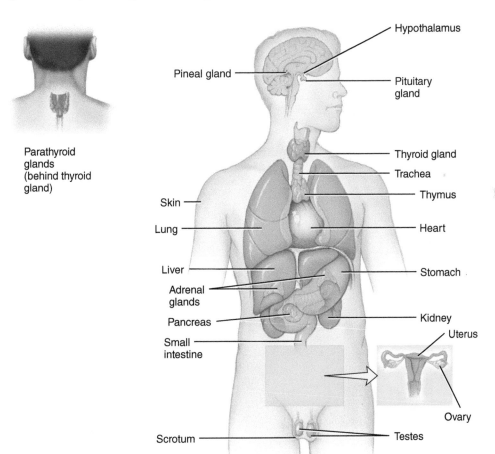

Figure 16.1 **Location of the endocrine organs.** *Source:* Tortora and Derrickson (2009). Reproduced with permission of John Wiley & Sons.

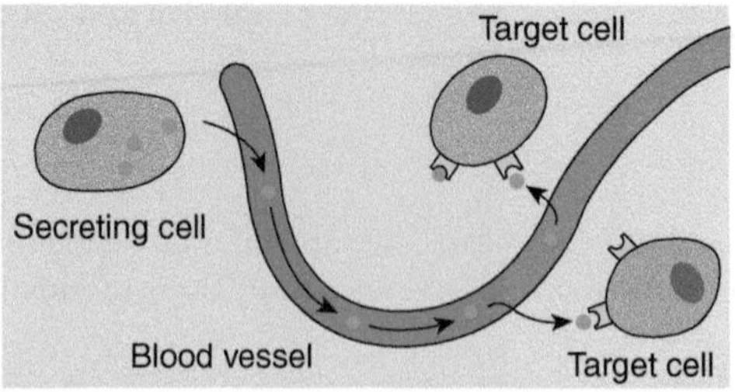

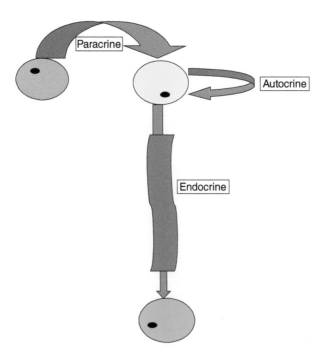

Figure 16.2 **Transportation of hormones in the blood.**

Endocrine, Paracrine, Exocrine and Autocrine

Many words in anatomy and physiology have a similar ending to other words used about the same processes or areas of the body (Figure 16.3). It is important to be aware of these as confusion can quickly take over.

Endocrine is usually used to refer to hormones that are secreted into the blood and have an effect on cells distant from those that released the hormone. However, many endocrine hormones are known to act locally and even on the cells that secrete them.

Paracrine refers to hormones that act locally and diffuse to the cells in the immediate neighbourhood to produce their action.

Autocrine refers to hormones that act on the cells that produce it.

Exocrine refers to glands/organs that secrete substances into ducts that eventually lead to the outside of the body (for instance, the sweat glands, the part of the pancreas that secretes digestive juices, the gallbladder).

436

Figure 16.3 **Endocrine, paracrine and autocrine.**

Hormones

Hormones are chemical messengers that are secreted into the blood or the extracellular fluid by one cell and have an effect on the functioning of other cells. Unlike the nervous system, which could be said to be based on wires (the neurones) like a telegraph, the endocrine system is like a radio broadcast. As it is with a radio broadcast, it is necessary for there to be a receiver in order for the hormonal message to be received and acted upon. As hormones circulate in the blood, they come into contact with virtually every cell in the body, but they only exert their specific effect on those cells that have receptors for that hormone (the target cells). Like a lock and key mechanism, only the right key (hormone) can unlock a particular lock (receptor) (see Figure 16.4).

Hormone receptors are either found within the target cell or on its surface (as in Figure 16.4). The site of the receptor is dependent on the type of hormone the receptor is for. Most hormones are made from amino acids, but some are made from cholesterol (the steroid hormones).

- Amino acid-based hormones cannot cross the cell membrane and thus their receptors are found on the cell wall. These hormones tend to exert their influence by activating enzymes and other molecules within the cell, which then affect the cell activity. This is often through a cascade of changes, with the activation of the enzyme or molecule being the first step. The best understood example of this is cyclic adenosine monophosphate.
- The steroid hormones can cross the cell membrane because they are small and lipid soluble and thus their receptors are found within the cell itself. These hormones usually exert their effect by stimulating the production of genes within the target cell. The genes then stimulate the synthesis of new proteins.
- One exception is thyroid hormone, which is not a steroid hormone but is lipid soluble and very small and can diffuse easily across the cell membrane into the cell.

437

The activation of a target cell depends on the concentration of the hormone in the blood, the number of receptors on the cell and the affinity of the receptor for the hormone. Changes in these factors can happen quickly in response to a change in stimuli.

The most important factor affecting the effect of a hormone on its target cell is its concentration in the blood and/or extracellular fluid. This concentration of a hormone at the target cell is determined by three factors:

- Rate of production of the hormone – this is the most highly regulated aspect of the endocrine system.
- Rate of delivery of the hormone – for instance, the blood flow to the organ or cell.
- Rate of destruction and elimination of the hormone (half-life). Hormones with a short half-life will rapidly drop in concentration once production decreases. If the half-life of the hormone is long, then the hormone will still be present in significant concentrations for some time after its production stops.

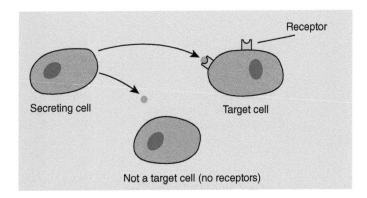

Figure 16.4 **Target cell and non-target cell.**

Changes in the concentration of hormones can be a rapid mechanism of control, especially the rate of production, but longer term adjustments to target cell sensitivity to a hormone will almost certainly include changes in the numbers of receptors as well. Changes in the number of receptors are known as upregulation and downregulation.

- Upregulation is the creation of more receptors in response to low circulating levels of a hormone; the cell becomes more responsive to the presence of the hormone in the blood.
- Downregulation is the reduction in the number of receptors and is often the response of a cell to prolonged periods of high circulating levels of a hormone; the cell becomes less responsive (desensitised) to a hormone.

The Transportation of Hormones

Most hormones are secreted into the circulating blood, though there is the exception of hormones that are released into a local circulatory system known as a portal circulation. The two portal circulations in the human body are those connecting the hypothalamus and the anterior pituitary gland and the hepatic portal circulation that merges to form the portal vein entering the liver.

The steroid hormones are mostly conveyed within the circulation by being bound to transport proteins, with less than 10% making up the 'free fraction' of the hormone (Jenkins and Tortora, 2013). In clinical placements you may have noticed that some blood tests are specifically targeted at measuring both the bound and free elements of a hormone; the most common of these are the thyroid function tests, which measure both bound thyroxine (T_4) and free T_4. Water-soluble hormones are conveyed in their free form in the blood.

Effects of Hormones

Hormones typically produce one of the following changes:

- changes in cell membrane permeability and/or the cell's electrical state (membrane potential) by opening or closing ion channels in the cell membrane;
- synthesis of proteins or regulatory molecules (such as enzymes) within the cell;
- enzyme activation or deactivation;
- causing secretory activity;
- stimulation of mitosis.

Control of Hormone Release

The creation and release of most hormones are preceded by a stimulus that can be internal or external; for instance, a rise in blood glucose levels or a cold environment. The further synthesis and release of hormones is then usually controlled by a negative feedback system. As can be seen in Figure 16.5, the influence of a stimulus, from inside or outside the body (in this case a rise in blood glucose levels), leads to hormone release (insulin); following this, some aspect of the target organ function then inhibits further reaction to the stimulus and thus further release of the hormone by the organ.

The initial stimulus for the release of a hormone is usually one of three types, though some organs respond to multiple stimuli (Marieb and Hoehn, 2015).

- **Humoral:** A response to changing levels of certain ions and nutrients in the blood. For example, parathyroid hormone is stimulated by falling blood levels of calcium ions.
- **Neural:** A response to direct nervous stimulation. Very few endocrine organs are directly stimulated by the nervous system. An example is increased activity in the sympathetic nervous system that directly stimulates the release of catecholamines (adrenaline and noradrenaline) from the adrenal medulla.
- **Hormonal:** A response to hormones released by other organs. Hormones that are released in response to hormonal stimuli are usually rhythmical in their release (that is, the levels rise and fall in a specific pattern). An example of hormonal control is the release of thyroid stimulating hormone (TSH) from the anterior pituitary gland directly stimulating the production and release of T_4 from the thyroid gland.

Destruction and Removal of Hormones

Hormones are very powerful and can have a large effect at even low concentrations; therefore, it is essential that active hormones are efficiently removed from the blood. Some hormones are rapidly broken down within the target cells. Most are inactivated by enzyme systems in the liver and kidneys and then excreted mostly in the urine, but some are excreted in the faeces.

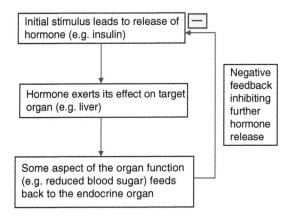

Figure 16.5 **The negative feedback system.** *Source:* Peate (2017). Reproduced with permission of John Wiley & Sons.

The Physiology of the Endocrine Organs

The Hypothalamus and the Pituitary Gland

The hypothalamus is a portion of the brain with a variety of functions. It is a small (about 4 g), cone-like structure that is directly connected to the pituitary gland by the pituitary stalk (or infundibulum). One of the most important functions of the hypothalamus is to link the nervous system to the endocrine system via the pituitary gland. Almost all hormone secretion by the pituitary gland is controlled by either hormonal or electrical signals from the hypothalamus (Figure 16.6).

The hypothalamus receives signals from virtually all the potential sources within the nervous system but is also under negative feedback control by the hormones regulated by the pituitary gland. Thus, when there is a low level of a hormone in the blood supplying the hypothalamus, this leads to the release of the appropriate releasing hormone or factor that stimulates the release of the hormone by the pituitary, which in turn stimulates the release of the appropriate hormone. As the level of the target hormone rises in the blood, this is detected by receptors in the hypothalamus and the stimulus for the release of the stimulating factor is removed and thus release of this factor is reduced. A classic example of this system is the release of thyrotropin releasing hormone (TRH) and the subsequent release of TSH by the anterior pituitary gland, which is described further on in this chapter.

The pituitary gland secretes at least nine major hormones and is the size and shape of a pea on a stalk. The pituitary gland is functionally and anatomically divided into two parts:

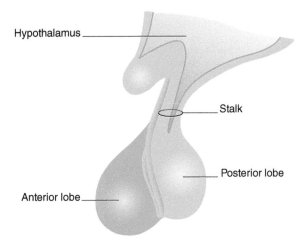

Figure 16.6 **The hypothalamus and pituitary gland.**

- The posterior lobe (neurohypophysis) is made up mostly of nerve fibres that originate in the hypothalamus and terminate on the surface of capillaries in the posterior lobe. The posterior lobe releases two hormones that it receives directly from the hypothalamus. In this sense it is in fact a storage area rather than a gland in the true sense of the term. The hypothalamus and the posterior pituitary are linked by a nerve bundle called the hypothalamic-hypophyseal tract.
- The anterior lobe (adenohypophysis) is much larger than the posterior lobe and partly surrounds the posterior lobe and the infundibulum. It is made up of glandular tissue and produces and releases several hormones. The hypothalamus and the anterior pituitary have no direct nerve connections but do have a vascular (blood vessel) connection known as the hypothalamo-hypophyseal portal system, whereby venous blood from the hypothalamus flows to the anterior lobe. Thus, control of the anterior pituitary is by releasing and inhibiting factors (or hormones) released by the hypothalamus.

Hormones that are secreted by the posterior pituitary are the following.

- **Oxytocin:** Oxytocin has an effect on uterine contraction in childbirth and is responsible for the 'let down' response in breastfeeding mothers (the release of milk in response to suckling). In men and non-pregnant women it appears to play a role in sexual arousal and orgasm (Jenkins and Tortora, 2013).
- **Antidiuretic hormone (ADH):** Under resting conditions, large quantities of ADH accumulate in the posterior pituitary; excitation by nervous impulses leads to the release of the ADH from where it is stored into the adjacent blood vessels. The effects of ADH are that it increases water retention by the kidneys by increasing the permeability of the collecting ducts in the kidneys. The secretion of ADH is stimulated:
  - by increased plasma osmolality – increased levels of certain substances in the plasma, such as sodium;
  - by decreased extracellular fluid volume;
  - by pain and other stressed states;
  - in response to certain drugs.

440

Clinical Considerations Syndrome of Inappropriate ADH Secretion (SIADH)

Though relatively rare, SIADH is a potentially life-threatening condition that causes a reduced blood sodium level. The pathophysiology varies, but one type is thought to be due to changes in the ability of the hypothalamus to detect a decrease in blood osmolality and thus ADH release is not reduced and the blood volume increases, reducing the concentration of sodium relative to the volume of blood. In the elderly it is thought that the cells of the hypothalamus increase ADH production with increasing age. Clinically detectable SIADH has many potential causes, including several commonly used medications (such as morphine, loop diuretics, angiotensin-converting enzyme inhibitors and many antidepressants), some neurological disorders, several types of cancer and hypothyroidism. It is the most common cause of hyponatraemia in critical care patients (Friedman and Cirulli, 2013) and is also common in the elderly.

The symptoms of SIADH includes loss of appetite, nausea, weakness, confusion and delirium. In the elderly, the diagnosis of SIADH can be late as one of the common presenting factors is altered mental states (including confusion) which can be mistakenly ascribed to many other factors or conditions such as dementia, infection and cerebrovascular events (Nelson and Robinson, 2012).

The diagnosis of SIADH includes the detection of a low blood sodium concentration with a normal blood volume (euvolaemia).

The treatment of SIADH involves fluid restriction, thus increasing relative sodium levels in the blood by reducing blood volume and where possible treating the cause. In cases requiring urgent treatment, hypertonic saline (3% saline) can be infused to temporarily increase the blood sodium level (Gross, 2012).

Hormones Released by the Anterior Pituitary Gland

Table 16.2 summarises the range of hormones released by the anterior pituitary gland and the releasing or inhibiting hormones (or factors) from the hypothalamus that influence this release.

There are five types of pituitary cell in the anterior lobe:

- somatotropes, which secrete growth hormones;
- lactotropes, which secrete prolactin;
- thyrotropes, which secrete TSH;
- gonadotropes, which secrete luteinising hormone (LH) and follicle-stimulating hormone (FSH);
- corticotropes, which secrete adrenocorticotropic hormone (ACTH).

Table 16.2 **Hormones released by the hypothalamus and the anterior pituitary gland.**

HYPOTHALAMUS	ANTERIOR PITUITARY GLAND	TARGET ORGAN OR TISSUES	ACTION
Growth-hormone-releasing factor	Growth hormone	Many (especially bones)	Stimulates growth of body cells
Growth-hormone-release-inhibiting factor	Growth hormone (inhibits release)	Many	
Thyroid-releasing hormone (TRH)	Thyroid-stimulating hormone (TSH)	Thyroid gland	Stimulates thyroid hormone release
Corticotropin-releasing hormone (CRH)	Adrenocorticotropic hormone (ACTH)	Adrenal cortex	Stimulates corticosteroid release
Prolactin-releasing hormone	Prolactin	Breasts	Stimulates milk production
Prolactin-inhibiting hormone	Prolactin (inhibits release)	Breasts	
Gonadotropin-releasing hormone	Follicle-stimulating hormone Luteinising hormone	Gonads	Various reproductive functions

Source: Peate (2017). Reproduced with permission of John Wiley & Sons.

Growth Hormone
Effects
As its name suggests, growth hormone promotes the growth of bone, cartilage and soft tissue by stimulating the production and release of insulin-like growth factor (IGF-1).

Regulation
Growth hormone release from the anterior pituitary is regulated by the release of growth-hormone-releasing hormone and growth-hormone-release-inhibiting hormone (somatostatin) by the hypothalamus. Both growth hormone and IGF-1 produce a negative feedback effect on the hypothalamus.

Prolactin
Effects
Prolactin stimulates the secretion of milk in the breast.

Regulation
Secretion is inhibited by the release of dopamine from the hypothalamus. Secretion can be intermittently increased by the release of prolactin-releasing hormone from the hypothalamus in response to the baby suckling at the breast.

Follicle-Stimulating Hormone and Luteinising Hormone (gonadotrophins)
Effects
In males, FSH stimulates sperm production. In females it leads to the early maturation of ovarian follicles and oestrogen secretion.

LH is responsible for the final maturation of the ovarian follicles and oestrogen secretion in females and in males it stimulates testosterone secretion.

Regulation
In males and females, LH and FSH production are regulated by the release of gonadotrophin-releasing hormone (GnRH). Testosterone and oestrogen exert a negative feedback effect on the release of GnRH from the hypothalamus.

Thyroid-Stimulating Hormone

Effects

TSH stimulates the activity of the cells of the thyroid gland leading to an increased production and secretion of T_4 and triiodothyronine (T_3).

Regulation

TSH is produced and released in response to the release of TRH from the hypothalamus. The hypothalamus can also inhibit the release of TSH through the action of somatostatin.

Free T_3 and T_4 in the blood have a direct negative feedback effect on the hypothalamus and the anterior pituitary gland.

Adrenocorticotrophic Hormone

Effects

ACTH stimulates the production of cortisol and androgens from the cortex of the adrenal gland. It also leads to the production of aldosterone in response to increased concentrations of potassium ions, increased angiotensin levels or decreased total body sodium.

Regulation

ACTH is secreted from the anterior pituitary in response to the secretion of corticotropin-releasing hormone (CRH) from the hypothalamus. Excitation of the hypothalamus by any form of stress leads to the release of CRH and the subsequent release of ACTH and then cortisol. Cortisol exerts a direct negative feedback on the hypothalamus and the anterior pituitary gland.

Episode of Care Adult

Mary is a 50-year-old lady who has come to see her GP. Mary has been reporting significant depression for which she has been prescribed antidepressants. Mary returns to the GP after one month for a review and whilst she feels somewhat better, the depression remains. On further questioning Mary reports increasing weight gain, especially in the face and on the back of the neck. At the same time, she has noticed excessive hair growth on her face and neck. She also reports that her skin is bruising easily and she is constantly tired.

The doctor suspects that Mary has Cushing's disease, which is a disease caused by excess levels of cortisol in the body, and refers her to an endocrinologist. There are several potential causes for Cushing's disease, with the most common being the long-term use of high-dose glucocorticoid medication. Mary does not take any steroids normally and this leads the endocrinologist to suspect that Mary may have a tumour that is causing the increased production of cortisol. Mary has bloods taken to measure her cortisol levels and a 24-hour urine analysis is carried out; both show elevated cortisol levels.

Magnetic resonance imaging shows that Mary has a tumour of her pituitary gland, which is causing an increased production of ACTH (corticotroph adenoma).

Mary is rapidly passed on to the care of a neurosurgeon for an operation known as transsphenoidal hypophysectomy (the removal of the pituitary gland via the nasal cavity). The procedure can remove part or all of the pituitary gland (Liubinas et al., 2011).

In Mary's case it was necessary to remove the whole gland. Following this procedure Mary will no longer have a pituitary gland and will no longer produce any of the pituitary hormones, including TRH and ACTH. The loss of TRH and ACTH production will mean there will be no stimulus for the thyroid gland and the adrenal glands to produce hormones, leading to the need for hormone replacement therapy for hypothyroidism (thyroxine) and hypoadrenalism (hydrocortisone and fludrocortisone). Follow up by Mary's GP found her depression to have improved significantly after surgery and her antidepressants were stopped.

In Cushing's disease a major depressive syndrome is seen in 50–70% of patients and often improves once the Cushing's disease is treated (Tang et al., 2013). Psychiatric disorders, especially depression, are a common finding in most patients with an endocrine disorder, with anxiety being the second most common finding. Traditionally depression and anxiety have been considered a consequence of diagnosis but increasingly it is being recognised that the endocrine disorders themselves may be the cause of psychiatric disturbances and treatment of the endocrine disorder will often improve any psychiatric symptoms (Sonino et al., 2015).

Multiple Choice Questions

1. Depression is associated with Cushing's disease in what percentage of cases.
   (a) 30–50
   (b) 50–70
   (c) 60–80
   (d) 70–90
2. Which medication can cause Cushing's disease?
   (a) antidepressants
   (b) mineralocorticoids
   (c) glucocorticoids
   (d) thyroxine
3. Mary has to collect a 24-hour urine collection, what is this used to test in this instance?
   (a) creatinine levels
   (b) thyroxine levels
   (c) urea levels
   (d) cortisol levels
4. Following removal of the pituitary gland, Mary will need to take which replacement therapy for hypothyroidism?
   (a) adrenaline
   (b) thyroxine
   (c) insulin
   (d) somatostatin
5. What medication will Mary need to take to replace one of the hormones missing due to hypoadrenalism?
   (a) adrenaline
   (b) calcium
   (c) hydrocortisone
   (d) prolactin

Skills in Practice Twenty-Four-Hour Urine Collection

Twenty-four-hour urine collections are undertaken for many reasons. For instance, in suspected Cushing's disease, a 24-hour collection of urine is undertaken to assess the excretion of cortisol in the urine. Whilst a simple test from the patient's point of view, it is important that the test is carried out correctly.

- Record all medications that the patient is taking, some medications can affect the test results (for instance if the patient is taking oestrogen or corticosteroids).
- The urine will be collected in a large container that may contain preservatives; it is therefore essential that the patient is informed not to pass urine directly into the container or touch the inside of the container as this may lead to skin contact with the preservative.
- Patients must use a clean receptacle every time they pass urine and to avoid contaminating the sample with faeces, menstrual blood, toilet paper or pubic hair.
- When the patient passes the first urine of the day (first thing in the morning) this urine is discarded and the time recorded (this is the time of the start of the test).
- All urine passed for the next 24 hours is then collected in the receptacle and the receptacle is normally kept in a cool area.
- Not collecting all the urine passed over 24 hours may affect the outcome of the test.
- At the point 24 hours are up (or just before) the patient should empty their bladder and add this to the collection. The final time should be noted, and the collection returned to the hospital laboratory.

The Thyroid Gland

The thyroid gland is a butterfly-shaped gland located in the front of the neck on the trachea just below the larynx (Figure 16.7). It is made up of two lobes joined by an isthmus (a narrow strip; isthmus = neck). The upper extremities of the lobes are known as the upper poles and the lower extremities the lower poles. Each

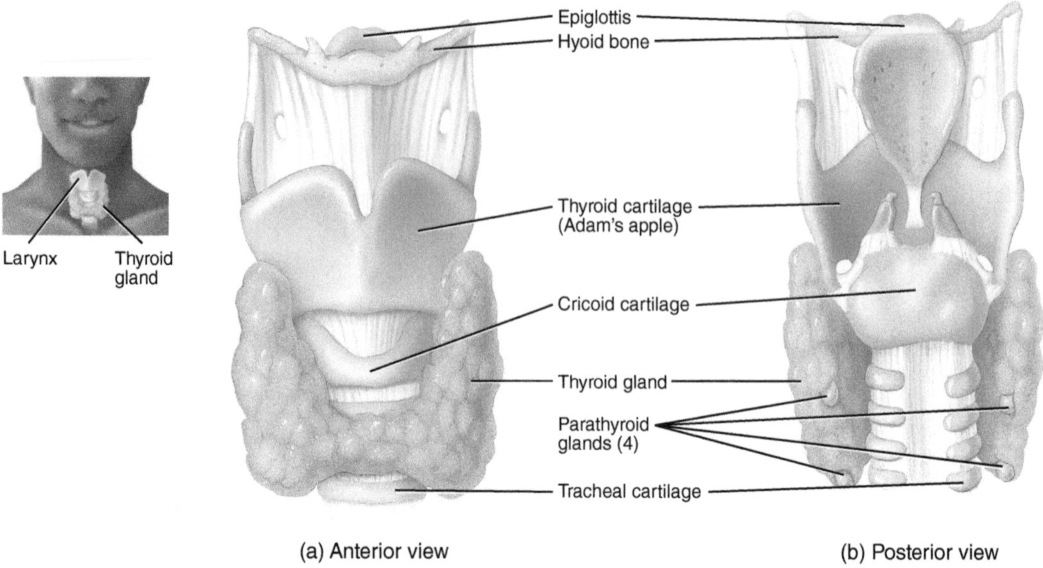

Figure 16.7 (a, b) Position of the thyroid gland and parathyroid glands. *Source:* Tortora and Derrickson (2009). Reproduced with permission of John Wiley & Sons.

lobe is made up of hollow, spherical follicles surrounded by capillaries. This leads to an abundant blood supply; although the thyroid gland accounts for 0.4% of the total body weight, it receives 2% of the circulating blood supply.

The follicles are comprised of a single layer of epithelial cells that form a cavity that contains thyroglobulin molecules with attached iodine molecules; the thyroid hormone is created from this. One unique factor of the thyroid gland is its ability to create and store large amounts of hormone; this can be up to 100 days of hormone supply (Hall and Guyton, 2016). The thyroid gland releases two forms of thyroid hormone: T_4 and T_3; both require iodine for their creation. Iodide taken in with the normal diet is concentrated by the thyroid gland and is changed in the follicle cells into iodine. This iodine is then linked to tyrosine molecules and these iodinated tyrosine molecules are then linked together to create T_3 and T_4. All the steps in thyroid hormone production are stimulated by TSH. T_4 is the primary hormone released by the thyroid gland; this is then converted into T_3 by the target cells. Most thyroid hormone is bound to transport proteins in the blood; very little is unbound (free) and T_3 is less firmly bound to transport proteins than is T_4.

Thyroid hormone affects virtually every cell in the body, except:

- the adult brain
- spleen
- testes
- uterus
- thyroid gland.

Both T_4 and T_3 easily cross the cell membrane and interact with receptors inside the cell. In the target cells, thyroid hormone stimulates enzymes that are involved with glucose oxidation. This is known as the calorigenic effect and its overall effects are:

- an increase in the basal metabolic rate;
- an increase in oxygen consumption by the cell;
- an increase in the production of body heat.

Basal metabolic rate is the amount of energy expended while at rest in a temperate environment (not hot or cold). The release of energy in this state is enough for the functioning of the vital organs. As basal metabolic rate is increased, so oxygen consumption is increased, as oxygen is required in the production of energy.

Thyroid hormone also has an important role in the maintenance of blood pressure as it stimulates an increase in the number of receptors in the walls of the blood vessels.

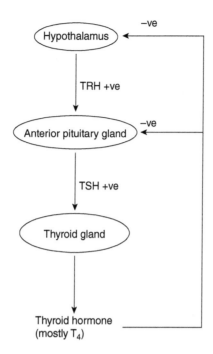

Figure 16.8 **Negative feedback control of thyroid hormone production.**

The control of the release of thyroid hormone is mediated by a negative feedback system that involves the hypothalamus and cascades through the pituitary gland (Figure 16.8).

Plasma levels of thyroid hormone are monitored in the hypothalamus and by cells in the anterior lobe of the pituitary gland. Increased levels of T_4 in the blood inhibit the release of TRH from the hypothalamus, thus reducing the stimulation for the release of TSH from the anterior pituitary gland. Thyroid hormones also have a direct negative feedback effect on the anterior pituitary gland. The effect of TSH on the thyroid gland is to promote the release of thyroid hormone into the blood; therefore, a reduction in TSH reduces the release of T_3 and T_4. A reduced level of T_4 in the blood reduces the negative feedback and thus there is an increase in the release of TRH, which leads to an increase in thyroid gland function. Conditions that increase the energy requirements of the body (such as pregnancy or prolonged cold) also stimulate the release of TRH from the hypothalamus and therefore lead to an increase in blood levels of thyroid hormone. In these situations, the stimulating conditions override the normal negative feedback system (Jenkins and Tortora, 2013). The negative feedback control of thyroid hormone can be likened to a central heating system. The hypothalamus and pituitary gland are the thermostat and the thyroid gland is the boiler. As the room temperature increases, the thermostat turns off the central heating boiler; when the temperature decreases, the thermostat turns the boiler on to increase the temperature.

The half-life of T_4 is approximately 7 days and the half-life of T_3 is 1 day. Thyroid hormones are broken down in the liver and the skeletal muscle and while much of the iodine is recycled, some is lost in the urine and the faeces. Therefore, there is a need for daily replacement of iodide in the diet.

Clinical Considerations Hypothyroidism and Hyperthyroidism

 A patient's blood level of thyroid hormone can be measured. Depending on whether the thyroid gland is overactive or underactive, different levels of hormones will be shown by the test. Generally, the patient would have their free T_4 and TSH levels assessed.

	TSH	FREE T_4
Hyperthyroidism	Reduced	Elevated
Hypothyroidism	Elevated	Reduced

In the case of a patient with an overactive thyroid gland (hyperthyroidism), free T_4 will often be elevated but TSH levels will be reduced as the levels of thyroid hormone will be exerting a negative feedback effect on the hypothalamus and the pituitary gland. Despite the reduced TSH levels and the negative feedback effect on the pituitary gland as well, hormone levels will remain elevated.

A patient with hypothyroidism (an underactive thyroid gland) will often present with a reduced free T_4 and an elevated TSH as the reduced hormone levels remove the negative feedback on the hypothalamus and the pituitary and thus TSH levels rise. The patient with a test results within normal ranges is called 'euthyroid'.

Sick euthyroid syndrome

During severe illness or starvation, the metabolic drive on the human body by the thyroid is reduced. The term 'sick euthyroid' is used in this condition since it represents a state of thyroid function appropriate for a sick individual; and it returns to normal with the return of good health.

T_3 is largely produced by target cell conversion of T_4. In the typical sick euthyroid patient, circulating T_3 is usually low but the total T_4 may be normal or even raised since there is reduced conversion to T_3. Conversely, T_4 may be low since the majority is carried on serum-binding proteins and their synthesis may be suppressed by severe illness. In these cases, the absence of a raised TSH excludes a diagnosis of primary hypothyroidism (McDermott, 2013).

Critically ill patients with sick euthyroid syndrome are known to have increased rates of mortality, but at present the routine testing of thyroid function in the critically ill is not recommended and should only be carried out when there is clinical suspicion of hypothyroidism (Economidou et al., 2011).

In addition to the thyroid epithelial cells there are C cells, which are found between the follicles and secrete calcitonin. Calcitonin is involved in the metabolism of calcium and phosphorus within the body. It decreases calcium levels in the blood by reducing the activity of osteoclasts (cells that 'digest' bone and thus release calcium and phosphorus into the blood); due to this action, calcitonin is used as a treatment for osteoporosis and may also have a future role in the treatment of osteoarthritis (Mero et al., 2014). Calcitonin also inhibits the reabsorption of calcium from urine in the kidneys.

Episode of Care Learning Disabilities

Daniel is a 28-year-old gentleman with Down syndrome. Daniel lives at home with his mother, father and sister in a semi-detached house. He attends a day centre Monday to Friday and enjoys a wide range of activities. Recently, his parents have noted that Daniel has become less interested in activities other than watching television and is reluctant to get out of bed in the morning. Daniel is gaining weight and appears to be constipated. On review, the GP is unsure if the symptoms being described are due to Daniel's Down syndrome. Lethargy, constipation and weight gain are common in patients with Down syndrome. The GP counsels Daniel and his family about getting exercise to lose weight and eating fibre. The GP also recognises these changes as possible signs of hypothyroidism and sends Daniel for a blood test (TFTs: thyroid function tests). The GP prescribes Daniel levothyroxine but warns him that it will be several weeks (if not months) before he feels completely better and in the meantime there would be a need for repeated blood tests to monitor his blood levels of T_4 to ensure that he is receiving the correct dose.

Levothyroxine is a synthetic version of the hormone T_4 and is generally free from side effects at the correct dose. Levothyroxine should be taken at the same time every day, preferably on an empty stomach. Where possible, patients are advised to take their levothyroxine an hour before breakfast.

In Europe the prevalence of hypothyroidism is between 0.2% and 5.3% (Chaker et al., 2017), however the prevalence in patients with Down's syndrome is estimated to be between 13% and 63% (Hardy et al., 2004). Several symptoms of hypothyroidism are also common in Down syndrome and thus the diagnosis of hypothyroidism is often missed in the patient with Down's syndrome. It is recommended that patients with Down syndrome are screened for hypothyroidism at birth and then every two years from then on (Prasher, 1999).

Multiple Choice Questions

1. The prevalence of hypothyroidism in patients with Down syndrome is:
    (a) the same as the general population
    (b) higher than the general population
    (c) lower than the general population
    (d) unknown

2. Patients with Down syndrome should be screened for hypothyroidism at birth and then:
   (a) every year
   (b) every two years
   (c) every five years
   (d) only if symptoms appear.
3. Levothyroxine should be taken:
   (a) with food
   (b) after food
   (c) before food
   (d) anytime
4. The blood test for diagnosing hypothyroidism is:
   (a) TFT
   (b) FBC
   (c) U&E
   (d) WBC
5. Levothyroxine is a synthetic version of:
   (a) T_2
   (b) T_3
   (c) T_4
   (d) T_5

Medicines Management Levothyroxine

Holly is a 24-year-old woman who has been experiencing symptoms of lethargy, a loss of appetite, weight gain and mild depression. Initially her GP decided her symptoms were due to Holly's lifestyle and advised Holly about getting sufficient rest and exercise. As the months went by the symptoms did not improve and Holly began to lose her hair. Holly's GP took blood and sent it to the local hospital for thyroid function testing. The results showed an increase in TSH and a decrease in free T_4, suggestive of hypothyroid disease.

The GP prescribed Holly levothyroxine but warned her that it would be several weeks (if not months) before she felt completely better and in the meantime there would be a need for repeated blood tests to monitor her blood levels of T_4 to ensure that she is receiving the correct dose.

Levothyroxine is a synthetic version of the hormone T_4 and is generally free from side effects at the correct dose. Levothyroxine should be taken at the same time every day, preferably on an empty stomach. Where possible, patients are advised to take their levothyroxine an hour before breakfast.

Holly should also be counselled that before she intends to become pregnant she should discuss this with her endocrinologist. Pre-conception measurement of thyroid replacement levels is advised as low levels of maternal T_4 in the first trimester are associated with intellectual impairment in the baby. Levothyroxine requirements increase by about 50% in pregnancy and the patient should be advised to increase their dose as soon as they are aware that they are pregnant (Weetman, 2013).

The Parathyroid Glands

The parathyroid glands (Figure 16.7) are small glands located on the back (posterior) of the thyroid gland. There are usually two pairs of glands, but the precise number varies and some patients have been reported to have up to four pairs (Marieb and Hoehn, 2015). The cells that create and secrete parathyroid hormone (parathyroid chief cells) are arranged in cords or nests around a dense capillary network. Parathyroid hormone is the single most important hormone for the control of the calcium balance in the body. Its major target cells are in the bones and the kidneys; it

- increases intestinal calcium absorption;
- stimulates renal calcium absorption;
- stimulates osteoclast activity and therefore reabsorption of calcium from the bones.

Physiologically, calcium is important in the transmission of nerve impulses, is involved in muscle contraction and is also required in the creation of clotting factors in the blood. The regulation of parathyroid hormone synthesis and secretion is in response to the levels of calcium in the blood, which is monitored by cells in the gland. A reduced blood calcium level leads to an increase in the synthesis and secretion of parathyroid hormone.

Calcitriol is a hormone released by the kidneys in response to a decrease in calcium ions in the blood; it is known to have some effect on parathyroid hormone secretion and inhibits the release of calcitonin. It also promotes the absorption of calcium from the gut and the reabsorption of calcium from the renal tubules. Parathyroid hormone is a known stimulus for the release of calcitriol, but when calcitriol levels achieve a high enough level its effect changes to that of inhibiting the release of parathyroid hormone. This prevents an uncontrollable increase in calcium in the blood.

The Adrenal Glands

The adrenal glands are complex, multifunctional organs whose secretions are essential for the maintenance of homeostasis. The two adrenal glands are found on the top of each of the two kidneys (Figure 16.9). The right gland is roughly triangular in shape and the left, which is commonly the larger of the two, is crescent-shaped. Both glands are encased in a connective tissue capsule and embedded in an area of fat. Adrenal glands are very vascular (have a rich blood supply from many blood vessels).

Functionally, each adrenal gland is actually two glands and is comprised of two major regions (Figure 16.10):

- adrenal medulla
- adrenal cortex.

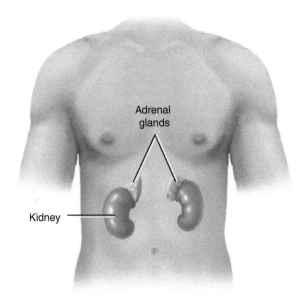

Figure 16.9 **Position of the adrenal glands.** *Source:* Tortora and Derrickson (2009). Reproduced with permission of John Wiley & Sons.

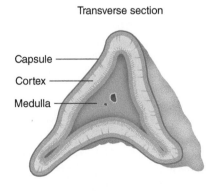

Figure 16.10 **Figure 16.10 Cross-section of an adrenal gland.** *Source:* Peate (2017). Reproduced with permission of John Wiley & Sons.

Adrenal Medulla

The adrenal medulla is the inner part of the adrenal gland; it makes up about 30% of the total mass of the adrenal gland. The function of the adrenal medulla is the secretion of catecholamines:

- adrenaline
- noradrenaline
- dopamine.

The adrenal medulla is mostly a modified, densely innervated, sympathetic ganglion made up of granule-containing cells. Within the adrenal medulla approximately 90% of the cells secrete adrenaline and the remaining 10% secrete noradrenaline. It is unclear which cells secrete dopamine at this time. The effects of the catecholamines are many and varied:

- they stimulate the nervous system;
- they have metabolic effects – for instance, glycogenolysis in the liver and skeletal muscle;
- they increase metabolic rate;
- they increase heart rate;
- they increase alertness – though adrenaline frequently evokes anxiety and fear;
- noradrenaline causes significant, widespread, vasoconstriction;
- adrenaline causes vasoconstriction in the skin and viscera but vasodilatation in skeletal muscles.

Although adrenaline and noradrenaline are essential for normal bodily functioning, adrenaline and the noradrenaline secreted by the adrenal medulla are not essential and serve only to intensify the effects of sympathetic nervous stimulation.

Secretion of catecholamines from the adrenal medulla is initiated by sympathetic nervous activity controlled by the hypothalamus and occurs in response to:

- pain
- anxiety
- excitement
- hypovolaemia
- hypoglycaemia.

The medulla receives its blood supply from the adrenal cortex rich in corticosteroids. These regulate the production of the enzymes that convert noradrenaline to adrenaline. Thus, an increase in corticosteroid production leads to an increased conversion of noradrenaline to adrenaline. With emergency stimulation of the hypothalamus there is a responding diffuse medullary activity preparing for fight or flight. Catecholamines have a very short half-life in the blood of less than 2 min as they are rapidly degraded by blood-borne enzymes.

Adrenal Cortex

The outer part of each adrenal gland is made up of three distinct functional layers (Figure 16.11). Each layer is involved in the production of steroid-based hormones (known collectively as the corticosteroids):

- zona glomerulosa – produces the mineralocorticoids;
- zona fasciculata – produces the glucocorticoids;
- zona reticularis – this zone is also involved in the production of glucocorticoids but also produces small amounts of adrenal sex hormones (the gonadocorticoids).

Mineralocorticoids

Mineralocorticoids are the group of hormones whose main function is the regulation of the concentration of the electrolytes in the blood. There are several known mineralocorticoids, but the most common is aldosterone, which accounts for 95% of all the mineralocorticoids synthesised and is also the most potent.

The effect of aldosterone is to reduce the excretion of sodium in the urine by regulating the reabsorption of sodium from the urine in the distal portion of the renal tubules. Sodium is in effect exchanged for potassium and hydrogen, which results in the renal excretion of potassium and acidic urine. Aldosterone also has an effect on the levels of water in the body and several other ions (including potassium, bicarbonate and chloride) due to the fact that their regulation is coupled to the regulation of sodium in the body. The control of aldosterone secretion is primarily related to the blood concentrations of sodium (Na+) and potassium (K+), the mean arterial blood pressure and blood volume. Increased concentrations of potassium, reduced blood concentrations of sodium and a reduction in blood pressure and/or blood volume all stimulate the release of aldosterone, while the opposite inhibits release (Figure 16.12). High blood levels of potassium are also known to have a direct effect on the adrenal cortex in the stimulation of aldosterone production and secretion.

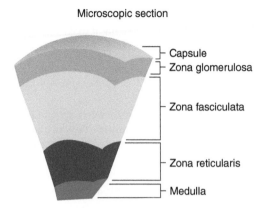

Microscopic section

- Capsule
- Zona glomerulosa
- Zona fasciculata
- Zona reticularis
- Medulla

Figure 16.11 **Cross-section of the adrenal cortex.** *Source:* Peate (2017). Reproduced with permission of John Wiley & Sons.

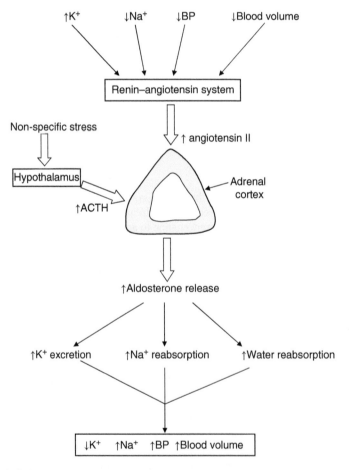

Figure 16.12 **Control of aldosterone secretion.** *Source:* Peate (2017). Reproduced with permission of John Wiley & Sons.

There are several mechanisms that regulate the release of aldosterone. The primary control mechanism is the production of angiotensin II by the renin-angiotensin system in response to reduced blood pressure in the kidneys or reduced sodium delivery to the distal tubules of the kidneys. Raised levels of potassium and reduced levels of sodium in the blood are also known to have a direct effect on the adrenal cortex and stimulate the release of mineralocorticoids. However, in response to a severe, non-specific stressor, hypothalamic release of CRH stimulates the increased release of ACTH. This increase in ACTH stimulates a slight increase in the release of aldosterone, leading to a slight increase in blood volume and pressure, which will help to maintain delivery of oxygen and nutrients to the tissues.

Glucocorticoids

There appears to be no cell within the body that does not have receptors for the glucocorticoid hormones. The glucocorticoid hormones have several effects:

- they influence the metabolism of most body cells;
- they promote glycogen storage in the liver;
- during fasting they stimulate the generation of glucose;
- they increase blood glucose levels;
- they are involved in providing resistance to stressors;
- they potentiate the vasoconstrictor effect of catecholamines;
- they decrease the permeability of vascular endothelium;
- they promote the repair of damaged tissues by promoting the breakdown of stored protein to create amino acids;
- they suppress the immune system;
- they suppress inflammatory processes.

The glucocorticoid hormones include:

- cortisol (hydrocortisone)
- cortisone
- corticosterone.

Only cortisol is secreted in any significant amounts. Cortisol is normally released in a rhythmical pattern, with most being released shortly after the person gets up from sleep and the lowest amount being released just before, and shortly after, sleep commences.

Cortisol release is stimulated by ACTH from the anterior pituitary gland. ACTH releases cholesterol from the cytoplasm in the cells, which is then converted and modified to create the steroid hormones. ACTH secretion is regulated by the release of CRH from the hypothalamus. Increasing levels of cortisol have a negative feedback effect on both the hypothalamus and the pituitary gland, inhibiting further release of both CRH and ACTH. However, this negative feedback system can be overridden by acute physiological stress (for instance, trauma, infection or haemorrhage) and mental stress. The increase in sympathetic nervous system activity in response to an acute stress triggers greater CRH release and thus there is a significant increase in subsequent cortisol production (Figure 16.13).

451

Clinical Considerations Glucocorticoid Steroids and Inflammatory Diseases

Synthetic glucocorticoid steroid hormones are used widely in health care for the suppression of inflammation in diseases such as arthritis, ulcerative colitis and acute severe asthma. However, after taking glucocorticoid steroids such as prednisolone for a significant length of time (except in asthma inhalers), steroid treatment should be gradually reduced, not stopped suddenly. Trials have shown that a short-term (5 days) course of high-dose prednisolone (60 mg) led to some suppression of ACTH production in children, but this did not require a tapering dose of steroids to prevent hypoadrenalism. However, it is felt that these patients should be counselled as to the potential symptoms of hypoadrenalism and to seek medical aid if these symptoms did appear (Crowley et al., 2014).

The constant intake of synthetic steroids for long-term treatment of inflammatory disease leads to a reduction in the production of steroids by the adrenal cortex (probably due to reduced CRH and ACTH secretion because of negative feedback to the hypothalamus and pituitary gland) and suddenly stopping steroid treatment may leave the patient with reduced levels of glucocorticoid steroids in their blood and may lead to a life-threatening hypoadrenal crisis. Thus, the patient will be advised to take a gradually reducing dose of steroids to allow the hypothalamus, pituitary gland and adrenal glands to respond to the reducing blood levels of steroids.

The need for adherence to the prescribed regimen of any course of steroid medication and advice on what to do in the event of gastrointestinal disease preventing the patient taking their steroids must be impressed on the patient. The patient should also carry a blue 'steroid card' at all times detailing the dose and type of steroid taken so that health care professionals can respond appropriately, even when the patient is unconscious.

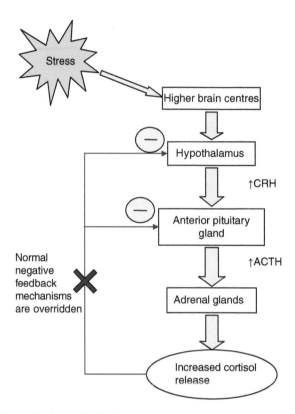

Figure 16.13 **Response of the endocrine system to stress.** *Source:* Peate (2017). Reproduced with permission of John Wiley & Sons.

Pancreas

The pancreas is an elongated organ and is found next to the first part of the small intestine. The pancreas is composed of two different types of tissues. The majority of the pancreas is made up of exocrine tissue and the associated ducts. This tissue produces and secretes a fluid rich with digestive enzymes into the small intestine. Scattered throughout the exocrine tissue are many small clusters of cells called islets of Langerhans (islets). These islets are the site of the endocrine cells of the pancreas. Each islet has three major cell types, each of which produces a different hormone:

- alpha cells, which secrete glucagon;
- beta cells, the most abundant of the three cell types and which secrete insulin;
- delta cells, which secrete somatostatin.

The different cell types within each islet are distributed in a set pattern, with the beta cells being the central portion of the islet, surrounded by alpha and delta cells. The islets are highly vascularised, ensuring rapid transit of the hormones into the bloodstream. Although the islets only account for 1–2% of the mass of the pancreas, they receive about 10–15% of the pancreatic blood flow. The pancreas is innervated by the parasympathetic and sympathetic nervous systems and it is clear that nervous stimulation influences the secretion of insulin and glucagon.

Medicines Management Type 2 Diabetes

George is a 56-year-old gentleman who has recently been diagnosed with type 2 diabetes. For the last few months he has noticed that he feels increasingly thirsty and is also constantly tired.

George has been reluctant to go to the GP as he does not feel that there is anything really wrong with him and he does not like to bother the doctor anyway. During a routine health screening the practice nurse carries out a dipstick test on George's urine and it is found that there is a significant level of glucose in it. The diagnosis is made of type 2 diabetes; in addition to being educated about lifestyle and dietary changes, George is prescribed metformin.

Metformin is an oral antidiabetic drug that is normally used as the first-line drug in the treatment of type 2 diabetes. It works by reducing the amount of glucose produced by the liver. In order to try to prevent the development of gastrointestinal side effects the GP has decided to start George on a relatively low dose of metformin and then to slowly increase the dose. If George is unable to tolerate metformin due to gastrointestinal side effects, current guidelines suggest a trial of extended absorption metformin (National Institute for Health and Care Excellence, 2017).

Insulin

Insulin is well known for its effect in reducing the blood glucose levels. It does this by:

- Facilitating the entry of glucose into muscle, adipose tissue and several other tissues. Note that the brain and the liver do not require insulin to facilitate the uptake of glucose.
- Stimulating the liver to store glucose in the form of glycogen.

However, as well as its effects on glucose, insulin is known to have an effect on protein and mineral metabolism. Finally, insulin has an effect on lipid metabolism. As has been noted, insulin promotes the synthesis of glycogen in the liver. As glycogen accumulation in the liver rises to higher levels (5% of the total liver mass), further glycogen synthesis is suppressed. Further uptake of glucose is then diverted by insulin into the production of fatty acids and insulin inhibits the breakdown of fat in adipose tissue and facilitates the production of triglycerides from glucose for further storage in these tissues.

From a whole-body perspective, insulin has a fat-sparing effect in that it promotes the use of glucose instead of fatty acids and stimulates the storage of fat in the adipose tissue.

The stimulation of insulin synthesis and secretion is primarily a response to a rise in blood glucose levels, but rises in blood levels of amino acids and fatty acids also have a stimulating effect. Some neural stimuli, for instance the sight and smell of food, also increase insulin secretion. The pancreas is innervated by the sympathetic and parasympathetic nervous systems and nervous stimulation clearly influences the secretion of insulin (and glucagon).

As blood glucose levels fall, there is a corresponding fall in the production and secretion of insulin. When insulin levels in the blood fall, glycogen synthesis in the liver reduces and enzymes that break down glycogen become active. The half-life of insulin is approximately 5 minutes and it is destroyed in the liver.

453

Skills in Practice Injecting Insulin with a Pen

Follow local policy on medicine administration (right patient, right time and so forth).
- Put a new needle on the pen (reusing needles causes more pain).
- Remove the cap from the needle.
- Hold the pen upright (needle uppermost) and dial 2–3 units of insulin and press the plunger. Watch for a steady stream of insulin, if a steady stream is not seen then repeat (carrying out an 'air shot' removes bubbles from the needle).
- Dial the correct (prescribed) dose.
- Pick an area of soft 'fatty' skin (top of the thigh, stomach, buttock), in thinner people it may be necessary to pinch a fold of skin to inject into.
- Hold the pen straight and push the needle into the skin.
- Push down the plunger slowly (pushing the plunger too fast can cause pain).
- Hold the pen in place for 10 seconds to ensure the whole dose is delivered.
- Dispose of the needle according to local policy.
- Return the insulin pen to safe storage.

Episode of Care Child

Thomas is a 14-year-old boy who was diagnosed with insulin dependent diabetes (type 1) at the age of 8. Since the onset of puberty, Thomas and his family have found that glucose control has become difficult with repeated episodes of hypoglycaemia and a constantly raised HbA1c (HbA1c is a blood test that shows the average blood glucose level over the period of 2–3 months before the test). Thomas' consultant recommends that as repeated insulin injections are not controlling Thomas' blood glucose effectively, he should consider the use of a continuous subcutaneous insulin infusion (CSII, otherwise known as an insulin pump).

Insulin pumps have been used in clinical practice for many years but the use in paediatric practice has only become more frequent in the last 10 years. NICE guidance (2008) recommends the use of an insulin pump in children over the age of 12 years if there are repeated hypoglycaemic events or HbA1c is consistently raised. The device is a pump unit with a reservoir of short acting insulin attached to a subcutaneous needle via a thin tube. The use of the pump allows for both timed delivery of insulin at different times of the day and allows the wearer to modify the immediate dose of insulin at any time. The use of pump therapy in children has been associated with a greater sense of control, greater satisfaction with treatment and a greater sense of freedom over diet and exercise (Hussain et al., 2017).

Discussions with Thomas covered the issues of Thomas being willing to wear the pump constantly (though it can be hidden under clothes in a special belt), troubleshooting problems with the pump of giving set/needle and the need to change the needle regularly.

Multiple Choice Questions

1. What are the benefits of an insulin pump for Thomas?
    (a) greater sense of control
    (b) freedom over diet
    (c) greater satisfaction
    (d) all of the above
2. What is one new activity Thomas will need to master to be independent with his pump?
    (a) how to hide the pump
    (b) troubleshooting problems with the giving set
    (c) topping up his insulin levels with subcutaneous injections
    (d) eating at set times in the day.
3. HbA1c is a test that measures the average blood glucose levels over:
    (a) 1–2 weeks
    (b) 2–3 weeks
    (c) 1–2 months
    (d) 2–3 months
4. Over what age does NICE suggest insulin pumps may be used?
    (a) 10 years old
    (b) 11 years old
    (c) 12 years old
    (d) 13 years old
5. Subcutaneous means:
    (a) under the skin
    (b) into the fat
    (c) into the muscle
    (d) into the vein

Medicines Management Insulin

There are more than 20 types of insulin available in four basic forms. Insulin types have three important factors to be considered when prescribing and using them:

1. how soon they start working (onset);
2. when they work the hardest (peak time);
3. how long they last in the body (duration).

The decision as to which insulin to prescribe a patient is based on multiple factors, including the patient's lifestyle and blood glucose levels.

On the ward, insulin is usually stored in the fridge, but cold insulin increases the pain of the injection and slows down the insulin absorption, so for better injection comfort and insulin efficiency it is advisable to take the insulin out of the refrigerator a minimum of 1 hour prior to injection.

Insulin Pens

Patients should be advised not to store opened insulin pens in the fridge (especially with the needle attached). Refrigerating a fluid leads to it contracting and warming it up causes it to expand. This is especially dangerous with cloudy insulins. Taking cloudy insulin from the fridge and allowing it to warm in a pen with needle attached can lead to the leakage of either the insulin or the inert carrier fluid, thus changing the strength of the insulin preparation. Leakage into the needle also leads to the formation of insulin crystals, which can block the needle and change the injection pressure or the amount injected.

Taking a pen (and needle) from the warm and putting it into the fridge leads to the contraction of the fluid and the development of air bubbles. Air bubbles are compressible and lengthen injection time. Even after the standard 10 seconds count, insulin can still be leaking from the needle when it is withdrawn.

Unopened pen cartridges are stored in a fridge, but once inserted into an insulin pen the pen should be kept out of the fridge. The insulin can be stored at room temperature for 28 days (NICE, 2016).

Premixed Insulins

When a patient (or nurse) is going to administer a cloudy, or premixed, insulin it is important that the pen or vial is rotated end over end 20 times (not shaken), otherwise the insulin may not be mixed correctly (Frid *et al.*, 2010). Research has shown that patients are often confused about this technique and the actual mixing of insulin by patients has a large variation that may be affecting glycaemic control (Frid *et al.*, 2010).

455

Clinical Considerations Hypoglycaemia

Hypoglycaemia is a constant worry in the patient with diabetes and as many hypoglycaemic episodes are associated with exercise, the fear of hypoglycaemia prevents many patients with diabetes from undertaking regular exercise (Kennedy et al, 2018). This is unfortunate, as exercise is one of the cornerstones in the prevention of diabetes-related complications and also aids in the control of diabetes by aiding weight loss and promoting vascular health (reducing heart attack and stroke risk).

Current guidelines suggest that the promotion of exercise in patients with both type 1 and type 2 diabetes should be associated with guidance on the management of blood glucose level changes linked with exercise. The patient should take their blood glucose before and after exercise and again several hours later. Patients with either very high or very low blood glucose should avoid exercising until the blood glucose has normalised (Kourtoglou, 2011). Patients using insulin therapy are advised to either omit the insulin dose prior to exercise or consume a carbohydrate load (such as a carbohydrate drink) before exercise; patients on medication regimens other than insulin are at a much lower risk of exercise hypoglycaemia and do not need to take this precaution (American Diabetes Association, 2019).

Any patient with diabetes who is considering exercise as part of their diabetes management should be encouraged, but they should always be advised to consult with their endocrinologist first for advice on the intensity and timing of exercise.

Glucagon

Glucagon has an important role in maintaining normal blood glucose levels, especially as the brain and neurones can only use glucose as a fuel.

Glucagon has the opposite effect on blood glucose levels to insulin (Figure 16.14); it:

- stimulates the breakdown of glycogen stored in the liver;
- activates hepatic gluconeogenesis (the creation of glucose from substrates such as amino acids);
- has a minor effect enhancing triglyceride breakdown in adipose tissue – providing fatty acid fuel for most cells and thus conserving glucose for the brain and neurones.

The production and secretion of glucagon are stimulated in response to a reduction in blood glucose concentrations and elevated blood levels of amino acids (for instance, after a protein-rich meal). It has also been found that glucagon levels in the blood rise in response to exercise, but it is unclear whether this is a response to the exercise itself or a response to the reduced blood glucose levels that exercise creates.

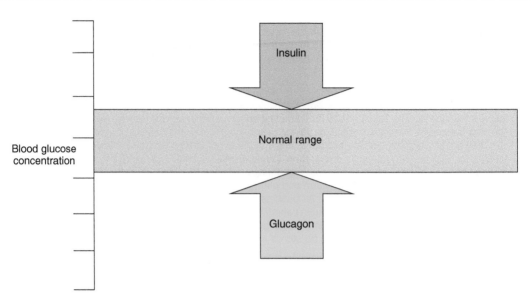

Figure 16.14 **Effects of insulin and glucagon on blood glucose concentrations.**

Glucagon production and secretion are inhibited when there is increased glucose levels in the blood; however, it is unknown whether this is a direct effect of the glucose levels or a response to rising levels of insulin, as insulin is known to inhibit the release of glucagon.

Somatostatin

Somatostatin is actually released by a broad range of tissues. Its physiological effect in the pancreas is to inhibit the release of insulin and glucagon; it does this in a paracrine fashion; that is, the hormone is released and has its effect locally. The exact mechanism of control of this hormone is unknown.

Conclusion

This chapter has introduced the reader to the endocrine system, a diverse system that is one of the two bodily systems necessary for the maintenance of homeostasis. While often working in close conjunction with the nervous system, the endocrine system is often responsible for the control of longer term processes. The major functions of the endocrine system are based on four main areas:

- the maintenance of homeostasis (especially electrolyte levels and fluid balance);
- metabolism;
- growth and development;
- responses to stress.

The secretion of hormones can be stimulated by nervous impulses, hormones or changes in the body levels of ions and nutrients; and further regulation of hormone release is then often controlled by negative feedback loops. Hormones can only have an effect on a cell if that cell has a receptor for the hormone; however, there appears to be virtually no cell within the body that is not affected by the endocrine system.

Glossary

Amino acid: Chemical compound that is the basic building block of proteins and enzymes.
Carbohydrate: A group of compounds (including starches and sugars) that are a major food source.
Catecholamines: A collective term for adrenaline, noradrenaline and dopamine.
Cortex: The outermost layer of an organ.
Corticosteroids: Steroid hormones released by the adrenal cortex, further divided into glucocorticoids and mineralocorticoids.
Cortisol: The major glucocorticoid steroid released by the adrenal gland.

Cytoplasm: The part of the cell enclosed within the cell membrane.

Downregulation: The reduction in the number of hormone receptors of a cell, often the response of a cell to prolonged periods of high circulating levels of a hormone.

Electrolytes: A group of chemical elements or compounds that includes sodium, potassium, calcium, chloride and bicarbonate.

Fatty acids: Dietary fats that have broken down into elements that can be absorbed into the blood.

Free T_4: Thyroxine in the blood that is not bound to proteins.

Ganglion: A mass, or group, of nerve cells.

Gland: Any organ in the body that secretes substances not related to its own, internal, functioning.

Glucocorticoids: A group of hormones that exert their major effect on the metabolism of carbohydrates.

Gluconeogenesis: Creation of new glucose from non-carbohydrate substrates.

Glycogen: A carbohydrate (complex sugar) made from glucose.

Glycogenolysis: Breakdown of glycogen to create glucose.

Hormonal stimulation: Stimulation of a gland that produces a change in the activity of that gland in response to hormones released by other organs.

Hormone: Chemical substance that is released into the blood by the endocrine system and has a physiological control over the function of cells or organs other than those that created it.

Humoral stimulation: Stimulation of a gland that produces a change in the activity of that gland in response to changing levels of certain ions and nutrients in the blood.

Hyperglycaemia: High blood levels of glucose.

Hypoglycaemia: Low blood levels of glucose.

Hypovolaemia: Low levels of fluid in the circulation.

Ion: An atom or group of atoms that carry an electrical charge.

Lipids: A group of organic compounds, including the fats, oils, waxes, sterols and triglycerides.

Medulla: The most internal part of an organ.

Mineralocorticoids: A group of hormones released by the adrenal glands that exert their effect on the electrolytes and water balance in the body.

Neural stimulation: Stimulation of a gland that produces a change in the activity of that gland in response to direct nervous activity.

Osmotic: The movement of water through a semipermeable barrier from an area of low concentration of a chemical to an area of high concentration of a chemical.

Osteoclasts: A type of cell that breaks down bone tissue and thus releases the calcium used to create bones.

Substrate: A molecule on which an enzyme acts.

Triglycerides: A form of fatty acid having three fatty acid components.

Upregulation: The increase of hormone receptors of a cell, usually in response to low circulating levels of a hormone.

457

References

American Diabetes Association (2019) Standards of medical care in diabetes – 2019. *Diabetes Care* **42**(Supplement 1): S11–S61.

Chaker, L., Bianco, A., Jonklaas, J., and Peeters, R. (2017) Seminar: Hypothyroidism. *The Lancet* **390**(10101): 1550–1562.

Crowley, R.K., Argese, N., Tomlinson, J.W. and Stewart, P.M. (2014) Central hypoadrenalism. *Journal of Clinical Endocrinology & Metabolism* **99**(11): 4027–4036.

Economidou, F., Douka, E., Tzanela, M., Nanas, S. and Kotanidou, A. (2011) Thyroid function during critical illness. *Hormones* **10**(2): 117–124.

Frid, A., Hirsch, L., Gaspar, R., Hicks, D., Kreugel, G., Liersch, J. and Strauss, K. (2010) New injection recommendations for patients with diabetes. *Diabetes & Metabolism* **36**: S3–S18.

Friedman, B. and Cirulli, J. (2013) Hyponatremia in critical care patients: frequency, outcome, characteristics and treatment with the vasopressin V2 receptor antagonist tolvaptan. *Journal of Critical Care* **28**(2): 219.e1–219.e12.

Gross, P. (2012) Clinical management of SIADH. *Therapeutic Advances in Endocrinology and Metabolism* **3**(2): 61–73. doi: 10.1177/2042018812437561.

Hall, J.E. and Guyton, A.C. (2016) *Guyton and Hall, Textbook of Medical Physiology* 13th edn. Philadelphia, PA: Elsevier Saunders.

Hardy, O., Worley, G., Lee, M. M., Chaing, S., Mackey, J., Crissman, B., & Kishnani, P. S. (2004) Hypothyroidism in Down syndrome: screening guidelines and testing methodology. *American Journal of Medical Genetics. Part A* **124A**(4): 436–437.

Hussain, T., Akle, M., Nagelkerke, N. and Deeb, A. (2017) Comparative study on treatment satisfaction and health perception in children and adolescents with type 1 diabetes mellitus on multiple daily injection of insulin, insulin pump and sensor-augmented pump therapy. *SAGE Open Medicine.* https://doi.org/10.1177/2050312117694938

Jenkins, G. and Tortora, G.J. (2013) *Anatomy and Physiology: From Science to Life* 3rd edn. Singapore: John Wiley & Sons.

Kennedy, A., Narendran, P., Andrews, R.C. for the EXTOD Group, *et al.* (2018) Attitudes and barriers to exercise in adults with a recent diagnosis of type 1 diabetes: a qualitative study of participants in the Exercise for Type 1 Diabetes (EXTOD) study *BMJ Open* **8**: e017813. doi: 10.1136/bmjopen-2017-017813

Kourtoglou, G.I. (2011) Insulin therapy and exercise. *Diabetes Research and Clinical Practice* **93**: S73–S77.

Liubinas, S.V., Porto, L.D. and Kaye, A.H. (2011) Management of recurrent Cushing's disease. *Journal of Clinical Neuroscience* **18**(1): 7–12.

McDermott, M.T. (2013) *Endocrine Secrets* 6th edn. Philadelphia, PA. Elsevier Health Sciences.

Marieb, E.N. and Hoehn, K. (2015) *Human Anatomy and Physiology* 10th edn. San Francisco, CA: Pearson Benjamin Cummings.

Mero, A., Campisi, M., Favero, M., Barbera, C., Secchieri, C., Dayer, J.M. and Pasut, G. (2014) A hyaluronic acid-salmon calcitonin conjugate for the local treatment of osteoarthritis: chondro-protective effect in a rabbit model of early OA. *Journal of Controlled Release* **187**: 30–38.

Peate, I. *(2017) Fundamentals of Applied Pathophysiology: An Essential Guide for Nursing Students*. 3rd edn. Oxford: John Wiley & Sons, Ltd.

Nelson, J.M. and Robinson, M.V. (2012) Hyponatremia in older adults presenting to the emergency department. *International Emergency Nursing* **20**(4): 251–254.

National Institute for Health and Care Excellence (2016) Clinical Knowledge Summary: Insulin therapy in type 1 diabetes. https://cks.nice.org.uk/insulin-therapy-in-type-1-diabetes#!scenario (accessed 7 June 2019).

National Institute for Health and Care Excellence (2017) Type 2 Diabetes in Adults: Management. NICE Guideline NG28. https://www.nice.org.uk/guidance/ng28/chapter/1-Recommendations#blood-glucose-management-2 (accessed 7 June 2019).

Prasher, V. (1999) Down syndrome and thyroid disorders: a review. *Down Syndrome Research and Practice* **6**(1): 25–42

Sonino, N., Guidi, J. and Fava, G. (2015) Psychological aspects of endocrine disease. *Journal of the Royal College of Physicians of Edinburgh* **45**: 55–59.

Tang, A., O'Sullivan, A. J., Diamond, T., Gerard, A. and Campbell, P. (2013). Psychiatric symptoms as a clinical presentation of Cushing's syndrome. *Annals of General Psychiatry* **12**(1):23. doi:10.1186/1744-859X-12-23

Tortora, G.J. and Derrickson, B.H. (2009) *Principles of Anatomy and Physiology* 12th edn. Hoboken, NJ: John Wiley & Sons, Inc.

Weetman, A. (2013) Current choice of treatment for hypo-and hyperthyroidism. *Prescriber* **24**(13–16): 23–33.

Further Reading

Addison's Disease Self Help Group

http://www.addisons.org.uk/

The Addison's Disease Self Help Group is a charity that aims to provide information about Addison's disease to patients, families and professionals. There are many publications on the site, including a guide specifically aimed at nurses.

British Thyroid Foundation

http://www.btf-thyroid.org/

The British Thyroid Foundation is a charity dedicated to helping people with thyroid disorders and their families. The website includes video stories of patient journeys and quick reference guides about thyroid diseases.

Diabetes UK

http://www.diabetes.org.uk/

Diabetes UK is the country's leading charity for people with diabetes. As well as providing information for patients and their families it is also a pressure group, campaigning both for better diabetes care and funding diabetes research.

Activities

Multiple Choice Questions

1. The receptors for amino acid-based hormones are found:
   (a) on the cell wall
   (b) inside the cell
   (c) inside the cell nucleus
   (d) none of the above

2. What stimulates the release of glucagon from the pancreas?
   (a) high levels of blood glucose
   (b) high levels of amino acids in the blood
   (c) high levels of calcium in the blood
   (d) high levels of sodium in the blood
3. Where in the body are the adrenal glands?
   (a) in the chest
   (b) behind the thyroid gland
   (c) next to the stomach
   (d) on top of the kidneys
4. The concentration of a hormone at the target cell is determined by:
   (a) the rate of hormone production
   (b) the rate of delivery of the hormone
   (c) the half-life of the hormone
   (d) all of the above
5. Adrenaline and noradrenaline are released in response to stimulation from:
   (a) the parasympathetic nervous system
   (b) the sympathetic nervous system
   (c) the enteric nervous system
   (d) somatic nervous system
6. The connection between the hypothalamus and the anterior pituitary gland is:
   (a) lymphatic
   (b) neural
   (c) vascular
   (d) humoral
7. The average person has how many parathyroid glands?
   (a) 2
   (b) 4
   (c) 6
   (d) 8
8. Thyroid hormone requires what to be produced?
   (a) amino acids
   (b) iodine
   (c) lipids
   (d) proteins
9. Which cells in the pancreas produce insulin?
   (a) alpha
   (b) beta
   (c) delta
   (d) gamma
10. ACTH is secreted by:
   (a) the posterior pituitary gland
   (b) the anterior pituitary gland
   (c) the hypothalamus
   (d) the adrenal gland
11. Gluconeogenesis is:
   (a) the creation of glucose from substrates such as amino acids
   (b) the breakdown of glycogen to create glucose
   (c) The creation of glycogen from glucose
   (d) The breakdown of glucose to create amino acids
12. Insulin can be stored at room temperature for:
   (a) 7 days
   (b) 14 days
   (c) 28 days
   (d) 56 days

13. Calcitonin
    (a) reduces calcium levels in the blood
    (b) increases calcium levels in the blood
    (c) encourages the reabsorption of calcium from the urine
    (d) encourages the excretion of calcium in the faeces
14. Which hormones increase the storage of glycogen into the liver?
    (a) insulin
    (b) glucocorticoids
    (c) neither insulin not glucocorticoids
    (d) both insulin and glucocorticoids
15. What does paracrine mean?
    (a) hormones that act on the cells that produce it
    (b) hormones that act locally and diffuse to the cells in the immediate neighbourhood to produce
        their action
    (c) substances secreted into ducts that eventually lead to the outside of the body
    (d) hormones that are secreted into the blood and have an effect on cells distant from those that
        released the hormone

Conditions

The following is a list of conditions that are associated with the endocrine system. Take some time and write notes about each of the conditions. You may make the notes taken from textbooks or other resources (e.g. people you work with in a clinical area), or you may make the notes as a result of people you have cared for. If you are making notes about people you have cared for, you must ensure that you adhere to the rules of confidentiality.

460

Addison's disease

Cushing's disease

Diabetes insipidus

Diabetes mellitus

Graves' disease

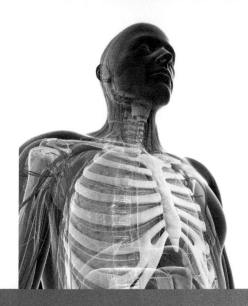

17

The Immune System

Janet G. Migliozzi

Test Your Prior Knowledge

- How do the T-helper and T-suppressor cells work together in helping to control the immune system?
- Which cells are involved in humoral immunity?
- Discuss the role of immunoglobulin E (IgE) in fighting infections?
- Identify the organs of the lymphatic system.
- What is meant by phagocytosis?

Learning Outcomes

After reading this chapter you will be able to:

- Describe and discuss the development of white blood cells and their roles in immunity.
- Explain how the immune system works to protect us from infections, listing the various barriers used to prevent infectious organisms from entering the body.
- Explain the process of phagocytosis and explain how inflammation works to protect the body.
- Describe and discuss cellular and humoral immunity.
- Explain the body's response to infection and the rationale for immunisations.

Visit the student companion website at www.wileyfundamentalseries.com/anatomy where you can test yourself using flashcards, multiple-choice questions and more. Instructor companion site at www.wiley.com/go/instructor/anatomy where instructors will find valuable materials such as PowerPoint slides and image bank designed to enhance your teaching.

Fundamentals of Anatomy and Physiology: For Nursing and Healthcare Students, Third Edition. Edited by Ian Peate and Suzanne Evans.
© 2020 John Wiley & Sons Ltd. Published 2020 by John Wiley & Sons Ltd.
Student companion website: www.wileyfundamentalseries.com/anatomy
Instructor companion website: www.wiley.com/go/instructor/anatomy

Body Map

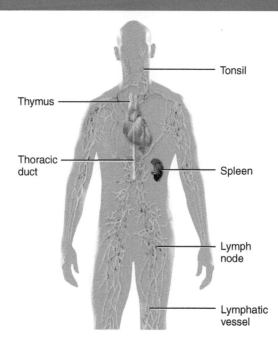

Tonsil

Thymus

Thoracic duct

Spleen

Lymph node

Lymphatic vessel

462

Introduction

Our bodies are continuously under attack from organisms that are out to destroy it. This may sound dramatic, but it is true. Infectious microorganisms, toxins and pollutants are some of the harmful substances from which it has to defend itself. Fortunately, the body has evolved and developed many defences to repel and destroy these harmful substances – this is what we call the immune system.

The immune system is a complicated and wonderful system that underpins so much of our understanding of disease and disease process, and not only those diseases caused by infectious microorganisms, but also many others, including cancer, arthritis, stress and so on.

This chapter will show what the body's immunological defences consist of and how they work together to give the body an opportunity of surviving the continuous and continuing assaults by microorganisms, toxins and other pollutants to which it is subjected.

Blood Cell Development

All our blood cells are descended from multipotent stem cells, which have the ability to switch to different types of cells. In terms of the immune system, the blood cells that form a substantial part of the immune system are the white blood cells, of which there are two major branches. One branch develops into the myeloid family of cells, which include the neutrophils and monocytes, the other branch develops into the lymphoid family of cells, made up of lymphocytes. Figure 17.1 shows the development of the white blood cells from the initial multipotent stem cell.

It can be seen from the family tree of blood cells that the myeloid family includes the macrophages (monocytes and tissue macrophages) and granulocytes (neutrophils, eosinophils and basophils). The lymphoid branch of white blood cells gives us T-lymphocytes and B-lymphocytes (with many of the B-lymphocytes developing into plasma cells). The myeloid branch also provides us with megakaryocytes (leading to platelets) and erythroid cells, which develop into erythrocytes (i.e. red blood cells). Red blood cells and platelets are discussed in Chapter 8.

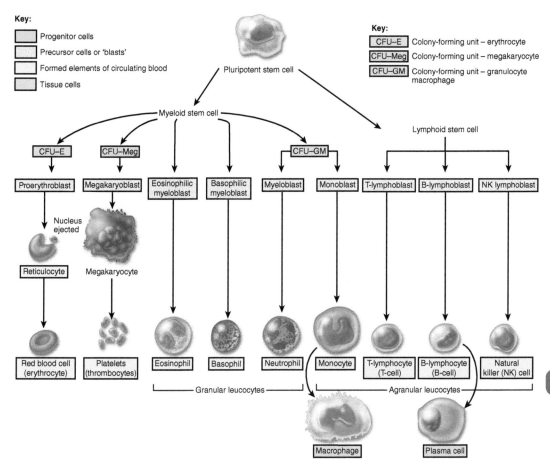

Key:
- Progenitor cells
- Precursor cells or 'blasts'
- Formed elements of circulating blood
- Tissue cells

Key:
- CFU–E   Colony-forming unit – erythrocyte
- CFU–Meg Colony-forming unit – megakaryocyte
- CFU–GM Colony-forming unit – granulocyte macrophage

Figure 17.1 **The development of blood cells.** *Source:* Tortora and Derrickson (2009). Reproduced with permission of John Wiley & Sons.

All the white blood cells commence initially in the bone marrow as stem cells, but, as they slowly mature through their various stages, they are found in different places around the body, including:

- the blood and lymph circulation
- the thymus
- the spleen
- the tonsils and other lymph nodes.

They also are found in all the mucosal membranes, such as the lining of the mouth and the gastrointestinal tract.

Organs of the Immune System

The main organs of the immune system are all part of the lymphatic system consisting of:

- the thymus
- the spleen
- the lymph nodes
- the lymphoid tissues scattered throughout the gastrointestinal, respiratory and urinary tracts.

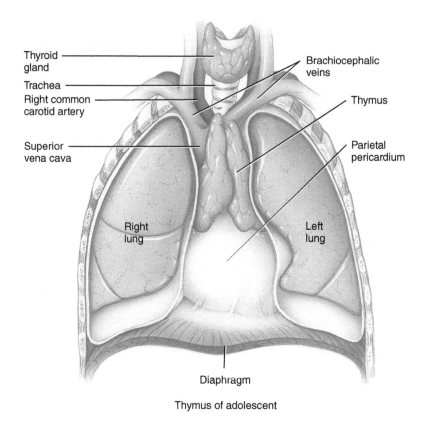

Thyroid gland

Trachea

Right common carotid artery

Superior vena cava

Brachiocephalic veins

Thymus

Parietal pericardium

Right lung

Left lung

Diaphragm

Thymus of adolescent

Figure 17.2 **Position of the thymus within the body.** *Source:* Tortora and Derrickson (2009). Reproduced with permission of John Wiley & Sons.

The Thymus

The thymus is located in the chest (Figure 17.2), in babies it is a large organ (relative to size) playing a major role in the development of competent immunological cells. It shrinks (atrophies) with age.

Within the thymus, certain blood stem cells mature and differentiate into various T-cell lymphocyte subclasses. In addition, they also acquire the ability to recognise and differentiate 'self' cells from 'non-self' cells – an important role in cell mediated responses to an antigen, the continued production of T cells throughout life and the development of an immunological memory.

'Self' cells originate and belong to the individual with that thymus, while 'non-self' cells come from outside of the individual such as from contact with viruses and bacteria.

The Lymphatic System

The lymphatic system is a specialised system of lymph vessels (similar to blood vessels) and lymph nodes. The lymphatic vessels contain lymph, a fluid which drains into the organs of the lymph system from nearby organs. This lymph originates from plasma leaking from the blood capillaries.

Lymphocytes migrate from the blood system by passing through the walls of the smallest venous capillaries in the lymph node. Lymphocytes spend only a few minutes in the bloodstream during each circuit of the body, but, in contrast, spend several hours in the lymphoid system.

The lymphatic system can be thought of as a parallel system to the blood circulatory system, but it does not have a pump like the heart, pumping blood around the body. Instead, the lymph is agitated around the body by a combination of the smooth muscular walls of the lymph vessels and the flexing and relaxing of striated muscle as an individual moves around.

The peripheral lymphatic system (Figure 17.3) is made up of lymphatic vessels and lymphatic capillaries, as well as encapsulated organs (i.e. organs that are situated within their own 'capsule').

These include:

- spleen
- tonsils
- lymph nodes.

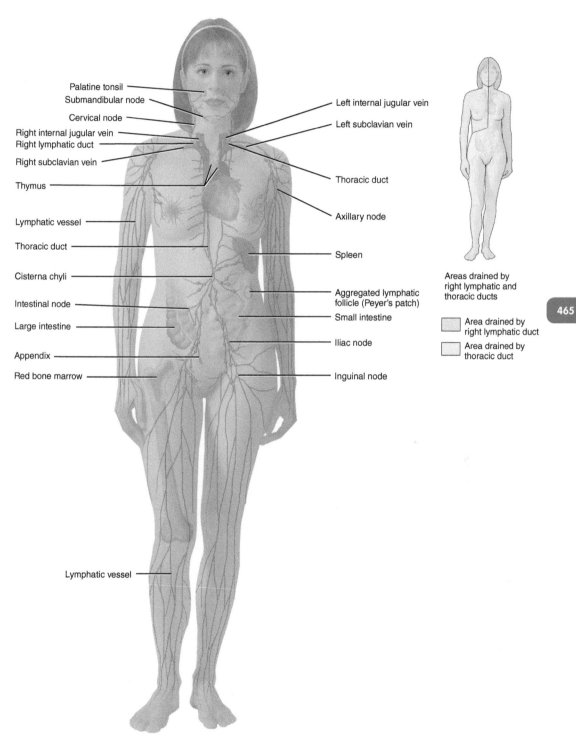

Figure 17.3 Principal components of the lymphatic system. *Source:* Tortora and Derrickson (2009). Reproduced with permission of John Wiley & Sons.

465

The lymphatic system also includes unencapsulated (not bound by a capsule, but more diffuse) lymphoid tissue in the gastrointestinal tract, the urogenital tract and the lungs.

The lymph vessels and capillaries form a network throughout the body and connect the tissues of the body to the lymphoid organs, such as the spleen, and the lymph nodes.

Lymphatic capillaries have some anatomical similarities to blood capillaries in that their walls consist of a layer of endothelial cells. However, lymphatic capillary walls do not have a basement membrane. This lack of a basement membrane allows substances of relatively large molecular size, such as plasma proteins, to enter the lymphatic capillaries between the cells of the capillary walls.

Lymph flows through the vessels by means of:

- muscle contraction in the limbs;
- the pulsing of arteries (caused by the beating of the heart);
- negative intrathoracic pressure (which draws up the lymph, as from a vacuum);
- the rhythmic contraction of the lymphatic vessels themselves.

The lymph eventually flows into two large lymph ducts. One is called the thoracic duct, and this receives lymph from:

- the lower limbs
- the digestive tract
- the left arm
- the left side of the thorax, head and neck.

The other large lymph vessel, the right lymphatic duct, receives lymph from:

- the right arm
- the right side of the head, neck and thorax.

The two lymph ducts then empty into the great veins in the neck, thus restoring fluid and proteins to the venous circulation.

Episodes of Care Child

Sally, a 14-year-old schoolgirl, has been sent home from school due to feeling unwell and complaining of a sore throat and a headache. Despite resting for 2 days at home and taking regular paracetamol, Sally is now feeling worse. Sally's mother takes her to see her GP and on examination it is found that Sally's cervical glands are swollen and she is finding it difficult to move her neck from side to side. She has a high temperature and is feeling tired and listless. A provisional diagnosis of glandular fever or infectious mononucleosis due to contact with the Epstein-Barr virus (EBV) is made.

EBV belongs to the herpes group of viruses and, once acquired, remains dormant in the body for the individual's lifetime. Confirmation of the virus is made by undertaking a blood test to look for antibodies to EBV commonly known as a monospot test – if positive, this indicates a current, recent or past exposure to EBV. EBV is a common illness that is easily contracted through close contact with saliva of an infected individual (hence also known as kissing disease) or using the utensils/crockery of an infected individual. In individuals with no other underlying disease, the illness is self-limiting and most sufferers will recover over a few weeks by resting, drinking plenty of fluids and taking simple painkillers to relieve symptoms. Due to the possibility of the virus causing an enlarged spleen and splenic rupture, sufferers are advised to avoid high contact sports for at least 6 months following the illness.

Multiple Choice Questions

1. EBV is usually transmitted through contact with_____ from infected persons:
   (a) synovial fluid
   (b) saliva
   (c) tears
   (d) urine
2. Infectious mononucleosis is caused by:
   (a) West Nile virus
   (b) Epstein-Barr virus
   (c) respiratory syncytial virus
   (d) cytomegaly virus

3. Lymphadenopathy is the:
   (a) clinical finding of infectious mononucleosis
   (b) haematological finding of infectious mononucleosis
   (c) immunological finding of infectious mononucleosis
   (d) not a finding of infectious mononucleosis
4. Heterophile antibodies is a
   (a) clinical finding of infectious mononucleosis
   (b) haematological finding of infectious mononucleosis
   (c) immunological finding of infectious mononucleosis
   (d) rare finding
5. Epstein-Barr (EB) virus has been implicated in the following malignancies except:
   (a) Hodgkin's disease
   (b) non-Hodgkin's lymphoma
   (c) nasopharyngeal carcinoma
   (d) multiple myeloma

Lymph Nodes

Lymph enters the lymph nodes from the afferent lymphatic vessels and from there it goes to the trabeculae. Afferent means 'leading towards'; therefore, in the case of lymph nodes, afferent vessels are those vessels that lead towards the lymph node.

The lymph node is made up of a mesh of cells – just like a net. The lymph at this stage contains antigens from infected cells and tissues. This lymph passes through this mesh in the lymph node and the antigens are trapped (Figure 17.4).

Antigens entering the body at any point are rapidly swept along the lymph vessels towards a lymphoid organ or lymph node.

Within the lymph node, B-cell lymphocytes are located in the primary lymphoid follicles as well as the secondary lymphoid follicles (which contain the germinal centres), and it is inside these germinal centres that the B-cells proliferate after encountering their specific antigen and its cooperating T-cell. The B-cells at the centre of the secondary lymphoid follicles are actively dividing, those at the periphery are antibody forming.

In addition, large numbers of phagocytic macrophages and plasma cells producing antibodies are found in the medulla of the gland. Macrophages and other antigen-presenting cells spend most of their lives migrating through the tissues until they encounter antigens. These are then phagocytosed (engulfed by phagocytes and 'eaten') and transported to the nearest lymph node.

Macrophages in the lymph node also encounter trapped antigens within the meshwork of reticular cells, and they phagocytose the dead cells and bacteria. The lymph that has destroyed the antigens in the lymph nodes then leaves through the efferent lymphatic vessel. Efferent means 'to lead away from'.

467

Clinical Considerations Secondary Immunodeficiencies

Secondary immunodeficiencies are disorders that, due to another illness, age, injury, environmental poisons or treatment, result in an increased susceptibility to infection. Almost all serious illnesses are associated with some impairment of one or more components of the immune system.

One of the major causes of immunodeficiency globally is protein deficiency due to malnutrition or to such disorders as Kwashiorkor disease. In developed countries, apart from HIV, the major causes of secondary immunodeficiencies are iatrogenic (i.e. caused by medical personnel/ treatment). These particularly include immunodeficiencies that occur following steroid or cytotoxic drug therapy for various diseases.

Someone with a secondary immunodeficiency will have a susceptibility to opportunistic infections, anorexia, diarrhoea and an increased risk of cancer.

Secondary immunodeficiencies are associated with a multitude of factors some of these include:

- infections – for example, HIV, hepatitis, measles, mumps, TB, congenital rubella, cytomegalovirus and infectious mononucleosis (glandular fever);
- medications – for example, steroids, cytotoxic drugs and immunosuppressive drugs, and even antibiotics, as well as alcohol, cocaine and heroin;
- stress – psychological and physical stress;

- malnutrition;
- cancers;
- autoimmune diseases;
- ageing;
- environmental chemicals;
- burns and other traumas;
- pregnancy;
- anaesthesia and surgery;
- radiation.

The treatment of secondary immunodeficiencies consists of removing or treating the cause (if possible) and supportive therapy. For example, if an infection is the cause, then the relevant antimicrobial drugs need to be given. If there is an iatrogenic cause, such as drugs or surgery, once these are stopped and recovery is under way the immune system will usually right itself. Similarly, if other diseases are causing the immunodeficiency, then they have to be tackled. If malnutrition is the cause, then the solving of the problem leading to malnutrition needs to take place.

Along with the elimination of the cause, supportive therapy is required to help to boost the immune system and to prevent infections. Drugs and nutrition, changes of lifestyle, and occasionally isolation may be necessary.

Secondary immunodeficiencies are often transient, and supportive therapy is usually only necessary until the cause has been dealt with and the immune system starts to recover. Unfortunately, however, there are some secondary immunodeficiencies to which this does not apply.

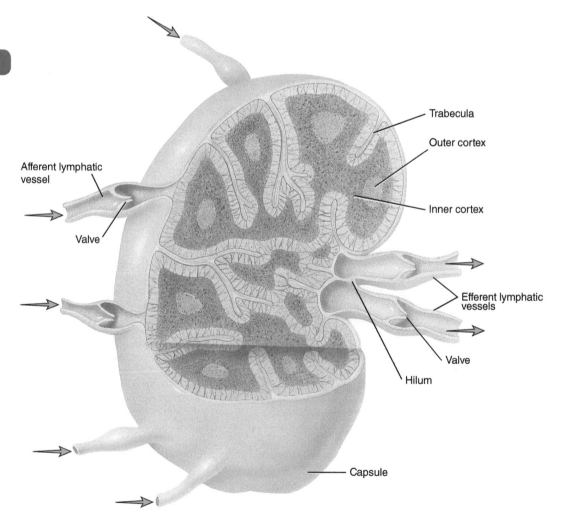

Figure 17.4 **Structure of a lymph node.** *Source:* Nair and Peate (2009). Reproduced with permission of John Wiley & Sons.

Lymphoid Tissue

As well as lymphatic vessels, the lymphatic system contains lymphoid tissue. This consists of lymph glands (i.e. lymph nodes), which are approximately the size and shape of a broad bean, and lymphoid tissue, found in specific organs, particularly:

- the spleen
- the bone marrow
- the lungs
- the liver
- other lymphoid tissue.

The Spleen

The spleen is situated just behind the stomach and is about the size of a fist. It collects antigen from the blood for presentation to phagocytes and lymphocytes, and also collects, and disposes of, dead red blood cells.

In summary, the lymphoid systems play a key role in the immune system by enabling lymphocytes to protect the tissues and vessels of the body from infectious microorganisms. It achieves this by holding micro-organisms in antigen 'traps' in the lymph nodes and other lymphoid organs, and it brings them into close proximity with other immune cells. This allow for the cell-to-cell communication required to recruit, direct and regulate a coordinated immune response. Lymph glands are the major centres for lymphocyte proliferation and antibody production, as well as for filtering the lymph.

Types of Immunity

There are two major types of immunity: the innate and the acquired.

Innate immunity is the immunity we possess at birth, so it is innate in all of us. On the other hand, acquired immunity is not present at birth; instead, it is something acquired as we go through life.

Innate immunity is the oldest type of immunity and is present in all creatures, whereas the second type of immunity, acquired immunity, is only found in more developed organisms, such as humans.

Another name for innate immunity is non-specific immunity. This means that these defences come into action no matter what infectious or non-self organism is trying to attack us; therefore, they are non-specific. Similarly, acquired immunity is also known as specific immunity because it responds to known specific organisms.

The Innate Immune System

Many parts of the body, as well as the white blood cells, combine to make up the innate immune system.

It is possible to categorise the innate immune system into four groups, although some parts may use more than one class of defence:

- physical barriers
- mechanical barriers
- chemical barriers
- blood cells.

Physical Barriers

These include the skin and mucosal membranes. The skin acts as a physical barrier to prevent infectious organisms and other matter from getting to the more 'at risk' and undefended organs within our body. However, not only is skin a physical barrier, it is also a chemical barrier, in that sweat produced from the skin is bactericidal (dangerous for bacteria). However, skin also has weak spots, namely the various orifices that connect the internal body to the outside, such as the mouth, nose, urethral opening and anus.

Mechanical Barriers

In this category are included cilia, coughing, sneezing and tears.

- Cilia are the tiny hairs found in the nose. They are constantly moving and they move dirt, microorganisms and mucus away to the adenoids (made of lymphatic tissue) where they can be dealt with.

- Sneezing and coughing work by expelling any microorganisms or irritants out of the body and into the external atmosphere. So, if someone has a cold or a cough and sneezes or coughs, millions of viruses are expelled into the atmosphere, which means that there are fewer viruses in that person's body to cause even worse problems. This is very effective for the infected person, but means that there are all these viruses in tiny droplets suspended in the air, just waiting for someone else to come along and breathe them in, thereby becoming infected themselves.
- Tears are also a mechanical barrier. Tears wash any dirt particles or microorganisms away from the eyes (like a windscreen washer in a car). Tears are also a chemical barrier because they contain a bactericidal enzyme known as lysozyme. Lysozyme will crop up quite a lot in the section on the innate immune system.

Chemical Barriers

Chemical barriers include tears, breast milk, sweat, saliva, acidic secretions, including stomach acid, and semen.

Most of these secretions contain either bactericidal enzymes, such as lysozyme, or antibodies. In addition, bacteria cannot survive in acidic secretions.

Blood Cells

As well as the previously mentioned defences, the innate system includes certain blood cells, namely leucocytes (white cells) and thrombocytes (platelets).

The white cells involved in the innate immune system are known as:

- neutrophils, make up 60% of the leucocytes in the body;
- monocytes and tissue macrophages, make up a total of 3% of leucocytes;
- eosinophils, make up only 1% of leucocytes;
- basophils, make up also only 1% of leucocytes.

The neutrophils, eosinophils and basophils are also known as granulocytes, because when seen through a powerful microscope they appear to be full of little granules (or grains). In fact these granules are vacuoles, or empty spaces, within the cells, and are very important when looking at one particular function of these white cells, namely phagocytosis.

Blood Cells of the Immune System

These, as mentioned previously, are the white blood cells. There are three main activities of the white blood cells:

- Phagocytosis – this is the destruction of infectious organisms/non-self matter by engulfing and then ingesting them/it. This will be explained a little later in this chapter.
- Cytotoxity – cyto means cell and toxicity means poisonous or, in immunological terms, 'lethal to'. So cytotoxity is the action that some types of white cell take in killing infectious organisms by damaging their cell membranes (see also complement system).
- Inflammation – white cells are very much involved in the response of body tissue to infection and injury.

There are many other roles that white cells play within the immune system, and these will be discussed throughout this chapter – Table 17.1 provides a summary of the blood cells and their role in the immune system.

The three main functions of the immune cells are as follows.

Table 17.1 Summary of blood cells and their roles within the immune system.

CELLS INVOLVED IN THE INNATE IMMUNE SYSTEM	
Natural killer cells	Kill (apoptosis) of virally infected cells
Neutrophils	Phagocytosis
Macrophages	Phagocytosis
Tissue mast cells	Release histamine and other inflammatory mediators

CELLS INVOLVED IN THE ADAPTIVE IMMUNE SYSTEM	
B lymphocytes	Produce plasma cells which secrete immunoglobulins (antibodies)
T lymphocytes	Release cytokines when activated, kill (apoptosis) virally infected cells

Phagocytosis

The cells that make up our innate immunity have two major functions: they are either phagocytes or mediator cells.

The phagocytes are cells that actually devour the infectious organisms that have managed to get through the other innate immune defences previously mentioned.

There are two types of phagocytes: mononuclear phagocytes and polymorphonuclear phagocytes.

Mononuclear phagocytes include monocytes and macrophages. They are called mononuclear because the nuclei of the cells are single round blobs (or spheres) when looked at through a microscope; in other words, they have a clearly defined single nucleus; neutrophils, on the other hand, make up the polymorphonuclear phagocytes.

When looked at through a microscope, the nuclei of neutrophils are seen as a blob which can take many shapes, hence poly (many) morpho (shape) nucleocyte (cell nucleus) – in other words, polymorphonucleocyte.

Episodes of Care Mental Health

Jerome is a 33-year-old who was recently diagnosed with paranoid schizophrenia and has been taking Clozapine for approximately 4 months. Jerome has recently complained of feeling feverish, unwell and having a productive cough – a recent blood test has indicated that Jerome's white blood cells (neutrophils) are low at 0.8×10^9/L. A low white blood cell count, known as neutropaenia, can occur for many reasons including exposure to certain toxins and through the use of certain medications.

Jerome has no other history of causative factors, therefore it is assumed that he has become neutropaenic due to the medication he is taking as psychotropic drugs, of which Clozapine is one, can cause bone marrow suppression consequently affecting the production of blood cells and leaving the person vulnerable to opportunistic infection. Other medications that can cause neutropaenia include:

- cancer treating drugs
- antibiotics – specifically penicillins, chloramphenicol and cephalosporins
- antifungals e.g. amphotericin
- psychotropics e.g. clozapine
- cardiovascular drugs, specifically antiarrhythmic agents.

Jerome was treated with antibiotics for his underlying chest infection and in order to prevent severe deterioration in his psychological state, commenced on Olanzapine as an alternative treatment to Clozapine. Ongoing and careful monitoring of Jerome's mental health and blood count was required to ensure early detection of any complications.

Multiple Choice Questions

1. Which one of the following is NOT true of neutropaenia:
   (a) it is caused by aspirin
   (b) it may be caused by a blood cancer
   (c) it is a cause of mouth ulcers
   (d) it is associated with systemic lupus erythematosus
2. Neutrophils can be found:
   (a) in the bone marrow
   (b) in the blood
   (c) in the tissues
   (d) all of the above
3. Antipsychotic medicines can:
   (a) suppress immunity
   (b) cause seizures
   (c) decrease blood pressure
   (d) all of the above
4. Schizophrenia:
   (a) is a type of psychosis
   (b) tends to run in families
   (c) can be triggered by drug abuse
   (d) all of the above
5. Neutropaenia:
   (a) can decrease susceptibility to infection
   (b) may manifest as a delay in wound healing
   (c) is commonly cause by a viral infection
   (d) is a genetic disorder

The role of a phagocytic cell is to phagocytose, or consume, any infectious organism or non-self matter that overcomes the external barriers. This process is known as phagocytosis, and it works as follows.

- Stage 1. A bacterium approaches a phagocyte – in this case a neutrophil (Figure 17.5). It is held in place by opsonins – complement factors or antibodies (immunoglobulins). Opsonins prepare the bacterium for being digested by the phagocyte by firmly holding the bacterium to the phagocyte so that it cannot escape.
- Stage 2. As the bacterium approaches the neutrophil, the neutrophil recognises that it is 'non-self' matter and it sends out pseudopodia (false arms) and starts to surround the bacterium (Figure 17.6).
- Stage 3. Once surrounded by the phagocyte, the bacterium comes into contact with the vacuoles (as mentioned above). A vacuole completely surrounds the bacterium and kills it, and then breaks it up by means of bactericidal enzymes such as lysozyme. The phagocyte then uses what it can from the bacterium for its own functions (growth, nutrition, etc.) and ejects the parts that it cannot use. This is the process of phagocytosis (Figure 17.7).

As well as bacteria, phagocytes also remove pus and other infected matter, as well as any other non-self matter that has found its way into the body.

Cytotoxicity

Cytotoxicity is the process of damage to or death of cells. Many substances are toxic to cells, including certain chemicals, components of the immune system, viruses and bacteria, and some types of venom (e.g. from certain snakes).

Within the immune system, T-cells that can kill other cells are known as cytotoxic T-cells, and produce proteins that play a role in the destruction of target cells. Cytotoxic T-cells (Tc cells) work by programming

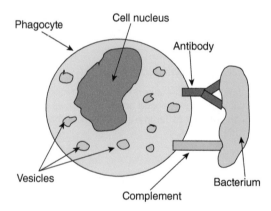

Figure 17.5 **Phagocytosis (stage 1).**

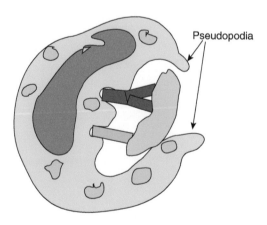

Figure 17.6 **Phagocytosis (stage 2).**

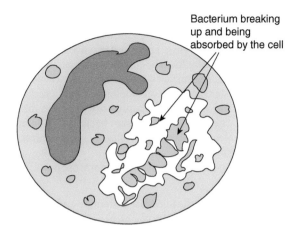

Bacterium breaking up and being absorbed by the cell

Figure 17.7 **Phagocytosis (stage 3).**

their target cells (often cells that have been infected by viruses, or even cancerous/pre-cancerous cells) to undergo apoptosis – otherwise known as cell suicide.

Inflammation

Inflammation is the body's immediate reaction to tissue injury or damage. This can be caused by:

- physical trauma
- intense heat
- irritating chemicals
- infection by viruses, fungi or bacteria (Marieb and Hoehn, 2018).

The inflammatory process involves the movement of white cells, complement and other plasma proteins into a site of infection or injury (Delves *et al.*, 2017).

There are four cardinal signs and symptoms of inflammation at the site of the injury:

swelling (also known as oedema):

- pain
- heat
- redness.

There may also be:

- nausea
- sweating
- raised pulse
- lowered blood pressure
- possibly loss of consciousness.

These last symptoms and signs are the body's response to pain and shock, but in terms of immunology, the first four signs and symptoms are the important ones, and that is why they are known as the 'four cardinal signs of inflammation'.

According to Helbert (2016), inflammation can be defined clinically as the presence of swelling, redness and pain. Although inflammation does cause pain and other problems, it actually has beneficial properties and effects. These are:

- the prevention of the spread to nearby tissues of infectious microorganisms and other damaging agents;
- the disposal of killed pathogens and cell debris;
- preparation for repair of the damage (Marieb and Hoehn, 2018).

Following injury or other damage to the body, three processes occur at the same time:

- Mast cell degranulation. Mast cells are tissue cells that contain granules in their cytoplasm. These granules contain, among other substances, serotonin and histamine, which are released into the tissues during the process of degranulation. These substances cause some of the signs and symptoms of inflammation, but they also work with the other two processes to provide the complete inflammatory signs and symptoms.

- The activation of four plasma protein systems. These systems are the complement system, the clotting system, the kinin system and immunoglobulins. The complement system consists of more than 30 proteins that are found in blood plasma and on cell surfaces. It works very closely with antibodies, and indeed is so called because the proteins in the system are seen to 'complement' antibodies in the destruction of bacteria. The complement system activates and assists the inflammatory and immune processes and plays a major role in the destruction of bacteria. The clotting system traps bacteria that have entered the wound and also interacts with platelets to stop any bleeding. The kinin system helps to control vascular permeability, while immunoglobulins help in the destruction of bacteria.
- The movement of phagocytic cells to the area in order to phagocytose bacteria or any other non-self debris in the wound (Figure 17.8).

Complement factors stimulate the mast cells to release histamine and other chemicals, which in turn can increase the permeability of blood vessels (Tortora *et al.*, 2015).

Other factors involved in vascular permeability are:

- cytokines (cell messengers), which promote inflammation and also attract white blood cells to the affected area (Marieb and Hoehn, 2018);
- kinins and prostaglandins, which are chemical messengers released from damaged and stressed tissue cells, phagocytes and lymphocytes.

All these factors – histamine, complement, cytokines and kinins – as well as having their own specific individual inflammatory roles, cause the small blood vessels in the area that has been damaged to dilate so that more blood is able to flow into the region surrounding the damaged area. This causes the redness and heat associated with inflammation (Marieb and Hoehn, 2018).

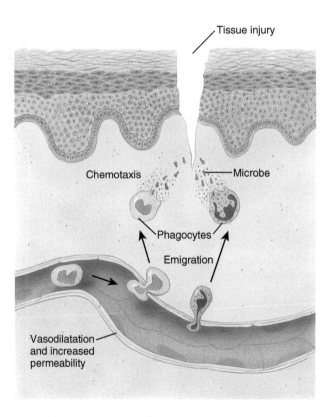

Figure 17.8 **Phagocytes migrate from blood to the site of tissue injury.** *Source:* Tortora and Derrickson (2014). Reproduced with permission of John Wiley & Sons.

Clinical Considerations Rheumatoid Disease

Rheumatoid disease is caused by an autoimmune reaction (this is body's immune system attacking the body's own cells), it is one of the commonest chronic inflammatory conditions. Some inflammatory cytokines have a key role to play in the pathogenesis of this disease. Rheumatoid arthritis is a common cause of disability, with one-third of patients likely to be severely disabled. The joint changes, which almost certainly represent an autoimmune reaction, consist of:

* inflammation
* erosion of cartilage and bone.

Autoimmune Diseases

Specific examples of autoimmune diseases include such diverse conditions as rheumatoid arthritis, type 1 diabetes mellitus, multiple sclerosis and systemic lupus erythromatosus (lupus). Autoimmune diseases affect 3% of the Western population and are found to be more common in people living in the more northerly latitudes. Almost all autoimmune diseases are more common in women; onset usually occurs between puberty and retirement. In addition, there tend to be clusters in families – not necessarily of the same disease, but of a tendency to an autoimmune disease.

Medicines Management Autoimmune Diseases

The drugs most frequently used in rheumatoid disease are disease-modifying anti-rheumatoid drugs (DMARDS) (these include, methotrexate, leflunomide, hydroxychloroquine and sulfasalazine) as well as non-steroidal anti-inflammatory drugs (NSAIDS). These drugs reduce the symptoms of rheumatoid disease, but do not prevent the progression of the disease.

Methotrexate is normally the first medicine given for rheumatoid arthritis, often alongside another DMARD and a short course of corticosteroids to relieve any pain. The drug may also be used in combination with the biological treatments. The common side effects of methotrexate can include:

475

* nausea
* loss of appetite
* a sore mouth
* diarrhoea
* headache
* hair loss.

The medication can also sometimes have an effect on the blood count and liver function. Other drugs that are used with this disease include:

* some immunosuppressants (drugs that suppress the immune system to try to prevent it attacking the body's own cells);
* steroids;
* anticytokine drugs – these are newer drugs and they have more specific action against the disease processes of rheumatoid disease.

Included within the category of DMARDs are a variety of drugs with different chemical structures and mechanisms of action. They can improve symptoms and reduce disease activity in rheumatoid arthritis. This can be measured by a reduction in:

* the number of swollen and tender joints
* the pain score
* the disability score.

However, there are doubts as to whether or not they halt the long-term progress of the disease.

Clinical Skills The Nurse's Role(s) in Assessing the Needs of a Patient with Multiple Sclerosis

Multiple sclerosis (MS) is an autoimmune disorder in which the myelin sheath surrounding and protecting the nerve fibres is damaged by the body's own immune system. This, in turn, leads to the damage of the underlying nerve fibres.

The signs and symptoms of MS are many and varied and depend upon which part of the central nervous system is affected, but potential symptoms can include problems with vision and balance, dizziness, fatigue, bladder and bowel problems, speech and swallowing difficulties, stiffness and/or spasms, and tremors, as well as memory, cognitive and emotional problems. It is also important for the nurse to know that there are different types of MS: new, relapsing, progressive and advanced forms.

Consequently, the role of the nurse is to ensure that they have a good knowledge of the signs, symptoms, cause and effects of MS, as well as knowledge of the patient. This knowledge will allow the nurse to help to provide explanations, initiate education of patients and families regarding MS, its treatment and prognosis, and to take part in (or refer for) counselling for patients and their families.

To be able to take on this role of guiding the patient and family with regards to this condition, nurses first of all must undertake a comprehensive assessment of the individual patient, looking at such areas as physical, cognitive, emotional, sensory effects and coping strategies, along with any problems concerning bowel and bladder functioning (and any sexual issues that may arise). These assessments must continually be updated throughout the course of the patient's life in order to ensure that the best physical, psychological, emotional and social support is always available and relevant for that patient and family. To that end, nurses need to have a knowledge and understanding of how various MS drugs work, and, with the medical team, ensure that the drug regimen is the most suitable for that patient in order to minimise the patient's MS symptoms and to ensure as good a quality of life as is possible. This will help to ensure that there is a better chance of patient compliance with the drug and other therapeutic regimens. Within this category, nurses must be aware of how any individual patient's condition responds to the therapies, as well as any side effects that may arise.

The nurse must also become an advocate for follow-up with the appropriate interdisciplinary health and social/psychological team that may be available.

Above all, the nurse needs to know the individual patients (and families) and to allow them to retain as much autonomy as possible in managing this disease, its effects and therapies; and to always keep in mind that this is a life-long condition for which – at the moment – there is no cure, and the patient and their family will always be aware of this fact.

476

These chemicals also increase the permeability of the capillary walls, which allows blood cells and protein-rich fluid to seep into the surrounding tissues, leading to oedema – the third of the classic signs of inflammation. Oedema performs three functions that are important to the healing of damaged tissue:

- the dilution of harmful substances in the area to make them less concentrated;
- the movement into the area of large quantities of oxygen and the nutrients necessary for the repair of any damage;
- the entry of clotting proteins to help seal off the damage (Marieb and Hoehn, 2018).

That leaves pain as the remaining classic sign of inflammation. Pain is caused partly by the pressure on the nerve endings as a result of the oedema in the tissues and partly by the release of bacterial toxins (Marieb and Hoehn, 2018).

Summary of Inflammation

Irrespective of cause, the timetable of a typical inflammatory response to tissue in injury is:
- Arterioles near the injury site constrict briefly.
- This vasoconstriction is followed by vasodilatation, increasing blood flow to the site of the injury (redness and heat).
- Dilatation of the arterioles at the injury site increases the pressure in the circulation.
- This increases the exudation of both plasma proteins and blood cells into the tissues in the area.
- Exudation causes oedema and swelling.
- The nerve endings in the area are stimulated, partly by pressure (pain).
- The clotting and kinin systems, along with platelets, move into the area and block any tissue damage by commencing the clotting process.
- White blood cells – phagocytes and lymphocytes – move into the area and start to destroy any infectious organisms in the vicinity of the trauma.
- These phagocytes and protein cells, along with the substances they produce, kill any bacteria or other microorganisms in the vicinity and remove the debris that results from the battle between the microorganisms and the immune system – this includes exudates and dead cells (pus).
- All these parts of the immune and blood systems remain in the area until tissue regeneration (repair) takes place – this is known as resolution.

Medicines Management New Therapies: Adalimumab

Adalimumab is a synthetic drug and is fundamentally a fully human anti-tumour necrosis factor alpha monoclonal antibody. In effect, it is a drug that is based upon the normal immune system. It is derived from synthetic antibodies that are programmed to target tumour necrosis factor alpha (TNFa). TNFa is a normal part of the human immune system, which, following an infection, allows for an increasing inflammatory reaction within the body as well as helping to mobilise the various cells of the immune system (e.g. lymphocytes) to fight the invading infectious microorganism.

Adalimumab is used as part of the drug therapy for people with autoimmune diseases such as rheumatoid arthritis. In an autoimmune condition, the body's own immune system attacks the body cells and tissues, because circulating levels of TNFa remain constantly high, whether or not there is an infection, and it is these high levels of TNFa that cause the immune cells to malfunction and so attack the body's own cells. Adalimumab blocks this TNFa production and consequently reduces the physical effects of rheumatoid arthritis, psoriasis and other autoimmune disorders.

The Acquired Immune System

Acquired immunity is the immunity that we acquire as we go through life – the acquired immune system is barely functioning when we are born, but is reliant upon the mother's own acquired immune system giving protection *in utero* – some of which (mainly certain immunoglobulins) remain within the infant for a short time post-natally. Another name for the acquired immune system is the specific immune system, because it is aimed at specific infectious organisms. It is very much based upon the white blood cells known as lymphocytes.

There are two types of acquired immunity: cell-mediated immunity and humoral immunity.

477

Cell-Mediated Immunity (T-cell Lymphocytes)

This type of immunity is known as cell-mediated immunity because the cells themselves destroy any invading antigens.

T-cell lymphocytes originate in the bone marrow, but, at a certain stage in their development, leave the bone marrow as immature lymphocytes. These immature lymphocytes find their way to the thymus, where they fully develop. In addition, they learn to recognise our own cells and so do not destroy these, but do destroy invading cells; for example, bacteria and viruses (see Figure 17.11). The thymus is situated in the chest. In babies it is a large organ (relative to size), but atrophies with age.

T-cell lymphocytes have different functions to perform within the acquired immune system, and the functions that they perform are dependent upon the differentiation they undergo within the thymus (Figure 17.9). Different types of T-cells carry different receptors on their surfaces, and these are known as clusters of definition (CDs) – so-called because the way in which these receptors are organised on the cell surface defines their role and function.

There are four classes of T-cell lymphocytes:

- T-cytotoxic lymphocytes
- T-helper lymphocytes
- T-suppressor lymphocytes
- T-memory lymphocytes.

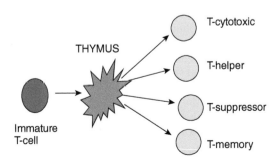

Figure 17.9 **Development and types of T-cell lymphocytes.**

The major functions performed by the T-cell lymphocytes are:

- cytotoxicity (cell destruction)
- control of the immune system
- memory.

Cytotoxicity (Cell Destruction)

This function is performed by the T-cytotoxic lymphocytes that possess the CD8 glycoprotein on their membrane. These cells mediate the direct cellular killing of target cells (Rote and Crippes Trask, 2018). The target cells may be virally infected cells, tumours or 'non-self' grafts, such as kidney transplants.

The T-cytotoxic lymphocytes bind to the target cell and release toxic substances into the target cell, which are capable of destroying it. If the target cell is a virally infected cell, that cell is destroyed, as are the viruses that have infected it. In this way the viruses are unable to go on to invade other cells.

Control of the Immune System

This is a task undertaken by the T-helper and T-suppressor lymphocytes working together.

T-helper cells are coated with CD4 proteins and they stimulate the immune system – both the acquired immune system and many parts of the innate immune system – to proliferate in response to infectious organisms (or other antigens) present in the body. There are two types of T-helper cell: type 1 T-helper cells and type 2 T-helper cells.

The body is usually very efficient at stimulating immune activity in response to an invasion by antigens, but there is a need for balances and checks to prevent the overstimulation of immunological activity, and this function is performed by the T-suppressor cells.

While many studies have identified T-suppressor cells, there appears to be no unique receptor marker for T-suppressor cells, and so immune suppression may actually be a task performed by a combination of T-helper and T-cytotoxic cells by means of a negative feedback mechanism (Male, 2013).

Memory

A special quality that the acquired immune system possesses is the ability to remember antigens – or, more specifically, the antigen receptors that have been previously detected by the immune system, and so produce a group of lymphocytes which can stimulate the parts of the immune system that are able to counter these antigens immediately if that antigen is detected in future infections. T-memory lymphocytes are responsible for a rapid response to further attacks by specific infectious microorganisms (Rote and McCance, 2018). This process is known as the secondary immune response and will be explained towards the end of this chapter (Figures 17.10 and 17.11).

Memory cells are long-lived and there is always a constant number of T-memory cells for a given antigen in circulation (Murphy and Weaver, 2016).

Humoral Immunity (B-cell Lymphocytes)

This second type of acquired immunity (which involves B-cell lymphocytes) is known as humoral immunity because the components effective in the immune system are soluble in fluids (and so is called humoral immunity).

B-cell lymphocytes originate and mature within the bone marrow.

As with the T-cell lymphocytes, the B-cells need to undergo a maturation process in which they have to survive a negative selection process. This is an attempt to ensure that the antigen receptors on their surface membrane do not display self-reactivity (i.e. do not react against our own cells) (Helbert, 2016).

During this process, those B-cell lymphocytes that are autoreactive to the host cells and tissues are destroyed, leaving only non-autoreactive naive lymphocytes behind, which will then be able to go on to the next stage of maturation and selection (Figure 17.10). This is a very important process, because if there should be any self-reactivity of the B-cells, as with T-cell self-reactivity, then autoimmunity may be the result.

The actual mechanism of the B-cell negative selection process within the bone marrow is similar to that process which is undergone by T-cells during their maturation and differentiation within the thymus (Figure 17.11). However, in addition, B-cells undergo a positive selection process in which those lymphocytes that are able to respond to non-self antigens are preserved, while those that are not are left to die. The B-cells

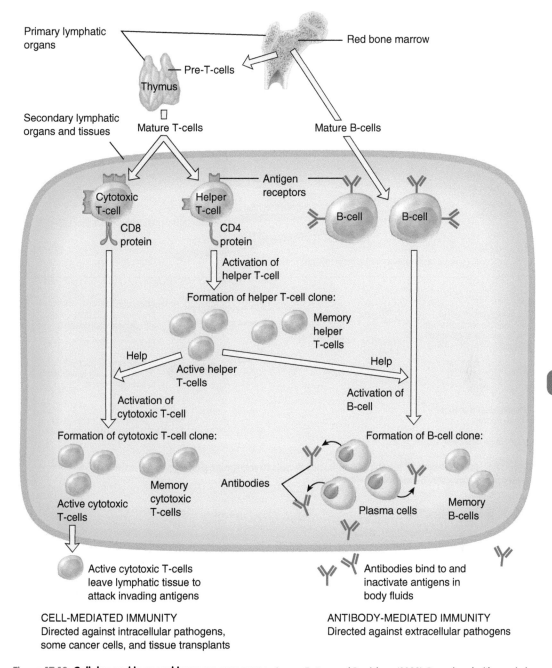

Figure 17.10 **Cellular and humoral immune responses.** *Source: Tortora and Derrickson (2009). Reproduced with permission of John Wiley & Sons.*

that have survived this negative selection find their way to the peripheral lymphoid organs, where they may encounter actual non-self antigens for which they have specificity. It is thought that more than 100,000,000 different antigens may be recognised by the B-cell lymphocytes.

Mature B-cells are of two types: B-memory cells (with a similar role to play as the T-memory cells) and antibody-secreting plasma cells.

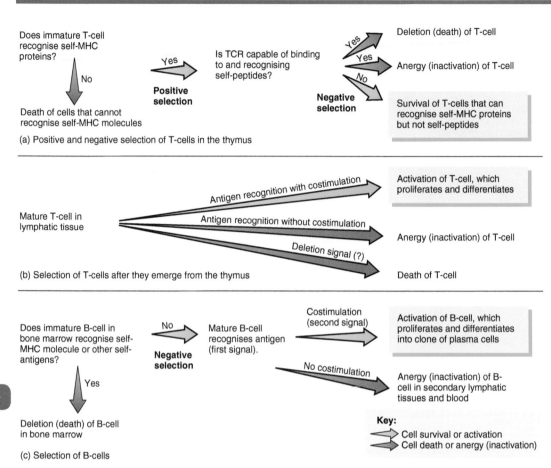

Figure 17.11 (a–c) Process of teaching T-cells and B-cells to recognise pathogens (infectious organisms). *Source:* Tortora and Derrickson (2009). Reproduced with permission of John Wiley & Sons.

Immunoglobulins (Antibodies)

The antibodies secreted by the plasma cells are also known as immunoglobulins, and their role is to act as mediators in the destruction of non-self antigens. These immunoglobulins are not responsible for the actual killing. Instead, they assist other components of the immune system in destroying non-self antigens.

There are five classes of immunoglobulin:

- IgG
- IgA
- IgM
- IgE
- IgD.

Immunoglobulin G

This is the most important class of immunoglobulins involved in the secondary immune response. It makes up about 75% of total serum immunoglobulin (Helbert, 2016), and it divides into four subclasses: IgG1, IgG2, IgG3 and IgG4.

Because it has a low molecular weight (i.e. it is very small), IgG is found within both the intravascular and extravascular areas of the body. This means that it can reach all parts of the body, and therefore its effects are far reaching. In particular, it plays a major role against blood-borne infective organisms as well as those invading the tissues.

The low molecular weight also means that IgG can cross the placental barrier to give a high degree of temporary passive immunity to the newborn child. This is important, because although maternal IgG disappears by the age of 9 months, by then the infant is usually producing its own IgG.

IgG helps the immune system in several ways (Helbert, 2016):

- it is important for activating the complement system;
- it can bind to macrophages, and so enhance phagocytosis;
- it binds to the T-cytotoxic cells and helps them in destroying infected cells;
- it binds to platelets and helps with the inflammatory response.

Immunoglobulin A

There are two types of IgA: 'serum' and 'secretory'. Serum IgA has similar roles to IgG.

Secretory IgA (SIgA) is most important because it is the major immunoglobulin found in external body secretions, such as saliva, breast milk, colostrum, tears, nasal secretions, sweat and the secretions of the respiratory tract and gastrointestinal tract.

As its name suggests, SIgA has a secretory component, which allows for the easy transfer of SIgA across the epithelial cells into various bodily secretions. It also helps to protect the IgA from the proteolytic (destruction of protein) attack mounted by enzymes that are themselves secreted by bacteria.

The main function of SIgA is to prevent antigens crossing the epithelium. In addition, SIgA can activate the complement system.

SIgA plays an important role in the protection of the host's body against respiratory, urinary and bowel infections. Also, because it is present in such large quantities in colostrum and breast milk, it performs a vital role in the prevention of neonatal gut infections – this is one of the reasons why breastfeeding is so heavily promoted (Rogier *et al.*, 2014).

481

Immunoglobulin M

IgM is the predominant antibody involved in the primary immune response (see 'Primary immune response' section), as well as being involved in the early stages of the secondary immune response.

It is very effective in activating the classic pathway of the complement system.

Because of its large size, IgM is restricted almost entirely to the intravascular (within blood vessels) spaces, and it is also often involved with any response by the immune system to complex, blood-borne infectious microorganisms (Helbert, 2016).

Immunoglobulin E

Only very small amounts of IgE are found in the body – in normal circumstances it makes up less than 0.01% of the total serum immunoglobulins, but is also found on the surfaces of mast cells and basophils because it has a very high avidity (binding potential) to tissue mast cells and circulatory basophils, and it is the binding of IgE to receptors on these cells in the presence of antigen that can trigger an allergic reaction.

This allergic reaction consists of:

- the activation of the mast cell
- the degranulation of the cell
- the release of mediators such as histamine.

Degranulation of the mast cell and release of histamine helps to cause an acute inflammatory response, which leads to the classic signs of allergic reactions, such as those seen in hay fever and asthma. IgE is also responsible for sensitising cells on mucosal surfaces, such as the conjunctival, nasal and bronchial mucosa. This gives rise to other symptoms of an allergy, including rhinitis and conjunctivitis (Helbert, 2016).

The main role of IgE in helping to maintain good health is that it can bind onto helminths and other intestinal worms and so lead to their destruction. Allergic reactions and autoimmune diseases are less common in areas where worm and parasitic infestation is rife. In societies where helminth infestation is rare, it is thought that the IgE then turns its attention to the cells of the body, and allergy/autoimmunity is a response to this.

As discussed IgE is a major factor in allergic reactions. However, it is known that allergic reactions (eczema, food allergies and so forth) are not as prevalent in countries where there is a high parasitic infestation, particularly in terms of intestinal nematodes and helminths, and particularly hookworm or ascaris. At the same time, in more developed countries with high levels of hygiene and general cleanliness, allergies are very much on the increase. It is this dichotomy that has persuaded researchers to think about helminth therapy to alleviate allergies (Alvarado et al., 2015; Wu et al., 2017). Indeed, there have been trials where patients with allergies have swallowed hookworm larvae (the maximum tolerated number being 10) and have reported improvements – although not enough to significantly improve allergic symptoms. However, because the treatment made some subjects 'feel better', they opted to remain in the treatment once the trial had ended. Although not proven as such, further trials may well take place in the future, and hookworm therapy may become one of the standard therapies for allergies.

Immunoglobulin D

There is little known about the functions of IgD. However, we do know that it is chiefly found on B-cell surface membranes and that it acts as a receptor molecule, but work is ongoing in trying to decipher and understand this particular immunoglobulin.

Role of Immunoglobulins

The primary function of an antibody is to bind phagocytes and other elements of the immune system to antigens by attaching to epitopes (or receptors) on the surface of the antigen (Figures 17.12 and 17.13); thus, the main functions of antibodies are to protect the host by (Rote and McCance, 2018):

- neutralising bacterial toxins;
- neutralising viruses;
- opsonising bacteria – opsonins are molecules that bind to non-self matter and to receptors on phagocytes, in this way acting as a bridge between the two and holding the non-self matter bound to the phagocytes (Male, 2013);
- activating components of the inflammatory response.

Antibodies rarely act in isolation. Instead, they join with other components of the immune system to destroy the infecting organisms.

A second role of the immunoglobulin is the neutralisation of bacterial toxins. These toxins are produced by the bacteria and make them more pathogenic (harmful), thus causing more harm to the host. When this happens, the immunoglobulins function as antitoxins.

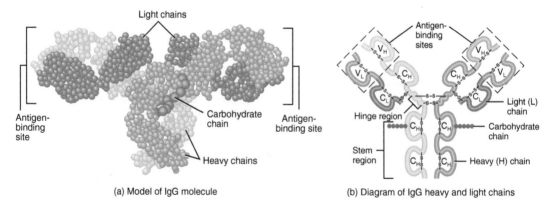

(a) Model of IgG molecule

(b) Diagram of IgG heavy and light chains

Figure 17.12 **(a, b) Model of an antibody (IgG).** *Source:* Tortora and Derrickson (2014). Reproduced with permission of John Wiley & Sons.

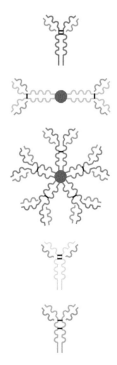

Figure 17.13 **Model of an antigen showing the epitopes (receptors).** Source: Tortora and Derrickson (2014). Reproduced with permission of John Wiley & Sons.

Similarly, the immunoglobulins neutralise viruses by binding to the viral surface receptors, so preventing them from binding to the host's cells, allowing the viruses then to be phagocytosed and so preventing the viruses from infecting cells of the body.

Immunoglobulins also activate components of the inflammatory response.

Medicine Management New Therapies: Immunoglobulin Therapy

Immunoglobulin therapy uses purified immunoglobulins (antibodies) taken from the blood of volunteer donors. It can be administered intramuscularly, intravenously or subcutaneously. It is particularly important for people with antibody or combined immunodeficiencies and has become essential for the management of these conditions. Immunoglobulin therapy has been available for patients with immunodeficiencies for many years, but in recent years the therapy has been found to be important for many other medical conditions, so that, no matter in what ward or clinic – or even at home – that a nurse is working, you will likely encounter this therapy at some time.

What is new about this therapy is that it can also be used for a huge number of medical conditions – and the list is growing continuously. The following are just a few of the conditions for which immunoglobulin therapy may be useful, or which are under review.

Immunological conditions:

Antibody deficiency	HIV
Combined immunodeficiency (T-and B-cells)	
Complement deficiencies	

Haematological/oncological conditions:

Various types of leukaemia	Aplastic anaemia
Haemophagocytic syndrome	
Idiopathic thrombocytopaenia purpura	

Infectious conditions:

Rheumatic fevers	Lyme disease
Recurrent otitis media	Chronic sinusitis

Neurologic conditions:

Alzheimer's disease	Encephalopathy
Epilepsy	Multiple sclerosis
Myeloma	

Rheumatological diseases:

Rheumatoid arthritis	Scleroderma
Kawasaki disease	Systemic lupus erythematosus

Other conditions:

Asthma	Atopic dermatitis
Cystic fibrosis	Diabetes mellitus
Sepsis and septic shock	Transplant rejection
Recurrent pregnancy loss or miscarriage	

Skills in Practice Education of Patients with Hypogammaglobulinaemia to Self-Administer Subcutaneous Immunoglobulin Therapy at Home

For chronic conditions, such as hypogammaglobulinaemia (low or absent B-lymphocytes leading to a lack of antibodies), the ability to self-treat at home leads to a better quality of life for the patient and family – because the patient is taking control of their condition and also there is less disruption to the patient's (and family's) lifestyle, as well as being more cost effective in terms of the health care professional's time. This then allows for more new or complex condition patients to be seen and monitored in a clinical setting. However, for this to be able to happen, some form of home therapy management needs to be put into place, and the first and most important is the ability of the nurse to teach the methods of subcutaneous treatment as well as monitoring of the ongoing treatment at home along with support of the patient and family. This requires the nurse to set up a teaching/training course once the patient has been deemed to be coping well with hospital/clinic-based treatment and after being assured that the patient (and/or a family member) has the desire, cognitive ability and manual dexterity to carry out this procedure at home. This is a new skill for many nurses and will require time and expertise to accomplish.

Protocols will have to be written and then agreed by the hospital/clinic before training can begin for this procedure to be undertaken by the patient/family at home.

First of all there is the home visit to ensure that the home environment and facilities available are suitable for this procedure to be carried out at home.

For training in self-administration of subcutaneous immunoglobulins, there are three steps during the training sessions for each patient – which may also include the family of the patient:

1. Nurse demonstration of the procedure.
2. The procedure carried out by the patient with the help of the nurse.
3. The patient carrying out self-administration on their own – validated by the nurse observing.

The whole training period can last for several weeks until the nurse is assured that the patient can safely cope at home.

Arrangements will need to be made for regular monitoring by the nurse of the situation to ensure that no problems occur, such as regular monitoring of the ongoing ability of the patient/family to carry out this procedure safely, as well as setting up a system of being able to be contacted to deal with questions or emergencies if/as they arise at home.

Natural Killer Cells

There is a further type of lymphocyte, which appears to express only the earliest markers of T-cell differentiation. These are known as null cells or NK (natural killer) cells. The NK cells do not bind antigens, nor are they induced to proliferate by contact with an antigen. Rather, they bind to chemical changes on the surfaces of virally infected cells or malignant cells, rather than antigen receptors (Rote and McCance, 2018).

Although they are lymphocytes, these cells are usually classified within the innate immune system.

Primary and Secondary Response to Infection

Finally, we will examine the immune system's response to infections. The one thing that really marks out the acquired immune system as special is its ability to 'remember' previous encounters with an antigen. Without this ability, each time an individual came into contact with a particular antigen there would be a risk of a serious, possibly fatal, illness. This immune memory is crucial because it allows the body to mount an immediate immune response to an antigen without waiting for the immune system to work out a way of destroying that antigen each time it infects us.

How does the immune system gain this memory of a specific antigen? There are two immune responses: the primary and secondary responses. The primary response occurs when the immune system first comes into contact with a new antigen (such as an infectious organism), and the secondary response occurs with all subsequent encounters with that same antigen.

Primary Immune Response

With the primary immune response, there is always a long time period before a response can be made. This is known as the 'lag' phase because the response lags some way behind the encounter with the antigen (Figure 17.14). During this time there are no detectable antibodies produced by the mature B-cell lymphocytes, but the immune system is working out how to destroy the antigen.

In the case of the primary immune response, the lag phase can take anything from 5 to 10 days before there has been sufficient production of antibodies to make a difference. During this period, the host can become very sick and may even die.

485

The major immunoglobulin class produced at this stage is IgM, and only small amounts of IgG are produced, but hopefully enough to destroy the antigen.

At the same time as the antigen is being destroyed, the memory cells are retaining a memory of this specific antigen and how to defeat it, and this memory will stay with the host for a long time. Each time the host is infected by that same antigen, the memory cells are reinforced.

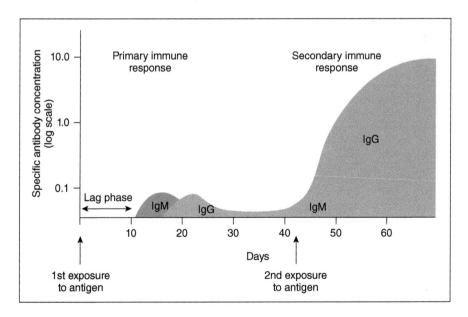

Figure 17.14 **Antibody responses to an infection.**

Clinical Considerations Hand Washing

 Hand washing is the single most important measure in preventing cross-infection. The technique employed involves thoroughly cleaning, rinsing and drying both hands. Hands are the principal route by which cross-infection occurs.

Effective hand washing remains an essential public health initiative. Hand washing is an essential aspect of any caregiver's repertoire of skills, and these skills must be mastered in order to provide all people with a safe environment. Those people with immunological deficiencies are at a particular risk of infection; and, as such, attention to scrupulous hand washing techniques must be carried out at all times.

All health care providers should strive to make hand washing an automatic behaviour that is performed by all in homes, schools and other environments. Families and carers who come into contact with those people with an immunological deficiency must adhere to effective hand washing. The key aim of effective hand washing is to prevent the spread of microorganisms between people or between other living things and people. Inanimate objects and surfaces, such as contaminated cutlery or clinical equipment, may put the health and well-being of an immunologically compromised person at risk.

Using the correct hand washing technique not only saves lives but can also save money. Poor hand washing practices can lead to urinary tract infections, bloodstream infections, respiratory infections and infection of incisional wounds. These infections are caused by the transfer of microorganisms from staff and families to vulnerable people, which could be prevented by using the correct hand washing procedures.

In all health care environments, hand washing is mandatory and must be carried out using established policies and procedures. There are a number of practices associated with hand hygiene – for example, using alcohol hand rubs and the act of physically washing the hands. The consequences of failing to use the correct procedure are many; the impact this can have on the health and well-being of the person you are caring for can be devastating.

Secondary Immune Response

If, at a later date, the same antigen infects the body again, because of the memory T-cell lymphocytes, the body is capable of mounting a secondary immune response that is much quicker. Because the memory cells are carrying their memory of this antigen, production of antibodies can take place very quickly, so that there is a very short lag phase.

In a secondary immune response, the major antibody class produced is IgG, although occasionally IgA or IgE may be produced depending upon the nature of the antigen and its route of entry (Helbert, 2016). IgG is produced in huge quantities very quickly, and therefore the response is very rapid and effective – often, the antigen is destroyed before any signs and symptoms appear.

Episodes of Care Learning Disabilities

Nathan is a 24-year-old with learning disabilities who lives independently with the help of a local support provider. His parents live nearby and visit him on a daily basis. Nathan has recently started working part time in a local garden centre and in his spare time enjoys playing football and attending a local social club. Nathan suffers with asthma which is normally well controlled with medication. However, of late, Nathan has presented to his GP with repeated asthma attacks, his most recent of which required hospitalisation and treatment.

An allergic reaction is an over-reaction by the immune system to an allergen. The most common anaphylactic reactions are to foods, insect stings, medications and latex. Allergy symptoms occur when the immune system reacts to one of these allergens and these symptoms can include skin rashes, itching, nausea, vomiting, breathlessness, swelling and pain. In Nathan's case, it was noted that his asthma symptoms had become worse since he had started working at the garden centre and his doctor considered it highly likely that increased exposure to plants and grasses at the garden centre was the trigger for this. Nathan was advised to ensure that he took an antihistamine before starting work and he was also commenced on an inhaler containing corticosteroid.

Multiple Choice Questions

1. Environmental risk factors for the development of asthma include:
   (a) socioeconomic status
   (b) allergen exposure
   (c) exposure to second-hand tobacco smoke at infancy
   (d) all the above

2. What is a common symptom of asthma?
   (a) wheezing
   (b) whistling
   (c) full breaths
   (d) snoring
3. People who only experience asthma symptoms at certain times of the year are said to have:
   (a) chronic rhinitis
   (b) seasonal asthma
   (c) atopic asthma
   (d) status asthmaticus
4. Symptoms associated with occupational asthma can include:
   (a) rhinitis and conjunctivitis
   (b) epistaxis and conjunctivitis
   (c) rhinitis, conjunctivitis, epistaxis and otorrhoea
   (d) none of the above
5. Which of the following is true:
   (a) everyone who has allergies has asthma. Allergens such as pollen, dust and pet dander cannot trigger asthma symptoms and asthma attacks in certain people
   (b) not everyone who has allergies has asthma, and not everyone with asthma has allergies. Allergens such as pollen, dust and pet dander can trigger asthma symptoms and asthma attacks in certain people
   (c) everyone who has allergies has asthma and everyone with asthma has will wheeze
   (d) allergens such as pollen, dust and pet dander will never trigger asthma symptoms and asthma attacks in those people who are aged over 18 years

Hypersensitivity

Whilst it is evident that the immune system provides protection for the individual, at times this ability may become compromised and an excessive or inappropriate immune response (or hypersensitivity reaction) can occur and this may prove life threatening. Types of hypersensitivity reactions are summarised in Table 17.2.

Table 17.2 **Types of hypersensitivity disorders.**

HYPERSENSITIVITY TYPE	ANTIBODIES/ CELLS INVOLVED	EFFECTOR CELLS	MEDIATORS	ASSOCIATED DISORDERS
I – immediate	IgE	Mast cells Basophils	Histamine	Anaphylaxis Allergic rhinitis Extrinsic asthma
II – cytotoxic	IgG IgM	Polymorphonuclear leukocytes	Complement K cells	Transfusion reactions Myasthenia gravis Graft rejection Haemolytic disease of the newborn
III – immune complex	IgG IgM	Polymorphonuclear leukocytes	Complement	Rheumatoid arthritis Systemic lupus erythematosus
IV – cell mediated	T cells	Mononuclear leukocytes	Lymphokines	Tuberculosis Contact dermatitis Protozoal or fungal infections Sarcoidosis

Anaphylaxis

Anaphylaxis is the most severe form of allergic reaction and requires prompt action. Anaphylaxis is a severe allergic response that can be triggered in sensitive individuals by substances such as penicillin, peanuts or latex rubber. Onset is usually sudden and in severe cases death may ensue in a matter of minutes if untreated. Anaphylaxis is classified as type I anaphylactic hypersensitivity. This occurs in those people with very high levels of IgE. When these people have been exposed to an allergen – for example, peanuts or penicillin – these high levels of antibody will activate mast cells and basophils that will then degranulate. Histamine is released and this constricts some smooth muscle, such as airway smooth muscle, vasodilation occurs and this increases vascular permeability. A type I reaction includes anaphylaxis where there is profound bronchoconstriction and shock due to the widespread vasodilation.

Immunisations

Immunisation, or vaccination, is either the process of transferring antibodies to an individual who is lacking them (passive immunisation) or the process of inducing an immune reaction in an individual (active immunisation). Immunisations induce the primary response by exposing the immune system to a vaccine that includes an infectious organism which is either inactivated (killed) or attenuated (weakened) so that it is no longer infectious but still possesses the receptors that can stimulate the immune system.

Passive immunisation

In passive immunisation, the individual is actually injected with the antibodies. There are two types of passive immunisation, which are natural and very common:

- The mother transfers IgG antibodies across the placenta to the foetus. Whatever organisms the mother is immune to, the newborn baby will also be immune to them.
- During breastfeeding, when the mother passes IgA antibodies to the baby in her colostrum and milk.

Passive immunisation is also short-lived and lasts only as long as it takes for these antibodies to be cleared from the body. This type of immunisation will not normally provoke an immune response in the recipient; therefore, there will be no immunological cover for subsequent exposure to that particular antigen.

Active Immunity

Active immunity is the process of presenting antigen to the immune system to induce an immune response to it. This is the type of immunity that takes advantage of the primary and secondary responses to immunity and is the basis for all the immunisations/vaccinations that we have throughout our lives.

A vaccine has to be able to stimulate both T-and B-cell lymphocytes to provide an immune response. If a vaccine is effective, it provides common immunity to a population.

Conclusion

This completes the chapter on the immune system. As you have learned, it is a very complex system, with each of the many components interacting with others to provide us with the protection that we need to survive in this very dangerous world. But, above all, hopefully you will be amazed and awestruck at its ability to fulfil its major role: that of keeping us safe from infections and other potential harm that could befall us.

What you must remember is that immunology is a dynamic subject. Research in the specialty is continually bringing us new knowledge, not only of the anatomy and physiology of the immune system, but also of disorders affected by it and of new therapies.

There is now so much progress being made in immunology that it is impossible to predict the future. But then, this is what makes immunology so exciting!

Glossary

Acquired immunity: Immunity that is acquired throughout life by coming into contact with many different infectious agents.

Active immunity: Immunity developed inside the body as a result of encountering infectious agents.

Antibodies: Also known as immunoglobulins, antibodies can recognise and attach to infectious agents and so provoke an immune response to these infectious agents. They are also opsonins.

Antigens: Anything that provokes an antibody response.

Atopy: A type of hypersensitivity that is linked to immunoglobulin E.

Bactericidal: The ability to kill bacteria.

Basophils: White blood cells that take part in the process of phagocytosis. Also involved in allergic/atopic reactions.

B-cell lymphocytes: Blood cells from which antibodies (immunoglobulins) develop. Part of the humoral immune system.

Bone marrow: The site in the body where most of the cells of the immune system are produced as immature stem cells.

Cell-mediated immunity: The type of acquired immunity generated by the T-cell **lymphocytes**.

Clotting system: The clotting of blood to reduce blood loss. Also involving thrombocytes (platelets).

Complement factors: A group of proteins that are involved in many of the immune processes (e.g. phagocytosis and inflammation). They are also opsonins.

Cytokines: Chemical messengers that affect the behaviour of other cells, including cells of the immune system.

Cytotoxicity: The process by which infectious microorganisms are killed or damaged (cyto = cell, toxicity = dangerous to).

Eosinophils: White blood cells involved in the destruction of parasitic worms, but also linked to hypersensitivity.

Epitopes: The parts of a cell that can bind to other cells (i.e. cell receptors).

Granulocytes: White blood cells that take part in the process of phagocytosis.

Humoral immunity: Another name for antibody immunity. This is the part of the acquired immune system that relies upon antibodies to help in the destruction of infectious agents.

Hypersensitivity: A heightened immune response that can cause allergies and atopic diseases.

Immunisation: The process of either transferring antibodies to someone (i.e. passive immunisation) or inducing an immune reaction naturally but safely (i.e. active immunity).

Immunity: The body's response to infection, damage or other diseases.

Immunoglobulins: Also known as antibodies, they are highly specialised protein molecules that hold onto foreign antigens to enable their destruction by other cells of the immune system.

Inflammation: The body's immediate reaction to tissue injury or damage.

Innate immunity: The immunity with which we are born.

Kinins: A specialist group of plasma proteins (i.e. proteins that circulate within blood plasma) and have a role to play in the process of inflammation.

Kinin system: The system in which kinins operate in order to activate and help inflammatory cells, such as neutrophils, to function properly as well as being involved in making the blood vessels more permeable to allow cells of the immune system to get to the area of inflammation or damage.

Leucocyte: Another term for a white blood cell (leuco = white, cyte = cell).

Lymph: A colourless liquid derived from blood.

Lymph nodes: Nodules within the lymphatic system that contain mesh traps which are able to trap antigens in order for them to be destroyed by antibodies and other components of the immune system.

Lymph vessels: These are similar to blood vessels, but they carry lymph, antigens (e.g. bacteria), antibodies and other components of the immune system, from the site of infection towards lymph nodes.

Lymphatic system: This shadows the blood system, but is very much involved in immunity. It consists of lymph vessels that contain lymph (which transports antigens and antibodies) and also lymph nodes and other lymphatic tissues (such as the tonsils and the spleen).

Lymphocyte: The major white blood cell of the acquired immune system.

Macrophage: Also known as a tissue macrophage, it is a white blood cell that takes part in the process of phagocytosis within the tissues as opposed to within the blood circulation.

Mast cells: Cells of connective tissue that are involved in the activation of the inflammatory response (inflammation).

Medulla: The central part of an organ.

Monocyte: A type of phagocytic white blood cell (known as a tissue macrophage once it migrates into the tissues).

Neutrophils: White blood cells that take part in the process of phagocytosis.

NK cells: Natural killer cells are a class of lymphocytes that are not specific to certain infectious agents and so are often classed with innate immunity as opposed to acquired immunity.

Null cells: Another name for the NK cells.

Oedema: A scientific term for swelling.

Opsonins: Substances that bind antigens to phagocytic cells, and so enhance the process of phagocytosis (e.g. complement factors and antibodies).

Passive immunity: The process of transferring antibodies to someone who is vulnerable to infections and cannot make their own active immunity.

Phagocyte: White blood cells that are able to ingest and destroy infectious microorganisms and other non-self matter, and include, among others, neutrophils and macrophages.

Phagocytosis: The ingestion and destruction of infectious microorganisms and other non-self matter by specialised cells (phagocytes).

Plasma cells: Cells that develop from B-cell lymphocytes and that produce antibodies.

Platelet: See thrombocyte.

Polymorphonuclear leucocytes: Also known as phagocytes, these are found in the blood.

Primary response: The immune response that occurs when we first come into contact with a new infectious agent.

Prostaglandins: Fatty acids that function as part of the inflammatory process (inflammation).

Pseudopodia: (Literal meaning = 'false arms'). These are finger-like projections that emerge from cells and, within immunity, they are very important in the process of phagocytosis.

Red blood cells: These cells carry oxygen from the lungs to the tissues.

Secondary response: The immune response that, following a successful primary immune response to a specific infectious agent, occurs every time we encounter that same specific infectious agent.

Spleen: Part of the lymphatic system, it functions to fight infections and to filter and clean blood. In addition, it serves as a blood reservoir.

Stem cells: Cells that have the potential to differentiate and mature into the different cells of the immune system.

T-cell lymphocytes: White blood cells that have many functions, including control of the acquired immune system and killing viruses. The major component of the cell-mediated immune system.

Thrombocyte: Another name for a platelet; it is important in the clotting process.

Thymus: The organ of the body where T-cell lymphocytes mature, distinguish between self and non-self cells and differentiate into various types of T-cells that each have different functions within the acquired immune system.

Tonsils: Lymph tissue that is situated within the oral region (the mouth) and helps to protect the respiratory and gastrointestinal tracts from infections.

Trabeculae: Connective tissue strands that help to form part of the framework of organs, so giving them rigidity.

References

Alvarado R., O'Brien B., Tanaka A., Dalton J. P., Donnelly S. (2015). A parasitic helminth-derived peptide that targets the macrophage lysosome is a novel therapeutic option for autoimmune disease. *Immunobiology* **220**: 262–269. 10.1016/j.imbio.2014.11.008 .

Delves, PJ., Martin, S.J., Burton, D.R. and Roitt, I.M. (2017) *Roitt's Essential Immunology*, 13th edn. Oxford; Blackwell Science.

Male, D. (2013) *Immunology: An Illustrated Outline*, 5th edn. London; Garland Science Publishing.

Marieb, E.N. and Hoehn, K. (2018) *Human Anatomy and Physiology*, 11th edn. San Francisco, CA: Pearson Benjamin Cummings.

Murphy, K. and Weaver C. (2016) *Janeway's Immunobiology*, 9th edn. New York: Garland Publishing.

Nair, M. and Peate, I. (2017) *Fundamentals of Applied Pathophysiology: An Essential Guide for Nursing Students*, 3rd edn. Oxford: John Wiley & Sons, Ltd.

Helbert, M. (2016) *Immunology for Medical Students*, 3rd edn. St Louis, MO: Mosby.

Rogier, E.W., Aubrey, L., Frantz, M. E., Bruno, C., Wedlund, L., Cohen, D.A., Stromberg, A.J., Kaetzel. C.S. (2014) Breast milk SLgA promotes intestinal homeostasis. *Proceedings of the National Academy of Sciences* **111** (8): 3074–3079; DOI:10.1073/pnas.1315792111

Rote, N.S. and Crippes Trask, B. (2018) Adaptive immunity. In McCance, K.L. and Huether, S.E. (eds), *Pathophysiology: The Biologic Basis for Disease in Adults and Children*, 8th edn. St Louis: Mosby.

Rote, N.S. and McCance K.L. (2018) Adaptive immunity. In: McCance, K.L. and Huether, S.E. (eds), *Pathophysiology: The Biologic Basis for Disease in Adults and Children*, 8th edn. St Louis: Mosby.

Tortora, G.J., Funke, B.R. and Case, C.L. (2015) *Microbiology: An Introduction*, 12th edn. San Francisco, CA: Pearson.

Wu, Z., Wang, L., Tang, Y. and Suyn, S. (2017) Parasite-derived proteins for the treatment of allergies and autoimmune diseases. *Frontiers in Microbiology* **8**: 2164. doi: 10.3389/fmicb.2017.02164. eCollection 2017.

Further Reading

Allergy UK
www.allergyuk.org
Offers support and advice to adults and children on all allergies and intolerances, including allergic conditions such as eczema, dermatitis, asthma, and so on.

Deficiency Foundation (IDF)
http://www.primaryimmune.org/
American immune deficiency organisation – much excellent information.

European Federation of Immunology Societies (EFIS)
http://www.efis.org/
An umbrella organisation for all European immunology societies.

INGID (International Nursing Group for Immunodeficiencies)
www.ingid.org
Contains excellent learning/teaching materials and information on immunology and immunodeficiencies.

UK Primary Immunodeficiency Network (UKPIN)
http://www.ukpin.org.uk/
Combines doctors, researchers and nurses.

Activities

Multiple Choice Questions
1. The two branches of white blood cells that form a major part of the immune system are:
   (a) lymphoid and myeloid
   (b) lymphoid and megakaryocytes
   (c) megakaryocytes and erythrophils
   (d) myeloid and macrophages
2. Immunoglobulins are produced by:
   (a) antibodies
   (b) plasma cells
   (c) T-cell lymphocytes
   (d) platelets
3. The specific immune system is also known as:
   (a) lymphatic immunity
   (b) mechanical immunity
   (c) innate immunity
   (d) acquired immunity

4. The spleen is the organ in which:
   (a) T-cells mature
   (b) immune cells learn to recognise 'non-self' cells
   (c) lymph nodes develop
   (d) dead red blood cells are disposed of

5. Immunoglobulin E:
   (a) triggers allergic reactions
   (b) activates the complement system
   (c) enhances phagocytosis
   (d) protects the body against respiratory infections

6. Natural killer (NK) cells are:
   (a) antibodies
   (b) erythrocytes
   (c) lymphocytes
   (d) opsonins

7. The primary response to infection:
   (a) builds on a memory of past infections
   (b) mainly concerns IgG antibodies
   (c) is a passive process
   (d) mainly concerns IgM antibodies

8. Immunisation is another name for:
   (a) immunoglobulin production and development
   (b) antibodies
   (c) vaccination
   (d) maturation of lymphocytes

9. Cytotoxicity is the process of:
   (a) cell memory
   (b) cell suppression
   (c) cell destruction
   (d) cell development

10. T-helper cells are:
    (a) coated with CD8 glycoproteins
    (b) coated with CD4 proteins
    (c) cytotoxic cells
    (d) inflammatory cells

11. Which immune cell is responsible for the quickest release of histamine that causes the red itchy welts associated with allergies?
    (a) lymphocyte
    (b) basophil
    (c) eosinophil
    (d) mast cell

12. What is the term used to describe white blood cells migrating toward a microorganism?
    (a) phagocytosis
    (b) chemotaxis
    (c) phototaxis
    (d) zeiosis

13. Which of these produces and secretes antibodies in the body?
    (a) virus
    (b) red blood cell
    (c) bacteria
    (d) plasma cell

14. What is a specific term for a bacterial or other foreign protein that initiates antibody production by the body?
    (a) complement
    (b) antigen
    (c) peptide
    (d) prion

15. Which of these cell types can play a primary role in attacking and killing cancer cells?
    (a) mast cell
    (b) cytotoxic T cell
    (c) red blood cell
    (d) platelet

True or False
1. Phagocytes are red blood cells.
2. The thymus is where immature T-cells mature.
3. Another name for an antibody is an immunoglobulin.
4. White blood cells are descended from omnipotent stem cells.
5. Macrophages include monocytes and granulocytes.
6. One branch of T-cells develop into plasma cells.
7. The spleen is a lymphatic organ.
8. The right lymphatic duct receives lymph from the right arm.
9. The lymphoid system enables lymphocytes to protect tissues from infections.
10. Sneezing is a physical barrier within the immune system.

Find Out More
1. What are the immunisation schedules for your country?
2. Find out the differences, in terms of cause, symptoms and treatment, between rheumatoid arthritis and osteoarthritis.
3. Explore the different methods of immunoglobulin therapy for people with primary immunodeficiency disorders.
4. Look at what medical conditions are treated by immunoglobulin therapy, other than primary immunodeficiencies.
5. What is anaphylaxis and how is it treated?
6. What are the differences between bacteria and viruses, and what are the differences between how these infectious conditions treated?
7. What is the normal treatment for a patient diagnosed with pulmonary tuberculosis (TB)?
8. Find out about and discuss the isolation policy for the hospital/health care centre, etc., that you are working in or have worked in as part of your nurse education.
9. How can nurses prevent infectious disease in hospitals and other health care institutions, as well as the home?
10. Find more out about the link between stress (physical, social, and psychological) and the immune system.

Conditions

The following is a list of conditions that are associated with the immune system. Take some time and write notes about each of the conditions. You may make the notes taken from textbooks or other resources (e.g. people you work with in a clinical area), or you may make the notes as a result of people you have cared for. If you are making notes about people you have cared for, you must ensure that you adhere to the rules of confidentiality.

Septicaemia

Myasthenia gravis

Pernicious anaemia	
Skin allergy	
Hay fever	
Coeliac disease	
Multiple sclerosis	
Tuberculosis	

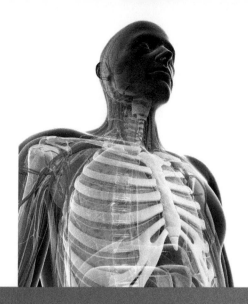

18

The Skin

Ian Peate

Test Your Prior Knowledge

- List the layers of the skin.
- What is the role of the skin in health?
- Describe three key functions of the skin?
- Discuss how the skin provides or helps to provide the body with various defence mechanisms.
- Ultraviolet light is said to be sometimes harmful to the skin, why is this?

Learning Outcomes

After reading this chapter you will be able to:

- Discuss the anatomy and physiology related to the skin.
- Describe the various functions associated with the skin.
- Discuss the structure and growth of the appendages.
- Explain how the skin functions as a homeostatic mechanism.
- Outline the factors that determine the skin colour.

Visit the student companion website at www.wileyfundamentalseries.com/anatomy where you can test yourself using flashcards, multiple-choice questions and more. Instructor companion site at www.wiley.com/go/instructor/anatomy where instructors will find valuable materials such as PowerPoint slides and image bank designed to enhance your teaching.

Fundamentals of Anatomy and Physiology: For Nursing and Healthcare Students, Third Edition. Edited by Ian Peate and Suzanne Evans.
© 2020 John Wiley & Sons Ltd. Published 2020 by John Wiley & Sons Ltd.
Student companion website: www.wileyfundamentalseries.com/anatomy
Instructor companion website: www.wiley.com/go/instructor/anatomy

Body Map

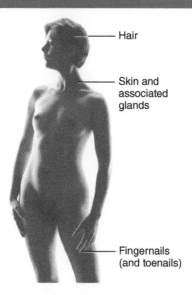

— Hair

— Skin and associated glands

— Fingernails (and toenails)

Introduction

The skin is sometimes known as the integumentary system and it protects the body in a number of ways; without skin and its protective mechanisms the human being would not survive. The skin is often the only organ of the body that is on show all of the time, and because of this the skin can reveal how we feel emotionally; for example, we may blush. It can also reveal how we are from a physiological perspective; for example, it can appear cyanosed. The skin is the organ that is the most commonly exposed to disease or infection; it is almost entirely waterproof.

This system has a number of homeostatic elements; for example, it can regulate body temperature and is often spoken of as the skin with appendages. The appendages are modifications of the skin. Waugh and Grant (2018) suggest that the average adult has 1.5–2 m² of skin and it weighs approximately 4.1 kg. The skin is twice as heavy as the brain. There are about 4.5 m blood vessels, 3.6 m nerves, 2.6 million sweat glands, 1500 sensory receptors and over 3 million cells that are continuously dying and being replaced. The skin receives nearly one-third of all blood that flows through the body (McLaughlin, 2018).

The skin plays an essential role in health and well-being. Any disturbance in skin can lead to physical and or psychological problems, and this in turn has the ability to impact on a person's quality of life. Just as a house needs bricks and mortar to act as a framework, the house would be of little value if it were not waterproof; using this analogy, the house also needs shelter from the environment, and in humans this job is carried out by the skin. The skin provides a defensive barrier, protecting the body from the elements as well as offering a defence against pathogens. It also has a number of other functions. The skin is made up of a superficial epidermis and a deeper structure called the dermis. Prior to discussing the functions of the skin, the next section will outline the structure of the skin.

Episodes of Care Learning Disabilities

Acne vulgaris is a disorder of the pilosebaceous follicles located in the face and upper trunk. At puberty, androgens increase the production of sebum from enlarged sebaceous glands; these become blocked and infected, causing an inflammatory reaction.

Karl is 15 years of age and has acne vulgaris; he also has moderate learning disabilities and struggles with anxiety and depression. The acne has impacted on his self-confidence, and his father reports that he has become withdrawn so much that he dreads going to school as his classmates tease him not only about his learning disability but also about his acne. Acne can cause severe psychological problems, undermining the person's self-assurance and self-esteem at a vulnerable time in their life. Karl's teachers reported that he is displaying a number of challenging behaviours that they have not seen in him before, he is angry and has occasional aggressive outbursts. Karl is often seen rubbing and scratching the skin lesions.

Follicles that are impacted and distended by incompletely desquamated keratinocytes and sebum are known as comedones. These can be open (blackheads) or closed (whiteheads). The inflammation causes papules, pustules and nodules to appear.

Acne is a mild and self-limiting condition; however, teenagers like Karl are very sensitive about it, and because of this it is essential to be empathetic as well as providing advice and reassurance. In Karl's case the condition was ongoing and he required referral to a dermatologist, who discussed treatment options with him and his parents and instigated topical and systemic treatment.

Karl was supported by his parents to apply his medication as prescribed and to take the prescribed antibiotics. Karl and his parents were advised to avoid over cleaning the skin as this can cause dryness and irritation. Twice daily washing with a gentle soap and fragrance-free cleanser is adequate for skin cleaning, acne is not caused by poor skin hygiene. It was explained to Karl that he should avoid picking and squeezing spots as this could increase the risk of scarring. It was also explained that the spots would not disappear overnight and that it could take some time for treatment to work and that when he applies the topical medication this can irritate the skin.

After 8 weeks, Karl's face was clearing up. He was informed that the spots were likely to come back and if so he should go back to see the GP where maintenance treatment may be considered.

Multiple Choice Questions

1. A comedone is:
   (a) an infected pilo sebaceous unit
   (b) a pore or hair follicle filled with skin debris, sebum and bacteria
   (c) a cyst
   (d) all of the above
2. A papule is:
   (a) a type of treatment for acne
   (b) a small tender pus-filled cavity
   (c) a small tender red bump
   (d) a large area of macerated skin
3. A main cause of acne is:
   (a) poor hygiene
   (b) excessive consumption of greasy foods
   (c) lack of exercise
   (d) excess oil production
4. Acne only effects:
   (a) pregnant women
   (b) adolescent boys
   (c) adolescent girls
   (d) none of the above
5. Stress:
   (a) can relieve acne
   (b) may make a person more prone to acne as a child
   (c) can exacerbate acne
   (d) is not a factor that is associated with acne

497

The Structure of Skin

According to Shier *et al.* (2016), the skin is one of the more versatile organs of the body. The skin is composed of two distinct regions: the dermis and the epidermis. The subcutaneous facia (sometimes referred to as the hypodermis) lies under the dermis (Colbert *et al.*, 2012); these masses of loose connective and adipose tissue attach to the skin and organs beneath; they are not part of the skin.

The Epidermis

The superficial and thinnest aspect of the skin, the epidermis, is the area of skin that can most commonly be seen. While the skin covers the whole of the body, there are several regional distinctions, and these are associated with flexibility, distribution and type of hair, density and types of gland, pigmentation, vascularity, innervations and thickness (Jenkins *et al.*, 2013). The thinnest part of the skin can be found on the eyelids; here, it is just 0.5 mm in thickness, whereas at the heel it is 4.0 mm thick.

The epidermis is made up of epithelium, called keratinised stratified squamous epithelium, and contains four key cell types (Figure 18.1):

- keratinocytes
- melanocytes
- Langerhans cells
- Merkel cells.

Keratinocytes

These cells are organised in four layers and are responsible for producing a protein called keratin. Keratin is a tough, fibrous protein that aids in the protection of the skin and tissues below from the heat, microorganisms and chemicals. The keratinocytes are also responsible for the production of the water-resistant properties of the skin, and act as a type of sealant that reduces water entry as well as water loss; they also prevent the entry of foreign matter.

Melanocytes

The developing embryo produces the pigment melanin from the melanocytes. Melanocytes are most profuse in the epidermis of the penis, nipples, the areola, face and limbs. Melanocytes have long, slender projections

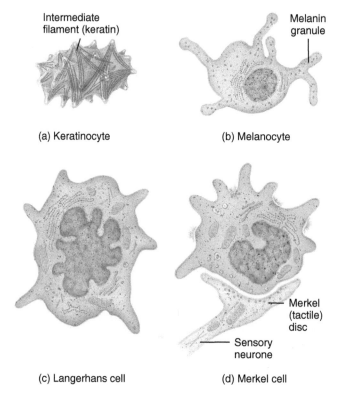

Figure 18.1 **(a–d) The types of cells in the epidermis.** *Source:* Tortora and Derrickson (2009). Reproduced with permission of John Wiley & Sons.

that extend between the keratinocytes and have the ability to transfer melanin granules. Melanin is responsible for the natural colour of a person's skin, and it helps to defend it from the damaging effects of the sun.

When skin has been exposed to a great deal of sun the melanocytes multiply the quantity of melanin in order to absorb more ultraviolet rays. This activity makes the skin darker, giving it a suntanned appearance. A suntan indicates that the skin has been harmed and is attempting to defend itself.

All people have about the same number of melanocytes; those people with brown or black skin have the same number of melanocytes but they make more of the pigment melanin. It is the amount of melanin produced and how it is distributed that results in a variation of skin colour. Brown or black skinned people have more natural protection from the harmful ultraviolet rays of the sun. Moles (sometimes called naevi) are a group or a cluster of melanocytes that lie close together. The majority of people with white skin have approximately 10–50 moles on their skin.

Skills in Practice Skin Biopsy

A skin biopsy is a procedure in which a sample of skin tissue is removed and this is then processed and examined under a microscope; it is usually undertaken to diagnose skin cancer or other skin conditions. There are several methods that may be used to obtain a skin sample; the method selected depends on the size and location of the abnormal area of skin (the skin lesion). When the specimen has been obtained, it is placed in a solution (such as formaldehyde) and sent to the laboratory where it is processed and examined.

An assessment of the patient is carried out prior to a skin biopsy being performed. There is no special preparation required before having the biopsy. The procedure must be explained and a consent form will need to be signed.

The skin is cleaned and a marker may be used to outline the edges of the skin sample. The procedure is undertaken using a sterile approach. A local anaesthetic is injected and the procedure is performed; sutures will not be needed in some cases (e.g. a shave biopsy). The biopsy site is then covered with a sterile dressing. In a punch biopsy there may be a need for sutures, and this will depend on the size of biopsy. In excision biopsy, pressure may be applied to the site until the bleeding stops; sutures are needed to close the wound.

After the procedure, specific instructions are given to the patient on how to care for the biopsy site. The biopsy site should be kept clean and dry until it has healed completely. The clinic or hospital where the biopsy took place should be contacted if the patient experiences excessive bleeding or drainage through the dressing. If there is increased tenderness, pain, redness or swelling at the biopsy site, then the dermatology nurse or doctor should be contacted.

499

Langerhans Cells

These cells are part of the immune system and arise from the red bone marrow (see Chapter 7 for a discussion on the red bone marrow), they migrate from the bone marrow to the epidermis and make up a small part of the epidermal cells. The Langerhans cells regulate immune reactions in the skin as a defence against microorganisms that invade it (Waugh and Grant, 2018); when the Langerhan cells are exposed to the sun they become very fragile and this impacts on their function.

The Langerhans cells are responsible for the processing of microbial antigens (helping to stimulate lymphocytes); their role is to assist other cells of the immune system in response to and recognition of microorganisms and destroy the invading microbes.

Merkel Cells

A Merkel cell has the ability to have contact with a flattened process of a sensory neurone (a synaptic contact); this is a structure called a tactile disc (sometimes this is called a Merkel disc). The Merkel cells and the tactile discs (the least numerous of cells on the epidermis) are capable of detecting touch sensations (Tortora and Derrickson, 2014).

Layers of the Epidermis

Just as there are two distinct layers of skin – the dermis and epidermis – there are also a number of distinct layers of keratinocytes. These layers are developed over time and form the epidermis. These layers are called strata and are microscopically visible (see Figure 18.2).

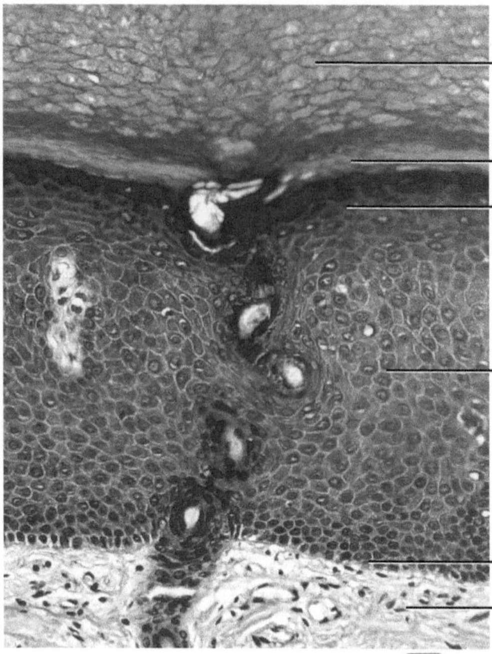

Superficial

Deep

Epidermis:
Stratum corneum

Stratum lucidum
Stratum granulosum

Stratum spinosum

Stratum basale
Dermis

LM 240x

Figure 18.2 **A microscopic perspective of the skin with the various strata.** *Source:* Tortora and Derrickson (2009). Reproduced with permission of John Wiley & Sons.

500

Table 18.1 **The layers of the epidermis.**

LAYER	LOCATION	DESCRIPTION
Stratum basale (sometimes called the basal cell layer)	The deepest layer	Cuboidal cells that are arranged as a single row; these divide and grow. The stratum basale also contains melanocytes
Stratum spinosum	Above the stratum basale and below the stratum granulosum	These keratinocytes are tightly packed, flat and have spine-like projections
Stratum granulosum	Under the stratum corneum	Flattened cells arranged in approximately three to five layers. Protect the body from losing fluid and also protect from harm. Compact brittle cells as they lose their nucleus
Stratum lucidum	When present, situated between the stratum corneum and the stratum granulosum	These cells are not present on the soles and palms. The cells have no nucleus and are tightly packed
Stratum corneum	The most superficial of layers	Several layers of keratinised, dead epithelial cells. These cells are flattened and have no nucleus

The superficial and deeper levels of the skin are:

- the stratum basale
- the stratum spinosum
- the stratum granulosum
- the stratum lucidum
- the stratum corneum.

These are now discussed separately, and Table 18.1 provides an overview of the layers of the epidermis.

Clinical Considerations Assisting with Personal Hygiene

Health care workers are required to demonstrate the knowledge, skills and an ability to meet people's needs related to personal and skin integrity and they must do this competently, with compassion and with due regard to dignity. One of the most important aspects of the role and function of the nurse and health care worker is to help people to attend to their personal hygiene when they are unable to do this. Washing a patient may be regarded a basic task that can be delegated to others; however, this important activity is a skilled activity that requires much thought as well as an assessment of the person being cared for. When assisting people with their hygiene needs, observe, assess and enhance skin and hygiene status and establish if there is any need for further support and intervention.

Understanding the anatomy and physiology of the skin and the complexities associated with this body system can help you offer high-quality care to those people you care for. When helping a person to maintain personal hygiene, take care and ensure that you use soaps and other toiletries that will not damage or potentially damage skin integrity. This will include ensuring that the person is not allergic to any of the products that have been chosen to wash and cleanse the skin. As far as is possible you should always ask the person if they are allergic to any toiletries or other skin products, as there are some people who are allergic to the chemicals found in soaps and cleansing products. This element of care provision requires you to be able to assess an individual's needs holistically.

You should bear in mind that when using some kinds of soap, this can have the same effect on the skin as swimming in the sea; the lather worked up by the soap when it is on the person's skin has a higher concentration of glycerine and as a result of this it can then draw out water from the epidermis. The product that has been chosen to clean the skin may have a harmful effect on the person's skin and this may potentially lead to the development of some skin conditions; for example, dermatitis and eczema.

Stratum Basale

The stratum basale rests on the basement membrane and is the deepest layer of the epidermis; this layer provides a definite border between the dermis and epidermis. This is made up of a single row of columnar keratinocytes. The cells (stem cells or mother cells) of the epidermis originate from this deep layer. New cells are being constantly produced; they are continually dividing (the constant regeneration of the skin), slowly pushing older cells (called daughter cells) up through the other layers of the epidermis until they reach the surface.

Stratum Spinosum

Above the stratum basale lies the stratum spinosum. The keratinocytes in this layer have spinelike projections (spinosum means thorn-like or prickly). The keratinocytes are tightly packed here. This tight packed arrangement provides strength and flexibility to the skin.

Stratum Granulosum

As the layers move towards the superficial level, the next layer is the stratum granulosum. There are between three and five layers of flattened keratinocytes in this aspect of the skin. These cells contain granules (hence the name stratum granulosum) that form a water-resistant lipid (lamellar granules), protecting the body from losing excess fluid and at the same time guarding against the entry of microbes. The flattening of the cells occurs as a result of pressure from below. The cells here undergo apoptosis; they lose their nucleus prior to dying, becoming compact and brittle as they move slowly up towards the surface; this process is known as keratinisation. The skin is now becoming tougher and stronger, getting ready to perform its protective function. This layer lies below the stratum lucidum.

Stratum Lucidum

Lying below the stratum corneum is the stratum lucidum, also known as the clear layer. There are five layers of flat dead cells here; this layer is not found on all aspects of the body, only on areas of thick skin; for example, the heels. The cells have no nucleus and are tightly packed, providing a barrier to fluid loss.

Stratum Corneum

This is the outer layer of the epidermis and is made up of a number (about 25) of scale-like layers that are dead and overlap with each other; the chief component of these dead cells is keratin; most of the fluid within these cells has been lost. The cells of the lower layers are composed of approximately 70% water, whereas this layer is made up of 20% fluid (Rizzo, 2006). These cells are very tough and horny. The surface is covered in lipids, which provide a protective barrier; this layer provides structural strength. Constant friction means that this layer is being continuously rubbed off (sloughed off).

There are other important functions associated with this layer, and these are in relation to a physical barrier to light and heat waves, microorganisms, chemicals and injury. The stratum corneum becomes thicker when it is exposed to strong sunlight, providing a barrier to ultraviolet rays. If the ultraviolet rays do reach the dermis, they will destroy the protein content of the skin, and this can lead to cancer of the skin.

Episodes of Care Mental Health

Most people enjoy the sunshine, but the sun also poses a real danger. Then sun can contribute to heat-related illnesses, for example, dehydration and heat stroke, the sun also emits powerful radiation as ultraviolet (UV) rays. Often referred to as ultraviolet A (UVA) and ultraviolet B (UVB), exposure to these emissions can result in sunburn, skin ageing and skin cancer. Exposure can also harm the eyes (contributing to cataracts) and the immune system (causing immunosuppression).

Photosensitivity is a side effect of a number of medications, including specific antibiotics and psychiatric drugs. By increasing the patient's sensitivity to light, then the damaging effects of the sun will be even more powerful. Most psychiatric medications will increase the body's sensitivity to the heat or sun. Photosensitivity is due to medications combining with proteins in the skin to form substances that react with direct light. Being in the sun for as little as 30 to 60 minutes can cause a variety of allergic skin rashes.

Kylma is 65-year-old patient who has been taking antipsychotic medication for bipolar disorder. Kylma has behavioural health conditions and taking psychotropic medications means that she is at a higher risk for heatstroke and heat-related illnesses. Antipsychotic medications can interfere with Kylma's ability to regulate heat and awareness that her body temperature is rising.

Effective methods to prevent heat exhaustion include drinking plenty of fluids, replacing salt and minerals that may be removed from heavy sweating, wearing loose light-coloured clothing, applying high factor sunscreen and staying cool indoors.

Other antipsychotics that can cause heat or sun sensitivity include:

- chlorpromazine
- clozapine
- prochlorperazine
- trifluoperazine
- haloperidol
- fluphenazine decanoate
- risperidone.

Multiple Choice Questions

1. Immunosuppression:
   (a) is associated with poor mental health
   (b) only affects people with HIV
   (c) is partial or complete suppression of the immune response of an individual
   (d) occurs only in the elderly
2. Photosensitivity is:
   (a) a term used to describe sensitivity to the ultraviolet rays from sunlight and other light sources.
   (b) an immune condition only affecting those people with leukaemia
   (c) a condition only experienced by those taking antipsychotic medication
   (d) an infectious disease
3. Which of the following is a common sign of heat exhaustion?
   (a) hyperactivity
   (b) constipation
   (c) headache
   (d) insomnia
4. Thermoregulation refers to:
   (a) an electrical dysfunction in the brain
   (b) hypothermia
   (c) hyperthermia
   (d) a process allowing the body to maintain its core internal temperature
5. Urticaria is:
   (a) an infection caused by mosquitos
   (b) a condition that causes heat stroke
   (c) a state of psychosis
   (d) a common cutaneous adverse reaction to antidepressant medication

The Dermis

The deepest part of the skin is called the dermis and lies directly below the epidermis; it is predominantly composed of dense connective tissue that contains collagen and elastic fibres. Embedded within the dermis are:

- blood vessels
- nerves
- lymph vessels
- smooth muscles
- sweat glands
- hair follicles
- sebaceous glands.

The elastic system associated with the dermis supports the components above, as well as allowing the skin to flex with movement and to return to its normal shape when at rest. The dermis can be divided into two layers:

- the papillary aspect
- the reticular aspect.

The surface area of the dermis is much increased as a result of the projectile-like papillary layers; the papillary layers connect the dermis to the epidermis. The fingerprints arise from this layer. The deeper aspect of the dermis is attached to the subcutaneous layer. Figure 18.3 shows the epidermis, the dermis and the subcutaneous layer.

The Papillary and Reticular Aspects

These aspects of the dermis, according to Tortora and Derrickson (2014), account for one-fifth of the total dermal layer, the superficial layer. The ridges caused by the papillary aspect are also known as friction ridges. These friction ridges can help the hand or foot grasp by increasing friction.

There is a capillary network within the papillary aspect. The dermal papillae also contain Meissner's corpuscles, and these are tactile receptors or touch receptors. The nerve endings here are sensitive to touch, as well as to sensations associated with warmth, coolness, pain and itching.

Attached to the subcutaneous layer are irregular, dense, connective tissues containing fibroblasts and collagen bundles, and coarse elastic fibre forms the reticular aspect. Other sensory receptors are found in this

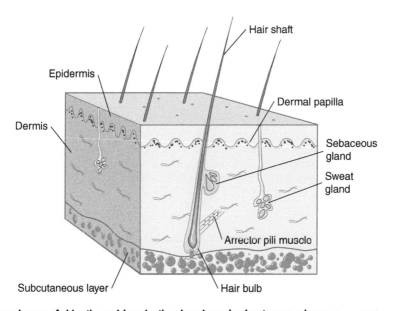

Figure 18.3 **Three layers of skin: the epidermis, the dermis and subcutaneous layer.** *Source:* Nair and Peate (2009). Reproduced with permission of John Wiley & Sons.

layer, for example, the Pacinian receptors for deep sensory pressure. This layer also contains sweat glands, lymph vessels, smooth muscle and hair follicles; these are called the accessory structures and are discussed next.

The Accessory Skin Structures

The accessory structures are also known as the appendages. The following accessory structures of the skin will be outlined in this section of the chapter:

- hair
- skin glands
- nails.

The Hair

Hair can be found on most surfaces of the body apart from the palms, soles and lips; the amount, its distribution, the colour and texture differ depending on location, gender, age and ethnic group. There are different types of hair, and the earliest type is distinctive at approximately the fifth month of foetal development. Known as lanugo, it is a very fine, downy, non-pigmented hair and covers the body of the foetus. Just prior to birth, the lanugo of the eyelashes, eyebrows and scalp is shed and replaced by coarse hair, longer in length and heavily pigmented.

The hair can play a part in a person's distinctive appearance. The colour of the hair is influenced by the melanocytes that are found within the hair bulb. A progressive decline in melanin results in hair that is grey in colour. Hair growth is determined by genetic and hormonal factors.

Hairs are growths of dead keratin; each hair is a thread of keratin and is formed from cells at the base of a single follicle (Timby, 2016). There are a number of functions associated with hair:

- sexual
- social
- thermoregulation
- protection.

The primary role of hair is to inhibit heat loss. The whole of the skin surface has hair follicles; every pore is an opening to a follicle, and these are located deep in the dermis on top of the subcutaneous layer. When heat leaves the body through the skin it becomes trapped in the air between the hairs. Each gland has attached to it a small collection of smooth muscle known as the arrector pili. These muscles contract and become erect in response to cold, fear and emotion. The contraction of the muscle can be seen on the skin in the form of 'goose bumps'.

Hair on the head can protect the scalp from the damaging effects of the sun. The hair on the eyelashes and eyebrows guards the eyes from foreign particles entering, and the hair situated in the nostrils helps to protect against the inhalation of foreign material (e.g. insects).

Sebaceous glands accompany the hair follicles, and sebum (a liquid substance) is exuded by these glands, supplying lubrication to the skin and at the same time ensuring that the skin and hair are waterproof as well as removing waste (e.g. old dead cells). Sebum is a slightly acidic substance and has antibacterial and antifungal properties (Boore et al., 2016). The distribution of the sebaceous glands differs. They are foremost on the scalp, face, upper torso and anogenital region, and these glands are at their most active during puberty, the manufacture of sebum is influenced by sex hormone levels. Figure 18.4 shows a pilosebaceous unit; this is made up of the follicle, the hair shaft, the sebaceous gland and the arrector pili.

The base of the onion-shaped bulb – the follicle – contains blood vessels, providing nourishment for the developing hair.

Skin Glands

There are a number of glands located within the skin; these can be thought of as mini-organs of the skin, which have a number of functions to fulfil. The sweat glands are coiled tubes composed of epithelial tissue and open out to pores that are located on the skin surface (see Figure 18.5). All of the glands have separate nerve and blood supplies; each secretes a slightly acidic fluid made up of water and salts.

There are two kinds of sweat gland: eccrine and apocrine.

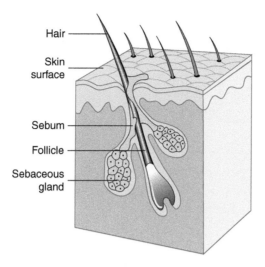

Figure 18.4 **A pilosebaceous unit.** *Source:* Nair and Peate (2009). Reproduced with permission of John Wiley & Sons.

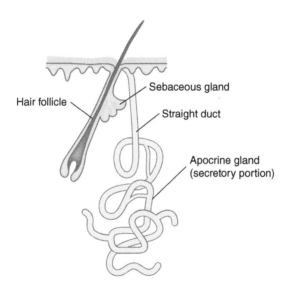

Figure 18.5 **A sweat gland.** *Source:* Nair and Peate (2009). Reproduced with permission of John Wiley & Sons.

Eccrine Glands

Reaction to heat and fear and the production of secretions by the eccrine glands occur in response to activity of the sympathetic nervous system. These types of gland are located all over the body; there are, however, sites on the body where they are more numerous; for example, the forehead, axillae, soles and palms.

The primary function of the eccrine glands is associated with thermoregulation. This is accomplished through the cooling effect of the evaporation of sweat on the surface of the skin. During hot weather, stress, exercise and pyrexia these glands produce more sweat.

Apocrine Glands

The apocrine glands are also coiled; there are not as many of these in comparison with the eccrine glands, and they are found in more localised sites, for example, the pubic and axillary areas, the nipples and perineum. The exact function of the apocrine glands is not fully understood. These glands are not fully active until the person reaches puberty; they are larger, deeper and produce thicker secretions than the eccrine glands. During periods of stress and when in a heightened emotional state these glands produce more sweat.

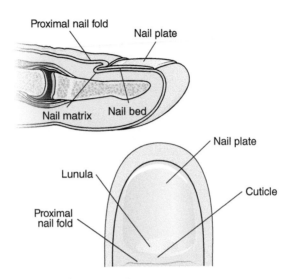

Figure 18.6 **The nail.** *Source:* Nair and Peate (2009). Reproduced with permission of John Wiley & Sons.

There are a number of modified types of apocrine glands (specialised types); for example, those that are seen on the eyelids, the cerumen-producing (ear wax) glands of the external auditory canal, and the milk-producing glands of the breasts.

The apocrine glands first develop on the soles and palms and then gradually appear all over the body. It is understood that they secrete pheromones; these are released into the external environment, enabling communication through the sense of smell with other members of the species, and this can provoke a number of reactions, including a sexual arousal reaction. A viscous material is excreted that results in body odour when activated by surface bacteria.

Nails

The nails provide a protective covering for the ends of the fingers and the toes. Nails are tightly packed, dead, hard, keratinised epidermal cells that form a clean, solid covering over the digits (see Figure 18.6).

The horn-like structure of the nails is a result of the concentrated amount of keratin present; there are no nerve endings in nails. Nails act as a counterforce to the fingertips, the fingertips have numerous nerve endings, permitting a person to receive information about objects that are touched.

The majority of the nail body is pink, a result of the blood capillaries lying underneath. The white crescent present at the proximal ends of the nail is known as the lunula and is formed by air mixed with keratin matrix. The size of the lunula varies with individuals. The cuticle (also called the eponychium) is stratum corneum extending over the proximal end of the nail body.

Fingernails grow faster than toenails; as a person ages, the growth of nails slows. Nail growth varies, on average they grow at a rate of 0.01 cm per day (1 cm per 100 days). Four to six months is required for fingernails to regrow completely; it takes toenails between 12 and 18 months for total regrowth. There are a number of factors that will influence the growth; for example, the age of the individual, the time of year, the amount of exercise undertaken, as well as hereditary factors. The growth of nails can be delayed by trauma and inflammation; changes in the integrity of the nails can be caused by injury or infection. In some cases, evidence of systemic diseases can be identified by the condition of the nails, for example, chronic cardiopulmonary disease or fungal infection (Timby, 2016; Fickertt-Wilson and Foret-Giddens, 2017).

> ### Episodes of Care Child
>
> Tinea pedis is also known as athlete's foot. This condition is a common fungal condition and is caused by a dermatophyte (a type of fungus). Dermatophytosis infections are caused by a group of fungi that invade and grow in dead keratin. These infections can also appear on the body (tinea corporis), the groin (tinea cruris), the hands (tinea manuum), the scalp (tinea capitis), the nails (tinea unguium) and the face (tinea faciei).

Most infections are passed on from person to person (anthropophilic), the infection can be passed on by animals (zoophilic).

Maya is a 12-year-old who has been selected to represent her school in the national basketball championships; the competitions take her all over the country and into Europe. Ever since Maya returned from a match in the north of the country six weeks ago she has experienced a problem with her feet itching. Whilst visiting the school nurse for her booster vaccinations, the school nurse asks Maya how the basketball is going, Maya tells the nurse how much she is enjoying it but, she says her itchy feet are driving her bonkers. The nurse asks Maya to explain.

Maya says that in her left foot, in between her toes it is itching like crazy and the bottom of her right foot is red and itchy and some of the skin is even peeling off. The nurse examines Maya's feet; interdigital involvement is present, the skin is macerated and is malodourous, she is able to make a diagnosis based on clinical examination and patient history. The nurse makes a diagnosis of tinea pedis and a note is given to Maya to let her patents know that she needs to make an appointment to see the practice nurse.

The practice nurse confirms the diagnosis and explains to Maya and her father what it is; Maya says she thought only boys could get athlete's foot, Maya is prescribed with a topical treatment that has to be applied to both feet including the soles of the feet as well as the interdigital spaces. Clotrimazole 1% cream was prescribed to be applied 2–3 times a day and continue for at least 4 weeks.

As recurrence of this condition is common, Maya and her father were advised to ensure that Maya keeps her feet well aerated by wearing breathable footwear and leaving shoes off around the home, she should ensure her feet (particularly in between the toes) are dried thoroughly when wet (dabbing as opposed to rubbing). A separate towel should be used for the feet and this should be regularly washed. Prophylactic treatment with topical antifungals can be used once to twice a week. Socks should be washed frequently, and shoes and trainers should be aired.

Maya should avoid scratching the affected skin as this can spread the infection to other parts of the body (cross infection). She should not walk around barefoot in places like changing rooms and showers, she should wear flip-flops. Never share towels, socks or shoes with others and do not wear the same pair of shoes for more than 2 days in a row.

Maya's father reminds Maya about applying the medication. After 2 weeks Maya tells her father that the itching has gone and her feet are less red, he tells Maya she must continue with the treatment for another 2 weeks as the practice nurse told them. After 4 weeks, the prescribed treatment is discontinued and Maya now uses antifungal talcum power.

507

Multiple Choice Questions

1. The term topical means:
   (a) a condition only found in the southern hemisphere
   (b) a medication taken via the mouth
   (c) applied directly to a part of the body
   (d) a type of hormone
2. A dermatophyte is:
   (a) a type of virus
   (b) a type of fungus
   (c) a type of bacteria
   (d) none of the above
3. What is ringworm:
   (a) a common fungal skin infection
   (b) a respiratory condition
   (c) a gastrointestinal infection
   (d) a condition that occurs after an animal bite
4. Pruritis only occurs in:
   (a) infection
   (b) ringworm
   (c) diabetes mellitus
   (d) none of the above
5. Which of the following is not an antifungal medication?
   (a) Cotrimoxizole
   (b) Nystatin
   (c) Caneston
   (d) Ketoconazole

> ### Skills in Practice Capillary Nail Bed Refill (Also Called the Nail Blanch Test)
>
> This is a non-invasive test that can be used to assess cardiovascular status and is performed on the nail bed as an indicator of tissue perfusion. The ambient environment should be warm.
>
> An explanation of the test is given to the patient; it should be explained that there will be minor pressure to the bed of the nail and this should not cause discomfort. If the person is using nail polish this must be removed prior to taking the test. It will not be possible to perform this activity if the person is wearing false or acrylic nails.
>
> Gently apply pressure to the nail bed until it turns white, indicating that the blood has been forced from the tissue (blanching). Once the tissue has blanched, pressure is removed. While the patient holds their hand above their heart, the nurse measures the time it takes for blood to return to the tissue. Return of blood is indicated by the nail turning back to a pink colour. If there is a good blood flow to the nail bed, a pink colour should return in less than 2 seconds after pressure is removed.
>
> Any abnormalities must be reported to the person in charge. The outcome of the test should be documented in the person's notes; at all times adhere to local policy and procedure.

The Functions of the Skin

A fundamental understanding of the structure of the skin allows the reader to begin to understand the numerous functions of the skin. These functions include:

- sensation
- thermoregulation
- protection
- excretion and absorption
- synthesis of vitamin D.

508

Sensation

There are several receptor sites on the skin that have the ability to sense change in the external environment with respect to temperature and pressure; these receptors throughout the skin are made up of a wide and varied range of nerve endings. The messages picked up in the skin are then usually transferred to the brain. Chapter 15 considers the senses in more detail.

Sensations that arise in the skin are known as cutaneous sensations; other sensations are those associated with vibration, tickling and irritations. There are some areas of the body that have more sensory receptors than others; for example, the lips, genitalia and tips of the fingers. The sensation of pain can signify actual or potential tissue injury.

> ### Medicines Management Use of Topical Steroids
>
>
> Topical steroids are used in addition to emollients (moisturisers) for treating skin conditions such as eczema. Topical steroids reduce skin inflammation, they are available as creams, ointments, gels, mousses and lotions; they work by reducing inflammation in the skin. Steroid medicines that reduce inflammation are also known as corticosteroids.
>
> They are generally grouped into four categories, depending on their strength: mild, moderate, potent and very potent. There are various brands and types in each category. Some mild corticosteroids can be bought over the counter at a pharmacy; however, stronger corticosteroids are prescription only. Hydrocortisone cream 1%, for example, is a commonly used steroid cream and is classified as a mild topical steroid. The greater the strength, the more effect it has on reducing inflammation but with this is also the greater risk of side effects with continued use. Creams are usually best to treat moist or weeping areas of skin. Ointments are usually best to treat areas of skin that are dry or thickened. Lotions may be useful to treat hairy areas, such as the scalp.
>
> It is usual to use the lowest strength topical steroid first. If there is no improvement after 3–7 days, a stronger topical steroid may be prescribed. For severe cases a stronger topical steroid may be prescribed from the outset. Occasionally, two or more preparations of different strengths are used at the same time, for example, a mild steroid for the face and a moderately strong steroid for patches of eczema on the

thicker skin of the arms or legs. A very strong topical steroid is often needed for eczema on the palms and soles of the feet of adults as these areas have thick skin.

In most cases, a course of treatment for 7–14 days is enough to clear a flare-up of eczema. In some cases, a longer course is needed. Many people with eczema may require a course of topical steroids to clear a flare-up. The frequency of flare-ups and the number of times a course of topical steroids is needed is dependent on patient needs.

Short courses of topical steroids are usually safe and cause no problems. Problems may arise if topical steroids are used for long periods, or if short courses of stronger steroids are often repeated. Side effects associated with mild topical steroids are uncommon. Side effects from topical steroids can either be local or systemic.

Thermoregulation

The skin has a role to play in homeostasis through thermoregulation, helping to keep the temperature of the body within narrow ranges, adapting and adjusting as a person engages in a number of different activities. Effective thermoregulation is essential for survival; temperature changes can influence alteration in enzyme function and, as such, can impact on the chemical make-up of cells. The skin acts as a temperature regulator through a range of complex and integrated activities.

Changes in the size of blood vessels in the skin can help to regulate temperature. As body temperature rises, so the blood vessels dilate – this is known as vasodilatation; this is a multifaceted bodily defence mechanism that is attempting to get hot blood from the deeper tissues beneath to the surface of the skin for cooling down: the surface of the skin is cooler as heat radiates away from the body. As this is happening, the sweat glands secrete water onto the surface of the skin. Evaporation occurs and, as a result of this, so too does cooling.

The opposite will occur when the person is in a cold environment. The blood vessels constrict – vasoconstriction – and blood stays closer to the core of the body, preserving heat.

The hair (as previously described) plays an important part in thermoregulation. Pockets of air are trapped in the hair when the arrector pili are stimulated to contract, making the hairs stand up. The trapped air causes insulation to occur, insulating the surrounding environment on the skin from the cooler atmosphere.

Medicines Management Transdermal Patches

 Transdermal drug administration (skin patch) provides consistent, continuous drug delivery through the skin into the bloodstream. When applying the medication the nurse should follow the manufacturer's instructions, adhere to local policy and procedure and:

- Follow the 'five rights' of drug administration.
- Provide privacy, perform hand hygiene and explain the procedure to the patient.
- Use gloves.
- If applicable, remove the old patch and dispose of it.
- Select a new site for the patch on a flat surface, such as the chest, back, flank or upper arm. Rotate sites throughout therapy.
- Ensure the skin is intact, non-irritated and non-irradiated.
- Avoid hairy areas if possible, or shave/cut excessive hair.
- If the site needs to be cleaned prior to application, use only clear water; let the skin dry completely.
- Open the packing carefully and remove the patch from its pouch and peel half of its protective liner. If the patch is damaged during opening, then throw it away and start again.
- Take care not to touch the sticky side of the patch. Place the adhesive side on the skin and then peel off the other half of the liner. Press the skin patch firmly with the palm of your hand for at least 30 seconds, making sure it adheres to the skin, particularly at the edges.
- Remove gloves and perform hand hygiene.
- Document the medication administration.

The patient can shower as usual and get the patch wet. However, the patch should not be kept under water for long periods of time as this this can cause it to loosen or fall off.

Advise the person not to use a heating pad on the body where wearing a patch. The heat can cause the patch to release its drug faster, this could result in overdose.

Patches should be stored as per manufacturer's instructions and they should be kept away from children.

Protection

There are many ways in which the skin protects the body, and a number of these have already been discussed; for example, the skin's ability to protect by the production of melanin against the harmful effects of ultraviolet light. Through its ability to intensify normal cell replacement when needed and the ability to shed dead skin and cause the migration of cells, the skin maintains the integrity of the body. Wound healing is an example of the skin's protective mechanism.

By eliminating waste products through the pores on the skin (and there are over 2 million of these), the skin can help to protect the body from a build-up of poisonous substances. The skin also has the ability to prevent body fluids from escaping, preventing dehydration and helping to regulate the amount of fluid through the content and volume of sweat produced. As a waterproof barrier, the skin can also ensure that harmful fluids in the environment are prevented from entering the body.

Clinical Considerations Dehydration

Many people in a number of care environments are prone to dehydration. The older person is particularly at risk, and your role is to prevent and to identify dehydration and to take actions to remedy any deficits; you will be required to assess, plan, implement and evaluate care.

Undertaking a safe and effective assessment of needs demands that you to use a variety of skills: you will be required to observe, measure and ask questions (Lapin, 2018). The skin can tell you much about the people you care for. You can make a diagnosis of dehydration by observing the skin of those in your care, although this is not and should not be used as the sole diagnostic tool. The classic signs of dehydration in older people include loss of skin recoil (also described as loss of skin turgor), increased thirst, reduced urinary output, tachycardia and hypotension; the person may also be confused. However, these signs are late signs of dehydration.

The skin may lack its normal elasticity and revert to its usual position slowly when gently pinched up into a fold, if lack of skin turgor is present. Normally, the skin springs right back into position in a hydrated person. Care must be taken not to harm the person when trying to make an assessment and diagnosis.

Sebum (an oily substance) secreted by the skin contains bacterial chemicals that have the ability to destroy surface bacteria. When sweat is produced, the acidic pH has the potential to hamper the proliferation of bacteria. Phagocytic macrophages present in the dermis have the ability to ingest and destroy viruses and bacteria that have penetrated the surface of the skin.

Clinical Considerations Occupational Dermatitis

The use of vinyl gloves (these are considered 'hypoallergenic') is believed to be safer than latex gloves and has increased. However, contact allergy to vinyl gloves is not rare and vinyl can also be responsible for dermatitis. Dermatitis can occur on any part of the body but the skin on the hands is the most commonly affected area. Wearing gloves for long periods, during clinical practice, for example, increases the risk of the health care worker developing occupational dermatitis; using the wrong type of glove for a particular task has the potential to cause the condition to develop and can also exacerbate an existing condition.

If the health care worker is concerned about occupational dermatitis, they should contact their occupational health services as soon as possible to seek advice. If the dermatitis does not resolve with treatment and modifications at work have been instigated, then a referral to a dermatologist for patch testing to identify or exclude sensitisers that may be causing the problem will be required.

Excretion and Absorption

Some elements of secretion and absorption have already been mentioned with respect to the skin's function in protecting the person. The skin has the ability to excrete substances from the body; sweat is composed of water, sodium, carbon dioxide, ammonia and urea. Jenkins *et al.* (2013) point out that the body (despite its almost waterproof nature) can excrete approximately 400 mL of water daily; those who lead a less active lifestyle will lose less, and a more active person will lose more.

The skin also has the ability to absorb substances from the environment. Materials are absorbed from the external environment into the body cells, and some of these substances when absorbed are toxic; for example, heavy metals such as lead and mercury. There are some therapeutic and non-therapeutic medications that can be absorbed through the skin. A number of fat-soluble vitamins – A, D, E and K – oxygen and carbon dioxide are also absorbed.

Medicines Management Administration of Medicines

There are some medications that you may be asked to administer via the skin. These include ointments, lotions, creams and gels. The application of medicines via the skin through an adhesive patch is also used in a number of care areas. All of these medicines are subject to the same rules and regulations associated with the administration of any medicine. Medicines applied to skin are often needed to treat skin conditions, and they are known as topical medications; they are administered externally onto the body as opposed to being ingested or injected.

Lotions are used to protect, soften and soothe and can provide relief from itching. Ointments are oil-based, and body heat causes them to melt after application; often, these medications are used to fight infection or relieve inflamed tissue. Gloves must be used when applying these medicines; they must be applied in thin, even layers unless the prescription states otherwise (Gawthorpe, 2018).

Most skin medications are provided for use in tubes; one tube must only be used for one person in order to prevent cross-infection. There are some skin medicines that must be sterile for use; when this is the case, after application, the leftover medication must be discarded.

When you are applying the medication, you must take care that you do not increase discomfort by using too much pressure or rubbing areas that are inflamed or causing the person pain.

Synthesis of Vitamin D

The skin is actively involved in the production and synthesis of vitamin D. For vitamin D to synthesise effectively, activation of a precursor molecule in the skin by ultraviolet rays in the sunlight (ultraviolet radiation) is required. Enzymes present in the kidneys and liver alter the molecules, producing calcitriol. Calcitriol (a hormone) assists in the absorption of calcium present in food in the intestines into the blood.

Conclusion

The skin is an exceptional organ and is also known as the integumentary system. There are a variety of diseases or injuries that can easily be observed on the surface of the skin; for example, a skin rash, the presence of jaundice or cyanosis. It is the largest organ in the body in weight and surface area (Hubert and Van Meter, 2018) The skin has the ability to reveal how we feel and what emotional state we may be in: humans blush, sweat and tremble. No other organ in the body is as easily looked over or palpated as the skin; the skin is also more easily exposed to injury, for example, infection and trauma.

This organ is the interface between the external and internal environments. The skin contributes to the homeostasis of the body, and the physical changes noted can point to homeostatic imbalance. The skin is also composed of the accessory structures, for example, the nails and a number of glands; these are sometimes called the appendages.

The skin has the ability to allow a person to experience pleasure, pain and other stimuli from the external environment.

Glossary

Absorption: Intake of fluids or other materials by cells of the skin.
Apocrine: A type of gland found in the skin, apocrine glands in the skin and eyelids are sweat glands.
Apoptosis: Death of a cell as signalled by the nuclei in a normally functioning cell.
Arrector pili: A microscopic muscle attached to hair follicles.

Calcitonin: A hormone that participates in calcium metabolism.
Cerumen: Ear wax secreted by ceruminous glands.
Collagen: A protein that is the main component of connective tissue.
Cutaneous: Relating to the skin.
Cyanosis: A bluish discolouration of the skin and mucous membranes.
Dermatitis: Inflammation of the skin.
Enzyme: A substance that accelerates chemical reactions.
Erythema: Redness.
Excretion: The process of elimination of waste products from the body.
Extrinsic: Originates externally.
Fascia: A fibrous membrane covering, supporting and separating muscles.
Hair: A thread-like structure produced by the hair follicles emerging from the dermis.
Homeostasis: The ability to maintain a constant internal environment.
Hyperkeratosis: Excess keratins are produced, resulting in thickening of the skin.
Innervation: Related to the supply of nerves.
Integumentary: The external covering of the body, relating to the skin.
Intrinsic: Originates internally.
Keratin: A tough, insoluble protein found in the hair and nails and other keratinised areas of the body.
Keratinise: To convert into keratin.
Lanugo: Fine, downy hair covering the foetus.
Lunula: The moon-shaped white area at the base of nails.
Maceration: Softening and breaking down of the skin.
Malodourous: Smelling unpleasant.
Melanin: Pigment found in some parts of the body, for example, the skin and hair.
Metabolism: A set of chemical reactions in the body required to maintain life.
Nail: A hard plate that is mainly composed of keratin.
Nodule: A growth of abnormal tissue.
Organ: A structure that is composed of two or more kinds of tissue with a specific function and a recognised shape.
Organism: A total living form.
Papule: A small pimple or swelling on the skin, often forming part of a rash.
Pathogen: A disease-producing microbe.
Phagocytosis: The act of destroying and ingesting microbes by phagocytes.
Pheromones: Chemicals that trigger an innate behavioural response in another.
Prognosis: A prediction about how a patient's disease will progress.
Proliferation: A rapid and repeated reproduction of new cells.
Prophylactic: Usually medication taken in order to prevent a disease
Pruritus: Itching.
Pustule: a small blister or pimple on the skin containing pus.
Sebum: An oily substance made of fat and the debris of fat-producing cells produced by the sebaceous glands.
Stratum: A layer.
Tactile: Pertaining to touch.
Thermoreceptor: A sensory receptor that has the ability to detect changes in heat.
Thermoregulation: Ability to regulate temperature.
Vasoconstriction: Reduction in the diameter of blood vessels.
Vasodilatation: Increase in diameter of blood vessels.

512

References

Boore, J., Cook, N. and Shepherd, A. (2016) *Essentials of Anatomy and Physiology for Nursing Practice*. London, Sage

Colbert, B.J., Ankney, J. and Lee, K.T. (2012) *Anatomy and Physiology for Health Professionals: An Interactive Journey*, 2nd edn. Upper Saddle River, NJ: Pearson.

Fickertt-Wilson, S. and Foret-Giddens, J. (2017) *Health Assessment for Nursing Practice* 6th edn. St Louis: Elsevier.

Gawthorpe, D.M. (2018) The principles of medicine administration and pharmacology. In Peate, I. and Wild, K. (eds), *Nursing Practice, Knowledge and Care*, 2nd edn. Oxford: John Wiley & Sons, Ltd; chapter 19 pp. 376–403.

Hubert and Van Meter (2018) *Gould's Pathophysiology for the Health Professions*, 6th edn. St Louis: Elsevier

Jenkins, G.W., Kemnitz, C.P. and Tortora, G.J. (2013) *Anatomy and Physiology: From Science to Life*, 3rd edn. Hoboken, NJ: John Wiley & Sons, Inc.

Lapin, M. (2018) The nursing process. In Peate, I. and Wild, K. (eds), *Nursing Practice, Knowledge and Care*, 2nd edn. Oxford: John Wiley & Sons, Ltd; chapter 6, pp. 111–128.

McLaughlin, M.F. (2018) Integumentary Issues. In Stannard, D. and Krenzischek, D.A (2018) *Perianesthesia Nursing Care*, 2nd edn. Burlington: Jones and Bartlett; pp 83–89.

Nair, M. and Peate, I. (2009) *Fundamentals of Applied Pathophysiology: An Essential Guide for Nursing Students*. Oxford: John Wiley & Sons, Ltd.

Rizzo D.C. (2006) *Delmar's Fundamentals of Anatomy and Physiology*, 2nd edn. New York: Thomson.

Shier, D., Butler, J. and Lewis, R. (2016) *Hole's Anatomy and Physiology*, 14th edn. Boston, MA: McGraw-Hill.

Timby, B.K. (2016) *Fundamental Nursing Skills and Concepts*, 11th edn. Philadelphia, PA: Wolters Kluwer Health.

Tortora, G.J. and Derrickson, B.H. (2009) *Principles of Anatomy and Physiology*, 12th edn. Hoboken, NJ: John Wiley & Sons, Inc.

Tortora, G.J. and Derrickson, B. (2014) *Principles of Anatomy and Physiology*, 14th edn. Hoboken, NJ: John Wiley & Sons, Inc.

Waugh, A. and Grant, A. (2018) *Ross and Wilson Anatomy and Physiology*, 13th edn. Edinburgh: Elsevier.

Further Reading

British Skin Foundation

http://www.britishskinfoundation.org.uk/SkinInformation/AtoZofSkindisease/Eczema.aspx. This organisation has a number of aims. They fund research to further understanding of the different types of skin disease, fundraise and campaign for change, institutionally and behaviorally for the good of those who have skin disease. They raise awareness and work with the community to encourage people to share their experiences with one another so they do not have to suffer in silence.

Changing Faces

https://www.changingfaces.org.uk

A UK charity for the 1.3 million people in the UK with a visible difference: a mark, scar or condition that makes them look different. Changing Faces provides advice, support and psychosocial services to children, young people and adults, challenging discrimination.

Psoriasis Association

https://www.psoriasis-association.org.uk

The Psoriasis Association works to help people whose lives are affected by psoriasis and psoriatic arthritis. They do this through research, information and raising awareness.

Activities

Multiple Choice Questions

1. How often (approximately) are the epidermal cells replaced? Every:
   (a) 30 days
   (b) 42 days
   (c) 15 days
   (d) 28 days
2. The skin is thickest on:
   (a) the lips
   (b) the earlobes
   (c) the hands
   (d) the nose
3. What is the name of the pigment that makes skin different colours?
   (a) melaena
   (b) melatonin
   (c) melonite
   (d) melanin

4. Hair follicles are made of:
   (a) sebum
   (b) sweat
   (c) keratin
   (d) muscle
5. The outermost layer of the skin is called:
   (a) the dermis
   (b) the epidermis
   (c) the muscularis
   (d) the subcutaneous
6. The skin does all of these except:
   (a) absorb sugar
   (b) protect the body
   (c) provide the sense of touch
   (d) help to thermoregulate
7. The word used when the skin has no melanin is:
   (a) aged
   (b) exhausted
   (c) eczema
   (d) albino
8. In what aspect of the skin are the cells that divide to form new cells?
   (a) the medulla
   (b) the follicle
   (c) the basal layers of the epidermis
   (d) the sebaceous glands
9. What will eventually happen to the cells of the epidermis?
   (a) they are reabsorbed
   (b) they become scars
   (c) they become infected
   (d) they die off and flake
10. The structures in the dermis that produce oil are called:
    (a) the sebaceous glands
    (b) the Merkel cells
    (c) the Meissner corpuscle
    (d) lamellar granules
11. The skin's natural oil is called:
    (a) arachis
    (b) sebum
    (c) serum
    (d) lanolin
12. The skin:
    (a) is the fastest healing organ in the body
    (b) has no nerve endings
    (c) is largest organ of the body
    (d) is heavier in men than women
13. Total healing of body piercings can take:
    (a) between 2 and 4 months
    (b) between 2 and 4 weeks
    (c) between 2 and 4 years
    (d) between 2 and 4 days
14. Goosebumps are caused by:
    (a) an immature immune system
    (b) the pilomotor reflex
    (c) the stimulation of the nerves
    (d) an increase in heart rate

15. Innervation relates to:
   (a) the lymphatic system
   (b) the blood supply
   (c) the nervous system
   (d) the feet

Find Out More

1. What are the names of the touch receptors?
2. Where does nail growth originate?
3. Describe the anatomical and physiological changes that occur when a person experiences goosebumps.
4. Name three potential complications of body piercing.
5. What procedures can be used to remove tattoos?
6. What is needed to activate vitamin D and why?
7. What is the role and function of the arrector pili?
8. Describe what happens to the skin when vasodilatation occurs.
9. Outline the processes involved as skin repairs itself after being damaged.
10. How does the skin and renal system work together to maintain homeostasis?

Conditions

The following is a list of conditions that are associated with the skin. Take some time and write notes about each of the conditions. You may make the notes taken from textbooks or other resources (e.g. people you work with in a clinical area), or you may make the notes as a result of people you have cared for. If you are making notes about people you have cared for, you must ensure that you adhere to the rules of confidentiality.

Tinea unguium

Skin cancer:
• Malignant melanoma
• Basal cell carcinoma (BCC)
• Squamous cell carcinoma (SCC)

Eczema

Human papillomavirus, types 1, 2, 4, 27 and 57

Burns:
• First degree
• Second degree
• Full thickness

Pressure sores

Normal Values

Haematology
Full blood count
Haemoglobin (males) 13.0–18.0 g dL^{-1}
Haemoglobin (females) 11.5–16.5 g dL^{-1}
Haematocrit (males) 0.40–0.52
Haematocrit (females) 0.36–0.47
MCV 80–96 fL
MCH 28–32 pg
MCHC 32–35 g dL^{-1}
White cell count $(4–11) \times 10^9$ L^{-1}

White Cell Differential
Neutrophils $1.5–7 \times 10^9$ L^{-1}
Lymphocytes $1.5–4 \times 10^9$ L^{-1}
Monocytes $0–0.8 \times 10^9$ L^{-1}
Eosinophils $0.04–0.4 \times 10^9$ L^{-1}
Basophils $0–0.1 \times 10^9$ L^{-1}
Platelet count $150–400 \times 10^9$ L^{-1}
Reticulocyte count $(25–85) \times 10^9$ L^{-1} or 0.5–2.4%

Erythrocyte Sedimentation Rate
Westergren
Under 50 years:
    Males 0–15 mm/1st hour
    Females 0–20 mm/1st hour
Over 50 years:
    Males 0–20 mm/1st hour
    Females 0–30 mm/1st hour

Plasma viscosity 1.50–1.72 mPa s^1 (at 25 °C)

Coagulation Screen
Prothrombin time 11.5–15.5 s
International normalised ratio <1.4
Activated partial thromboplastin time 30–40 s
Fibrinogen 1.8–5.4 g L^{-1}
Bleeding time 3–8 min

Fundamentals of Anatomy and Physiology: For Nursing and Healthcare Students, Third Edition. Edited by Ian Peate and Suzanne Evans.
© 2020 John Wiley & Sons Ltd. Published 2020 by John Wiley & Sons Ltd.
Student companion website: www.wileyfundamentalseries.com/anatomy
Instructor companion website: www.wiley.com/go/instructor/anatomy

Coagulation Factors
Factors II, V, VII, VIII, IX, X, XI, XII 50–150 IU dL^{-1}
Factor V Leiden Present or not
Von Willebrand factor 45–150 IU dL^{-1}
Von Willebrand factor antigen 50–150 IU dL^{-1}
Protein C 80–135 IU dL^{-1}
Protein S 80–120 IU dL^{-1}
Antithrombin III 80–120 IU dL^{-1}
Activated protein C resistance 2.12–4.0
Fibrin degradation products <100 mg L^{-1}
D-dimer screen <0.5 mg L^{-1}

Haematinics
Serum iron 12–30 µmol L^{-1}
Serum iron-binding capacity 45–75 µmol L^{-1}
Serum ferritin 15–300 µg L^{-1}
Serum transferrin 2.0–4.0 g L^{-1}
Serum B$_{12}$ 160–760 ng L^{-1}
Serum folate 2.0–11.0 µg L^{-1}
Red cell folate 160–640 µg L^{-1}
Serum haptoglobin 0.13–1.63 g L^{-1}

Haemoglobin Electrophoresis
Haemoglobin A >95%
Haemoglobin A2 2–3%
Haemoglobin F <2%

Chemistry
Serum sodium 137–144 mmol L^{-1}
Serum potassium 3.5–4.9 mmol L^{-1}
Serum chloride 95–107 mmol L^{-1}
Serum bicarbonate 20–28 mmol L^{-1}
Anion gap 12–16 mmol L^{-1}
Serum urea 2.5–7.5 mmol L^{-1}
Serum creatinine 60–110 µmol L^{-1}
Serum corrected calcium 2.2–2.6 mmol L^{-1}
Serum phosphate 0.8–1.4 mmol L^{-1}
Serum total protein 61–76 g L^{-1}
Serum albumin 37–49 g L^{-1}
Serum total bilirubin 1–22 µmol L^{-1}
Serum conjugated bilirubin 0–3.4 µmol L^{-1}
Serum alanine aminotransferase 5–35 U L^{-1}
Serum aspartate aminotransferase 1–31 U L^{-1}
Serum alkaline phosphatase 45–105 U L^{-1} (over 14 years)
Serum gamma glutamyl transferase 4–35 U L^{-1} (<50 U L^{-1} in males)
Serum lactate dehydrogenase 10–250 U L^{-1}
Serum creatine kinase (males) 24–195 U L^{-1}
Serum creatine kinase (females) 24–170 U L^{-1}
Creatine kinase MB fraction <5%
Serum troponin I 0-0.4 µg L^{-1}
Serum troponin T 0–0.1 µg L^{-1}
Serum copper 12–26 µmol L^{-1}
Serum caeruloplasmin 200–350 mg L^{-1}
Serum aluminium 0-10 µg L^{-1}

Serum magnesium 0.75–1.05 mmol L^{-1}
Serum zinc 6–25 µmol L^{-1}
Serum urate (males) 0.23–0.46 mmol L^{-1}
Serum urate (females) 0.19–0.36 mmol L^{-1}
Plasma lactate 0.6–1.8 mmol L^{-1}
Plasma ammonia 12–55 µmol L^{-1}
Serum angiotensin-converting enzyme 25–82 U L^{-1}
Fasting plasma glucose 3.0–6.0 mmol L^{-1}
Haemoglobin A1 C 3.8–6.4%
Fructosamine <285 µmo L^{-1}
Serum amylase 60–180 U L^{-1}
Plasma osmolality 278–305 mosmol kg^{-1}

Urine
Albumin/creatinine ratio (untimed specimen) <3.5 mg $mmol^{-1}$ (males)
  <2.5 mg $mmol^{-1}$ (females)

Lipids and Lipoproteins
Target levels will vary depending on the patient's overall cardiovascular risk assessment
Serum cholesterol <5.2 mmol L^{-1}
Serum LDL cholesterol <3.36 mmol L^{-1}
Serum HDL cholesterol >1.55 mmol L^{-1}
Fasting serum triglyceride 0.45–1.69 mmol L^{-1}

Blood Gases (Breathing Air At Sea Level)
Blood H^+ 35–45 nmol L^{-1}
pH 7.36–7.44
PaO_2 11.3–12.6 kPa
$PaCO_2$ 4.7–6.0 kPa
Base excess ±2 mmol L^{-1}

Carboxyhaemoglobin
Non-smoker <2%
Smoker 3–15%

Immunology/Rheumatology
Complement C3 65–190 mg dL^{-1}
Complement C4 15–50 mg dL^{-1}
Total haemolytic (CH50) 150–250 U L^{-1}
Serum C-reactive protein <10 mg L^{-1}

Serum Immunoglobulins
IgG 6.0–13.0 g L^{-1}
IgA 0.8–3.0 g L^{-1}
IgM 0.4–2.5 g L^{-1}
IgE <120 kU L^{-1}
Serum β_2-microglobulin <3 mg L^{-1}

Cerebrospinal Fluid
Opening pressure 50–180 mmH_2O
Total protein 0.15–0.45 g L^{-1}
Albumin 0.066–0.442 g L^{-1}
Chloride 116–122 mmol L^{-1}
Glucose 3.3–4.4 mmol L^{-1}

Lactate 1–2 mmol L^{-1}
Cell count ≤5 mL^{-1}

Differential
Lymphocytes 60–70%
Monocytes 30–50%
Neutrophils None
IgG/ALB ≤0.26
IgG index ≤0.88

Urine
Glomerular filtration rate 70–140 mL min^{-1}
Total protein <0.2g/24 h
Albumin <30 mg/24 h
Calcium 2.5–7.5 mmol/24 h
Urobilinogen 1.7–5.9 µmol/24 h
Coproporphyrin <300 nmol/24 h
Uroporphyrin 6–24 nmol/24 h
δ-Aminolevulinate 8–53 µmol/24 h
5-Hydroxyindoleacetic acid 10–47 µmol/24h
Osmolality 350–1000 mosmol kg^{-1}

Faeces
Nitrogen 70–140 mmol/24 h
Urobilinogen 50–500 µmol/24 h
Fat (on normal diet) <7 g/24 h

The values listed here are generalisations. Each laboratory will have its own specific reference ranges.

Answers

Chapter 1 Basic Scientific Principles of Physiology

Activities

Multiple Choice Questions

1. (d); **2.** (b); **3.** (d); **4.** (c); **5.** (b); **6.** (a); **7.** (d); **8.** (a); **9.** (c); **10.** (c); **11.** (d); **12.** (d); **13.** (c); **14.** (a); **15.** (c).

True or false

1. False – an ion has a net charge and is not therefore electrically neutral.
2. True
3. True
4. True
5. False – Lipids are organic molecules.
6. True

Chapter 2 Cells, Cellular Compartments, Transport Systems, Fluid Movement Between Compartments

Episodes of Care

Adult, Hyponatraemia Multiple choice questions:
1. (a); **2.** (b); **3.** (a); **4.** (c); **5.** (b).

Episodes of Care

Adult, Burns Multiple choice questions:
1. (b); **2.** (c); **3.** (c); **4.** (c); **5.** (c).

Activities

Multiple Choice Questions

1. (c); **2.** (c); **3.** (b); **4.** (a); **5.** (d); **6.** (c); **7.** (a); **8.** (b); **9.** (c); **10.** (c); **11.** (c); **12.** (d); **13.** (b); **14.** (c); **15.** (c).

True or False

1. False – molecules move from where they are at high concentration to where they are at a lower concentration.
2. True
3. True
4. True
5. False – sodium is the principal extracellular ion

Fundamentals of Anatomy and Physiology: For Nursing and Healthcare Students, Third Edition. Edited by Ian Peate and Suzanne Evans.
© 2020 John Wiley & Sons Ltd. Published 2020 by John Wiley & Sons Ltd.
Student companion website: www.wileyfundamentalseries.com/anatomy
Instructor companion website: www.wiley.com/go/instructor/anatomy

6. True
7. False – it is a lower than normal sodium level
8. False – it is an isotonic solution
9. True

Chemical Symbols

Potassium	K^+
Sodum	Na^+
Bicarbonate	HCO_3^-
Chloride	Cl^-
Organic phosphate	PO_4^{3-}
Sulfate	SO_4^{2-}
Calcium	Ca^{2+}

Chapter 3 Genetics

Episodes of Care
Learning disability, Turner syndrome Multiple choice questions:
1. (a); 2. (d); 3. (c); 4. (a); 5. (c).

Episodes of Care
Mental health, Schizophrenia Multiple choice questions:
1. (a); 2. (c); 3. (d); 4. (a); 5. (b).

Episodes of Care
Child, Acute lymphoblastic leukaemia Multiple choice questions:
1. (b); 2. (c); 3. (a); 4. (d); 5. (c).

Activities
Multiple Choice Questions
1. (d); 2. (b); 3. (b); 4. (b); 5. (b); 6. (a); 7. (c); 8. (d); 9. (b); 10. (c); 11. (c); 12. (d); 13. (b); 14. (b); 15. (b).

True or False
1. True
2. False – the phenotype would be determined by the dominant allele
3. True
4. False – hydrogen bonds hold the two strands together
5. True

Chapter 4 Tissue

Activities
Multiple choice questions
1. (c); 2. (a); 3. (a); 4. (b); 5. (a); 6. (a); 7. (b); 8. (c); 9. (a); 10. (a); 11. (c); 12. (b); 13. (b); 14. (a); 15. (a).

Chapter 5 Embryology

Episodes of Care
Adult, Foetal alcohol syndrome (FAS) Multiple choice questions
1. (a); 2. (d. All statements are true); 3. (a); 4. (b); 5. (a).

Episodes of Care
Adult, Pre-term birth Multiple choice questions
1. (b); **2.** (b); **3.** (a); **4.** (d. All statements are true); **5.** (f).

Episodes of Care
Adult, Gestational diabetes Multiple choice questions
1. (b); **2.** (a); **3.** (b); **4.** (e); **5.** (d. All statements are true).

Episodes of Care
Learning disabilities, Down syndrome Multiple choice questions
1. (a); **2.** (b); **3.** (a); **4.** (a); **5.** (b)

Activities
Multiple Choice Questions
1. (a); **2.** (b); **3.** (a); **4.** (c); **5.** (b); **6.** (a); **7.** (b); **8.** (a); **9.** (c); **10.** (a); **11.** (a); **12.** (c); **13.** (a); **14.** (b); **15.** (c).

Chapter 6 The Muscular System

Episodes of Care
Child, Muscular dystrophy Multiple choice questions:
1. (b); **2.** (c); **3.** (a); **4.** (a); **5.** (d).

Episodes of Care
Adult, Fibromyalgia Multiple choice questions:
1. (b); **2.** (d. All statements are true); **3.** (c); **4.** (c); **5.** (d. All statements are true).

Episodes of Care
Child, Soft tissue injuries Multiple choice questions:
1. (c); **2.** (c); **3.** (d. All statements are true); **4.** (b); **5.** (d. All statements are true).

Activities
Multiple Choice Questions
1. (a); **2.** (c); **3.** (c); **4.** (d); **5.** (a); **6.** (d); **7.** (a); **8.** (d); **9.** (c); **10.** (c); **11.** (b); **12.** (c); **13.** (c); **14.** (c); **15.** (b).

Chapter 7 The Skeletal System

Episodes of Care
Mental health, Musculoskeletal disorders Multiple choice questions:
1. (b); **2.** (d. All statements are true); **3.** (c); **4.** (a); **5.** (b).

Episodes of Care
Child, Perthes' disease Multiple choice questions:
1. (d); **2.** (b); **3.** (c); **4.** (a); **5.** (d. both (a) and (b) are true).

Episodes of Care
Adult, Hip surgery Multiple choice questions:
1. (d); **2.** (c); **3.** (a); **4.** (a); **5.** (c).

Episodes of Care
Learning disabilities Multiple choice questions:
1. (b); **2.** (a); **3.** (b); **4.** (d); **5.** (d. All statements are true).

Activities
Multiple Choice Questions
1. (b); 2. (c); 3. (c); 4. (a); 5. (c); 6. (d); 7 (a); 8. (d); 9. (c); 10. (b); 11. (b); 12. (a); 13. (c); 14. (a); 15. (d).

True or False
1. True
2. False – babies have more bones than adults
3. True
4. False – the ribs protect the organs in the chest cavity
5. False – red bone marrow produces blood cells
6. False – male bones tend to be larger and therefore heavier
7. False – the patella is located between the femur and the tibia
8. True
9. True
10. False – the appendicular skeleton has many more bones than the axial.

Chapter 8 The Circulatory System

Episodes of Care
Child, Thalassaemia minor Multiple choice questions:
1. (a); 2. (b); 3. (b); 4. (b); 5. (c).

Episodes of care
Learning disabilities, haemophilia Multiple choice questions:
1. (d); 2. (b); 3. (c); 4. (d); 5. (a).

Episodes of care
Mental health, Hodgkin disease Multiple choice questions:
1. (b); 2. (b); 3. (a); 4. (b); 5. (c).

Activities
Multiple Choice Questions
1. (c); 2. (a); 3. (d); 4. (b); 5. (a); 6. (c); 7 (d); 8. (b); 9. (c); 10. (a); 11. (b); 12. (b); 13. (d); 14. (c); 15. (b).

Chapter 9 The Cardiac System

Episodes of Care
Child, Hypertrophic cardiomyopathy Multiple choice questions:
1. (b); 2. (b); 3. (d. All statements are true); 4. (a); 5. (b).

Episodes of Care
Learning disabilities, Congenital heart defects Multiple choice questions:
1. (a); 2. (d. All statements are true); 3. (c); 4. (b); 5. (b).

Episodes of Care
Mental health, Recurrent chest pain Multiple choice questions:
1. (d. All statements are true); 2. (a); 3. (c); 4. (c); 5. (d. All statements are true).

Activities
Multiple Choice Questions
1. (b); 2. (c); 3. (b); 4. (c); 5. (d); 6. (a); 7 (d); 8. (d); 9. (b); 10. (b); 11. (b); 12. (a); 13. (c); 14. (b); 15. (c).

Chapter 10 The Digestive System

Episodes of Care
Learning disabilities, Dysphagia Multiple choice questions:
1. (b); 2. (d. All statements are true); 3. (b); 4. (c); 5. (d. All statements are true).

Episodes of Care
Mental health, Anxiety Multiple choice questions:
1. (c); 2. (b); 3. (d); 4. (b); 5. (d. All statements are true).

Episodes of Care
Child, Inflammatory bowel diseases Multiple choice questions:
1. (c); 2. (d. All statements are true); 3. (d. All statements are true).; 4. (a); 5. (d).

Activities
Multiple Choice Questions
1. (d); 2. (b); 3. (b); 4. (c); 5. (d. All statements are true); 6. (a); 7 (d); 8. (a); 9. (d); 10. (a); 11. (b); 12. (a); 13. (b); 14. (d); 15. (b).

True or false
1. True
2. False
3. False
4. True
5. True
6. False
7. True
8. False
9. False
10. False

Chapter 11 The Renal System

Episodes of Care
Learning disabilities, Acute kidney injury Multiple choice questions:
1. (a); 2. (c); 3. (c); 4. (b) and (c); 5. (b).

Episodes of Care
Child, Urinary infection Multiple choice questions:
1. (c); 2. (b); 3. (d); 4. (b); 5. (a).

Episodes of Care
Adult, Chronic kidney disease Multiple choice questions:
1. (c); 2. (b); 3. (c); 4. (d. All statements are true); 5. (a).

Activities
Multiple Choice Questions
1. (c); 2. (b); 3. (a); 4. (d); 5. (c); 6. (a); 7 (a); 8. (c); 9. (b); 10. (c); 11. (a); 12. (d); 13. (a); 14. (b); 15. (a).

Chapter 12 The Respiratory System

Episodes of Care
Child, Asthma Multiple choice questions:
1. (d. All statements are true); 2. (c); 3. (b); 4. (c); 5. (d).

Episodes of Care
Learning disabilities, Pneumonia Multiple choice questions:
1. (d); 2. (d. All statements are true); 3. (b); 4. (c); 5. (d).

Episodes of Care
Mental health, COPD Multiple choice questions:
1. (a); 2. (c); 3. (d. All statements are true); 4. (c); 5. (d. All statements are true).

Activities
Multiple Choice Questions
1. (c); 2. (a); 3. (a); 4. (b); 5. (a); 6. (c); 7 (a); 8. (d. All statements are true); 9. (d); 10. (a); 11. (b); 12. (d. All statements are true); 13. (c); 14. (d. All statements are true); 15. (c).

Chapter 13 The Reproductive Systems

Episodes of Care
Child, Testicular torsion Multiple choice questions:
1. (b); 2. (d); 3. (c); 4. (d); 5. (c).

Episodes of Care
Learning disabilities, Sexual health Multiple choice questions:
1. (b); 2. (d); 3. (d. All statements are true); 4. (b); 5. (a).

Episodes of Care
Adult, Genital piercing Multiple choice questions:
1. (b); 2. (c); 3. (d. All statements are true); 4. (b); 5. (a).

Episodes of Care
Adult, Ectopic pregnancy Multiple choice questions:
1. (d. All statements are true); 2. (d); 3. (a); 4. (d); 5. (a).

Activities
Multiple Choice Questions
1. (b); 2. (a); 3. (a); 4. (d); 5. (d); 6. (d); 7. (d); 8. (c); 9. (b); 10. (c); 11. (a); 12. (d); 13. (a); 14. (d); 15. (b).

Chapter 14 The Nervous System

Episodes of Care
Child, Epilepsy Multiple choice questions:
1. (b); 2. (d. All statements are true); 3. (a); 4. (b); 5. (d).

Episodes of Care
Mental health, Alzheimer's disease Multiple choice questions:
1. (c); 2. (b); 3. (b); 4. (d. All statements are true); 5. (d)

Episodes of Care
Learning disabilities, Spinal cord injury Multiple choice questions:
1. (c); 2. (b); 3. (c and d); 4. (a and b); 5. (d).

Activities
Multiple Choice Questions
1. (c); 2. (a); 3. (c); 4. (a); 5. (c); 6. (c); 7 (c); 8. (a); 9. (b); 10. (b and c); 11. (b); 12. (d); 13. (c); 14. (a); 15. (a).

Chapter 15 The Senses

Episodes of Care
Mental Health, Dry mouth Multiple choice questions:
1. (d. All statements are true); **2.** (a); **3.** (b); **4.** (c); **5.** (d).

Episodes of Care
Learning disabilities, Hearing loss Multiple choice questions:
1. (c); **2.** (a); **3.** (b); **4.** (d); **5.** (b).

Episodes of Care
Adult, Age related macular degeneration Multiple choice questions:
1. (c); **2.** (d); **3.** (a); **4.** (b); **5.** (d. All statements are true).

Activities
Multiple Choice Questions
1. (c); **2.** (a); **3.** (c); **4.** (a); **5.** (c); **6.** (a); **7.** (d); **8.** (b); **9.** (d); **10.** (c); **11.** (b); **12.** (c); **13.** (b); **14.** (b); **15.** (d).

Chapter 16 The Endocrine System

Episodes of Care
Adult, Cushing's disease Multiple choice questions:
1. (b); **2.** (c); **3.** (d); **4.** (b); **5.** (c).

Episodes of Care
Learning disabilities, Hypothyroidism Multiple choice questions:
1. (b); **2.** (b); **3.** (c); **4.** (a); **5.** (c).

Episodes of Care
Child, Insulin pumps Multiple choice questions:
1. (d. All statements are true); **2.** (b); **3.** (d); **4.** (c); **5.** (a).

Activities
Multiple Choice Questions
1. (a); **2.** (b); **3.** (d); **4.** (d); **5.** (b); **6.** (c); **7.** (b); **8.** (b); **9.** (b); **10.** (b); **11.** (a); **12.** (c); **13.** (a); **14.** (d); **15.** (b).

Chapter 17 The Immune System

Episodes of Care
Child, Epstein-Barr virus Multiple choice questions:
1. (b); **2.** (b); **3.** (a); **4.** (b); **5.** (d).

Episodes of Care
Mental health, Neutropaenia Multiple choice questions:
1. (a); **2.** (d. All statements are true); **3.** (d. All statements are true); **4.** (d. All statements are true); **5.** (b).

Episodes of Care
Learning Disability, Allergic reaction Multiple choice questions:
1. (d. All statements are true); **2.** (a); **3.** (b); **4.** (a); **5.** (b).

Activities
Multiple Choice Questions
1. (a); 2. (b); 3. (d); 4. (d); 5. (a); 6. (c); 7. (d); 8. (c); 9. (c); 10. (b); 11. (d); 12. (b); 13. (d); 14. (b); 15. (b).

True or False
1. False – phagocytes are white blood cells
2. True
3. True
4. False – they are descended from multipotent stem cells
5. False – it is monocytes and tissue macrophages that are included within the family of macrophages
6. False – it is some of the B-cells that develop into plasma cells
7. True
8. True
9. True
10. False – sneezing is a mechanical barrier

Chapter 18 The Skin

Episodes of Care
Learning disabilities, Acne vulgaris Multiple choice questions:
1. (b); 2. (c); 3. (d); 4. (d); 5. (c).

Episodes of Care
Mental health, Photosensitivity Multiple choice questions:
1. (c); 2. (a); 3. (c); 4. (d); 5. (d).

Episodes of Care
Child, Tinea pedis Multiple choice questions:
1. (c); 2. (b); 3. (a); 4. (d); 5. (a).

Activities
Multiple Choice Questions
1. (d); 2. (c); 3. (d); 4. (c); 5. (b); 6. (a); 7. (d); 8. (c); 9. (d); 10. (a); 11. (b); 12. (c); 13. (a); 14. (b); 15. (c).

Index

Page locators in **bold** indicate tables. Page locators in *italics* indicate figures. This index uses letter-by-letter alphabetization.

20/20 vision, 427

ABO system, 197–198, *197*, **198**
absorption
   selective reabsorption, 293–294, **293**
   skin, 510–511
   tubular reabsorption and secretion, 295–296
absorptive cells, 260
ABVD therapy, 207
accessory skin structures, 504–508
   hair, 504, *505*, 509
   nails, 506–508
   sweat glands, 504–506, *505*, 510–511
ACE *see* angiotensin-converting enzyme
acetylcholine (ACh), 127–128, 375
acetylcholine esterase (AChE), 127–129
ACh *see* acetylcholine
AChE *see* acetylcholine esterase
acidity *see* pH
acne vulgaris, 495–496
acquired immunity, 477–479
   cell-mediated immunity, 477–478, *477*, *479–480*
   control of the immune system, 478
   cytotoxicity, 478
   humoral immunity, 478–479, *479–480*
   memory, 478
ACTH *see* adrenocorticotrophic hormone
action potentials, 372–374, *373*
activated partial thromboplastin time (APTT), 195–196
active immunisation, 488
active transport, 29–30, *30*, 293–294
acute compartment syndrome, 126
acute kidney injury (AKI), 283–284, 286–287
acute lymphoblastic leukaemia (ALL), 71–72
acute spinal cord compression, 389
adalimumab, 477
ADD *see* attention deficit disorder
adenosine deaminase deficiency severe combined
   immunodeficiency, 64

adenosine triphosphate/diphosphate (ATP/ADP)
   cell biology, 30
   digestive system, 270
   muscular system, 124–126, 130, *131*
   respiratory system, 330, *331*
ADH *see* antidiuretic hormone
adipocytes, 84
ADP *see* adenosine triphosphate/diphosphate
adrenal glands, 448–452, *448*
   adrenal cortex, 449, *449*
   adrenal medulla, 449
   glucocorticoids, 451, *452*
   mineralocorticoids, 449–451, *450*
adrenaline, 236, 239, 449
adrenocorticotrophic hormone (ACTH), 442–443,
   450–451
aerobic respiration, 130–133
afferent nerves, 406
afterload, 237
ageing
   muscular system, 146
   renal system, 291, 296
   sensory system, 422–423
   skeletal system, 174
age-related macular degeneration (AMD), 422–423
ageusia, 408
airway resistance, 320
AKI *see* acute kidney injury
aldosterone, 295, 449–450, *450*
alkalinity *see* pH
ALL *see* acute lymphoblastic leukaemia
alleles, 51–52
allergy
   hypersensitivity and anaphylaxis, 486–488, **487**
   immune system, 481–482, 486–487
   reproductive systems, 358
Alzheimer's disease, 375–376
AMD *see* age-related macular degeneration
amino acid-based hormones, 437

ampulla, 413, *414*
anabolic steroids, 130
anaemia, 187, 188–189
anaerobic respiration, 130
anaesthesia, 110, **110–111**
analgesia
    embryology, 110, **110–111**
    nervous system, 389
anaphylaxis, 486–487, 488
androgens, 348, 352
angiogram, 226
angiotensin, 290, 295
angiotensin-converting enzyme (ACE) inhibitors,
        286, 291
anosmia, 403–404
ANP *see* atrial natriuretic peptide
antibiotics
    immune system, 468
    sensory system, 410–411
    skin, 507
antibodies *see* immunoglobulins
anticoagulants, 196
anticonvulsants, 392
antidepressants
    endocrine system, 442–443
    nervous system, 387
    sensory system, 406–407
antidiuretic hormone (ADH)
    circulatory system, 184
    endocrine system, 440
    renal system, 289, 295, 296
antigens, 467, 469, 477–481, *479*, *482*, 484–486, 488
antihistamines, 486–487
antipsychotics
    cardiac system, 225–226
    sensory system, 407
    skin, 502
anxiety/stress
    digestive system, 259
    endocrine system, 451, *452*
    respiratory system, 324
apocrine glands, 505–506
appendicitis, 267
appendicular skeleton, 165, *166*, **167**
appetite, 406, 408
APPT activated partial prothrombin time
arterial blood gas, 328
arteries
    cardiac system, 223–224, *224*, **224**
    circulatory system, 199, *199–201*, **201**
    renal system, 292
    respiratory system, 316
arthrotec, 174
asthma, 314–316, 322, 486–487
astrocytes, 376
athlete's foot, 506–507
atomic structure, 4–5, *5–6*
ATP *see* adenosine triphosphate/diphosphate
atria, 221, 228–231, *228–229*, 233–236
atrial natriuretic peptide (ANP), 295–296

atrioventricular (AV) node, 229–231, 233–236
atrophic vaginitis, 356–357
attention deficit disorder (ADD), 196–197
auscultation, 221–223, *223*
autoimmune disease, 475–476, 481
autonomic nervous system, 370, 389–392
    cardiac system, 237
    parasympathetic division, 391, *391*, **392**
    sympathetic division, 390–391, *390*, **392**
autosomal dominant inheritance, 62–63, *63*, 66, *66*
autosomal recessive inheritance, 63–66, *66*
autosomes, 51–52
AV *see* atrioventricular
axial skeleton, 165, *166*, **167**
axons, 370, 402, 424, 428

bacterial toxins, 482
balance, 412–416, *414–415*
ball and socket joints, 172
bariatric surgery, 269
baroreceptors, 237–239, *238*
bases *see* pH
basophils, 192, *193*
benzodiazepines, 382
bile, 260–261, 264–266, *265*
biopsy, 499
bisphosphonates, 156
bladder *see* urinary bladder
blastocyst, 101–102
bleeding times, 195–196
blood
    cell biology, 34–35, *35*, 462–463, *463*
    cells of the blood, 182, *183*
    circulatory system, 182
    coagulation/clotting, 185, 194–197, **195**
    components of blood, 182, *183*
    formation of blood cells, 186, *186*
    functions of blood, 184–186, 191
    haemostasis, 194
    immune system, 462–463, *463*, 470–477, **470**, *472–474*
    physiological principles, 10–11, *10–11*
    plasma, 184, **185**
    platelets, 194
    properties of blood, 184
    red blood cells, 186–191, *186–188*, *190*
    renal system, 290, 292–296, **293**, *294*
    skeletal system, 153–154
    tissue, 87–88
    white blood cells, 186, *186*, 191–193, *192–193*, 463,
        470–477, **470**, *472–474*
blood gas analysis, 328
blood groups, 68, 197–198, *197*, **198**
blood lipids, 14
blood pressure
    cell biology, 36
    circulatory system, 202–203
    control of arterial blood pressure, 203
    endocrine system, 444
    physiological factors regulating blood pressure, 202
    renal system, 286–287

blood supply
    cardiac system, 223–228, *224–225*, **224**, *227–229*
    circulatory system, 198–201, *199–202*, **201**
    muscular system, 126
    renal system, 292
    respiratory system, 316, *317*
    skin, 509
blood transfusion, 198
B-lymphocytes *see* humoral immunity
body fluids
    composition, 31–32, **32**
    electrolyte and water balance, 32–34, **32–33**
    fluid compartments in the body, 31, *31*
    fluid movement between compartments, 34–37, *35*
    intravenous fluids/electrolytes, 38–39
body movements
    muscular system, 121, 133–136, **145**
    physiological principles, 2
    skeletal system, 153, 170–174, **172–173**
body posture, 121
body temperature *see* thermoregulation
bone
    as a tissue, 87, 152, 154–156, **155**
    axial and appendicular skeleton, 165, *166*, **167**
    formation, 158, *159*
    fractures, 164–165, *164*
    growth, 159–161, *160–161*
    remodelling, 161–163
    renal system, 290
    shapes, 165–169, *168–171*
bone marrow
    circulatory system, 186, *186*, 188
    renal system, 290
    skeletal system, 153–154
bony labyrinth, 412, 416
botulism, 127
Bowman's capsule, 287–288, *288*, 292–293
Boyle's law, 317–318, **317**, *318*
brain, 379–383
    brainstem, 381
    cerebellum, 382
    cerebrum, 380–381, *381*
    circle of Willis, 379, *379*
    diencephalon, 381
    limbic system and reticular function, 382
    structures of the brain, 379–380, *380*
brainstem, *324*, 381
breast examination, 359
breasts, 358–359, *358*
breathing *see* pulmonary ventilation/breathing
brittle bone disease, 154
bronchial secretions, 312
bronchial tree, 312–313, *313*
bundle of His, 230–231
burns, 36–37

calcitonin, 446, 448
calcitriol, 290, 448, 511
calcium channel blockers, 226
calcium homeostasis, 152, 154

callus formation, 164
cannulae *see* catheterisation
capillaries
    cell biology, 34–35, *35*
    circulatory system, *199–200*, 201, *202*
    renal system, 292, *294*
capillary nail bed refill, 508
carbamazepine, 392
carbohydrates, 13, 270
cardiac action potential, 220, *220*
cardiac muscle, 91, *91*, **120**, 121, 217–218, *218*, 229
cardiac output (CO), 236, 328
cardiac system, 215–244
    activities and learning, 242–244
    auscultation for heart sounds, 221–223, *223*
    blood flow through the heart, 228, *228–229*
    blood supply to the heart, 223–227, *224–225*, **224**, *227*
    body map, 216
    cardiac cycle, 233–236, *234–235*
    electrical pathways of the heart, 229–232, *230*,
        232–233
    factors affecting cardiac output, 236
    heart chambers, 220–221, *220*
    heart wall, 217–220, *218*
    physiological functions, 216
    regulation of heart rate, 237–239, *238*
    regulation of stroke volume, 236–237
    size and location of the heart, 216, *217*
    structures of the heart, 217–223, *218*, *220*, *223*
cardiovascular centre, 237–239, *238*
cardiovascular performance, 146
cartilage, 87, *88*, 156–158
cartilaginous joints, 170
catheterisation
    cardiac system, 225–226
    circulatory system, 201
    respiratory system, 312
CCK *see* cholecystokinin
cell biology, 23–43
    active transport, 29–30, *30*
    activities and learning, 40–43
    bulk transport across the cell membrane, 37–39, *38*
    cell cycle, *58–59*, 189, *190*
    cell membrane structure, 25, *26*
    cells of the blood, 462–463, *463*
    circulatory system, 182, *183*, 186–193, *186–188*, *190*,
        192–193
    communication between cells, 30–31
    composition of body fluids, 31–32, **32**
    digestive system, 256–257, *256*, 260, *261*
    electrolyte and water balance, 32–34, **32–33**
    endocrine system, 437–438, *437*, 452
    facilitated diffusion, 28–29, *29*
    fluid compartments in the body, 31, *31*
    fluid movement between compartments, 34–37, *35*
    genetics, *46*, 56–57, *58–59*
    immune system, 462–463, *463*, 470–485, **470**
    mitochondrial energy production, 30
    nervous system, 370, 376
    osmosis, 28, *29*, 33

cell biology (*cont'd*)
    passive transport/simple diffusion, 26–27, *27*
    sensory system, 422–424
    skeletal system, 153–156, **155**
    skin, 498–499, *498*
    structure of cells, 24–25, *25*
    tissue, 78, 83–84, **85**, 92
    transport of substances across the cell membrane, 26–30
    types of cells, 24, *24*
    see also embryology
cell-mediated immunity, 477–478, *477*, *479–480*
central adaptation, 402
central nervous system, 369
cerebellum, 382
cerebrospinal fluid (CSF), 376–379
cerebrum, 380–381, *381*
cervix, 357
CF *see* cystic fibrosis
chemical elements, 4
chemotherapy, 207, 208–209, 257
chest drains, 313
chest pain, 221–222, 225–226
CHF *see* congestive heart failure
chief cells, 256
childhood rickets, 154
cholecystokinin (CCK), 257, 260, 263, 266, **268**
cholesterol
    cardiac system, 237
    digestive system, 270
    physiological principles, 14
chondrocytes, 159
choroid, 421
chromatin, 47
chromosomes, 49–52, *50–51*
    disorders of chromosomes, 70–71
    inheritance, 60–61, *62–63*, *66–68*
    learning disability, 47–48
    transference of genes, 56–60, *60*
    types, 47
chronic kidney disease (CKD), 290, 297–298
chronic obstructive pulmonary disease (COPD), 316, 322–323, 326
chyme, 255, 260–261
cilia, 469
ciliary body, 421
ciliated epithelium, 79, *81–82*
circle of Willis, 379, *379*
circulatory system, 181–213
    activities and learning, 211–213
    blood groups, 197–198, *197*, **198**
    blood pressure, 202–203
    blood vessels, 198–201, *199–202*, **201**
    body map, 182
    cells of the blood, 182, *183*
    coagulation/clotting, 185, 194–197, **195**
    components of blood, 182, *183*
    erythropoietin/erythropoiesis, 188–189, *190*
    formation of blood cells, 186, *186*
    functions of blood, 184–186, 191

    haemostasis, 194
    lymphatic organs, 207–209
    lymphatic system, 203–207, *204–206*
    physiological functions, 182
    plasma, 184, **185**
    platelets, 194
    properties of blood, 184
    red blood cells, 186–191, *186–188*, *190*
    transport of respiratory gases, 184, 191
    white blood cells, 186, *186*, 191–193, *192–193*
citalopram, 387
CKD *see* chronic kidney disease
CL *see* corpus luteum
clicks, 222
clitoris, 357
Clostridium botulinum, 127
clozapine, 225–226, 471
CO *see* cardiac output
coagulation/clotting
    cardiac system, 227, *227*
    circulatory system, 185, 194–197, **195**
    immune system, 474, 476
cochlea, 412, 416, *416–417*
collagen fibres, 85–87
collapsed lung *see* pneumothorax
collecting ducts, 289, 293
columnar epithelium, 78–81, *79*, *81–82*
compact bone, 152, *153*
compartment syndrome, 126
complement system, 474
concussion, 382
condyloid joints, 173
cones, 421–424
congenital heart defects, 221–222
congenital myotonic dystrophy, 125–126
congestive heart failure (CHF), 30
connective tissue, 83–88
    bone, 87, 154–156
    cartilage, 87, *88*, 156–157
    cell biology, 83–84, **85**
    composition and structure, 83–85, *85–86*, **86**
    connective tissue proper, 85–87
    functions, **86**
    ligaments, 157
    liquid connective tissue, 87–88
    loose/dense connective tissue, 86–87
    tendons, 157
constipation, 267
contraception and sexual health
    breast examination, 359
    genital piercings, 358
    intrauterine device, 355, *356*
    learning disabilities, 351
    oral contraceptive pill, 354
    vaginal swabs, 357
contractility, 236
contrast dyes, 290
COPD *see* chronic obstructive pulmonary disease
coronary arteries, 223–224, *224*, **224**
corpus luteum (CL), 98, 352

corticosteroids
  immune system, 475, 486
  respiratory system, 316
  skin, 508–509
corticotropin-releasing hormone (CRH), 442, 450–451
cortisol, 442–443, 451, *452*
coughing, 470
covalent bonds, 8, *8*
COX *see* cyclooxygenase
cranial nerves
  peripheral nervous system, 383, *384*, **385**
  sensory system, 406, 416, 418
creatine phosphate, 130
Creon, 263
CRH *see* corticotropin-releasing hormone
Crohn's disease, 263–264
cryptorchidism, 345
CSF *see* cerebrospinal fluid
CTL *see* cytotoxic T-lymphocytes
cuboidal epithelium, 78–79, *79*, 80–81, *81*, *83*
culture samples, 292
cumulus–oocyte complex, 98, 100
Cushing's disease, 442–443
cutaneous membranes, 89–90
cyclooxygenase (COX), 389
cystic fibrosis (CF), 64, 263
cystitis, 300
cytokines, 474–475
cytotoxic T-lymphocytes (CTL), 472–473, 478

Dalton's law, 317–318, **317**
DCT *see* distal convoluted tubule
decibel (dB) levels, 418
deglutition *see* swallowing
dehydration, 36, 510
dendrites, 370
depression
  endocrine system, 442–443
  nervous system, 387–388
  respiratory system, 322–323
  sensory system, 406–407
dermatophytosis, 506–507
dermis, 503–504, *503*
  papillary and reticular aspects, 503–504
desmopressin, 196–197
diabetes
  embryology, 113
  endocrine system, 452–454
  tissue repair, 92
diabetic nephropathy, 291
dialysis, 297–298
diastole, 233–236
diclofenac, 174
diencephalon, 381
diet and nutrition
  balanced diet: the food pyramid, 268–269, *269*
  carbohydrates, 270
  digestive system, 250–252, 256–257, 261–262, 268–272, *269*, **271–273**
  endocrine system, 444, 452–453, 455

fats, 270
minerals, 272, **273**
nutrient groups, 269
nutrients, 268
physiological principles, 2, 3
proteins, 270–271
renal system, 296
vitamins, 271, **271–272**
water, 270
diffusion
  active transport, 29–30, *30*
  facilitated diffusion, 28–29, *29*
  mitochondrial energy production, 30
  osmosis, 28, *29*
  renal system, 293
  respiratory system, 325
  simple diffusion, 26–27, *27*
digestive system, 245–279
  activities and learning, 276–279
  body map, 246
  gallbladder, *262*, 266
  gastric glands and cells, 256–257, *256*, *258*
  hormones, 256–257, 260, 263, 266, **268**
  large intestine, 266–267, *266*
  liver and the production of bile, *262*, 264–266, *265*
  mouth/oral cavity, 247–250, *248–250*
  nutrition, chemical digestion, and metabolism, 268–272, *269*, **271–273**
  oesophagus, 251, 252–253, *253*
  organisation and anatomical features, 246, *247*
  pancreas, 262–264, *262*
  pharynx, 250–252, *251*
  physiological functions, 246
  small intestine, 260–262, *260–261*
  stomach, 255–259, *255–256*, *258*
  structure of the digestive tract, 254–255, *254*
digoxin, 30, 231
diploid cells, 58
disease-modifying anti-rheumatoid drugs (DMARD), 475
distal convoluted tubule (DCT), 289, 293
diltiazem, 226
DMARD *see* disease-modifying anti-rheumatoid drugs
DNA, 47–48
  chromosomes, 47, 49–52, *50–51*
  double helix structure, 48–49, *49–50*
  from DNA to proteins, 52–56, *53–55*
  inheritance, 61
  transference of genes, 56–60, *57–60*
dopamine, 375, 449
downregulation, 438
Down syndrome
  cardiac system, 221–222
  embryology, 113–114, *114*
  endocrine system, 446–447
  genetics, 70–71
  renal system, 286–287
  respiratory system, 320–321
  sensory system, 409–410
dropsy *see* oedema
dry mouth, 406–407

Duchenne muscular dystrophy, 67, 125–126
dysgeusia, 408
dysphagia, 251–252

ears
    ear wax and infections, 409–411
    inner ear, 412, *413*
    middle ear, 411–412
    outer ear, 408
    structure of the ear, 408–412, *409*
    see also equilibrium and hearing
EBV *see* Epstein-Barr virus
eccrine glands, 505
ECF *see* extracellular fluids
ECG *see* electrocardiography
ECM *see* extracellular matrix
ectopic pregnancy, 111, 360–361
eczema, 508–509
ED *see* erectile dysfunction
EDV *see* end diastolic volume
EEG *see* electroencephalogram
efferent fibres, 369
efferent nerves, 372
ejaculatory duct, 346–347
elastic cartilage, 87, 156
elastic fibres, 85–87
electrical pathways of the heart, 229–232, *230, 232–233*
electrocardiography (ECG)
    cardiac cycle, 235, *235*
    correct lead placement, 232, *233*
electroencephalogram (EEG), 374, 375
electrolytes
    cell biology, 32–34, **32–33**
    intravenous fluids/electrolytes, 38–39
    physiological principles, 9–10
    renal system, 289–290, 293–296, **293**
electromyography (EMG), 129
embryology, 97–118
    activities and learning, 117–118
    complications of pregnancy, 111–115, *114–115*
    concepts and definitions, 98, *98*
    differentiation of embryonic or germ layers, 104–105, *105–106*
    early placental formation, 102, *104*
    fertilisation, 100, *101*
    hormones of the menstrual cycle, 98, *99*
    implantation, 102, *103*
    late gestation and birth/second and third trimesters, 108–110, *109*, **110–111**
    oocyte maturation and ovulation, 98, *99*
    pain relief during labour, 110, **110–111**
    post-implantation development/first trimester, 104–108, *105–107*
    pre-implantation development, 100–102, *101*
    sperm maturation, 99–100, *100*
    timings, 98
EMG *see* electromyography
end diastolic volume (EDV), 234, 236–237
endocardium, *218*, 220, 223
endochondral ossification, 158–161, *159–161*

endocrine system, 433–460
    activities and learning, 458–460
    adrenal glands, 448–452, *448, 450, 452*
    body map, 434
    control of hormone release, 438, *439*
    destruction and removal of hormones, 438
    effects of hormones, 438
    hormones, 435–438, *436–438*
    hypothalamus and pituitary gland, 439–443, *439*, **441**
    nervous system, **434**
    organisation and anatomical features, 434–435
    organs of the endocrine system, 435–436, *435–436*
    pancreas, 452–456, *456*
    paracrine/autocrine/exocrine, 436, *436*
    parathyroid glands, *444*, 447–448
    physiological functions, 434, **434**, 439–456
    thyroid gland, 443–447, *444–445*
    transportation of hormones, 438
endocytosis, 37, *38*
endometrium, 354, *355*, **355**, 359–360
energy production
    cell biology, 30
    digestive system, 270
    genetics, 56
    muscular system, 121, 124–126, 130, *131*
    respiratory system, 330, *331*
enteral feeding, 256–257
enteroendocrine cells, 256, 260
eosinophils, 192, *192*
ependymal cells, 376
epidermis, 498–502
    cells in the epidermis, 498–499, *498*
    layers of the epidermis, 499–502, *500*, **500**
epididymis, 346
epilepsy, 374, 392
epiphyseal plate, 158–159, *160*
epithalamus, 381
epithelial tissue, 78–82
    composition and structure, 78–79, *79*
    functions, 78
    glandular epithelium, 82, *84*
    respiratory system, 309
    sensory system, 400
    simple epithelium, 78–79, *80–82*
    stratified epithelium, 80–81, *82–83*
Epstein-Barr virus (EBV), 466–467
equilibrium and hearing, 408–418
    equilibrium, 412–416, *414–415*
    hearing, 416–418, *416–417*
    hearing loss and ototoxicity, 409–411, 418
    structure of the ear, 408–412, *409, 413*
erectile dysfunction (ED), 348
ERV *see* expiratory reserve volume
erythema, 473–475
erythrocytes, 328
erythropoietin/erythropoiesis, 188–189, *190*, 290
ethics, 351
excretion
    circulatory system, 185
    digestive system, 267

physiological principles, 2
  renal system, 282, **293**, 294–295, *294*, 300–301
  skin, 510–511
exercise/physical activity
  cardiac system, 225–226, 236
  endocrine system, 453, 455
exocrine glands, 82, *84*
exocytosis, 37, *38*
exothermic reactions, 12
expiratory reserve volume (ERV), 321–322
external respiration, 324–327, *325*
  factors influencing diffusion, 325
  gaseous exchange, 324–325, *325*, *331*
  oxygen therapy, 326–327
  sputum, 326
  ventilation and perfusion, 327
extracellular fluids (ECF)
  composition, 31–32, **32**
  fluid movement between compartments, 34–35
extracellular matrix (ECM), 84
eyes *see* sight/vision

facilitated diffusion, 28–29, *29*
faeces, 267
Fallopian tubes, 354
FAS *see* foetal alcohol syndrome
fast glycolytic fibres, 126
fast oxidative–glycolytic fibres, 126
fats/lipids
  cholesterol, 14, 237, 270
  digestive system, 270
  fatty acids, 13, *14*
  physiological principles, 13–14, *14–15*
  triglycerides, 13, *14*
FBC *see* full blood count
female reproductive system, 348–361
  breasts, 358–359, *358*
  cervix, 357
  corpus luteum, 352
  external genitalia/vulva, 357–358
  Fallopian tubes, 354
  hormonal control of female reproduction, 352–354, 356–361
  oogenesis and follicular development, 350–351, *352–353*
  organisation and anatomical features, 348–349, *350*
  ovarian and uterine cycles, 359–361, *360*
  ovaries, 349–350
  uterus, 354, *355*, **355**
  vagina, 356–357
female urethra, 300–301, *302*
fertilisation, 100, *101*
fibres
  effects of ageing, 146
  microanatomy of skeletal muscle fibre, 123–126, *125*, **126**
  tissue, 85–87
  types of muscle fibres, 126
fibrocartilage, 87, 156–157
fibromyalgia, 131–133
fibrosis, 92, 146

fibrous joints, 170
fibrous tunic, 420–421
Fick's law, **317**, 325
filtration, 292–293
flat bones, 168, *170*
flixonase, 401–402
fluid balance, 184, 285, 290
fluid compartments, 31, *31*, 34–37, *35*
fluid therapy, 184, 185–186
fluoxetine, 406–407
focal length, 425–426, *425*
Foetal alcohol spectrum disorder (FASD), 107–108
folic acid, 189
follicle-stimulating hormone (FSH), 98, 350–351, 441
follicular development, 350–351, *353*
food *see* nutrition
food pyramid, 268, *269*
foot ulcers, 92
force of contraction, 236
FSH *see* follicle-stimulating hormone
full blood count (FBC), 195

gallbladder, *262*, 266
gametes
  embryology, 98
  genetics, 56–57, *62*
  reproductive systems, 340, 350
ganglion cells, 424, 428
gaseous exchange, 324–325, *325*, *331*
gastric glands and cells, 256–257, *256*, *258*
gastrin, 257, 266, **268**
gastrulation, 104–105, *105*
g cells, 256
gender determination, 66–67, *67*
gene crossover, 59–60, *60*
generalised anxiety disorder, 259
gene replacement therapy, 64
genetic counselling, 64–65
genetics, 45–76
  activities and learning, 74–76
  anatomical map, *46*
  autosomal dominant inheritance and ill health, 62–63, *63*
  autosomal recessive inheritance and ill health, 63–64
  chromosomes, 49–52, *50–51*
  concepts and definitions, 46
  disorders of chromosomes, 70–71
  DNA and RNA, 47–48
  DNA double helix, 48–49, *49–50*
  from DNA to proteins, 52–56, *53–55*
  inheritance, 60–69, *62–63*, *66–68*
  Mendelian inheritance, 60–61, *62*
  morbidity and mortality of dominant versus recessive disorders, 66
  non-Mendelian (complex) inheritance, 68–69
  spontaneous mutation, 70
  transcription, 52–53, *53*
  transference of genes, 56–60, *57–60*
  translation, 53–54, *54–55*
  X-linked recessive disorders, 66–67, *67–68*

genetic screening of newborns, 68–69, 70
genital piercings, 358
geriatrics *see* ageing
germ layers, 104–105, *106*
gestational diabetes, 113
glandular epithelium, 82, *84*
glaucoma, 424
gliding joints, 173
glomerular filtration, 292–293
glucagon, 455–456, *456*
glucocorticoids, 401–402, 451, *452*
glucose, 35, 270
glycogen/glycolysis, 130, 453
glycosaminoglycans, 84
GnRH *see* gonadotrophin-releasing hormone
goblet cells, 260
gonadotrophin-releasing hormone (GnRH), 348
gout, 154
Graafian follicles, 350–351
granulation tissue, 92
granulocytes, 462
ground substance, 84
growth, 2
growth hormone, 441
gustatory pathway, 406
Guthrie test, 70

haemoglobin
    circulatory system, 187–188, *188*
    respiratory system, 328, *329*, 330
haemophilia, 67, 196–197
haemopoiesis, 153–154
haemostasis, 194
hair, 504, *505*, 509
hair cells, 413–417, *415*
hand washing, 486
HbA1c blood test, 454
hCG *see* human chorionic gonadotropin
HCM *see* hypertrophic cardiomyopathy
HDL *see* high density lipoprotein
hearing *see* equilibrium and hearing
heart *see* cardiac system
heart murmurs, 222
heart rate (HR), 236, 237–239, *238*
heel prick test, 70
helminth therapy, 482
helper T-lymphocytes, 478
Henry's law, **317**
heparin, 196
hepatocytes, 264
high density lipoprotein (HDL), 14
hinge joints, 172
HOCM see hypertrophic obstructive cardiomyopathy
Hodgkin disease/Hodgkin lymphoma, 207, 208–209
homeostasis
    circulatory system, 182, 184, 194
    digestive system, 268, 273
    endocrine system, 434
    haemostasis, 194
    physiological principles, 15–16

renal system, 282
skeletal system, 152, 154
tissue, 78
hormone replacement therapy (HRT), 356–357
hormones
    adrenal glands, 448–451, *450*, *452*
    cardiac system, 236, 239
    cell biology, 33, **33**
    control of hormone release, 438, *439*
    destruction and removal, 438
    digestive system, 256–257, 260, 263, 266, **268**
    effects, 438
    embryology, 98, *99*
    endocrine system, 435–438, *436–438*
    hypothalamus and pituitary gland, 439–443, *439*, **441**
    parathyroid glands, 447–448
    renal system, 290, 295–296
    reproductive systems, 343, 348, *349*, 350–354, 356–361
    thyroid gland, 444–447, *445*
    transportation, 438
HR *see* heart rate
HRT *see* hormone replacement therapy
human chorionic gonadotropin (hCG), 102
humoral immunity, 478–479, *479–480*
Huntington's disease, 66
hyaline cartilage, 87, 156, 158
hydrogen bonding, 9, *9*
hydrostatic pressure, 34–35, *35*
hypercapnia, 326, 330
hypercholesterolaemia, 237
hyperopia, 426–427, *427*
hypersensitivity, 487–488, **487**
hyperthyroidism, 445–446
hypertrophic cardiomyopathy (HCM), 219
hypertrophic obstructive cardiomyopathy (HOCM), 219
hypoadrenalism, 451–452
hypogammaglobulinaemia, 484
hypogeusia, 408
hypoglycaemia, 454, 455
hyponatraemia, 33–34, 440
hypothalamus, 381, 439–443, *439*, **441**
hypothyroidism, 445–447
hypotonic fluids, 289
hypoxaemia, 326–328, 330
hypoxia, 328, **329**

ICD *see* implantable cardioverter-defibrillator
ICF *see* intracellular fluids
ICP *see* intracranial pressure
IM *see* intramuscular
immune system, 461–494
    acquired immunity, 477–479, *477*, *479–480*
    activities and learning, 491–494
    anaphylaxis, 486–487, 488
    blood cell development, 462–463, *463*
    body map, 462
    cell-mediated immunity, 477–478, *477*
    cytotoxicity, 472–473, 478
    humoral immunity, 478–479, *479–480*
    hypersensitivity, 487–488, **487**

immunisation/vaccination, 488
immunodeficiency, 64, 467–468
immunoglobulins, 474, 480–487, *482–483*
inflammation, 473–477, *474*
innate immunity, 469–477
lymphatic system, 464–469, *465*
lymph nodes, 467–468, *468*
lymphoid tissue, 469
natural killer cells, 484–485
organs of the immune system, 463–469
phagocytosis, 467, 471–472, *472–473*
physical/mechanical/chemical barriers, 469–470
physiological functions, 462
primary and secondary response to infection,
    485–487, *485*
spleen, 469
thymus, 464, *464*
types of immunity, 469
white blood cells, 463, 470–477, **470**, *472–474*
immunoglobulins, 474, 480–487
immunoglobulin A, 481, 486
immunoglobulin D, 482
immunoglobulin E, 481–482, 486
immunoglobulin G, 480–481, *482*, 485–486
immunoglobulin M, 481, 485
immunoglobulin therapy, 483–484
primary and secondary response to infection,
    485–487, *485*
role of immunoglobulins, 482–483, *482–483*
implantable cardioverter-defibrillator (ICD), 129, 219
implantation, 102, *103*
infections
    circulatory system, 185
    immune system, 466–468, 471–472, *472–473*, 480,
        481–487, *485*
    muscular system, 127
    nervous system, 377
    renal system, 291, 299–300
    reproductive systems, 351, 357–358
    respiratory system, 320–321, 326
    sensory system, 409–411
    skin, 506–507
    tissue, 90, 92
inflammation
    digestive system, 263–264
    endocrine system, 451–452
    immune system, 473–477, *474*
    respiratory system, 314–316, 320–321
    sensory system, 410
    skeletal system, 174
    skin, 508–509
inhalers, 314–315
inheritance, 60–69
    autosomal dominant inheritance and ill health,
        62–63, *63*
    autosomal recessive inheritance and ill health, 63–64
    constructing a family pedigree, 65, *66*
    gene replacement therapy, 64
    genetic counselling, 64–65
    Mendelian inheritance, 60–61, *62*

morbidity and mortality of dominant versus recessive
        disorders, 66
    non-Mendelian (complex) inheritance, 68–69
    X-linked recessive disorders, 66–67, *67–68*
innate immunity
    cytotoxicity, 472–473
    inflammation, 473–477, *474*
    phagocytosis, 467, 471–472, *472–473*
    physical/mechanical/chemical barriers,
        469–470
    white blood cells, 470–477, **470**, *472–474*
inspiratory reserve volume (IRV), 321–322
insulin, 453–455, *456*
internal respiration, 330, *331*
intracellular fluids (ICF)
    composition, 31–32, **32**
    fluid movement between compartments, 34–35
intracranial pressure (ICP), 379
intramuscular (IM) injection, 123
intra-ocular pressure (IOP), 424
intrauterine device (IUD), 355, *356*
intravenous (IV) cannulae/catheters, 201
intravenous (IV) fluids/electrolytes, cell biology,
        38–39, 185–186
ionic bonds, 6–7, *7*
IOP *see* intra-ocular pressure
iris, 421
iron deficiency anaemia, 187
irregular bones, 168, *171*
IRV *see* inspiratory reserve volume
islets of Langerhans, 452
isotonic fluids, 184, 289
IUD *see* intrauterine device
IV *see* intravenous

joints
    muscular system, 121
    skeletal system, 170–174, **172–173**

karyotype, 50–51, *51*
keratinocytes, 498, *498*
kidneys
    blood supply to the kidney, 292
    external structures, 282–283, *284*
    functions of the kidneys, 290
    internal structures, 284, *285–286*
    nephrons, 287–290, *288*, 294–295, *294*
    renal system, 282–292
kinin system, 474
knee reconstruction, 158

labia majora/minora, 357
lacrimal apparatus, 419–420, *419*
lactulose, 267
lamina propria, 400
Langerhans cells, *498*, 499
large intestine, 266–267, *266*
laryngopharynx, 250, 309
larynx, 310–311, *312*
LDL *see* low density lipoprotein

learning disabilities
  cardiac system, 221–222
  circulatory system, 196–197
  digestive system, 251–252
  embryology, 113–114, *114*
  endocrine system, 446–447
  genetics, 47–48
  immune system, 486–487
  nervous system, 387–388
  renal system, 286–287
  reproductive systems, 351
  respiratory system, 320–321
  sensory system, 409–410
  skeletal system, 164–165
  skin, 495–496
leucocytes, 291
levothyroxine, 446–447
Leydig cells, 343
LH *see* luteinising hormone
lifestyle *see* diet and nutrition; exercise/physical activity
ligaments, 157
limbic system, 382
lipids *see* fats/lipids
liver, *262*, 264–266, *265*
lobules, 313, *314*
long bones, 166-167, *168*
loop of Henle, 289, 293
low density lipoprotein (LDL), 14
lower respiratory tract (LRT), 310–316
  bronchial tree, 312–313, *313*
  gross anatomy, 310, *311*
  larynx, 310–311, *312*
  lobules, 313, *314*
  trachea, 311
lumbar puncture, 378–379
lung compliance, 319–320
lung volumes and capacities, 321–323, *321*, **322**
luteinising hormone (LH)
  embryology, 98
  endocrine system, 441
  reproductive systems, 348, 350–351
lymphatic system, 203–207, *204*
  immune system, 464–469, *465*
  lymph, 87–88, 203, 466
  lymphatic organs, 207–209
  lymph capillaries and large lymph vessels, 203, *205*, 464–466
  lymph nodes, 203–205, *206*, 467–468, *468*
  lymphoid tissue, 87–88, 469
  spleen, 469
lymphocytes
  circulatory system, 193, *193*
  immune system, 462, 464, 467, 472–473, 477–479, *477*, *479–480*
lysozyme, 470

macrophages, 84, 462, 467
magnetic resonance imaging (MRI), 5
male reproductive system, 340–348
  epididymis, 346
  hormonal control of male reproduction, 348, *349*

organisation and anatomical features, 340–341, *341*
  penis, 347–348, *347*
  scrotum, 341–343, *342*
  seminal vesicles and prostate gland, 347
  sperm, 99–100, *100*, 345, *346*
  spermatogenesis, 344–345, *345*
  testes, 342–343, *342*, *344*, 345
  vas deferens, spermatic cord and ejaculatory duct, 346–347
male urethra, 300, *301*
mammary glands *see* breasts
mast cells
  degranulation, 473–474, 481
  tissue, 84
medulla oblongata, 381
medullary cavity, 152, 161, *161*
meiosis, 56–57, 58–59, 98
melanocytes, 498–499, *498*
membranes
  cell biology, 25, 26–30, *26*, 37–39, *38*
  immune system, 469
  tissue, 89–90, *89*
membranous labyrinth, 412
memory T-lymphocytes, 478
Mendelian inheritance, 60–61, *62*
meninges, 376–377, *378*
meningitis, 377
menopause, 356–357
menstruation/menstrual cycle, 98, *99*, 359–361, *360*
mental health
  cardiac system, 225–226
  circulatory system, 208–209
  digestive system, 259
  endocrine system, 442–443
  genetics, 69
  immune system, 471
  nervous system, 375–376, 387–388
  respiratory system, 322–323
  sensory system, 406–407
  skeletal system, 157–158
  skin, 502
Merkel cells, *498*, 499
messenger RNA (mRNA), 52–56, *53–55*
metabolic rate, 444
metformin, 453
MI *see* myocardial infarction
microglia, 376
microsuction, 409, 411
micturition, 301
midazolam, 382
midbrain, 381
mild traumatic brain injury, 382
mineralocorticoids, 449–451, *450*
minerals, 272, **273**
miscarriage, 111
misoprostol, 174
mitochondria, 30, 56
mitosis, 56–58
monocytes, 192, *193*
monospot test, 466
mons pubis, 357

morula, 101
motor function
    cerebrum, 380
    cranial nerves, 383, *384*, **385**
    peripheral nervous system, 369–374, *371, 373*
    spinal nerves, 384–386, *386–388*
motor nerve testing, 129
motor unit, 127, *127*
mouth/oral cavity
    digestive system, 247–250, *248–250*
    oral hygiene, 250
    respiratory system, 308–309
MRI *see* magnetic resonance imaging
mRNA *see* messenger RNA
MS *see* multiple sclerosis
mucous membranes, 89–90, 469
mucous neck cells, 256
multiple sclerosis (MS), 372, 475–476
muscular dystrophy, 67, 125–126
muscular system, 119–150
    activities and learning, 147–150
    aerobic respiration, 130–133
    blood supply, 126
    body map, 120
    body movements, 121, 133–136, **145**
    composition of skeletal muscle tissue, 122
    contraction and relaxation of skeletal muscle, 127–129,
        127–128
    effects of ageing, 146
    energy sources for muscle contraction, 130, *131*
    functions, 121
    gross anatomy of skeletal muscles, 122–123, *123*
    microanatomy of skeletal muscle fibre, 123–126, *125*, **126**
    muscle fatigue/fibromyalgia, 131–133
    organisation of the skeletal muscular system, 133–146,
        134–136, *137–144*, **145**
    respiratory system, 318, *319*
    types of muscle fibres, 126
    types of muscle tissue, 90–91, *90–91*, 120–121, **120**
myelin sheath, 370–371
myocardial infarction (MI), 227, *227*, 237
myocardium, 217–218, *218*
myocytes, 217–218, *218*
myofibrils, 125
myometrium, 354, *355*, **355**
myopia, 426–427, *426*

nails, 506–508
Na, /K, *see* sodium-potassium
nasal cavity, 308–309
nasogastric tubes, 256
nasojejunal tubes, 256
nasopharynx, 250, 309
natural killer (NK) cells, 484–485
nausea and vomiting, 257
nematode therapy, 482
neoplasms
    chemotherapy, 207, 208–209, 257
    circulatory system, 207, 208–209
    genetics, 71–72
    radiotherapy, 208–209

nephrons
    Bowman's capsule, 287–288, *288*
    collecting ducts, 289
    distal convoluted tubule, 289
    excretion, 294–295, *294*
    loop of Henle, 289
    proximal convoluted tubule, 288–289
    renal system, 287–290, *288*, 294–295, *294*
nephrotoxicity, 291
nerve conduction studies, 129
nervous system, 367–397
    activities and learning, 395–397
    autonomic nervous system, 370, 389–392, *390–391*, **392**
    body map, 368
    brain, 379–383, *379–381*
    central nervous system, 369
    cerebrospinal fluid, 376–379
    endocrine system, **434**
    meninges, 376–377, *378*
    motor division of the peripheral nervous system,
        369–374, *371, 373*
    neuroglia, 376, *377*
    neurotransmitters, 374–376
    organisation and anatomical features, 368, *369*
    peripheral nervous system, 383–389, *384*, **385**, *386–388*
    physiological functions, 368
    sensory division of the peripheral nervous system,
        368–369
    sensory system, 406, 416, 418, 424, 428
    tissue, 91–92, *92*
neural tunic, 421–425, *422*
neuroglia, 91–92, 376, *377*
neurones
    muscular system, 127, *127*
    nervous system, 370, *371*, 372, 376
    sensory system, 424
    tissue, 91–92, *92*
neurotransmitters, 374–376, 406, 413
neurulation, 105, *106*
neutropaenia, 471–472
neutrophils, 191–192, *192*
nitrates, 291
nitrous oxide/oxygen, 110
NK *see* natural killer
nodal cells, 231
noise exposure, 418
non-ciliated epithelium, 79, *81*
non-keratinised epithelium, 80, *82*
non-Mendelian (complex) inheritance, 68–69
non-steroidal anti-inflammatory drugs (NSAID), 174, 291
noradrenaline, 448–449
norepinephrine, 375
NSAID *see* non-steroidal anti-inflammatory drugs
nutrition *see* diet and nutrition

obesity
    cardiac system, 222, 225–226
    digestive system, 269, 271, 272
occupational dermatitis, 510
ondansetron, 257
oedema, 206–207, 473, 476

oesophagus, 251, 252–253, *253*
oestrogen, 350, 352–354, 356–357, 359–360
olanzapine, 471
olfaction/sense of smell, 400–404
   gross and microscopic anatomy, 400, *401*
   olfactory discrimination and anosmia,
     402–404
   olfactory pathway, 402, *403*
   olfactory receptors, 400–401
   respiratory system, 309
oligodendrocytes, 376
omeprazole, 253, 259
oogenesis, 98, *99*, 350–351, *352*
opportunistic health promotion, 226
optic nerve, 424, 428
oral cavity *see* mouth/oral cavity
oral contraceptive pill, 354
organ control/protection, 121, 152–153
organic molecules, 12–15, *14–15*
organ of Corti, 416–417, *417*
oropharynx, 250, 309
osmosis/osmolality
   cell biology, 28, *29*, 33–35, *33*
   circulatory system, 184
   renal system, 289, 293
osmotic pressure, 34–35, *35*
ossification, 158–161, *159–161*
osteoarthritis, 174
osteoblasts, 154, 155, 159–161
osteoclasts, 154–156, 161
osteocytes, 154, 155
osteogenesis imperfecta, 154
osteoporosis, 154, 156
otitis media, 409–410
otolith, 413–414, *415*
ototoxicity, 418
ovarian cycle, 359–361, *360*
ovaries, 349–350
oxygen debt, 130
oxygen requirements, 4
oxygen therapy, 326–327
oxyhaemoglobin dissociation curve, 328, *329*, 330
oxytocin, 440

pacemakers, 129, 231, *232*
paediatrics
   cardiac system, 219–220
   circulatory system, 188–189
   digestive system, 263–264
   embryology, 107–108
   endocrine system, 454
   genetics, 71–72
   immune system, 466–467
   muscular system, 125–126, 145–146
   nervous system, 374
   renal system, 291
   reproductive systems, 342–343, 345
   respiratory system, 314–315
   skeletal system, 162
   skin, 506–507

pain
   immune system, 473, 476
   nervous system, 389
   reproductive systems, 342–343, 360–361
   skeletal system, 157–158, 162–163, 174
   see also analgesia
palate, 248, *248*
palpation, 359
pancreas, 452–456, *456*
   digestive system, 262–264, *262*
   glucagon, 455–456, *456*
   insulin, 453–455, *456*
   somatostatin, 456
pancreatic insufficiency, 263
paneth cells, 260
panic attacks, 389
paracetamol, 389
paranoid schizophrenia, 471
parasitic infestation, 481–482
parasympathetic nervous system, 391, *391*, **392**
parathyroid glands, *444*, 447–448
parathyroid hormone, 447–448
parenchymal cells, 92
parietal cells, 256
parietal pleura, 312–313
Parkinson's disease, 403–404
passive immunisation, 488
passive transport, 26–27, *27*
patella, 168, *171*
patient assessment, 488
PCI *see* percutaneous coronary intervention
peak expiratory flow rate (PEFR), 323
pedigree, 65, *66*
PEFR *see* peak expiratory flow rate
PEG *see* percutaneous endoscopic gastrostomy
PEJ *see* percutaneous endoscopic jejunostomy
penis, 347–348, *347*
percutaneous coronary intervention (PCI), 227, *227*
percutaneous endoscopic gastrostomy (PEG) tubes, 257
percutaneous endoscopic jejunostomy (PEJ) tubes, 257
pericardium, 217, *218*
perimetrium, 354, *355*, **355**
peripheral nervous system, 383–389
   cranial nerves, 383, *384*, **385**
   motor division, 369–374, *371*, *373*
   sensory division, 368–369
   spinal cord/nerves, 383–389, *386–388*
peristalsis, 251, *253*
peritonitis, 90
personal hygiene, 501
Perthes disease, 162–163
pH
   circulatory system, 184
   physiological principles, 10–11, *10–11*
   renal system, 293–296
   respiratory system, 330
phagocytosis
   cell biology, 37, *38*
   immune system, 467, 471–472, *472–473*
pharyngeal arches, 105, *107*

pharynx, 250–252, *251*, 309
phenylketonuria (PKU), 63, *63*, 68–70
phenytoin, 383
Philadelphia chromosome, 71–72
phospholipids, 14, *15*
photoreceptor cells, 421–424
photosensitivity, 502
physiological principles, 1–21
    acids and bases, 10–11, *10–11*
    activities and learning, 19–21
    bodily requirements, 3–4
    characteristics of life, 2
    chemical equations, 11–12, *12*
    chemical reactions and chemical bonds, 6–10, *7–9*
    homeostasis, 15–16
    levels of organisation, 2, *3*
    life at the chemical level, 4–5, *5–6*
    organic molecules, 12–15, *14–15*
    units of measurement, 16, **16–18**
pinocytosis, 37, *38*
pituitary gland, 439–443, *439*, **441**
pivot joints, 172
PKU *see* phenylketonuria
placenta, 102, *104*
plasma
    circulatory system, 184, **185**
    immune system, 474
    tissue, 84
platelet aggregation, 194, 195
pneumonia, 320–321
pneumotaxic centre, 324
pneumothorax, 90, 312–313
polarisation/depolarisation, 372, *373*
polar molecules, 8–9, *9*
polypharmacy, 296
pons, 381
post-implantation embryonic development, 104–108,
    105–107
pre-eclampsia, 112
pregnancy tests, 102
pre-implantation embryonic development, 100–102, *101*
preload, 236
prenatal monitoring, 109
presbyopia, 426–427
pre-term birth, 112
primary blast cells, 84, **85**
progesterone, 350, 352–354, 359–360
prolactin, 358, 441
prostaglandins
    eye drops, 424
    immune system, 474
    skeletal system, 174
prostate gland, 347
proteins
    digestive system, 270–271
    genetics, 52–56, *53–55*
    physiological principles, 15
    transcription, 52–53, *53*
    translation, 53–54, *54–55*
prothrombin time, 195

proximal convoluted tubule, 288–289, 293
pseudostratified epithelium, 79, *82*
pulmonary ventilation/breathing, 316–324
    control of breathing, 323–324, *324*
    lung volumes and capacities, 321–323, *321*, **322**
    mechanics of breathing, 316–318, *318–319*, **318**
    work of breathing, 319–321
pulse oximetry, 328
punnet square, 63–64, *63*, 67, *67*
pyridostigmine, 129

radiotherapy, 208–209
RBC *see* red blood cells
recombination, 59–60, *60*
red blood cells (RBC)
    circulatory system, 186–191, *186–188*, *190*
    renal system, 290
refraction, 425–426, *425*
refractory period, 374
renal system, 281–305
    activities and learning, 304–305
    blood supply to the kidney, 292
    body map, 282
    composition of urine, 296–298, **297**
    external structures of the kidneys, 282–283, *284*
    formation of urine, 292–296, **293**, *294*
    functions of the kidneys, 290
    internal structures of the kidneys, 284, *285–286*
    kidneys, 282–292
    micturition, 301
    nephrons, 287–290, *288*, 294–295, *294*
    organs of the renal system, 282, *283*
    physiological functions, 282
    ureters, 298, *298*
    urethra, 300–301, *301–302*
    urinary bladder, 299–300
renin, 290
repetitive strain injury (RSI), 145
replacement hip surgery, 163
reproductive systems, 339–366
    activities and learning, 364–366
    body map, 340
    breasts, 358–359, *358*
    cervix, 357
    corpus luteum, 352
    epididymis, 346
    external genitalia/vulva, 357–358
    Fallopian tubes, 354
    female reproductive system, 348–361, *350*
    genetics, 56
    hormonal control of female reproduction, 352–354,
        356–361
    hormonal control of male reproduction, 348
    male reproductive system, 340–348, *341*
    oogenesis and follicular development, 350–351,
        352–353
    organisation and anatomical features, 340–341, *341*,
        348–349, *350*
    ovaries, 349–350
    penis, 347–348, *347*

reproductive systems (*cont'd*)
  physiological functions, 340–341
  physiological principles, 2
  scrotum, 341–343, *342*
  seminal vesicles and prostate gland, 347
  sperm, 345, *346*
  spermatogenesis, 344–345, *345*
  testes, 342–343, *342, 344,* 345
  uterus, 354, *355,* **355**
  vagina, 356–357
  vas deferens, spermatic cord and ejaculatory duct,
    346–347
residual volume (RV), 321–322
respiratory system, 307–337
  activities and learning, 335–337
  aerobic/anaerobic respiration for muscle activity,
    130–133
  blood supply, 316, *317*
  body map, 307
  external respiration, 324–327, *325, 331*
  internal respiration, 330, *331*
  lower respiratory tract, 310–316, *311–314*
  lung volumes and capacities, 321–323, *321,* **322**
  organisation and anatomical features, 308, *309*
  phases of respiration and the gas laws, 316–318,
    317, *318*
  physiological functions, 308
  physiological principles, 2
  pulmonary ventilation/breathing, 316–324, *318–319,*
    318, *321,* **322,** *324*
  respiratory rate, 324
  transport of gases, 327–330, **327,** *329,* **329**
  upper respiratory tract, 308–309, *310*
reticular fibres, 85–87
reticular function, 382
retina, 421–425, *422*
reversible reactions, 12
rhabdomyolysis, 122
rhesus factor (Rh) system, 197–198
rheumatoid disease, 475
ribosomal RNA (rRNA), 53–54, *55*
RICE principle, 145
rickets, 154
RNA, 47–48, 52–56, *53–55*
rods, 421–424
rRNA *see* ribosomal RNA
RSI *see* repetitive strain injury
rubs, 222
RV *see* residual volume

SA *see* sinoatrial
saddle joints, 173
salbutamol, 315
salivary glands, 249–250, *250*
saltatory conduction, 373
sarcolemma, 123–124, 127
sarcomeres, 125
sarcoplasm, 124–125
satellite cells, 376
scar tissue, 92, 164

schizophrenia
  cardiac system, 225–226
  genetics, 69
  immune system, 471
Schwann cells, 376
SCI *see* spinal cord injury
scrotum, 341–343, *342*
sebaceous glands/sebum, 504, 510
secondary immunodeficiency, 467–468
secretin, 257, 260, 263, **268**
seizures *see* epilepsy
selective reabsorption, 293–294, **293**
selective serotonin reuptake inhibitors (SSRI), 387
seminal vesicles, 347
seminiferous tubules, 343, *344*
sensitivity, 2
sensory nerve testing, 129
sensory system, 399–432
  activities and learning, 430–432
  cerebrum, 380–381
  cranial nerves, 383, *384,* **385**
  equilibrium, 412–416, *414–415*
  hearing, 416–418, *416–417*
  lacrimal apparatus, 419–420, *419*
  motor division of the peripheral nervous system, 372
  olfaction/sense of smell, 400–404, *401, 403*
  physiological functions, 399
  sensory division of the peripheral nervous system,
    368–369
  sight/vision, 419–428, *419–420, 422, 425–427*
  skin, 508–509
  spinal nerves, 384–386, *386–388*
  structure of the ear, 408–412, *409, 413*
  structure of the eye, 420–424, *420*
  taste, 404–408, *405*
serous membranes, 89–90
Sertoli cells, 343
sesamoid bones, 168, *171*
sex chromosomes, 47, 50
  transference of genes, 60
  X-linked recessive disorders, 66–67, *67–68*
sexual health *see* contraception and sexual health
short bones, 167, *169*
SIADH *see* syndrome of inappropriate ADH secretion
sick euthyroid syndrome, 446
sight/vision, 419–428
  chambers of the eye, 424
  fibrous tunic, 420–421
  focusing images onto the retina, 425
  lacrimal apparatus, 419–420, *419*
  myopia, hyperopia, and presbyopia, 426–427, *426–427*
  neural tunic/retina, 421–424, *422*
  processing of visual information, 428
  refraction and focal length, 425–426, *425*
  structure of the eye, 420–424, *420*
  vascular tunic/uvea, 421
  wall of the eye, 420
sildenafil, 348
simple epithelium, 78–79, *80–82*
sinoatrial (SA) node, 229–231, 237

SI units, 16, **16–18**
skeletal muscle
  blood supply, 126
  composition, 122
  contraction and relaxation, 127–129, *127–128*
  gross anatomy, 122–123, *123*
  microanatomy of skeletal muscle fibre, 123–126, *125*, **126**
  organisation of the skeletal muscular system, 133–146, **134–136**, *137–144*, **145**
  tissue types, 90, *90*, **120**, 121–129
  types of muscle fibres, 126
skeletal system, 151–179
  activities and learning, 176–179
  axial and appendicular skeleton, 165, *166*, **167**
  body map, 152
  bone as a tissue, 87, 152, 154–156, **155**
  bone formation, 158, *159*
  bone fractures, 164–165, *164*
  bone growth, 159–161, *160–161*
  bone remodelling, 161–163
  bone shapes, 165–169, *168–171*
  factors affecting bone density, 155, **155**
  functions, 152–154
  joints, 170–174, **172–173**
  other connective tissues, 156–158
skin, 495–515
  accessory skin structures, 504–508
  activities and learning, 513–515
  body map, 495
  dermis, 503–504, *503*
  disorders, 495–496, 506–507
  epidermis, 498–502, *498*, *500*, **500**
  excretion and absorption, 510–511
  functions, 508–511
  hair, 504, *505*, 509
  immune system, 469
  layers of the epidermis, 499–502, *500*, **500**
  nails, 506–508
  papillary and reticular aspects, 503–504
  physiological functions, 495
  protective functions, 510
  sensation, 508–509
  structure and anatomical features, 496–508, *503*
  sweat glands, 504–506, *505*, 510–511
  synthesis of vitamin D, 511
  thermoregulation, 502, 505, 509
  topical application of medicines, 508–509, 511
SLE *see* systemic lupus erythematosus
slow oxidative fibres, 126
SMA *see* spinal muscular atrophy
small intestine, 260–262, *260–261*
smoking, 225–226
smooth muscle, 91, *91*, 120, **120**
sneezing, 470
Snellen chart, *427*
sodium-potassium (Na+/K+) pump, 30, *30*
soft tissue injuries, 145–146
somatic cells, *59*
somatic nervous system, 369

somatostatin, 456
spermatic cord, 346–347
spermatogenesis, 344, *345*
spermatozoa, 99–100, *100*, 345, *346*
sperm cells, 343
spinal cord injury (SCI), 387–388
spinal cord/nerves, 383–389, *385–388*
spinal muscular atrophy (SMA), 70
spindle fibres, 57–58
spirometry, 323
spleen, 207, 469
spongy bone, 152, *153*
spontaneous mutation, 70
sprains, 145–146
sputum, 326
squamous epithelium, 78–81, *79–80*, *82*
SSRI *see* selective serotonin reuptake inhibitors
statins, 237, 456
stents, 227, *227*
steroids
  anabolic steroids, 130
  corticosteroids, 316, 475, 486, 508–509
  endocrine system, 437–438
  glucocorticoids, 401–402, 451, *452*
  physiological principles, 14
stillbirth, 111
stomach, 255–259, *255–256*, *258*
strains, 145–146
stratified epithelium, 80–81, *82–83*
stroke volume (SV), 236–237
stromal cells, 92
suction catheters, 312
sunlight, 4, 502, 510
supportive therapy, 468
suppressor T-lymphocytes, 478
surface mucous cells, 256
surfactants, 320
SV *see* stroke volume
swallowing, 251, *251*
sweat glands, 504–506, *505*, 510–511
sympathetic nervous system, 390–391, *390*
syndrome of inappropriate ADH secretion (SIADH), 440
synovial joints, 170–172, **172–173**
synovial membranes, 89–90, *89*
systemic lupus erythematosus (SLE), 291
systole, 233–236

taste, 404–408, *405*
  disorders of taste, 406–408
  five basic tastes, 404, 406
  gustatory pathway, 406
  taste buds/papillae, 404, *405*
  taste receptor, 404–406
T-cells *see* cell-mediated immunity
tears, 470
teeth, 248, *248–249*
tender point examination sites, 132
tendons, 157
testes, 342–343, *342*, *344*, 345
testicular torsion, 342–343

testosterone, 343, 348, *349*
thalamus, 381
thalassaemia minor, 188–189
thermoregulation
  circulatory system, 184
  immune system, 473–475
  muscular system, 121
  skin, 502, 505, 509
thorax, 316–318
three-lead cardiac monitoring, 232
three-parent babies, 56
thrombolysis, 227
thymus, 208, 464, *464*
thyroid gland, 443–447, *444–445*
thyroid hormone, 437–438, 444–447
thyroid-stimulating hormone (TSH), 438, 442, 444–446
thyrotropin releasing hormone (TRH), 439, 442–443, 445
thyroxine, 236, 239
tinnitus, 418
tissue, 77–95
  activities and learning, 94–95
  bone as a tissue, 87, 152, 154–156, **155**
  cell biology, 78, 83–84, **85**, 92
  connective tissue, 83–88, *85–86*, **85–86**, *88*, 154–158
  epithelial tissue, 78–82, *79–84*
  glandular epithelium, 82, *84*
  membranes, 89–90, *89*
  muscle tissue, 90–91, *90–91*, 120–122, **120**
  nervous tissue, 91–92, *92*
  simple epithelium, 78–79, *80–82*
  stratified epithelium, 80–81, *82–83*
  tissue repair, 92
TLC *see* total lung capacity
TNFα *see* tumour necrosis factor alpha
tongue
  digestive system, 247–248, *248*
  sensory system, 404, *405*
tonometry, 424
tonsils, 309
topical application of medicines, 508–509, 511
total lung capacity (TLC), 321–322
trabecular bone, 152, *153*
trachea, 311
tracheostomy, 312
transcription, 52–53, *53*
transdermal patches, 509
transfer RNA (tRNA), 53–54, *55*
transitional epithelium, 81, *83*
translation, 53–54, *54–55*
transport
  acid–base balance, 330
  active transport, 29–30, *30*, 293–294
  bulk transport across the cell membrane, 37–39, *38*
  carbon dioxide, 330
  circulatory system, 184, 191, 198–201, *199–202*, **201**
  endocrine system, 438
  hypoxia and hypoxaemia, 328, **329**
  oxygen, 328, *329*, **329**
  passive transport, 26–27, *27*
  respiratory system, 327–330
  terminology and definitions, **327**

transverse tubules, 123–124
trauma
  nervous system, 382, 387–388
  sensory system, 403–404
TRH *see* thyrotropin releasing hormone
triglycerides, 13, *14*
Trisomy 21 *see* Down syndrome
tRNA *see* transfer RNA
trophoblast cells, 101–102
TSH *see* thyroid-stimulating hormone
tubular reabsorption and secretion, 295–296
tumour necrosis factor alpha (TNFα), 477
Turner syndrome, 47–48
twenty-four-hour urine collection, 443

ulceration, 92
ultrasound, 114–115, *115*
ultraviolet (UV) light, 4, 502, 510
undescended testes, 345
units of measurement, 16, **16–18**
upper respiratory tract (URT), 308–309, *310*
upregulation, 438
ureters, 298, *298*
urethra, 300–301, *301–302*
uric acid, 154
urinary bladder, 299–300
urinary system *see* renal system
urinary tract infection (UTI), 291, 299–300
urine
  characteristics of normal urine, 296
  composition, 296–298, **297**
  excretion, **293**, 294–295, *294*
  filtration, 292–293
  hormonal control of tubular reabsorption and
    secretion, 295–296
  selective reabsorption, 293–294, **293**
  urinalysis, 291, 292, 443
URT *see* upper respiratory tract
uterine cycle, 359–361, *360*
uterus, 354, *355*, **355**
UTI *see* urinary tract infection
uvea, 421

vaccination, 488
vagina, 356–357
vaginal swabs, 357
valve stenosis, 222
valvular incompetence, 221–222
vascular tunic, 421
vas deferens, 346–347
vasoconstriction, 194
veins
  circulatory system, 199, *199–201*, **201**
  respiratory system, 316
ventilation and perfusion, 327
ventricles
  cardiac system, 221, 228–231, *228–229*, 233–236
  nervous system, 377–379, *378*
vertebrae, 168, *171*
visceral pleura, 312–313
visceral tissue *see* smooth muscle

vision *see* sight/vision
vitamins, 271, **271–272**, 511
vulva, 357–358

wall of the eye, 420
warfarin, 196
water
    bodily requirements, 3
    chemical equations, 11–12, *12*
    circulatory system, 184
    digestive system, 270

electrolyte and water balance, 32–34, **32–33**
    hydrogen bonding, 9, *9*
white blood cells (WBC)
    circulatory system, 186, *186*, 191–193, *192–193*
    immune system, 463, 470–477, **470**, *472–474*
    tissue, 84
xerostomia, 406–407

X-linked recessive disorders, 66–67, *67–68*

zona pellucida, 100, *101*